Clinical Massage Therapy

ASSESSMENT AND TREATMENT OF ORTHOPEDIC CONDITIONS

Clinical Massage Therapy

ASSESSMENT AND TREATMENT OF ORTHOPEDIC CONDITIONS

Steven E. Jurch, MA, ATC, LMT

*Medical University of South Carolina and
Trident Technical College
Charleston, South Carolina*

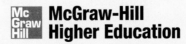

McGraw-Hill
Higher Education

Boston   Burr Ridge, IL   Dubuque, IA   New York   San Francisco   St. Louis
Bangkok   Bogotá   Caracas   Kuala Lumpur   Lisbon   London   Madrid   Mexico City
Milan   Montreal   New Delhi   Santiago   Seoul   Singapore   Sydney   Taipei   Toronto

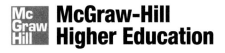
McGraw-Hill
Higher Education

ISBN   978-0-07-351093-4
MHID   0-07-351093-9

Vice President/Editor in Chief: *Elizabeth Haefele*
Vice President/Director of Marketing: *John E. Biernat*
Developmental Editor: *Connie Kuhl*
Marketing Manager: *Kelly Curran*
Lead Media Producer: *Damian Moshak*
Director, Editing/Design/Production: *Jess Ann Kosic*
Project Manager: *Marlena Pechan*
Senior Production Supervisor: *Janean A. Utley*
Designer: *Marianna Kinigakis*
Senior Photo Research Coordinator: *Carrie K. Burger*
Media Project Manager: *Mark A. S. Dierker*
Typeface: *10/12 Melior*
Compositor: *Electronic Publishing Services Inc., NYC*
Printer: *R. R. Donnelley*

Photo Credits

Figure 1.1: © Bettmann/Corbis; **1.2**: © Brown Brothers; **3.2a**: © Ed Reschke; **3.2b-c**: © The Mc-
Graw-Hill Companies, Inc./Photo by Dr. Alvin Telser; **4.1**: © Vol. 1 PhotoDisc/Getty; **5.2, 5.4,
5.6, 6.3a-b**: © The McGraw-Hill Companies, Inc./Joe DeGrandis, photographer; **7.18**: © The Mc-
Graw-Hill Companies, Inc./Timothy L. Vacula, photographer; **8.5, 8.18, 10.2a-b**: © The McGraw-
Hill Companies, Inc./Joe DeGrandis, photographer; **All Other Photographs:** © The McGraw-Hill
Companies, Inc./Jack Alterman, photographer.

Library of Congress Cataloging-in-Publication Data

Jurch, Steven E.

 Clinical massage therapy : assessment and treatment of orthopedic conditions / Steven E.
Jurch.
   p. ; cm.
 Includes bibliographical references and index.
 ISBN-13: 978-0-07-351093-4 (alk. paper)
 ISBN-10: 0-07-351093-9 (alk. paper)
 1. Massage therapy. 2. Orthopedics. I. Title.
 [DNLM: 1. Massage--methods. 2. Musculoskeletal Diseases--therapy. WB 537 J955c 2009]
RM721.J87 2009
615.8'22--dc22   2007039928

Dedication

To my wife, Jennifer, for her continuous love and support
throughout this process and for being my "in house"
editor and sounding board.

To my children, Owen and Molly, for providing me with
the motivation for this project.

To my parents, for helping me understand the value
of education.

About the Author

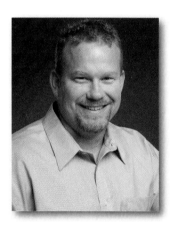

Steven Jurch, MA, ATC, LMT
Medical University of South Carolina, Charleston
Trident Technical College, Charleston, South Carolina

Steve has been involved in the health care industry for the past 15 years in numerous capacities ranging from a practitioner to a program director. Originally from Brandon, Florida, Steve began his education at Florida State University, receiving a bachelor's degree in Nutrition and Fitness. Along the way, he developed an interest in massage therapy after encountering some therapists working with athletes at a triathlon. After he completed his studies at Florida State, he attended Suncoast School of Massage Therapy in Tampa, Florida, and specialized in Sports Massage. Enjoying his work with athletes, Steve entered a 2-year internship program at the University of Tampa to receive his certification as an Athletic Trainer. During this time he was able to put his massage therapy skills into practice on a daily basis with the athletes as part of their rehabilitation programs. While he was at the university, he was chosen to work as an athletic-trainer intern with the Tampa Bay Buccaneers and eventually became the massage therapist for the team. To further his education in sports medicine, Steve went to Murray State University and worked as a graduate assistant for the football, women's basketball, and baseball teams while receiving his master's degree in Health, Physical Education, and Recreation, with an emphasis in Human Performance. Once he completed his degree, he took the position of head football trainer at Wingate University, where he also taught courses and supervised student athletic trainers.

Given an opportunity to move to Charleston, South Carolina, Steve took a job with a physical therapy group before beginning to teach at Trident Technical College in the Massage Therapy program. He took over the program as its coordinator in the first few months. Rewriting the entire curriculum, Steve spent 8 years as the coordinator before stepping down to pursue other opportunities. He still remains on staff as an adjunct instructor and also is an adjunct faculty member at the Medical University of South Carolina, teaching in its doctorate-level Physical Therapy and master's-level Occupational Therapy programs.

In addition to his teaching, Steve is the founder of the Wellness Education and Research Alliance and the owner of the Center for Therapeutic Massage. His years of education and experience working with college, professional, and international athletes both as a massage therapist and as an athletic trainer give him a unique perspective in the profession. Throughout his career, Steve has had the opportunity to work in exciting and challenging settings. In addition to working with the Buccaneers, he acted as the massage therapist for the Tampa Bay Rowdies professional soccer team and was involved in arena football, jai alai, professional ballet, and college athletics. Since his relocation, Steve has become a pioneer in the massage therapy field in Charleston. His approach to massage has provided unique opportunities for him and his business. The Center for Therapeutic Massage is the official massage therapy provider for the College of Charleston athletic teams and continues to work with U.S. Soccer to provide massage and athletic training coverage for its national soccer teams. Numerous local and visiting teams have utilized its services such as the NY Red Bulls and DC United of the MLS, the NBA Washington Wizards, and the players of the WTA at the Family Circle Cup Tournament.

Steve, his wife Jennifer, and their two children Owen and Molly enjoy the wonderful lifestyle of the Lowcountry, and through all of his efforts, Steve hopes to continuously enrich the profession of massage therapy.

Brief Contents

Contents

Preface

FROM THE AUTHOR

As an educator, one of my goals in writing this book was to create an educational tool for massage therapists that will instruct at the appropriate level while subsequently meeting the needs of the profession as the required competency level rises. With dual certifications in athletic training and massage therapy, I have the privilege of actively working in both professions. My experience has given me unique insights relative to the growing needs of massage education, and I continually strive to improve the quality and standards of the profession both inside and outside the classroom.

Experience has shown me that many massage therapists possess excellent hands-on skills yet still need additional training in assessing and treating the intricacies of orthopedic conditions. Conversely, many therapists who have advanced training in treating orthopedic pathologies often lack the knowledge and skill of effective soft tissue application. While many texts on orthopedic assessment in massage are technically sound, some lack information when it comes to describing how to address specific medical conditions. This text seeks to fill in some of the blanks.

While this book focuses on the clinical aspects of massage therapy, it's been my experience that utilizing a variety of techniques, when applied with specific intent, achieves the best results. Therefore, throughout this text students are encouraged to tailor the information to suit each patient's specific needs.

In my opinion, there are two primary components of clinical massage: knowledge and assessment. First, a clinical massage therapist must have advanced knowledge of anatomy and physiology. Such knowledge will aid the therapist in determining when treatment is appropriate and when it is necessary to refer patients to other health care providers. Second, to determine the best course of treatment, a therapist must be able to skillfully assess a condition. Assessment includes everything from taking a client's history, palpating the tissue, and administering special tests to then incorporating all the results into a treatment plan using well-developed clinical reasoning skills. I have written this text with these two primary components in mind.

As massage therapy continues to grow and become accepted as a form of preventive and restorative health care, particularly in the treatment of musculoskeletal dysfunction, the demand for highly skilled therapists who can tackle such pathologic conditions has grown as well. It is my belief that massage therapists can make a significant contribution to the preventive medicine movement. And while manual therapy is not the only tool available in preventive health care, it is a significant piece of the puzzle for an improved quality of life. My hope is that this text will contribute to the continuing growth of this dynamic form of health care.

ORGANIZATION AND STRUCTURE

Written primarily for the massage therapy profession, this text allows individual instructors to have the freedom and flexibility of either using it at its intended advanced level or tailoring it to their specific needs in the classroom. As an advanced examination of clinical orthopedic massage therapy, the text addresses the body's tissues and offers a systematic approach to applying various techniques in relation to specific orthopedic conditions. Its initial review of basic techniques serves to enhance one's existing knowledge of massage, thereby offering a platform of skills on which to build; it also offers fresh insight into the practice of massage as a whole. While the book introduces techniques that are modifications of common strokes, it does not identify any single technique as the "be-all and end-all" for every ailment. In fact, it allows for a broader application of the information by encouraging individual therapists to customize treatments based on their patients' specific needs. The four-step treatment outline allows therapists to utilize their strengths within the protocol by using their techniques of choice; however, a suggested method of treatment is always included for those with less clinical experience.

The text is divided into two main parts. While it is not intended to offer a comprehensive review of every massage therapy technique, Part I does review some basic components, including the importance of manual therapy and its place in health care; a working definition of clinical massage; basic equipment needs, draping techniques, proper body mechanics, and correct stroke application; and theory and principles of advanced techniques. Connective tissue massage encompasses a wide range of application methods; therefore, several of the major theories are covered, as well as the theory of trigger-point therapy. Also covered are advanced strokes, the use of active and passive motion, and various stretching techniques.

Part II begins by presenting a systematic approach to treating orthopedic conditions. It discusses the importance of having a focused approach on the condition and then addressing compensatory concerns. It then discusses proper assessment techniques and the steps necessary to make a prudent and proper treatment decision, including taking a history, determining the mechanism of the injury, and performing manual muscle testing and orthopedic assessments. Part II also addresses common conditions in various regions of the body, all of which were chosen because they are effectively treated through soft tissue therapies. This part also covers all the relevant information necessary for dealing with a specific condition, including topics such as anatomy and physiology, the client history, proper orthopedic assessments, and stretching. Finally, Part II reviews the treatment of general conditions for which massage takes on a supportive role and focuses on compensatory issues.

FEATURES OF THE TEXT

Generally, the more senses involved in the instruction process, the better students retain the material. Therefore, the book offers support materials that are designed to appeal to students with a wide range of learning styles. Among these features are:

- Logically organized chapters, which allow for easy progression through the material
- Full-color photos and illustrations of the featured techniques and body structures
- A hardbound spiral cover, which allows the book to lie flat for easy reference while the reader is studying or doing practical applications
- Key terms listed at the beginning of the chapters that introduce important concepts
- User-friendly, at-a-glance marginal definitions
- Practical tips containing important information that engages the reader and provokes critical thinking
- A consistent organizational chapter format in Part II for effective learning
- Clear references throughout the chapters that assist readers in finding material located elsewhere in the text
- Chapter objectives at the start of each chapter that offer a preview of the chapter's material
- Review Questions at the end of each chapter
- Critical-Thinking Questions at the end of each chapter that encourage students to troubleshoot multiple scenarios and engage in discussion
- Quick Reference Tables at the end of each chapter in Part II that summarize key points covered in the chapter
- Links at the OLC to supplemental education materials

ONLINE LEARNING CENTER
(www.mhhe.com/jurchclinical)

The Online Learning Center (OLC) consists of three sections: Information Center, Instructor Center, and Student Center. The Information Center has sections of the student text, including a sample chapter.

The Student Center also has sections of the student text, along with a mixed quiz for each chapter, the Glossary from the book, and games for enhanced learning.

The Instructor Center contains the Instructor's Manual for this text, which includes an overview of and introduction to the material to aid instructors with its incorporation into the curriculum. The manual also includes extended chapter outlines, sample course outlines, curriculum suggestions, sample lesson plans, teaching strategies/instructor tips, learning activities, and answers to the questions in the text.

Also for the instructor are PowerPoint presentations for each chapter; an image bank of the text's illustrations, which can be printed and used as handouts; and EZ Test questions for each chapter.

McGraw-Hill's EZ Test is a flexible and easy-to-use electronic testing program. The program allows instructors to create tests from book-specific items. It accommodates a wide range of question types, and instructors may add their own questions, as well. Instructors can also create multiple versions of the test, and any test can be exported for use with course management systems such as WebCT, BlackBoard, and PageOut. EZ Test Online is a new service that gives instructors a place online where they can easily administer EZ Test–created exams and quizzes. The program is available for both PC and Macintosh operating systems.

ACKNOWLEDGMENTS

The creation of this book has been a distinct privilege and the culmination of my education and experiences to date, and it would not have been possible without the numerous people I have encountered throughout my life. To all those who have influenced the development of this text, I say thank you. In particular, I would like to thank Kim Morris, for giving me the opportunity that has opened numerous doors and led me to some of the best experiences of my life; my massage therapy instructors, in particular Fran Cegalka and Angie Bitting, who instilled a passion in me for the profession and opened my eyes to its possibilities; Robinlee Hackney, for helping me realize my potential; Graham Solomons for his guidance and advice; Hughie O'Malley, for providing me the opportunity to work with and learn from the best; George Stamathis, for helping me get this project off the ground; my photographer, Jack Alterman, for lending his creative genius to this project; John Di Giovanni and all the models, for donating their bodies to the cause; Alisa Whitt, for lending her expertise in research; my editor, Rebecca Razo, for honing my words to help them deliver their message; Connie Kuhl, for keeping me on task and helping me navigate through this project; the entire production team at McGraw-Hill, without whom none of this would have been possible; and, finally, all my instructors, colleagues, and students, who continually challenged me to elevate the profession of massage therapy.

Reviewer Acknowledgments

Lynne Anderson, BA Soc. Science/Holistic Health, LMT, NCTMB
High Tech Institute
Kansas City, MO

Lurana S. Bain, LMT
Elgin Community College
Elgin, IL

Mary Berger, BA, CMT
Kirtland Community College
Roscommon, MI

Bernice L. Bicknase
Ivy Tech Community College of Indiana
Fort Wayne, IN

Jennifer L. Bierbower, CNMT, LMT, NCBTMB, BA
Southeastern School of Neuromuscular and Massage Therapy, Inc.
N. Charleston, SC

Raymond J. Bishop, Jr., PhD
Certified Advanced Rolfer
The Center for Inner Knowing
Sandy Springs, GA

Monique Blake
Keiser Career College
Miami Lakes, FL

Susan L. Bova, NCBTMB
Massage Therapy Program Coordinator
Certified Master Medical Massage Therapist
Penn Commercial
Washington, PA

Gregory John Brink
University of Pittsburgh
Titusville, PA

Susan E. Brock, LMT, NMT
Academy of Healing Arts
Macon, GA

Duane D. Brooks, MS, ATC
New Orleans Saints
Metairie, LA

Rebecca Buell
McIntosh College
Dover, NH

Michelle Burns, BSN, BS Alt. Med, LMT, MTI
Advanced Holistic Healing Arts
Austin, TX

Nathan Butryn
Boulder College of Massage
Boulder, CO

Nancy Mezick Cavender, MM, LMT, LNMT
Rising Spirit Institute of Natural Health
Atlanta, GA

Fran Cegelka
Institute of Therapeutic Massage and Movement
Nashville, TN

Mark L. Dennis, III, LMT
Director of Student Services
Southern Massage Institute
Collierville, TN

Jennifer M. DiBlasio, AST ACMT, CHT
Career Training Academy, Inc.
New Kensington, PA

Cindi Gill
Body Business School of Massage Therapy
Durant, OK

Jocelyn Granger
Ann Arbor Institute of Massage Therapy
Ann Arbor, MI

Jeanne S. Griebel, LMT, NCETMB
Director of Massage
Capri College
Dubuque, IA

Holly Huzar, LMT
Center for Natural Wellness School of Massage Therapy
Albany, NY

Marc H. Kalmanson, MSN, ARNP, LMT, C.Ht., RYT
Holistic Health Care Consultants
Keystone Heights, FL

Joel Lindau
Cambridge College
Aurora, CO

Theresa Lowe, LMT, NCTMB
Hesser College
Manchester, NH

Mary A. McCluskey
Wisconsin School of Massage Therapy
Germantown, WI

Tara G. McManaway, M.Div., LPC ALPS(WV), LMT (WV), CMT (MD)
College of Southern Maryland
La Plata, MD

Lisa Mertz, PhD, LMT
Queensborough Community College
Bayside, NY

Maralynne D. Mitcham, PhD, OTR/L, FAOTA
Professor and Director, Occupational Therapy Education Program
Medical University of South Carolina
Charleston, SC

Adam C. Nance, LMT
International Academy of Massage Therapy
Colorado Springs, CO

Jay Nelson, LMT, LMP (member ABMP, NCBTMB)
Inner Journey Healing Arts Center
Hillsboro, OR

Deborah Ochsner
Institute of Business and Medical Careers
Fort Collins, CO

David J. Razo
American Career College
Anaheim, CA

Dr. Grace Reischman, BA, DC, LMBT
South Piedmont Community College
Monroe, NC

Suann Schuster, MA/LMP
Great Lakes Institute of Technology
Erie, PA

Sandy Scott, NCRMT-CCI
Director of Massage Program, TCL and Lead Instructor
South Carolina Massage & Esthetics Institute
Beaufort, SC

Missy Sheldon
Keiser University
Lakeland, FL

Cheryl Siniakin, PhD, LMTI, NCTMB
Director of the Associate-in-Science Degree in Massage
Therapy Program
Community College of Allegheny County, Allegheny
Campus
Pittsburgh, PA

Matthew Sorlie, LMP
Director of Education
Cortiva Institute, Brian Utting School of Massage
Seattle, WA

Tina A. Sorrell, RMT, LMT, MTI, NCTMB
American Institute of Allied Health
Lewisville, TX

Michael A. Sullivan, BS, CMT
Assistant Professor and Program Coordinator,
Therapeutic Massage
Anne Arundel Community College
Arnold, MD

Brad Welker, DC
Central Oregon Community College
Bend, OR

Kim Woodcock, NCBTMB
Program Director, Massage Therapy
McCann School of Business and Technology
Sunbury, PA

Walkthrough

chapter 9

Conditions of the Hip and Knee

Every chapter opens with a Chapter Outline, Objectives, Key Terms, and an Introduction that help prepare students for the learning experience.

chapter outline

chapter objectives

At the conclusion of this chapter, the reader will understand:

- bony anatomy of the region
- how to locate the bony landmarks and soft tissue structures of the region
- where to find the muscles, and the origins, insertions, and actions of the region
- how to assess the movement and determine the range of motion for the region
- how to perform manual muscle testing to the region
- how to recognize dermatome patterns for the region
- trigger-point location and referral patterns for the region
- the following elements of each condition discussed:
  - background and characteristics
  - specific questions to ask
  - what orthopedic tests should be performed
  - how to treat the connective tissue, trigger points, and muscles
  - flexibility concerns

KEY TERMS

acetabulum
angle of inclination
anteversion
chondromalacia patella
iliotibial band friction syndrome (ITBFS)
ligamentum teres

meralgia paresthetica
patellar tendonosis
patellofemoral pain syndrome (PFPS)
piriformis syndrome
quadriceps angle (Q angle)
screw-home mechanism

Introduction

The hip and the knee compose an important part of the lower extremity. While constructed differently, they are interrelated and dysfunction in one can affect the other. The hip and the knee provide a stable foundation that allows the upper body and the trunk to perform activity. Since humans interact with their surroundings through bipedal locomotion, limitations in either of these regions can be devastating.

The hip's strong, bony stability helps protect it from injury. It is one of the body's two ball-and-socket joints, and it is one of the largest and most stable joints in the body. During locomotion, however, the hip can be subjected to forces that are four to seven times the body's weight, thus making the joint vulnerable to stress-related injuries (Anderson et al., 2000). While injuries to the hip are not as common as injuries to the lower extremities, the overall prevalence of hip pain in adults has increased over time (Paluska, 2005). Yet 30% of hip-related pain still remains without a clear etiology.

There are three reasons why it is difficult to determine the origin of hip pain:

1. The joint is not superficial. Pain may be felt across a broader region, making it more difficult to determine which structures are involved.
2. Hip pain is often referred from the surrounding structures, and dysfunction in the sacrum, the lumbar spine, and the groin can all refer pain into the hip.
3. There is debate as to the specific topographic area that can be defined as the "hip" (Birrell et al., 2005).

Not surprisingly, the prevalence of hip pain depends largely on the assessment methods used, and, unfortunately, no gold standard of assessment exists.

Quite different from the hip, the knee is prone to traumatic injury because of its anatomy. It is located at the ends of the two longest bones in the body, the femur and tibia, which act as two long lever arms, exposing the joint to large torques. Because these two long bones are stacked on one another, the knee has to rely on soft tissue structures, such as ligaments and muscles, to provide stability. This intricate balance between static and dynamic structures makes the knee a complicated area to assess. All the relevant structures must be considered, including related areas that may refer pain into the knee, such as the lumbar spine, hip, and ankle.

Entire texts are written on the pathology of the hip and knee. While this chapter is not a comprehensive review of these regions, it does provide a thorough assessment of the dysfunctions and some of the more common pathologies in the regions. In addition, this chapter covers:

- Specific bony landmarks for palpation
- Soft tissue structures, including the muscles of the region
- The movements of the region, and basic biomechanics of the hip and knee
- Manual muscle tests for the hip and knee
- Dermatome and trigger-point referral patterns for the involved muscles
- Some common causes of dysfunction, and how to assess and treat them using soft tissue therapy

Dynamic color illustrations and photographs enhance learning.

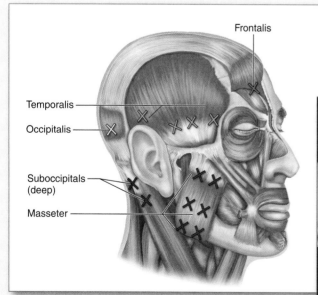

Frontalis
Temporalis
Occipitalis
Suboccipitals (deep)
Masseter

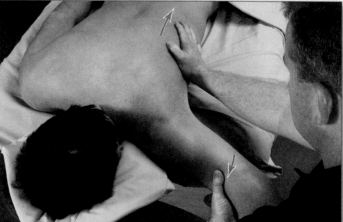

Table 6-8 Orthopedic Tests for SIJ Dysfunction

Orthopedic Test	How to Perform
Gillet's (sacral fixation) test (This is a mobility test.)	Have the client stand directly in front of you, facing away. Place your thumbs on the PSIS on both sides, and have the client fully flex one thigh to the chest while standing on one leg. The PSIS on the flexed side should move in an inferior direction. If it does not move or moves in a superior direction, it indicates a hypomobile joint or a "blocked" joint; this is a positive test.
Sacroiliac compression (gapping) test (This is a pain provocation test.)	Client is in the supine position. Place your hands cross-armed on the ASIS, and repeatedly apply a downward and outward pressure to the ASIS as if you were trying to spread the two iliums apart. Unilateral pain in the posterior leg, the PSIS, or the gluteals may indicate an anterior sprain to the SIJ. Pain elsewhere may indicate the involvement of other structures.
Patrick's (Faber's) test (This is a pain provocation test.)	Client is in a supine position. Place the outside of the foot and ankle of the involved leg on the knee of the contralateral leg, and let it fall out to the side. Place one hand on the knee of the involved leg and the other hand on the ASIS of the uninvolved leg. Stabilize the ASIS, and apply pressure to the bent knee. Pain in the SIJ of the involved side may indicate pathology and is considered a positive test.
Gaenslen's test 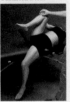 (This is a pain provocation test.)	Client is in the supine position close enough to the edge of the table that the hip extends beyond the edge. Have the client draw both legs up to the chest and slowly lower one into extension. Pain in the SIJ of the extended leg is considered a positive test and may indicate pathology. *Note:* If the client cannot lie in the supine position, place him or her on the side and draw the bottom leg up to the chest; have the client hold the position. Bring the top leg into hyperextension while stabilizing the pelvis. Pain in the SIJ is considered a positive test.

Chapter 6 Conditions of the Lumbar Spine and Sacrum 199

Tables within each chapter help summarize important information.

"It is a good, straightforward writing on the basic and useful information needed to plan a treatment." *Nancy Cavender, Rising Spirit Institute of Natural Health, Atlanta, GA*

iliotibial band friction syndrome (ITBFS) A common overuse injury caused by excessive friction between the distal iliotibial band and the lateral condyle of the femur, resulting in inflammation and pain.

Marginal definitions provide easy reference to the important terms within each chapter.

Practical Tip boxes give students important information to expand on concepts or enhance the treatment of conditions.

Practical Tip

The primary goal in treating contusions is to remove the excess blood and fluid from the area as quickly as possible to provide the optimal environment for healing.

SUMMARY

"For a treatment to work, it must be specific" (Kraft, 2003). Formulating a treatment plan is an ongoing process for each client. It involves a constant sequence of assessing, treating, reassessing, and either continuing with the same treatments or trying something different. This requires that therapists continually use all of their resources to provide the most effective therapy possible. This chapter has discussed the components of gathering information to create a treatment plan. In order to know how to heal, the therapist must first understand the types of tissue involved, the ways injuries can occur, and the injury process itself. Information must be gathered from the client that will contribute to the overall picture of the problem. This information is gathered in several different ways, ranging from verbal questioning to manual assessment techniques. When an injury occurs, other structures may be affected far away from the injury site. The methods of assessing the kinetic chain and determining the level of compensation were discussed in this chapter. Once the necessary information is obtained, various me[...]
sented in the chapter help assemble it into useful patterns and [...]
treatment plan.

The key points in each Chapter Summary help students retain what was just learned.

REVIEW QUESTIONS

1. How large are the forces that the hip is subjected to during locomotion?
2. What is the angle of inclination?
3. What is the purpose of a labrum in the joint?
4. What is the strongest ligament in the body?
5. What is the function of the ligamentum teres?
6. What are the functions of the menisci?
7. What are the six orientations of the sciatic nerve in relation to the piriformis?
8. What is a classic symptom of iliotibial band friction syndrome?
9. What is the "movie theater sign"?
10. What is the difference between true and functional leg-length discrepancies?
11. Why does the degeneration of the articular cartilage in chondromalacia not cause pain?
12. What is the Q angle, and how is it measured?

Review and Critical-Thinking Questions at the end of every chapter reinforce the concepts learned in the chapter.

QUICK REFERENCE TABLES

Bony Structures of the Lumbar Spine

Lamina groove	Groove on either side of the spinous processes from the cervical region to the sacral region.
Umbilicus	Known as the belly button and lies at the level of L3-L4.
L4-L5 interspace	L4-L5 interspace should line up with the top of the iliac crest.
Iliac crest	Place the palms of your hands in the flank area just below the ribs, and press down and in. You should feel the top of the crests.
Transverse processes L1-L5	Directly lateral to their spinous processes. Make sure you are lateral to the musculature. The longest and easiest to find is L3. Use the L4-L5 interspace to locate L4 and the rest of the segments. L1 is more difficult to locate as it is partially covered by the 12th rib. L5 is also difficult, as it is covered by the iliac crest.
Iliac tubercle	From the top of the crests, move anteriorly to find this tubercle. It is the widest point on the crests.
Anterior superior iliac spine (ASIS)	Most anterior part of the crest. Have the client lie supine, and place the palms of your hands on the front of his or her hips.
Anterior inferior iliac spine (AIIS)	From ASIS, move inferiorly about ½ inch. You won't be able to directly palpate this structure.
Pubic crest	Place your fingertips in the umbilicus. Rest your hand in an inferior direction on the abdomen. Slowly press down and in; the heel of your hand will hit a bony ledge.
Pubic symphysis	Once you find the crest, there is a joint directly in the middle.
Pubic tubercles	On either edge of the pubic crest are small bumps.
Anterior transverse processes of lumbar spine	Have the client flex the knees to soften the abdomen. Use the umbilicus and ASIS as reference points. Starting at the ASIS, slide into the tissue until you reach the lateral edge of the rectus abdominus. Once there, direct pressure downward.

QUICK REFERENCE TABLE

Quick Reference Tables summarize information discussed in the chapter in a quick and easy format.

"The Quick Reference Tables make the material easier to follow."
Michael Sullivan, Anne Arundel Community College, Arnold, MD

part I

General Principles

chapter 1

Introduction to Clinical Massage

chapter outline

chapter objectives

At the conclusion of this chapter, the reader will understand:

- basic history and evolution of massage therapy
- the three classifications of touch therapy
- differences between orthopedic and medical massage
- components of clinical massage according to the author

key terms

clinical massage
clinical reasoning
manual therapy

massage therapy
medical massage
orthopedic massage
sensitivity

specificity
Swedish Movement System

Introduction

In order to discuss clinical massage, we must first remind ourselves where massage has come from and understand the importance touch has had in the realm of health care. This chapter begins by giving a brief history of massage therapy and discussing different types of touch therapy. It then discusses two popular systems of clinically relevant massage, listing their major objectives and principles. The components of clinical massage are introduced in this chapter and expanded on throughout the remainder of the text. The basis of treatment—putting all the components involved in clinical massage together—closes out the chapter, stressing the importance of understanding why, when, and to what extent the techniques of clinical massage are applied.

HISTORY OF MASSAGE THERAPY

Manual therapy has been used since the beginning of recorded history. "Medicine was essentially touch therapies before the advent of drugs" (Field, 2002). Early cave paintings depict people engaged in massage, and Hippocrates, the founder of modern medicine, placed great value on the practice: "The physician must be skilled in many things and particularly friction" (Hippocrates from Mochlicon, 1928) (Fig. 1-1).

The age of modern massage and manual therapy took shape thanks in large part to Swedish physiologist Pehr Henrik Ling (Fig. 1-2). In the early nineteenth century, Ling combined gymnastics, exercise, and manual therapy to develop the **Swedish Movement System** The practice rapidly gained popularity, making its way to the United States in 1856. Soon, the Swedish Movement System and the practice of manual therapy began

manual therapy
The diagnosis and treatment of ailments of various etiologies through hands-on intervention.

Swedish Movement System Developed by Pehr Henrik Ling, a combination of massage, gymnastics, and exercise used in the treatment of disease and injury.

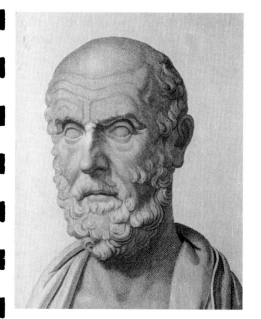

Figure 1-1 Hippocrates of Cos (c. 460 B.C.–c. 370 B.C.).

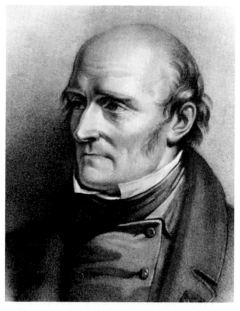

Figure 1-2 Pehr Henrik Ling (1776–1839).

growing in new directions, eventually expanding to both traditional and nontraditional health care settings.

Massage began to wane from the American medical model around the 1940s at the time of the pharmaceutical revolution; however, several countries, such as China, Japan, Russia, and Germany, continued to use massage as a form of health care. Today, many countries still consider massage therapy a form of medical treatment and include it in the national health insurance (Field, 2002). Although this has not always been the case in the United States, massage has recently started to reemerge in the American health care setting.

Defining Touch Therapy

As numerous techniques for assessing and treating musculoskeletal disorders have evolved, the terms massage therapy and manual therapy have held different meanings for different people (Rivett, 1999). According to DiFabio, soft tissue manipulation, massage, manual traction, joint manipulation, and joint mobilization all encompass massage therapy (DiFabio, 1992). Yet with more than 75 varying types of massage and bodywork, and with myriad terms to describe the practice, massage therapy can seem difficult to define. Generally, however, **massage therapy** is defined as the manual manipulation of the body's soft tissues for therapeutic purposes.

There are three classifications of touch therapy: energy methods, manipulative therapies, and amalgams (combinations of both) (Field, 2002). It is important to note, however, that no single system of touch can treat every problem. A good therapist will utilize a variety of techniques, along with well-developed clinical-reasoning, critical-thinking, and interpersonal skills to determine the most appropriate course of treatment.

Additionally, therapists should aim to involve their clients in the healing process. Empowering clients to take an active role in their own health care is a fundamental principle in preventive medicine.

The remainder of this text examines the use of massage therapy for treating orthopedic conditions through utilization of various tools within a massage therapist's scope of practice, including assessment, soft tissue manipulation, manual traction, and joint mobilization.

SYSTEMS OF CLINICALLY RELEVANT MASSAGE

As massage has moved further into the realm of acceptance as a health care modality, various systems of treatment have evolved to meet the needs of the public. Forms of therapeutic massage, including clinical, medical, and orthopedic massage, utilize advanced techniques that are usually outside the general population's normal understanding of massage therapy.

Medical Massage

Medical massage is applied to a specific area of the body on the basis of the pathology of the patient's chief complaint. It is not a general massage treatment (Lawton, 2002). Rather, it uses a system of patient care and treatment

---

📖 **massage therapy**
The manual manipulation of the soft tissues of the body for therapeutic purposes.

⭐ **Practical Tip**

Involve clients in their treatment as much as possible. The more the clients understand, the more quickly they will heal.

📖 **medical massage**
A system of manually applied techniques designed to reduce pain, establish normal tissue tension, create a positive tissue environment, and normalize the movement of the musculoskeletal system.

that is based on the medical model. Much like training for other health care professions, medical-massage training involves the thorough study of the structure and function of the human body; this creates the foundation for "problem-based education," which means that the training is centered on the treatment of the patient. In other words, the therapist's education is based on the characteristics of the pathology and the application of massage techniques directed at that pathology. Each problem is addressed on the basis of its pathology, and the body is assessed part by part.

Medical massage is not a full-body massage. Instead, massage techniques and protocols are applied in stages that attempt to correct a specific pathology and achieve four important clinical objectives: reduce inflammation, restore a normal soft tissue environment, establish a normal range of motion, and find improvements in the patient's complaints.

Objectives of Medical Massage

1. Reduce inflammatory process
2. Restore normal soft tissue environment
3. Establish normal range of motion
4. Find improvements in patient complaints

Orthopedic Massage

Orthopedic massage involves therapeutic assessment, manipulation, and movement of locomotor soft tissues to reduce pain and dysfunction. Orthopedic massage uses a more varied approach of techniques and systems and incorporates a broad spectrum of methods and tactics to treat soft tissue dysfunction (Lowe, 2003). Orthopedic massage also requires an advanced understanding of the body and how it functions; therefore, massage therapists must possess specialized knowledge, skills, and abilities, as well as understand how to use specific massage techniques to determine the most appropriate and effective method of treatment.

There are four components of orthopedic massage. The first is orthopedic assessment, wherein the practitioner must assess the nature of the condition and understand the physiological characteristics of the problem. Next, the therapist must match the physiology of the injury to the treatment. Since no single massage technique can treat every complaint, for the most effective results, the pathology of the injury should match the physiologic effects of the technique. The third component is treatment adaptability. Since each client is different, the therapist must tailor treatment to each client and take care not to fall into a routine based simply on the condition. Lastly, the therapist must understand the rehabilitation process: that the body heals at different rates depending on the individual and type of tissue involved.

There are four steps in the rehabilitation protocol. The first is to normalize the soft tissue dysfunction, which can be achieved through various modalities based on the tissues. The next step is to improve flexibility through appropriate stretching techniques. The last two steps are to restore proper movement patterns and to strengthen and condition the area.

orthopedic massage
A combination of therapeutic assessment, manipulation, and movement of locomotor soft tissues to reduce pain and dysfunction.

Objectives of Orthopedic Massage

1. Conduct orthopedic assessment
2. Match physiology of injury to treatment
3. Adapt or modify treatments to best fit individual clients
4. Understand the rehabilitation protocol
   - Normalize soft tissue dysfunction
   - Improve flexibility
   - Restore proper movement
   - Restore proper strength

COMPONENTS OF CLINICAL MASSAGE

Like medical massage and orthopedic massage, **clinical massage** is also tailored to the individual. While there is a systematic order to working on the various tissues, therapists should adapt their knowledge and skill to fit each situation. The process of treating specific musculoskeletal disorders begins first with knowing what not to treat. As therapists, we must be able to recognize situations that are outside our scope of practice, and we must know when we should modify treatments or when the use of modalities other than massage may be more beneficial. In order to accomplish this, we must have a foundation of knowledge on which to build.

Components of Clinical Massage

The foundation of clinical massage includes several components:

1. Advanced knowledge of anatomy and physiology
2. Proficient palpation skills
3. Competent assessment ability (special tests)
4. Detailed history
5. Visual observation

Advanced Knowledge of Anatomy and Physiology

The first component of clinical massage is an advanced working knowledge of the anatomy and physiology of the body, particularly the musculoskeletal system. This is especially important considering that up to 30 percent of visits to primary care physicians in the United States are due to musculoskeletal disorders (DiCaprio, 2003). Advanced anatomy and physiology knowledge includes understanding the biomechanics of the body and how its dysfunction contributes to the development of pathologies. Without this knowledge, moving on to and comprehending more advanced concepts is impossible. How can we treat the body if we don't know how it works?

The fact is that a fundamental knowledge of the musculoskeletal system is necessary regardless of the medical discipline one practices. However, a 1998 study showed that medical students are not getting the necessary education to gain proficiency in this area of medicine. Eighty-five medical school graduates took a basic musculoskeletal competency exam, in which a passing score of 73 was certified by 124 chairpersons of various orthopedic medicine departments around the country. A staggering 82 percent of those who took the test did not pass (DiCaprio, 2003).

While massage therapists are not held to the same standards as physicians, it is crucial for them to possess advanced knowledge when it comes to the musculoskeletal system. Indeed, with growing evidence supporting the efficacy of massage, therapists should consider themselves soft tissue specialists (Jull, 2002), whose primary goal is to assist in the elimination of pain through the correction of dysfunction in the body.

Proficient Palpation Skills

Therapists must be proficient at palpation, since palpation skills are vital to assessing a condition. Many approaches to manual therapy depend on the validity of palpatory findings. Treatment is guided by a therapist's knowledge of the body's structures and ability to differentiate them, as well as the ability to determine muscle-fiber direction and identify temperature differences; therefore, therapists who are not proficient in palpation will be unable to provide effective treatment.

A common problem with palpation is *competency*, which is the mastery of a relevant body of knowledge, skills, and behaviors. Several studies have shown that a strong foundation in clinical assessment combined with professional experience leads to greater reliability and accuracy in palpation.

Competent Assessment Ability (Special Tests)

As therapists develop their skills, they become increasingly proficient at creating an assessment. Performing special tests, including the assessment of active and passive ranges of motion, manual muscle tests, and specific orthopedic tests, is an essential component of this skill set. Yet the role of assessment in the profession of massage is often misunderstood because therapists do not diagnose. Diagnosing involves labeling a symptom or group of symptoms, which is clearly outside the therapist's scope of practice. Assessment, however, helps the therapist gather information, which, in turn, guides treatment. In addition, a great deal of information about a client's condition comes from special tests, which are one of the most accurate ways to assess the function of the body's locomotor tissues.

A therapist's success lies in his or her ability to administer assessment tests properly; simply performing regional tests correctly isn't enough. Therapists must consider sensitivity and specificity when analyzing test results.

Sensitivity is the percentage of clients who have the condition and also show a positive result. A test's sensitivity demonstrates how accurate the test is at identifying when the condition is present. **Specificity** represents the percentage of clients who show a negative result but who do not have the condition. This determines whether the test shows a negative result. If a test has a high sensitivity and is accurate in identifying a condition

sensitivity
The percentage of subjects tested who have the condition and show a positive result.

specificity
The percentage of subjects who show a negative result but who do not have the condition.

but has a low specificity and is therefore unable to distinguish between those who have the condition and those who don't, then additional information gathered during the assessment will help determine the course of treatment. Knowledge regarding which tests have the highest levels of both sensitivity and specificity will help identify the client's problem.

In addition to providing information, assessment tests facilitate communication between health care providers about the condition, and this subsequently improves the client's continuity of care.

Detailed History and Visual Observation

The final components of clinical massage are taking a detailed history and conducting a visual observation of the client.

The first and most important step in creating a treatment plan is to thoroughly interview the client. An interview provides vital information about the client's condition and helps determine the mechanism of injury. It will also guide every other step of the assessment, from what structures to palpate to which orthopedic tests to perform. There exists an important synergy between the client's history and the assessment. Understanding the history of a condition is useless without having a knowledge base on which to draw and the ability to apply the skills required. Likewise, having the necessary skill set but failing to gather a client history is equally useless.

Visual observation correlates to a therapist's knowledge of anatomy and physiology in order to recognize what is normal and abnormal, based on each individual. Although this skill seems simple, it often takes years of experience to master.

ASSEMBLING THE PIECES

Using clinical massage to treat a condition is similar to using a recipe to cook a meal: The ingredients are combined in a specific order, and following the steps of the recipe exactly as they are written will produce a favorable result. Remember, however, that not everyone will enjoy the meal to the same extent because individual tastes vary. One person may like more spices, while another may prefer fewer. A good chef discusses individual tastes with his or her patrons and adjusts the ingredients as necessary.

Clinical massage takes the same approach. The recipe directs the order of the treatment components, which are the connective tissue, trigger points, muscle inconsistencies, and range-of-motion restrictions. The ingredients encompass the massage therapist's knowledge and skills. The therapist talks with the client to gather information and then draws on his or her experience to determine the best way, and in what proportion, to apply the treatment that will produce the most benefit. One person may require additional connective tissue work, while another may need more flexibility training. There are many protocols that give step-by-step instructions on which stroke to use and in what direction. While these may generally produce positive results, every person is unique and treatment must be customized to the individual.

Clinical Reasoning

Massage therapists learn how to adjust the recipe to the needs of the client through **clinical reasoning**. A therapist might have the biggest bag of tricks in the profession, but picking through them one by one is a shotgun approach to treatment.

Clinical reasoning involves taking the separate details of the subject and organizing them into usable patterns. All too often, therapists memorize techniques and then blindly apply them. Memorization is helpful but only when the techniques are used in the proper context. According to Bloom's Taxonomy of Educational Objectives, there are six levels of increasing cognitive complexity (see Table 1-1).

The first three levels—knowledge, comprehension, and application—involve learning the techniques. While these levels are important, they may not help much in the clinical setting. In order to elevate treatment beyond the learning stage, the therapist must practice the three higher levels—analysis, synthesis, and evaluation. To some extent, these levels are developed through experience, which is why experienced practitioners respond differently to information than do novice practitioners.

Massage modality notwithstanding, a fundamental characteristic of a successful therapist is a greater understanding of how the body functions. As we know, massage therapy involves much more than spreading lubricant on a client in a series of strokes for a designated period of time. It is essential to understand why, when, and to what extent we apply specific techniques, as well as how they affect the body.

clinical reasoning
The process of taking separate details of the subject, analyzing and evaluating the information, and organizing it into usable patterns that can be applied to the treatment.

Table 1-1 Bloom's Taxonomy of Educational Objectives

1. Knowledge	4. Analysis
2. Comprehension	5. Synthesis
3. Application	6. Evaluation

SUMMARY

This chapter has looked at the history and various systems of clinical massage, discussing their basic theories and objectives. Once the components of clinical massage have been collected, the therapist uses a very important clinical-reasoning process to ensure that those components are put together in a way that produces the most effective results possible.

REVIEW QUESTIONS

1. What are the three classifications of touch therapy?
2. What are the objectives of medical and orthopedic massage?
3. What are the components of clinical massage, as described in the text?
4. What is the difference between sensitivity and specificity when dealing with orthopedic assessments?

CRITICAL-THINKING QUESTIONS

1. Should people take more responsibility for their own health? Why?
2. Should a massage therapist know how to perform clinical massage? Why?
3. Discuss why the critical-thinking process is important in the development of a treatment plan.

chapter 2

Review of the Basics

chapter outline

chapter objectives

At the conclusion of this chapter, the reader will understand:

- selecting a table
- factors for selecting lubricant
- positioning of clients in the prone, supine, and side-lying positions
- draping of clients in the prone, supine, and side-lying positions
- basic principles of body mechanics
- two main stances used in massage
- elements of massage strokes
- the five basic Swedish massage strokes

key terms

body mechanics
effleurage
ergonomics
friction
petrissage
repetitive motion injury
tapotment
vibration

11

Introduction   This chapter reviews some basic equipment and skills necessary to succeed in the massage therapy profession. It covers criteria for choosing a massage table; lubricants and their uses; client positioning techniques and corresponding draping methods; proper body mechanics; the two primary stances; basic Swedish massage techniques; and repetitive motion injuries, their causes, and techniques for their prevention.

TOOLS OF THE TRADE

There are several questions to consider when choosing massage equipment:

ergonomics The scientific study of the relationship of anatomy and physiology to the work of humans.

1. *Is the equipment ergonomically supportive?* **Ergonomics** is the scientific study of the relationship of anatomy and physiology to the work of humans. We must be able to adjust the environment and equipment to support the alignment and balance of the body during activity (Salvo, 2003).
2. *Does the equipment enhance the client's comfort?* Equipment should make the therapist's job easier by facilitating the relaxation of the client.
3. *Is the equipment a wise investment?* Is it durable, quality equipment for the price? Is the equipment really necessary?

When you are assessing equipment for purchase, it is wise to garner the opinions of other experienced massage therapists.

Massage Tables

Choosing a table is largely based on the type of work to be performed. Therefore, this section focuses on tables suitable for clinical massage. Although table features vary among manufacturers, there are some universal variables:

- *Frame:* Table frames are made of wood or aluminum, and there is little difference in quality between the two. The major advantage of aluminum over wood is weight and ease of adjustability. Regardless of the frame, the table should be strong enough to support the weight of both the therapist and the client.
- *Height:* Depending on the style, a table's height can range from 17 to 34 inches and is usually adjustable in ½-inch increments. Adapting the height of the table to each situation is vital in maintaining proper mechanics and avoiding injury. To determine proper height, stand next to the table with your arms by your side. In this position, your fingertips should barely brush the top of the table; however, it's also fine if your fingers are just short of the table. In clinical massage, it is better to have the table slightly lower.
- A common mistake among therapists is failing to adjust the height of the table for individual clients. Therapists use their body weight more

efficiently and avoid injury when the massage table is adjusted properly; therefore, the therapist must know when adjusting the height is necessary. Variables include how high on the table the client's body is when he or she is lying down and how he or she is positioned during treatment.

- *Width:* Generally, massage tables are between 28 and 31 inches wide. Appropriate width depends on the massage therapist's height but can also be affected by the size of the client. A shorter therapist will need a narrower table, while a taller therapist can work with a wider table.
- *Length:* Length is the least important factor in selecting a table. Generally, tables measure 72 to 73 inches long, but the face cradle will add 10 to 12 inches and bolsters will shorten the length of the client.
- *Accessories:* The most important massage table accessory is the face cradle, which should be fully adjustable to a variety of angles. Another important accessory is a rolling stool, which enables the therapist to move around the client with ease.

<aside>
Practical Tip

When choosing a height range for your table, set the table as high as it will go to determine whether you will ever use it at that height. If not, consider a lower table range.
</aside>

Lubricants

In clinical massage, lubricant allows minimal to unhindered glide over the client's body, depending on the tissue being addressed. Some factors to consider when selecting lubricant include how long it lasts, the amount of glide it has, its cost, whether it will stain clothing or linen, if it nourishes the skin, if it has medicinal properties, and if it could cause allergic reactions.

For connective tissue and trigger-point work, select a lubricant that is somewhat tacky and provides very little glide, such as cocoa butter. When focusing on general treatment of the muscles, use something that allows more glide over the tissues, such as oil, lotion, or cream.

When deciding how much lubricant to use, consider factors such as how emollient the lubricant is, whether the client has dry skin, the amount of the client's body hair, and the objective of the massage. Starting with less lubricant is better; more can be added as necessary (Salvo, 2003).

POSITIONING

Often overlooked, the way in which a therapist positions the client can dramatically alter the quality of the massage. Clinical massage is usually goal-specific and performed on a particular region of the body. This usually involves the client's direct participation. Consider these factors when determining client position:

1. The client should be as comfortable as possible.
2. The client's body should be properly aligned.
3. The client's position should facilitate efficient and effective access to the area of concern.
4. The client's position should be adjusted based on his or her physical limitations and individual situation.

Once treatment has started, do not be afraid to reposition the client as necessary.

Prone Positioning

In the prone position, the client's neck should be in a neutral position in the face cradle. Heavier clients or large-chested female clients may need additional support between the chest and face cradle. Use a small bolster or a rolled-up towel, and place it horizontally on the table to provide support.

A client with a low-back condition may benefit from a pillow placed across the front of the pelvis to reduce the lordotic curve in the spine. Providing bolstered support underneath the feet or simply hanging the feet off the end of the table is also beneficial and can increase a client's comfort.

Supine Positioning

In the supine position, supporting the neck with a rolled-up towel, a small bolster, or the face cradle pad will help keep the neck in a neutral position. A bolster or pillow behind the back of the knees offers additional support, although the amount of support necessary will vary from client to client. Additional support for the feet, legs, or arms may be required, depending on the situation.

Side-Lying Positioning

The side-lying position is great for clinical massage purposes. It is especially important to adjust the table's height to accommodate this position.

The key to effectively using a side-lying position is to ensure the stability of the client. The client should feel secure during the session and not as though he or she might fall off the table. Ensure appropriate side-lying positioning through the following steps:

- Have the client move his or her back near the edge of the table.
- Straighten the client's bottom leg, and place the top leg over a pillow or pillows. Use enough pillows so that the top leg is parallel to the table. This keeps the client from rolling forward and keeps the hip from rotating.
- Have the client hug another pillow to support the top arm and shoulder.
- Place a pillow underneath the head to keep the neck aligned.

Practical Tip

Since the client will be resting higher on the table, lower the table's height to accommodate a side-lying position.

PRINCIPLES AND PURPOSES OF DRAPING

While this section does not provide comprehensive descriptions of every draping method, it includes specific techniques geared for clinical massage treatments. Draping is a simple concept, yet its implications are huge. Proper draping helps establish a client's trust and confidence in his or her therapist.

Since clinical massage involves frequently changing the client's position, an option is to have the client wear a minimal garment (bathing suit top, tube top, running shorts, etc.) to decrease the possibility of unwanted exposure. The purposes of draping remain the same regardless of the work performed. They include defining the area of work, creating a professional atmosphere, protecting the client's modesty, and keeping the client warm.

Therapists should be proficient in draping using both a sheet and a towel. Sheet draping typically consists of a twin fitted sheet, a twin top sheet, and a pillowcase. Towels used for draping should be full bath size. It is wise to have both sheets and towels available to accommodate any situation. Adhere to the following principles when draping:

1. Discuss draping with the client prior to the start of the session, informing him or her of the draping possibilities even if you are unsure about the position(s) you will use during the session. This will give the client a sense of security and prevent unwelcome surprises to the client.

2. If the client is wearing undergarments, tuck the drape into the garments and slide them down to the appropriate level before undraping the area. This prevents lubricant from getting on the clothes and keeps the drape in the appropriate position.

3. If it becomes necessary to treat an area in close proximity to a sensitive area on the body, drape so that only the direct area of treatment is exposed. Inform the client of your intentions, and be sensitive to his or her comfort level. Use discretion and err on the side of caution in your draping practices.

4. Enlist the help of the client as necessary. Ask the client to secure the drape when you are working around sensitive areas.

5. When turning the client over, secure the drape to the table to prevent unwanted exposure.

Prone-Position Draping Techniques

Sheet

Undrape the back to the level of the posterior superior iliac spine or the top of the natal cleft (Fig. 2-1). If the client is wearing undergarments, tuck the drape in the back and along the sides and slide the garments down to the appropriate level before peeling the drape back.

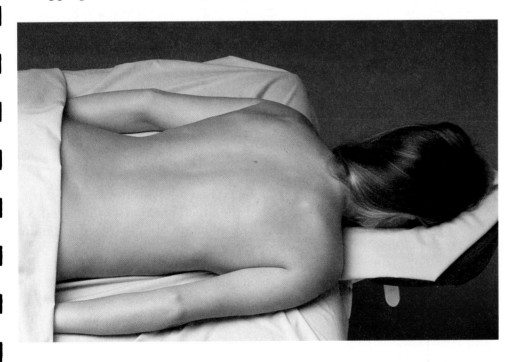

Figure 2-1 Prone back drape. Tuck drape into undergarments if necessary.

Figure 2-2 Prone leg drape. Tuck drape and fold free edge back so that only the treated leg is exposed.

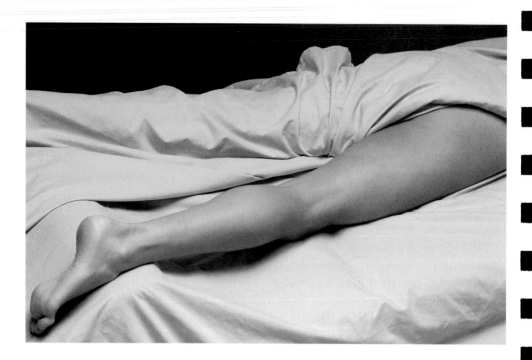

To drape the leg:

1. Expose the foot and lower leg and move the leg closer to the therapist, supporting it under the foot and at the knee.
2. With the hand closest to the client's head, pick up some of the drape at the midthigh. With the other hand, tuck the drape under the opposite leg about halfway up the thigh, angling the drape up toward the opposite side of the hip.
3. Fold the free edge of the drape back so that only the treated leg is exposed (Fig. 2-2).

To work higher up on the thigh at the pelvis, use the same procedure, but stand on the opposite side of the client and tuck the drape under the treatment thigh, aiming your hand toward the hip you are going to work on. Drape the hip as part of either the back or the leg.

- *As part of the back:* Pin the drape in the center at the top of the natal cleft, and fold it back toward the hip.
- *As part of the leg:* Tuck the drape on the side on which you are working. Fold the drape up and over the hip, being careful not to expose the natal cleft.

Towel

Using a towel to drape can take practice since it is smaller than a sheet. Before the client gets on the table, fold the towel in an accordion fashion and place it on the table at hip level. For female clients, place an additional towel across the table at chest level.

Once the client is on the table and has pulled the towel across the hips, adjust the drape lengthwise to cover the entire body. To expose the back down to the hips, use the sheet method described above.

Drape the legs using the sheet method as well, even though you will not have additional material to tuck.

To drape the leg:

1. Expose the leg and secure the free edge of the towel under the treatment leg. If the towel is not large enough to cover the entire body, use an additional towel to cover any exposed areas not being worked on.

To turn the client over:

1. Adjust the towel to the horizontal position along the body, and pin the towel against the table.
2. For female clients, pull the far edge of the chest-level towel over the back.
3. Roll the client away from you; the drapes will cover as they need to.

Supine-Position Draping Techniques

Sheet

To drape the chest and abdomen of a male client, tuck the drape into any garments as necessary and fold the sheet back to the level of the anterior superior iliac spine.

For female clients:

1. Place a towel on top of the sheet across the chest area.
2. Holding the towel in place, slowly slide the sheet out from under the towel.
3. Once you have pulled the sheet past the bottom edge of the towel, tuck the drape into any garments and fold the sheet back to the level of the anterior superior iliac spine (Fig. 2-3).

If necessary, ask the client to secure the top drape while you slide the sheet out. To access different parts of the chest and abdomen, fold the free edges of the towel, taking care not to expose the breasts.

Leg draping in the supine position is similar to that in the prone position:

1. Using a pillow or bolster under the knees, expose the foot and move the leg closer to you, supporting it under the knee and at the ankle.

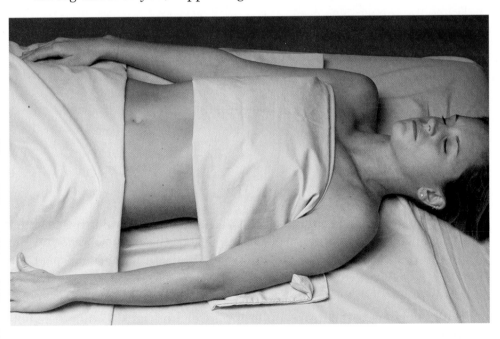

Figure 2-3 Chest and abdomen drape for a female client in the supine position.

Figure 2-4 Supine leg drape. Tuck drape and fold free edge back so that only the treated leg is exposed.

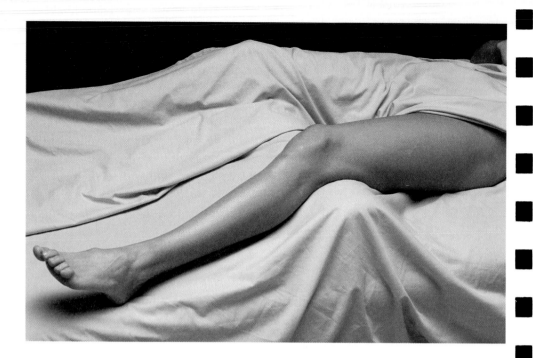

2. Pick up some of the drape at the midthigh level with the hand closest to the client's head. With the other hand, tuck the drape under the opposite leg about halfway up the thigh, angling the drape up toward the opposite side of the hip.
3. Fold the free edge of the drape back so that only the treated leg is exposed (Fig. 2-4).

Leg draping in the supine position should be easier than in the prone position because of the gap created by the bolster under the knees. If you are working up higher on the thigh, tuck the drape under the leg of the side on which you are working. For both legs, peel the free edge of the drape back and conform it to the thigh, being careful not to cause unwanted exposure.

Towel

Towel-drape a male client using the same techniques as described for the prone position. If you used a towel to drape a female client in the prone position, peel the drape back to access the part of the chest you are going to treat. If you did not, use the sheet draping technique described above. For leg draping of clients of either gender, use the techniques described for the prone position.

Side-Lying-Position Draping Techniques

In clinical massage, an option is to have clients in the side-lying position wear minimal garments. For male clients, tuck the drape in around the pillows to the level of the anterior superior iliac spine and then peel the drape back as necessary.

For female clients:

1. Pull a portion of the drape up to hip level, and tuck it under the bottom side.

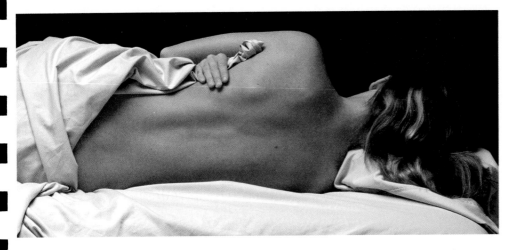

2. Have the client use her bottom hand to secure the drape along her top side.
3. Peel the sheet back to her hand. You should have access to the entire back, arm, and neck (Fig. 2-5).

Drape the legs using the following steps for either gender:

1. Expose the top foot up to the knee.
2. Slide the free edge of the drape at the knee directly up the lateral side of the thigh.
3. As you move the drape up, tuck it lightly around the thigh to temporarily secure it and avoid any unwanted exposure (Fig. 2-6).

Figure 2-6 Side-lying leg drape.

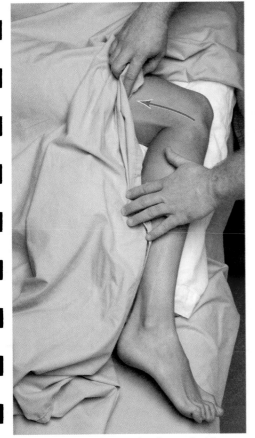

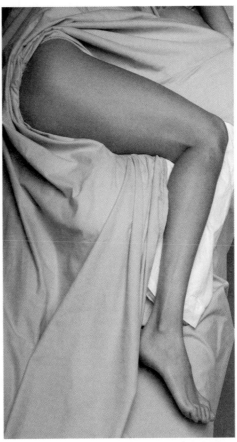

(a) Slide directly up the lateral side of the thigh

(b) Once the hip and leg are exposed, tuck the drape to secure.

4. Once the hip and leg are exposed, tuck the drape in between the thigh and the pillow to secure.

BODY MECHANICS AND STANCES

Body mechanics are the proper use of postural techniques to deliver massage therapy with the highest level of efficiency while causing the least amount of strain to the practitioner. Proper body mechanics can influence the application of massage, as well as decrease fatigue and discomfort and help prevent repetitive motion injuries to the practitioner.

Principles of Body Mechanics

There are five basic principles of body mechanics:

1. *Strength:* Massage requires strength for assisting clients on and off the table and performing the massage.
2. *Stamina:* Massage therapists must have enough stamina to see several clients over the course of a single day.
3. *Breathing:* Proper breathing helps therapists relax and keep a steady pace, as well as fuel the muscles and enhance mental and physical health.
4. *Stability:* Therapists must move from a stable base. The legs are two and a half times stronger than the upper body and provide much more stability. Proper body mechanics will transfer the force from the lower body to the upper body and then to the client.
5. *Balance:* In combination with stability, balance helps therapists overcome the forces of gravity. The more balanced a therapist is, the less energy he or she will expend during the massage.

Using proper body mechanics also includes utilizing other parts of the body to perform massage strokes. Fingers and thumbs should be aligned with the rest of the body and supported. This reduces wear and tear on the joint. Forearms, elbows, massage tools, and even knees are common substitutes for the hands and thumbs when extra pressure is required. Understanding how to use these body parts in combination with the other components of body mechanics can significantly enhance the longevity of a therapist's career.

Stances

There are two main stances used in the application of massage therapy: front/archer and straddle/horse. While both can be used to apply all the strokes, each stance is recommended in specific situations.

The following principles relative to these stances will help ensure proper alignment:

1. *Keep the low back straight.* Bend the knees and not the waist to lower the body to reach the client. Bending at the waist puts unwanted stress on the lumbar spine and changes the center of gravity responsible for maintaining balance.

---

body mechanics
The proper use of postural techniques to deliver massage therapy with the highest level of efficiency, while causing the least amount of strain to the practitioner.

Practical Tip
Always work within your limits, even if you use proper body mechanics. Overworking yourself will only lead to the breakdown of the body.

2. *Maintain a constant distance between the hands and the abdomen* by imagining a rod connecting the hands to the umbilicus. This will prevent overreaching in front or behind during stroke application, forcing you to move around the client during the massage.
3. *Keep a proper distance from the client.* This is accomplished by keeping the elbows almost straight but not locked during the stroke. Stay far enough away from the table and client so that there are minimal wrinkles on the dorsal side of your wrist from too much extension at the joint.
4. *Remember that the movement and pressure of the stroke comes from your body weight.* Keeping your elbows straight ensures that the force is transferred to the client. Pressure from leaning on the client and sinking into the legs will propel you along the client's body.

Front/Archer

Use the front/archer stance when motion along the client's body is required. To perform a stroke using this stance:

1. Place your feet parallel to the table, pointed at a 45° angle to the table.
2. Place your hands on the client, bending your front knee to reach the client, being mindful of the wrinkles in your wrists and the distance between your hands and umbilicus. Keep the lumbar spine straight.
3. Keeping your shoulders relaxed and back leg straight, sink into your front leg and let your hands slide along the client (Fig. 2-7) until you reach the end of the body part or your body mechanics begin to become compromised.
4. Once the stroke has ended, bend your back knee. This will lower your center of gravity and start your body moving backward. Push off with

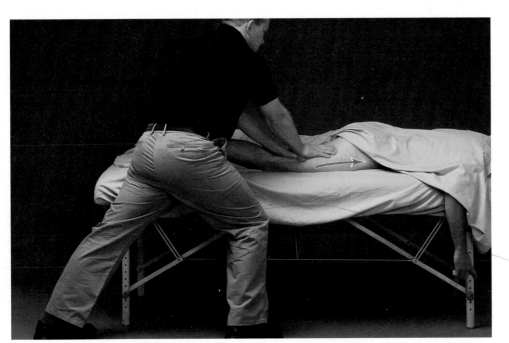

Figure 2-7 Performance of effleurage stroke in the front stance. Bend front knee to reach client. Sink into your front leg, and let your hands slide along the client.

Figure 2-8 Performing the return stroke in the front stance. Bend your back knee and push off with your front leg while returning your hands along the client.

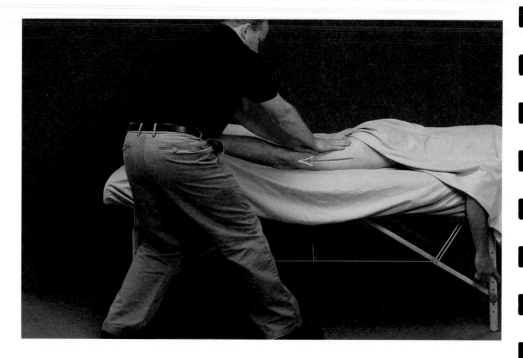

your front leg while returning your hands along the client (Fig. 2-8). Keep your lumbar spine straight and at a constant distance between your hands and stomach on the return stroke.

If you wish to continue the stroke along the client without returning:

1. When you reach the end of the stroke, instead of bending the back knee, bring the back foot up to meet the front foot.
2. Continue moving along the client with both feet together until you start to reach too far with your hands.
3. Step forward with your front leg while you continue the stroke.

Straddle/Horse

Use the straddle/horse stance when little or no movement along the client is necessary or when you must reach across the client's body. Some of the principles we saw in the front stance are also applied here (Fig. 2-9).

1. Stand facing the table with your feet perpendicular to the table and at least shoulder width apart.
2. Bend the knees to lower yourself to the client, keeping the lumbar spine straight.
3. Perform the stroke keeping the knees bent, the low back straight, and wrinkles in the wrist to a minimum.

MASSAGE STROKES

Effects of Massage Strokes

When massage techniques are applied to the body, they can affect it through two different response pathways. Mechanical responses to techniques occur as a direct result of the manipulation of the tissues from components such

Part I General Principles

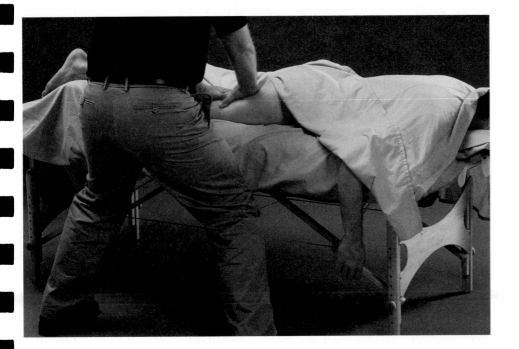

as pressure, range of motion, and the pushing, pulling, lifting, compressing, and twisting of the tissue. Changes to the body as a result of these effects include increased circulation to the area, changes in fluid movement, increased pliability of the tissue, and reduction of adhesions. The other type of response is called a *reflexive response* and is the result of changes directed through the nervous system. When the nerves in the area are stimulated, they create a response either locally or systemically. Examples of reflexive responses include the reduction of blood pressure through the increased diameter of blood vessels, the decreased arousal of the sympathetic nervous system, and changes in hormone levels. While these responses are discussed separately, they are closely related and often occur simultaneously.

Elements of Application

Five basic strokes form the foundation of Swedish massage. From this foundation, parts of the strokes are modified to create advanced techniques. Regardless of the technique, however, there are several basic elements relevant to stroke application:

1. *Intention:* The primary element of stroke application, which drives the other stroke components. It is based on a plan of action or desired outcome.
2. *Pressure:* The amount of force applied to the tissue. Pressure can be a difficult element to master, and sensing the amount of pressure that a client can tolerate takes years of experience; however, there are a few general rules of thumb:
   * The more pressure used, the slower the stroke should be. This allows the client's body time to adjust.
   * The smaller the surface used to apply the stroke, the slower the stroke should be. A smaller surface area (e.g., the thumb versus the palm) transfers more pressure than does a larger surface.

- The harder the body part used to apply the stroke, the slower the stroke should be. A bony surface (e.g., the elbow versus the palm) transfers more pressure than does a surface with more soft tissue.

3. *Depth:* The distance traveled into the body's tissue. Depth is related to pressure and is controlled by the client. A therapist can use as much pressure as he or she wants; however, it will be effective only if the client allows penetration of the tissue. A client tensing his or her muscles, for example, can diminish the effectiveness of the stroke.

4. *Excursion:* The distance traveled over the body in one stroke. It is based on whether the therapist chooses to treat a whole region of the body, a single muscle, or a restricted area within a muscle.

5. *Rhythm:* The repetition or regularity of the massage movements.

6. *Continuity:* The flow of the strokes and the transition from one stroke to the next. Continuity is related to rhythm.

7. *Duration:* The length of time spent massaging a certain area.

8. *Sequence:* The combination and arrangement of strokes. Sequence is based on the plan of care.

9. *Speed:* How fast or slow a massage movement is. Both fast and slow movements have specific effects on the body. As a general rule:
   - Fast movements are stimulatory in nature, while slow movements are relaxing.
   - The client should be able to follow the therapist's movements across his or her body.
   - Speed can affect the therapist's palpation ability.

The elements of massage stroke application are listed in Table 2-1.

Table 2-1   Elements of Massage Stroke Application

Intention	Pressure
Depth	Excursion
Rhythm	Continuity
Duration	Sequence
Speed	

Swedish Massage Strokes

Effleurage

Effleurage is the most widely used stroke in massage therapy. It is also known as the *gliding stroke* and is extremely versatile. It is often the first and last stroke applied and can be used on any body surface. Some of its uses are listed in Table 2-2.

There are many variations of this stroke, but the basic gliding stroke is applied while the therapist is in the front stance. The hand placed in front should be on the same side as the leg that is forward, with the heel of the front hand placed in the web space of the back hand. It is important

effleurage The most widely used stroke in massage therapy. It has several uses, including applying lubricant, warming up the tissue, assessing the condition of the tissue. Also known as *gliding stroke*.

Table 2-2 Uses of Effleurage

Introducing the client to the therapist's touch

Applying lubricant

Warming up the superficial tissue

Assessing the condition of the tissue

Transitioning between strokes when moving around the body

Breaking from a more specific technique

Moving blood and lymph

Soothing or stimulating an area

to conform the hands to the body part being worked. Apply the stroke using the technique described above for the front stance. Effleurage can be applied using the palm, fist, fingers, forearms, thumb, and elbows.

Depending on the intention or the body part, there are variations of effleurage:

1. *One-handed:* Used for small areas such as the neck, hands, and feet.
2. *Two-handed:* Performed with hands side by side; generally used for the back.
3. *Shingling:* Performed by using one hand followed immediately by the other hand in an alternating fashion.
4. *Nerve/feather:* Performed by tracing lightly over the skin; primarily used as a finishing stroke.

All effleurage strokes should be applied in a centripetal direction when appropriate. This stroke has a powerful impact on venous blood flow and should be used to encourage the return of blood to the heart.

Petrissage

Also known as the *kneading stroke,* **petrissage** has multiple uses, some of which are listed in Table 2-3. Petrissage is usually applied to areas where

petrissage A stroke that is applied by kneading the tissues to wring out the waste products and bring in new blood flow.

Table 2-3 Uses of Petrissage

Flushing the tissues of the body in order to "milk" or "wring out" the muscle

Removing metabolic waste and drawing in new blood, improving tissue nutrition

Separating the muscle fibers to reduce adhesions

Stretching and broadening the tissue

Improving tissue pliability

Stimulating the nervous system

more tissue exists, such as the legs and arms; however, it can be applied in some form to the entire body. There are hybrids of this stroke, but traditional petrissage is performed as follows:

1. Arrange the hand in a C formation, and conform it to the body part.
2. Compress the tissue, grasp it, lift it off the body, and repeat in a smooth, rhythmic manner.
3. To avoid pinching the client, do not slide.
4. Have minimal space between your hand and the tissue.
5. Once you have worked an area, move along the body part and repeat.

This technique can be applied using one hand for smaller areas or two hands for larger areas. If using two hands, alternate them: When one hand is compressing and squeezing the tissue, the other is lifting it off the body.

Friction

friction The most specific Swedish stroke. The skin is secured and the tissue underneath is moved in various directions depending on the intent. It is typically used around joints, bony areas, and specific restrictions within the muscles.

Friction is the most specific of Swedish stroke techniques. Because it is effective at increasing circulation, it is typically used in areas that do not get a lot of blood flow; however, it can be applied anywhere on the body. Friction does not involve sliding or gliding along the tissue, so lubricant is not generally used. Rather, it is necessary to secure the skin and move the tissue underneath. Friction can be applied superficially or deeply, depending on the intent. It is typically used around joints, bony areas, or specific restrictions and adhesions in the muscles and tendons. Some of its uses are listed in Table 2-4.

Table 2-4 Uses of Friction

Generating heat

Breaking up adhesions and scar tissue

Increasing circulation

Dilating capillaries

Reducing joint stiffness

Stimulating a healing response

To perform this stroke, use any body part that is suitable for the area on which you are working, typically a thumb or braced finger, and secure the skin moving only the tissue underneath. Press downward and move in different directions depending on the desired outcome. Some of the variations include:

1. *Parallel friction:* Applied along the same direction as the fibers in the tissue being worked.
2. *Cross-fiber friction:* Applied perpendicular to the fiber direction of the tissue.

3. *Circular friction:* Applied by moving in a circular direction after the skin has been secured.
4. *Multidirectional friction:* Applied in multiple directions once the skin is secured. This is beneficial for working on scars because of the random pattern in which the fibers are laid down.

Tapotment

Most people are familiar with percussion, or **tapotment.** Percussion involves simultaneous or alternating striking movements, delivered with the hands, fingertips, palms, or loose fists. Its uses are listed in Table 2-5.

There are several variations of this stroke, all of which should be applied rhythmically, beginning slowly with a light touch and gradually increasing speed and depth. Percussion methods include:

1. *Hacking:* This is the "karate chop" stroke portrayed in television and movies. It is delivered with the hands vertical, making sure the hands and wrists are relaxed, using the ulnar side of the pinky finger, alternating hands to produce a rhythm.
2. *Beating:* This stroke is performed using a loose fist and striking the client with the ulnar side of the hand. Beating is typically used on more muscular areas such as the gluteals and legs. It is important to be mindful of the pressure and alternate the fists in a pattern during application.
3. *Cupping:* This stroke is used primarily to loosen congestion in the chest. Forming a *C* with the hand, strike the client's thoracic region with the edges of the cupped hand, producing a "horse-hoof" sound. It is important to remain aware of the mechanical effect of this stroke and take breaks to allow for clearing of the lungs. It is a good idea to perform some soothing strokes after cupping to help relax the client.

tapotment A stroke that involves striking movements using various parts of the hand. Its uses include stimulating or relaxing the nervous system, increasing local blood flow, and mechanically loosening phlegm in the respiratory system. Also known as *percussion.*

Table 2-5 Uses of Tapotment

Stimulating the nervous system
Increasing local blood flow
Decreasing pain through the gate theory
Desensitizing nerve endings in an area
Mechanically loosening phlegm in the respiratory system
Relaxing the nervous system if done for an extended period of time

Vibration

Vibration is defined as a shaking, quivering, trembling, or rocking motion applied to the body using hands, fingers, or tools. There are three categories

vibration A shaking, quivering, trembling, or rocking motion applied using the hands, fingers, or tools.

of vibration: fine, gross, and rocking. Each is applied in a different manner, but the effects of all are the same and are listed in Table 2-6.

Fine vibration involves using the fingertips to apply a quivering or trembling motion to the body. The therapist can remain in one location or move along the body.

Gross vibration is sometimes referred to as *jostling,* wherein the therapist grasps the muscle belly and shakes it rather vigorously back and forth. Moving the limbs can also create slack in the muscle where gross vibration is applied in order to increase the intensity. A variation on gross vibration incorporates traction. It is performed by grasping the limb and applying slight axial traction while shaking the limb gently.

Rocking is similar to jostling, the difference being that the whole body is rocked at once. Starting at one end of the body or in the middle, rock the body back and forth until fluid movement is achieved. Move alongside the client until the entire body is incorporated.

Table 2-6 Uses of Vibration

Enhances relaxation

Increases circulation

Relieves pain

Stimulates proprioceptive mechanisms in the muscle

Reduces sensitivity of trigger points and tender points

Stimulates peristalsis in the large intestine

REPETITIVE MOTION INJURIES

In the massage profession, therapists are born possessing the tools necessary to perform the job: their hands and other body parts. Therapists generally do not have to make a huge investment in equipment to do the work; however, there is a downside to this. Unlike the case with other trades, if a therapist's "tools" wear out or break, they cannot be replaced.

The most common reason therapists leave the profession is repetitive motion injury. To ensure long and successful careers, therapists must make taking care of their bodies a priority.

Signs and Symptoms

📖 **repetitive motion injury** An injury that results from an accumulation of micro-traumas related to inefficient biomechanics, poor posture, incorrect work habits, or constant motion.

A **repetitive motion injury** results from an accumulation of micro-traumas related to inefficient biomechanics, poor posture, incorrect work habits, or constant motion (Salvo, 2003). Initial symptoms are related to the inflammatory response and can include pain, swelling, heat, and redness.

As the condition progresses, increased muscle tone, trigger-point formation, muscle imbalances, and nerve entrapment can occur. One would assume that massage therapists would be able to identify an injury in its early stages and reverse its effects, but this is not as easy as it sounds. Repetitive motion injuries take time to manifest. By the time the pain presents, the therapist may have already incorporated improper body mechanics into normal activities—and it is not always easy to break a bad habit.

Practical Tip

Repetitive motion injuries take time to develop, so be sure to always use proper mechanics.

Prevention Tips

Taking precautions to prevent the onset of repetitive motion injuries is the best way to keep them from occurring. Ways to reduce the onset of repetitive motion injuries are listed in Table 2-7.

Table 2-7 Ways to Reduce Repetitive Motion Injuries

Using various types of strokes

Scheduling periods of rest between clients

Stretching between appointments

Adjusting the massage table to an appropriate height

Avoiding too much sustained pressure

Maintaining a personal level of physical fitness

Using proper body mechanics

Getting regular massages

SUMMARY

Understanding the basics of massage therapy can prevent many unwanted consequences of performing massage incorrectly or with the wrong equipment. The primary equipment, such as the table and lubricants, were discussed along with selection criteria for both. Client positioning and draping were reviewed to ensure the most effective and comfortable treatment possible. The fundamental principles of body mechanics and how they relate to the use of the two primary stances in massage therapy were addressed so that the therapist does not incur any detrimental effects of performing therapy. The last section of this chapter explained the basic Swedish massage strokes used in the profession and discussed the elements of their application as well as the benefits of using each. A therapist must have a strong understanding of the basic principles of massage therapy in order to be able to effectively apply the advanced techniques covered later in this text.

REVIEW QUESTIONS

1. What are some considerations when purchasing a table?
2. What are some considerations when selecting a lubricant?

3. How is a client placed in the prone, supine, and side-lying positions?

4. What are the purposes of draping?

5. What are the proper draping techniques for a client in the prone, supine, and side-lying positions?

6. What are the basic principles of body mechanics?

7. What are the two main stances used in massage? How are they done?

8. What are the elements of application for massage strokes?

9. What are the five basic massage strokes? How are they applied? When are they used?

10. How does a therapist reduce the chances of incurring a repetitive motion injury?

CRITICAL-THINKING QUESTIONS

1. How does a client's size influence the height of the massage table?

2. What are some reasons to avoid using a lot of lubricant when working on connective tissue?

3. How does client positioning assist with the therapist's body mechanics?

4. What are some reasons that therapists leave the profession?

chapter 3

Advanced Concepts

chapter outline

chapter objectives

At the conclusion of this chapter, the reader will understand:

- components and functions of fibrous connective tissue
- difference between loose and dense fibrous connective tissue
- how and why connective tissue changes in response to stress
- history, theory, and application of the connective tissue massage techniques discussed
- history of myofascial trigger points
- normal contraction cycle of a muscle fiber
- causes and characteristics of myofascial trigger points
- pathophysiology of a trigger point
- how to treat a trigger point using noninvasive techniques
- how and when to perform the advanced strokes discussed
- uses and benefits of stretching, and reasons people don't stretch
- what research says about stretching
- theory and application of the stretching methods discussed

key terms

contraction knots

convergence projection theory

fibroblasts

flexibility

integrated hypothesis

Law of Facilitation

piezoelectric charge

postisometric relaxation

reciprocal inhibition

tensegrity system

Introduction   We have looked at the importance of building a strong foundation of basic massage techniques. While those techniques can be applied across any massage treatment, they are typically used in Swedish massage or as complements to other types of manual therapy.

In the area of clinical massage, we as massage therapists must have an advanced level of skill. In order to provide effective treatment, a therapist must be able to identify varying aspects of the client's condition, as well as properly incorporate advanced manual therapy methods into a plan of care. In this chapter, we discuss several advanced techniques that will also be applied as part of a treatment sequence later in the book.

CONNECTIVE TISSUE MASSAGE

Connective tissue massage takes on many different forms depending on the style applied. One of its principal uses is to elongate connective tissue that may be restricting motion. All connective tissue massage applications focus on the same tissue; therefore, more than one style may fit a particular condition. Additionally, one style is not necessarily better than another.

What Is Connective Tissue?

According to Saladin, "A tissue is composed of cells and matrix, and the matrix is composed of fibers and ground substance" (Saladin, 2005). When it comes to different types of tissue, connective tissue takes many forms, such as bone, blood, and adipose tissue. One type of dense connective tissue known as *fascia* is the most abundant and widely distributed tissue in the body. It is the first tissue that forms during embryonic development, and it is an integral part of every body structure. As a general rule, connective tissue cells take up less space than the ground substance and bind the body's structures together. They create an environment for all the other "stuff" that holds the body together and produce a shared environment for the body's cells.

Connective tissue is often described as the organ of "form." Every muscle, muscular fascicle, microfibril, and cell is surrounded by fascia, which can exert pressure of over 2000 pounds per square inch. Ultimately, it is the connective tissue that determines the length and function of muscles. It can take on many different forms and falls into three broad categories: fibrous, supportive, and fluid. This discussion focuses on fibrous connective tissue.

Components of Fibrous Connective Tissue

fibroblasts Large, flat cells that produce the fibers and ground substance that form the matrix of the tissue.

All tissue is made up of cells suspended in a ground substance. For fibrous connective tissue, the primary cells that are involved are called **fibroblasts**. Fibroblasts produce several kinds of fibers and the ground substance that create the matrix of connective tissue (Fig. 3-1).

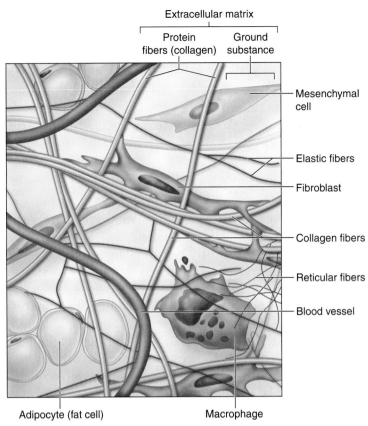

Extracellular matrix

Protein fibers (collagen) — Ground substance

Mesenchymal cell

Elastic fibers

Fibroblast

Collagen fibers

Reticular fibers

Blood vessel

Adipocyte (fat cell)   Macrophage

Figure 3-1 Fibrous connective tissue.

Fibers: Connective tissue fibers are made of protein and divided into three types: collagen, elastin, and reticular (Fig. 3-2).

1. *Collagen:* Made of collagen, this fiber makes up about 25% of the body's protein; it is extremely strong and resists stretching.

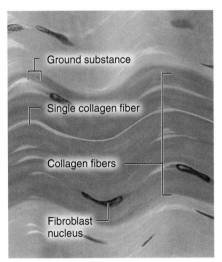

Ground substance

Single collagen fiber

Collagen fibers

Fibroblast nucleus

Ground substance

Fibroblast nucleus

Elastic fibers

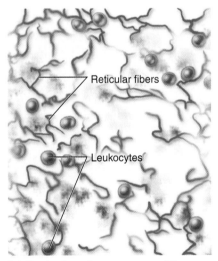

Reticular fibers

Leukocytes

(a) Collagen–extremely strong and resists stretching.

(b) Elastin–thinner and more flexible than collagen fiber.

(c) Reticular–forms spongelike frameworks for organs.

Figure 3-2 Connective tissue fibers.

2. *Elastin:* This fiber, made of a protein called *elastin,* is thinner and more flexible than collagen fiber; it recoils like an elastic band.
3. *Reticular:* Reticular fiber is a thinner, immature version of collagen fiber; it forms spongelike frameworks for different organs.

Ground substance: The various types of connective tissue fibers create a lot of free spaces in the tissue, which are filled by a gelatinous, rubbery material known as *ground substance.* Ground substance consists of large protein and carbohydrate molecules called *glycosaminoglycans* (primarily hyaluronic acid), *proteoglycans,* and *adhesive glycoproteins.* These proteins allow the easy distribution of metabolites, create part of the immune-system barrier, and form the "glue" that holds the cells together.

Fibers and ground substance are the primary components of connective tissue, no matter where the tissue is located. The many different types of connective tissue are created by varying the percentages of the different fibers and their orientation. Think of connective tissue as a gelatin mold with various materials suspended in it. The gelatin is the ground substance. When heated, the gelatin becomes fluidlike and pliable; however, it is strengthened and stabilized when material is added. For example, collagen fibers, which are very stiff, are similar to matchstick carrots. Adding matchstick carrots to the gelatin would strengthen it. Elastin fibers, in contrast, are similar to cooked spaghetti. Cooked spaghetti, which is more flexible than matchstick carrots, adds elasticity to the gelatin. The more carrots added to the gelatin in relation to spaghetti, the stiffer and stronger the gelatin mold becomes. Conversely, a higher percentage of spaghetti would add stability to the gelatin, while still allowing flexibility.

These varying combinations of fibers divide fibrous connective tissue into two categories: loose connective tissue and dense connective tissue.

Loose connective tissue has a higher ratio of ground substance to fibers. It contains all the different types of fibers and is categorized into areolar, reticular, and adipose tissue. Loose connective tissue comprises everything from fat cells and blood-vessel coverings to structural framework for spongy organs.

Dense connective tissue has a higher ratio of fibers to ground substance; it is categorized as regular and irregular. Dense regular connective tissue is much more closely packed with collagen fibers that are oriented in a parallel fashion, making it a perfect match for tendons and ligaments. Dense irregular connective tissue is packed with collagen fibers that are oriented in random directions. This allows the fiber to resist stresses from multiple directions. It is commonly found binding the dermis to the underlying tissue and the surrounding bones, nerves, and organs.

Connective Tissue and Its Relation to Massage Therapy

How does connective tissue relate to massage therapy? One unique property of connective tissue is its ability to modify its structure based on the demands placed on it. This can affect everything from the exchange of nutrients and waste products at the cellular level to the functioning of different structures within the body.

How does the body know to respond to changes? There is something in the body called a **piezoelectric charge**, which occurs when stress is transmitted through a material. When the material is deformed due to the stress, a small charge is released. In connective tissue, the cells register this charge and respond by changing or modifying the intracellular elements in the area.

One example of this process is the change in bone density as the result of weight-bearing activity. The stress placed on the bone creates extra support through the depositing of minerals, which add strength to the area. The connective tissue's response to demands can also be applied to the fibrous network.

For example, many people adopt an incorrect forward-head, rounded-shoulder posture position, which puts a tremendous amount of stress on the muscles supporting the head and neck. As a result, these muscles are not able to perform the function for which they were designed—that is, to contract and relax in succession. Instead, they are forced into a constant state of contraction, acting as straps. This strain creates a piezoelectric charge across the muscles. In response to the charge and the demands on the area, fibroblasts secrete additional collagen fibers that orient themselves along the line of tension to strengthen the straps. This new congested matrix subsequently affects the nourishment of the muscle, resulting in weakness, reduced function, and increased toxicity.

Fortunately, this process also works in reverse. The therapist must start by restoring normal function to the connective tissue in the area. Because this tissue is so integral to the function of the body, it must be addressed first; this will allow the other body tissues to expand as they are treated. Fascia has a symbiotic relationship with all the other tissues. When fascia is ignored, other treatments become less effective.

In order to reverse the process, reduce the tension on the muscle, reabsorb the additional fascia, and restore function to the area, there are two primary objectives:

1. The tissue must be reopened. This will restore normal muscle function, reconnect the sensory motor system, and restore fluid flow for tissue nutrition.
2. The lines of tension that caused the initial increased stress must be reduced.

As massage therapists, we have the ability to effect great change in the body through fascial work; moreover, there are several different approaches to working with this tissue.

Types of Connective Tissue Massage

Bindegewebsmassage

The *Bindegewebsmassage* technique is considered the precursor to all other types of fascial work. It was discovered in 1928, much by accident, by German physiotherapist Elizabeth Dicke. Dicke suffered from endarteritis obliterans, a vascular disease that causes severe arterial insufficiency. Her condition was so dire that at the time of her discovery, she was awaiting amputation of her leg. Dicke massaged her low back and gluteals

piezoelectric charge The ability of an inorganic or organic substance to generate an electric charge from pure mechanical deformation.

to ease the pain. Since the location was not easily accessible, the strokes she applied included a series of pulling and stretching movements. As she worked, she noticed that the tissue in the region was hard and thickened. The strokes created cutting and tingling sensations and a feeling of warmth. To her surprise, the circulation in her lower extremities began to improve, as did a digestive problem she had been experiencing. After her release from the hospital, Dicke spent the rest of her career researching this new technique.

Theory Bindegewebsmassage is based on a series of reflex zones and the interface of the connective tissue with the somatic and autonomic nervous systems as they correlate to the zones. The technique has been referred to as a reflex or neural therapy as well as a manual therapy because it uses the nervous system to bring about a cure. The tissue changes Dicke observed corresponded to skin zones identified by Dr. Head in 1898. These viscerocutaneous reflexes occur in dermatomes that share the same nerve root as the associated organ. The reflexes are present between the dermis and the hypodermis in the acute phase and between the dermis and the fascia in chronic conditions. Any irritation of a structure within a spinal segment facilitates the synapses within it, and this alters the activity of any other structures that share the segment. For example, dysfunction with the heart will cause a detectable change to the skin in the heart zone, as well as any structures along the segment.

Application In Bindegewebsmassage, the initial assessment requires a holistic interview to determine the extent of the autonomic imbalance. The more zones involved, the greater the imbalance. Palpate the zones by pressing, lifting, and pulling the skin, looking for asymmetry between the sides. Once the affected zones have been identified, start with the lower zones and use the tips or pads of the middle and ring fingers to pull away from the restriction; this creates the trademark "cutting" sensation. Take out the slack in the superficial tissue to allow stimulation at the proper depth. The stimulus should be within the client's tolerance level. Application requires a high level of sensitivity on the therapist's part to adjust treatment as necessary.

Structural Integration (Rolfing)

Structural Integration was developed by biochemist Ida Rolf. Born in New York City in 1896, Rolf received her PhD from Columbia University. During the 1920s, Dr. Rolf, whose primary interest was the study of the movement and function of connective tissue, was a research associate at the Rockefeller Institute. During her time there, she began to investigate homeopathy, the Alexander Technique, yoga, and osteopathy. On the basis of her studies, Rolf experimented with hands-on techniques and discovered that she could effect significant change in the human body. Over time, Rolf developed a 10-session system of touch that she termed "Structural Integration" (known today as *Rolfing*) for its relevance to how the body's structure affects its function. Rolf began teaching Structural Integration and eventually established the Rolf Institute of Structural Integration in 1971, now located in Boulder, Colorado.

Theory Rolfing restructures the connective tissue of the body, thereby realigning the physical construct. It is based on two central concepts:

1. Generally, the human body is out of alignment with gravity. Once the body moves out of alignment, gravity stresses it to a greater extent than normal. Reestablishing the balance between the two systems allows for better functioning.
2. The body's shape is created by the fascial web that can be molded. Structural Integration can reshape body structure by applying systematic pressure to tight tissues.

Rolfing seeks to align the body to its original state. When muscles are out of balance, the body compensates by adjusting to a new—usually incorrect—position, which is eventually "set" in the body as normal. If the body sets the wrong position, it starts a chain of dysfunction, thereby disrupting the entire system. The application of proper strokes and pressure will soften the fascia, allowing it to become pliable and returning it to its natural balance.

Application The fascia is manipulated using the fingers, hands, knuckles, elbows, and even knees. Treatments are between 60 and 90 minutes and performed over 10 sessions. The 10-session protocol is broken down into three phases:

1. *Superficial:* The first three sessions focus on the surface layers of the fascia. The diaphragm and rib cage are typically addressed first.
2. *Core:* Sessions 4 through 7 involve deeper layers of muscle and fascia.
3. *Integrative:* The last three sessions combine the work of the two earlier phases.

During Rolfing's infancy, sessions could cause a significant amount of discomfort to a client. As the technique evolved, therapists have emphasized communication with their clients in order to achieve maximum results with the least amount of discomfort possible. The level of discomfort can depend on how severe the past trauma was, how long the restrictions in the body have been present, or whether there are any emotional components involved. It is important to note, however, that while treatment may be uncomfortable, it should never be unbearable.

Myofascial Release

Whereas the integration of connective tissue work as part of a holistic approach to health care dates back to the beginning of osteopathy and Rolfing, *myofascial release* is a relatively new concept. Based on the Latin words *myo* for "muscle" and *fascia* for "band," this technique was created in the 1970s at Michigan State University. Over the past three decades, myofascial release has gained credibility and popularity thanks to physical therapists such as John Barnes, whose work in advancing and refining the technique has brought it to the forefront of manual therapy.

Theory Myofascial release is based on the concept that poor posture, injury, stress, and illness throw the body out of alignment. Once out of alignment, abnormal pressure is placed on the fascial network of the body, creating a "snag in the fascial sweater," which, over time, snowballs and causes adhesions, eventually resulting in adaptive tissue restrictions similar to the concentric layers of an onion. Tissues become tighter and eventually restrict the body's ability to move, making it susceptible to injury. Myofascial release works to free disruptions in the fascial network through the application of a gentle, sustained force to the restriction. The release increases space and mobility and restores balance between the body and gravity. This balance subsequently enables the body's self-correcting mechanisms to alleviate symptoms and restore proper functioning.

Application Begin with a visual analysis of the client's posture at rest and in motion, and conduct a hands-on assessment of the fascial system to evaluate areas of tightness. Once they are identified, manipulate the areas using the fingertips, hands, knuckles, or arms, starting superficially and then working into the deeper layers of the fascia. Pressure is gentle, comfortable, and relaxing. The pressure is applied in the direction of the muscle fibers and is held until the tissue "releases" or softens. The release relieves the pressure on various other structures, including the bones, muscles, joints, vessels, and nerves. The myofascial stretch can be held for between 1 and 2 minutes and sometimes up to 5. Repeat the process until the tissue is fully released. The same process is used to address the deeper layers.

The frequency of treatment is based on the individual as well as the type and severity of the condition. Myofascial release should be incorporated as part of a comprehensive treatment program that includes exercise, flexibility training, movement-awareness techniques, mobilization and muscle-energy techniques, and instruction in body mechanics. As with other types of connective tissue work, there is often an emotional component that accompanies myofascial release that may contribute to a client's physical issues; therefore, therapists may want to refer a client to counseling to help facilitate emotional healing, if necessary.

Kinesis Myofascial Integration

Thomas Myers developed *Kinesis Myofascial Integration* based on patterns of structural relationships in the body's fascia. This approach examines the musculoskeletal system in global patterns, which Myers calls "anatomy trains," rather than as a group of isolated structures. This system of treatment stemmed from his 25 years of experience as a certified Rolfer (Myers trained directly under Ida Rolf) and from his various academic roles at the Rolf Institute, which ranged from faculty member to chair of the Rolf Institute's Fascial Anatomy Faculty.

As we know, connective tissue is an endless web. Various conditions can be treated through massage applied to areas far from where the primary complaint is located. The logical question, however, is how these areas are connected. Myers began investigating the synergistic relationships of stringing muscles, bones, and other tissues together through myofascial meridians instead of separating them further and examining their roles individually. The concept of interlinked relationships is not new and has been investigated since the 1930s. While these relationships, which were discovered long ago, are based on functional connections, anatomy trains are based on fascial connections.

Theory The muscles operate both on an individual basis and as functionally integrated bodywide continuities within the fascial network (Myers, 2002). There are traceable "tracks" of connective tissue that develop as a result of strain, tension, compensations, and fixations. The purpose of Kinesis Myofascial Integration is to reverse strain patterns residing in the body's locomotor system and to subsequently restore balance, alignment, length, and ease of movement. Once these patterns are recognized, they can be easily treated to enhance overall movement and body function. While the term *meridians* usually refers to energetic lines of transmission, these connective tissue tracks can be referred to as *myofascial meridians*, which are based on lines of pull that transmit strain and movement throughout the body.

A strong underlying concept within the anatomy train model is the view of the musculoskeletal system as a **tensegrity system**. The term *tensegrity* is an invention: a shortened version of the phrase *tension integrity,* coined by the designer R. Buckminster Fuller (Myers, 2003). Tensegrity, at its essence, is a synergy between push and pull. These opposing forces should be looked at not as opposites but as complements to each other that can always be found together. Tensegrity's premise contends that structures maintain their integrity by balancing the continuous tensile forces within them, rather than leaning on compressive forces. Tensegrity structures offer the maximum amount of strength in relation to the amount of material.

When a compression structure is stressed too much, it breaks down only in the area that is stressed. This creates an isolated dysfunction that does not necessarily affect the rest of the structure and is easily corrected. When a tensegrity structure is overloaded, it also breaks down but not necessarily at the location of the stress. Because the structure distributes the load over its entirety, it will give at a point that may be far away from the load. In essence, a tensegrity structure can adjust to the strain and will become more stable as more stress is placed on it.

If we apply this concept to the body, the myofascial meridians are the main structures that tensile strain runs through. The goal is to balance the strain along these tracks and allow the bones and muscle to "float" within the fascia.

Application Kinesis Myofascial Integration generally consists of 12 sessions of deep, slow myofascial manipulation, together with movement re-education. While this technique is similar to Rolfing's multiple-session protocol, it is different through its use of the myofascial meridians as its basis. The structures along the lines are worked in different orders depending on the client. As long as the tracks are addressed in the correct order, any Structural Integration technique can be applied. As with Rolfing, there are three treatment sequences:

1. *Superficial:* Sessions 1 through 4 consist of treating the superficial front and back lines, the lateral line, and balancing the spiral line.
2. *Core:* Sessions 5 through 8 consist of treating the deep front line and balancing the lateral line.
3. *Integration:* The last four sessions consist of balancing the lines around the body.

tensegrity system A system wherein structures stabilize themselves by balancing the counteracting forces of compression and tension.

Connective Tissue Therapy

Connective tissue therapy is a general system of massage subscribed to by Florida massage therapist Pete Whitridge. Whitridge has been a massage therapist since 1988 and has spent time teaching in various institutions as well as serving both with the Florida State Massage Therapy Association and on the Florida Board of Massage. An essential element of this method is the knowledge of the muscles and their fiber directions, origins, insertions, and actions. Connective tissue therapy provides a foundation for the application of the strokes discussed later in the text.

Theory The web of connective tissue becomes restricted due to a variety of factors. As restrictions develop, other structures become compressed, inhibited, and congested. Since a large part of connective tissue is a gellike matrix, its form can be altered through pressure and heat to relieve restrictions. The focus of this work is to change the consistency of the matrix and redistribute the fascia to its original position, thereby creating more space within the tissue. By adding space to the body, all aspects of proper body function, from tissue metabolism to the uninhibited movement of the muscles and joints, can occur. The superficial layers are addressed first to create space, which allows access to the deeper layers.

The pressure and heat are applied through the therapist's touch. If the consistency of the tissue is not changing as needed, incorporating the active movement of the targeted muscles can generate additional heat, This will cause the release of heat from the inside out and allow the gel matrix to become more fluidlike. Passive motion can also be incorporated; this adds additional pressure by pulling the tissue underneath the therapist's hand, helping to "iron out" the fascia. Some components of this work include the following:

- *Use as little lubricant as possible.* It is necessary to be able to feel the connective tissue.
- *No pain, no pain.* The application of this technique should not be painful. Pain causes the body to engage its sympathetic nervous system, which creates a counterproductive environment for the work.
- *Work slowly.* Working slowly allows the client to provide real-time feedback and gives him or her time to adjust to the technique.
- *Add movement.* Movement helps encourage the tissues to "let go."
- *Treat the client, not the condition.* Be flexible with techniques, and base treatment on the situation presented.

Application Start by working the superficial fascial layers over the general region of complaint, followed by the deeper layers in the same area and any secondary areas. Basic principles include the following:

1. *Assess the tissues* (Fig. 3-3):
   - *Cranial to caudal:* Place your hands or fingers on the area you are addressing. Push and pull the tissue cranially and caudally to determine the direction in which it moves more easily.

> ⭐ **Practical Tip**
>
> Visualizing the changing consistency of the tissue can help a therapist focus on the intent of the work.

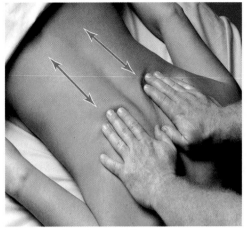
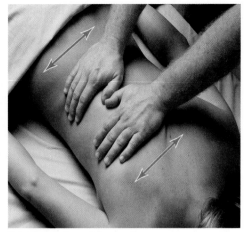

Figure 3-3 Assessment of superficial connective tissue.

(a) Cranial and caudal   (b) Medial and lateral

- *Medial to lateral:* Place your hands on the client, and move the tissue back and forth in a horizontal direction. Determine the direction in which the tissue moves more easily.
- *Diagonals:* Place your hands on the client in different orientations, and move the tissue back and forth to determine the direction of resistance.

2. *Push into the resistance.* For each direction assessed, engage the fascia in the direction of the restriction, sinking and softening into the tissue until it releases. The tissue will feel as though it "gives way," and you will begin to slide along the tissue. Pressure should be at an oblique angle between 30° and 45° and should not cause the client pain.

3. *Define the individual muscles.* Once the superficial fascia has been released, separate the borders of the adjacent muscles in the area of complaint (Fig. 3-4) and move your fingertips or thumbs along the fiber direction to strip out the fascia covering the muscles. Movement can be in one direction or in opposite directions using two fingers.

4. *Look for localized restrictions.* Apply miniversions of the lengthening and defining strokes used in the superficial-release section to individualized areas of restriction within the muscle.

5. *Incorporate adjunct techniques.* Utilize active and passive movement in areas that won't release. Do not neglect the antagonist muscles; when they are engaged, the agonist muscles shut off.

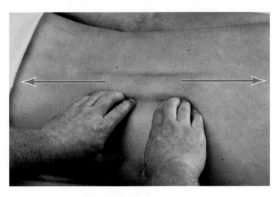

Figure 3-4 Separate the borders to identify individual muscles in the area.

- *Active:* Engage the tissues, either superficial or deep, with the stroke. Have the client contract the muscle on which you are working or its antagonist (Fig. 3-5). Try both ipsilateral and contralateral muscles until you find one that works. There is no one right way for everybody. This works for general regions as well as individual muscles.
- *Passive:* Engage the tissue in the direction of the restriction, and move the limb or tissue in an opposite direction to create countertension (Fig. 3-6). This works well for regional as well as specific areas.
- *Isometric contractions:* When working with tendons or scars within the muscle, place a directional force through the tissue along its fiber direction. This will help align the collagen fibers in a more functional pattern. A gentle isometric contraction of the involved muscle during the stroke will facilitate this.

This technique can be applied anywhere on the body as long as the therapist knows the muscles' locations and their origins, insertions, actions, and

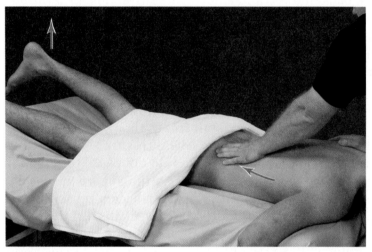

Figure 3-5 Actively engage the muscles in the area to help the tissue release.

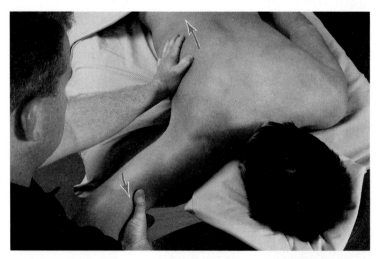

Figure 3-6 Push the tissue in one direction while moving the limb in the opposite direction to encourage the tissue to release.

fiber directions. While it is important to modify the approach based on the needs of the individual, therapists should not be afraid to create a personalized way to apply these techniques. Do what feels right for each particular client, and encourage feedback during the session. The more connection between a therapist and client, the more effective the therapy will be.

TRIGGER-POINT THERAPY

This section examines another important component of clinical massage: myofascial trigger points, including history, definitions, pathophysiology, and treatment.

The wear and tear on muscle tissue from daily activity is often a primary source of dysfunction in the body. The skeletal muscles account for nearly 50% of the body's weight—that's 200 muscle pairs, or 400 total muscles, vulnerable to developing trigger points that are capable of producing significant pain.

History

While documentation about the existence of myofascial trigger points has been around for some time, our understanding of them has evolved piece by piece. Because of their uncharacteristic presentation, they have been "discovered" numerous times and given a variety of names: In 1900, Adler described trigger points as muscular rheumatism, and a 1915 text characterized the presence of trigger points as fibrositis. The first true book about trigger points was written in 1931 in Germany and titled *Myogelosis*. In it, the authors noted that these conditions were treated effectively using manual therapy. The modern theory of myofascial trigger points emerged in 1942 thanks to Janet Travell. Between 1942 and 1993, Travell wrote over 15 papers and 4 books on the subject. The following section is based on her work.

Definitions

Understanding the terms listed below will help facilitate further understanding of myofascial trigger points.

1. *Active myofascial trigger point:* A point that generally causes complaint. It is tender, restricts range of motion, inhibits muscle strength, re-creates pain on compression, produces a local twitch response, and refers to a general reference zone.
2. *Attachment trigger point:* A point that lies at the musculotendinous junction and is caused by the tension characteristic of the taut band produced by the central point.
3. *Central myofascial trigger point:* A point located near the center of the muscle belly and associated with the dysfunctional motor end plate.
4. *Essential pain zone:* A region of referred pain produced by an active trigger point.
5. *Latent myofascial trigger point:* A point that demonstrates the same characteristics as an active point but exhibits pain and other symptoms only when palpated.

6. *Local twitch response:* A contraction of localized muscle fibers in a taut band around a trigger point, in response to stimulation of that trigger point.

7. *Motor end plate:* The area where the terminal branch of a motor neuron contacts the skeletal muscle fiber.

8. *Myofascial trigger point* (clinical definition): A hyperirritable spot in a skeletal muscle that is associated with a hypersensitive palpable nodule in a taut band. This spot is painful on compression and can give rise to referred pain, tenderness, motor dysfunction, and autonomic phenomena.

9. *Satellite myofascial trigger point:* A central point induced either neurologically or mechanically by the activity of another trigger point.

10. *Snapping palpation:* Similar to plucking a guitar string, palpation that is done by placing a fingertip at a right angle to the fiber direction of a tense band and then suddenly pressing down while drawing the finger back and rolling the band under the finger.

11. *Spillover pain zone:* An area beyond the essential pain zone in which pain is experienced by some clients due to a greater hyperirritability of a trigger point.

12. *Zone of reference:* The specific region of the body where the referral caused by the trigger point is observed.

Background

Each muscle is subdivided into smaller and smaller units, each surrounded by its own connective tissue membrane, until it reaches its functional unit: the muscle fiber (Fig. 3-7).

The muscle fiber is encased by a membrane called the *sarcolemma* and comprises long protein bundles called myofibrils. *Myofibrils* consist of different types of filaments that have various functions. The two main filaments, actin and myosin, are known as the *contractile proteins;* they shorten the muscle fiber.

The myofibrils are segmented along their length into units known as *sarcomeres* and are separated by what is called a *Z line.* Each sarcomere contains both actin and myosin and is considered the functional contractile unit of the muscle fiber. Each muscle fiber is innervated by a motor end plate that branches off the motor nerve. This end plate creates the neuromuscular junction with the fiber and is vital to muscle contraction.

Two other components essential to muscle contraction are acetylcholine and calcium. *Acetylcholine* is a neurotransmitter that is released by the motor end plate as a result of a nerve impulse. It is picked up by the sarcolemma and causes it to depolarize. This depolarization results in the release of stored calcium into the muscle fiber through a network of tubules. It is the presence of calcium that causes a reaction between the actin and myosin fibers and shortens the sarcomere. The cumulative effect of each sarcomere's shortening results in an overall change in the muscle's length.

Once the contraction is over, the calcium is pumped out of the muscle fiber in an active process using adenosine triphosphate (ATP). Since calcium is no longer present to cause the reaction between actin and myosin, the bond is broken and the sarcomere returns to its normal resting length, relaxing the muscle.

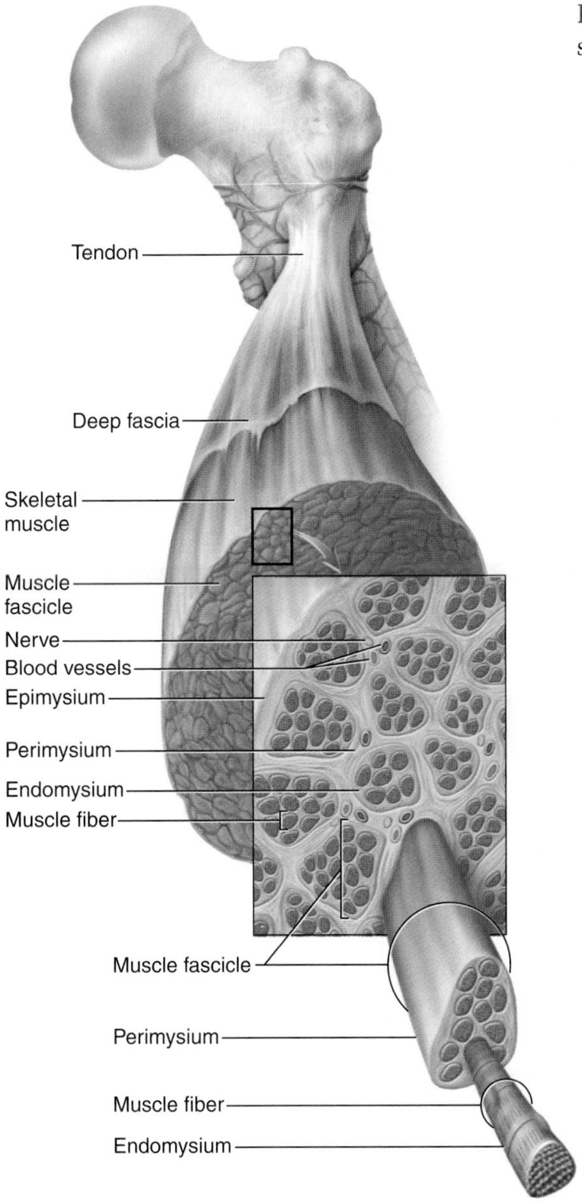

Figure 3-7 Organization of skeletal muscle.

Tendon

Deep fascia

Skeletal muscle

Muscle fascicle

Nerve

Blood vessels

Epimysium

Perimysium

Endomysium

Muscle fiber

Muscle fascicle

Perimysium

Muscle fiber

Endomysium

Causes

"Few adults make it through life without experiencing musculoskeletal pain" (Simons, 2004). Although exact figures are not known, studies have shown that trigger points were the primary cause of musculoskeletal pain in 74% of patients at a community medical center, 85% at a pain center, and 55% at a dental clinic (Fryer, 2005).

Trigger points typically arise as the result of three types of muscle overload:

- *Acute:* Excessive or unusual activity
- *Sustained:* Postural stresses, structural abnormalities, a muscle left in a shortened position for an extended period of time
- *Repetitive:* Repeated movement, especially with biomechanical faults

These types of muscle overload can occur in a variety of settings, such as occupational and athletic settings, as well as result from underlying pathologies. Additionally, muscle overload is not always physiologic; both psychological and emotional stresses can cause overload to an area.

Typically, trigger-point formation starts with an inactive point in healthy tissue. Over time, the point evolves into a latent trigger point. As acute, sustained, or repetitive stress continues, the trigger point eventually becomes active. Emotional distress, diseased organs and joints, and other points can activate trigger points, as well. However, the process works in both directions: Trigger points can revert to inactive or latent status with rest and the removal of the perpetuating factors. This cycle can repeat itself for years.

Characteristics

Whereas nerve problems cause tingling and numbness, and vascular dysfunction causes throbbing pain, trigger-point discomfort is manifested as steady, deep, and aching pain.

We have seen the definition of an active trigger point as a hyperirritable nodule within a taut band that exhibits a local twitch response and refers pain to a distance. Some of the physical findings and symptoms of trigger points include:

- Increased muscle tension
- Decreased range of motion
- Discomfort with lengthening
- Decreased force production

Latent trigger points are prevalent in both symptomatic and asymptomatic people. They transform easily into active points through minor muscle overloads; moreover, they exhibit the same characteristics as active points but elicit pain and referrals only when compressed. Attachment trigger points appear as a result of increased tension along the taut band at the musculotendinous junction. They are painful and resist stretch and vigorous contraction. Satellite points develop due to the physical effects of the tension or referral patterns of active points.

Clients with active points will complain of a poorly localized, general aching in the muscles and joints. Both motor and autonomic functions can be disturbed by trigger points, and some are listed in Table 3-1.

convergence projection theory The theory that each sensory neuron has multiple branches. When pain arises in unexpected areas of the body, it sensitizes some of the other branches and the pain is projected to those other areas.

The referred pain commonly associated with trigger points is explained by the **convergence projection theory**, which states that each sensory neuron has connections with more than one body part. It is normally expected that painful stimuli will come from only one of those areas. When pain arises in unexpected parts of the body, it is misinterpreted as coming from the usual recognized site of pain and it spills over and sensitizes adjacent areas of the spinal cord. These newly sensitized areas project the pain into an expanded region of pain.

Another characteristic of trigger points is their distinct palpable quality. The taut band described earlier results from increased tension in the shortened sarcomeres. It feels like a cord and can range in size depending on the severity of the trigger point. In some cases, several trigger points can be so close together that several different bands seem to merge.

Table 3-1 Motor and Autonomic Disturbances from Trigger
Points

Motor Disturbances	Autonomic Disturbances
Spasm of other muscles	Abnormal sweating
Weakness	Watery eyes
Loss of coordination in the involved muscle	Excessive salivation
Increased fatigue in the involved muscle	Pilomotor activities
	Dizziness
	Tinnitus
	Intestinal and digestive disturbance

There are two basic methods of palpating a trigger point and band: *flat palpation,* which uses the fingertip to locate the band and then move along its length to reveal the trigger point, and *pincer palpation,* which is performed by grasping the belly of a muscle between the thumb and fingers and rolling it back and forth to locate the bands and the trigger point. When palpated at the trigger point, the band can elicit a unique characteristic called a *twitch response.* It is a visual jerk of the muscle and occurs as a result of snapping palpation, direct pressure, and needle penetration. These combined characteristics create the criteria for assessing the presence of a trigger point. Table 3-2 lists the criteria for a trigger point.

Table 3-2 Trigger-Point Criteria

Palpable taut band
Localized tender nodule
Referred pain (active point)
Limited range of motion
Local twitch response
Reproduction of symptoms of complaint

Pathophysiology

What happens to the muscle to cause a trigger point? Unfortunately, there is no gold standard for the pathology behind trigger points. The current etiology is known as the **integrated hypothesis** (Simons, 2004) because it combines two widely accepted theories: energy crisis theory and motor

integrated hypothesis The theory that a central myofascial trigger point consists of several muscle fibers that are demonstrating regional sarcomere shortening due to an excessive and uninterrupted release of acetylcholine through a positive feedback loop.

end-plate hypothesis. The integrated hypothesis postulates that a central myofascial trigger point consists of several muscle fibers that are demonstrating regional sarcomere shortening due to an excessive and uninterrupted release of acetylcholine through a positive feedback loop.

Formation of a Trigger Point

1. Muscle overload causes an abnormal release of acetylcholine from dysfunctional motor end plates.
2. This release causes the influx of calcium into regional sarcomeres around the area of the end plates, resulting in localized contraction of the affected sarcomeres.
3. Because of the sarcomere contraction, there is an increase in the tension of the muscle fiber. This tension creates **contraction knots** in the short sarcomeres, with the contraction knots evolving into the trigger point. The lengthening of the rest of the sarcomeres causes attachment trigger points to develop, contributing to the taut band. The combination of contraction knots and lengthened sarcomeres, referred to as the *trigger-point complex,* constitutes the taut band in several adjacent fibers.
4. Trigger-point complexes that occur in multiple fibers cause an increase in the metabolic demand in the area due to the resources needed to maintain the sustained contraction; this also compromises circulation, which produces local ischemia.
5. The local hypoxia causes an energy crisis that results in the reduction of available ATP and the release of sensitizing substances, which sensitize the local nociceptor pathways. The end result is pain.
6. Because of the reduction in available ATP, the pumps that are responsible for removing the calcium that stops the contraction cannot function, and the cycle perpetuates (Fig. 3-8).

Treatment

Trigger-point therapy is divided into invasive and noninvasive modalities.

Invasive

1. Anesthetic injection
2. Botulinum toxin injection
3. Dry needling

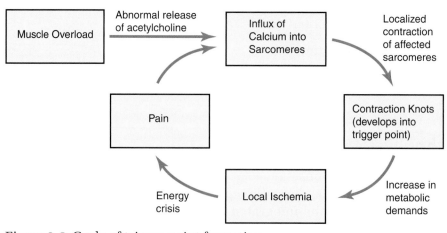

Figure 3-8 Cycle of trigger-point formation.

contraction knots Knots that are formed as a result of the localized contracted sarcomeres. The more sarcomeres involved, the larger the knot.

Noninvasive

1. Stretching
2. Transcutaneous electrical nerve stimulation (TENS)
3. Ultrasound
4. Laser
5. Manual pressure release

Since this is a textbook on clinical massage, we will discuss manual therapy approaches to treatment, specifically digital pressure and stretching.

The goal of treatment is to release the sarcomere contraction. To use the manual pressure release, locate the point and apply pressure to a tolerable level for the client (usually a range of 7 out of 10 on a standard 10-point pain scale). Maintain pressure until the tissue releases or softens; then increase pressure to reach the tolerable level again. Repeat until the nodule is no longer palpable or the complaints have diminished. Since trigger points can consist of multiple fibers, change the angle of pressure to make sure all the fibers are addressed. Maintain pressure for 30 to 90 seconds, depending on the client. Ninety-second holds produce the best results, but 30 seconds is sufficient to induce change. The technique works because digital pressure flattens out the contraction knots and helps the sarcomeres return to their original length. This return breaks the cycle and allows the fiber to relax.

Both passive and active stretching techniques can be used alone or in conjunction with manual pressure to treat trigger points. Since the goal is to return the sarcomeres to their normal resting length, stretching is a desired approach to treatment.

Passive Stretching

1. Take up slack in the muscle by stretching it to the point of beginning resistance or discomfort.
2. Have the client perform a gentle (10% of maximum) isometric contraction for 10 seconds.
3. As the client relaxes, lengthen the muscle to take up any additional slack that was created.
4. Repeat the process until there is no more possible release because the joint has reached its end range.

This type of stretching takes advantage of the neuromuscular principle of **postisometric relaxation**. A recovery phase immediately following the muscle contraction prevents the muscle from contracting again.

Active Stretching

1. Follow the same steps as those in passive stretching until the point of contraction.
2. Once the client relaxes, have the client actively engage the antagonist muscle to the one he or she contracted, to the new point of resistance or discomfort.
3. Repeat until there is no more possible release.

> **Practical Tip**
>
> When treating trigger points, vary the angles of treatment to address all the fibers involved.

> 📖 **postisometric relaxation** After an isometric contraction, a latency period that occurs that prevents the muscle from contracting again too rapidly. This is attributed to the repolarization of the muscle fibers.

In addition to using postcontraction relaxation, this process utilizes another nervous system principle called **reciprocal inhibition**, which states that for a muscle to move, its antagonist must relax.

Using one of these two stretching techniques in conjunction with manual pressure is more effective than using either method by itself.

ADVANCED STROKES

Therapists wishing to expand beyond traditional Swedish massage will want to incorporate advanced therapeutic strokes into their practices; all of these strokes can be adapted to any situation and applied to any region on the body. As with any technique, therapists should always take care to use proper body mechanics to reduce chances of injury.

Deep Parallel Stripping

Deep parallel stripping is a modification of effleurage, the most widely used stroke in Swedish massage. It provides the same benefits as regular effleurage with the addition of specificity. It requires an advanced level of skill to know how to palpate the tissue and apply the correct amount of pressure. Deep parallel stripping can be used to strip out entire individual muscles from one end to the other or to treat specific taut bands when deactivating trigger points.

As with effleurage, use a broad surface such as the palm or forearm or a small surface such as a thumb, finger, or pressure tool to apply the stroke. Perform the stroke along the fiber direction at a pressure level close to the client's discomfort threshold. Generally, a broader application is used first to prepare the tissue for any specific work to follow.

Compression

Compression has different names depending on the factors of its application. Trigger-point therapy, acupressure, neuromuscular therapy, and shiatsu all use variations of compression. It can be applied using a large surface area such as the palm of the hand, fist, or forearm or a small surface area such as a thumb, a fingertip, or the tip of the elbow. The rate of application varies depending on the desired results. A rapid succession of compression strokes may be used to stimulate the area and increase local circulation, by creating a pumping action. When applied slowly in a static fashion, compression may be used to treat a trigger point or an area of hypertonicity. The direction of pressure can be changed to affect the intent of the stroke. Various positional holds can be performed using compression in this manner. Pressure can also be applied using a variety of tools for either a broad or a specific application.

To perform compression, determine the intent and method of application based on the situation, and apply pressure to the client's tolerance level using proper body mechanics. The duration of the pressure varies with the intent.

Perpendicular Compressive Effleurage

Muscle activity consists of a broadening phase and lengthening phase. When the sarcomeres of a muscle fiber shorten during a contraction, they broaden and increase in size. To function properly, a muscle must be able to shorten completely. Injury or inactivity can cause the actin and myosin fibers to stick together, inhibiting their ability to slide past each other when contracting. Applying perpendicular compressive effleurage can break up unwanted bonds between the filaments and help restore normal function by separating the muscle fibers and breaking up adhesions within the muscle. Since there is a compression component to the stroke, it will also increase local circulation to the area.

Perpendicular compressive effleurage is performed by applying heavy pressure, to the client's tolerance level, with palms or fists for a large area or fingers or thumbs for a small area (Fig. 3-9). While maintaining constant pressure, slowly slide your hands perpendicular to the fiber direction of the muscle or area on which you are working.

To rapidly bring blood to the area, lift the tissue up off the bone during the return stroke to encourage a change in circulation. This is sometimes referred to as *lifting and broadening.* It is a variation of the stroke with a quicker pace and lighter pressure, which does not cause the client discomfort.

Cross-Fiber Fanning

Cross-fiber fanning is a cross between effleurage and compression broadening. It is used to increase circulation, reduce muscle tension, and separate adhered muscle fibers. It is usually applied to a small, specific area using the thumb.

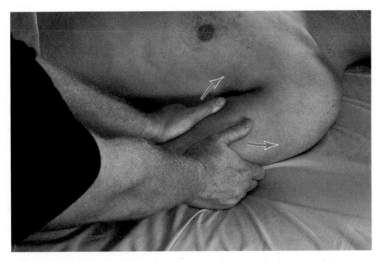

Figure 3-9 Perpendicular compressive effleurage. Slide hands perpendicular to the fiber direction.

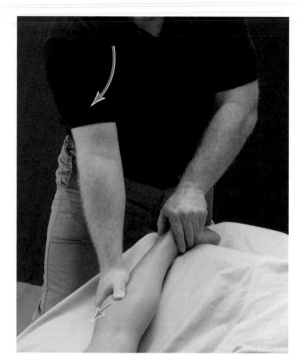

Figure 3-10 Cross-fiber fanning. Keep the thumb stationary, and perform the movement from the shoulder.

Place the length of your thumb on the area parallel to the fibers (Fig. 3-10). Adjust pressure to fit the situation, and move your thumb perpendicular to the tissue. It is important to keep the thumb stationary and perform the movement from the shoulder to prevent an overuse injury.

Incorporating Movement

The pain associated with musculoskeletal disorders is a challenging problem for any health care provider. Musculoskeletal dysfunction can occur for a variety of reasons and is identified by the following characteristics:

- As pain increases, motor-unit discharges decrease.
- Synergistic muscles related to the dysfunctional muscle demonstrate decreased motor-unit discharge.
- Endurance levels decrease. As muscles fatigue, the load is shifted to unaffected muscles, increasing their burden.
- EMG activity decreases.
- Blood vessels can be compressed with a muscle contraction of only 30% of maximum force.
- Proprioceptive functioning decreases.
- Adaptive shortening causes stretch weakness.
- Muscle imbalances lead to changed motor programming in the CNS.
- The pain-spasm-pain cycle perpetuates.

So how does movement remedy these characteristics? The main principle deals with movement reeducation. When pain occurs in the body, after a period of time, the brain shuts off communication with the affected area to avoid the sensation; however, faulty movement patterns created as a result of the original dysfunction remain. Incorporating passive and active movement with massage strokes reconnects the broken link of communication between the nervous system and the muscle. The **Law of Facilitation** states that when an impulse passes through a specific set of neurons to the exclusion of others, it generally takes the same course on a future occasion; each time the impulse traverses this path, resistance is less. When the link is reconnected, movement reestablishes its correct pattern, causing the body to facilitate a new neuron pathway and remove the dysfunction.

There are additional benefits to incorporating movement, as well:

1. Shortening a muscle during a stroke can help desensitize a trigger point or reduce the restriction that is created by the added tension when it is lengthened. This increases the client's comfort level during treatment, making the treatment more effective.
2. Passively lengthening a muscle under the pressure of a stroke will mobilize connective tissue and effectively "pull the muscle" under the stroke. This is more comfortable for the client because the therapist

Law of Facilitation The principle that when an impulse passes through a specific set of neurons to the exclusion of others, it generally takes the same course on a future occasion; each time it traverses this path, resistance is less.

can control the speed at which the tissue is lengthened and maintain the pain threshold more effectively.

3. Employing active movement during strokes works in several ways:
   a. Deep fascia is mobilized better and more quickly because heat is generated internally and externally, and this helps the matrix change to a fluid state faster.
   b. The pressure is intensified for the client due to the contraction of the muscle.
   c. Connective tissue restrictions are broken up more effectively.
   d. The client is able to control the stroke better and maintain the threshold level to increase the effectiveness.

Passive Movement with Compression

Perform the stroke by compressing an area of the muscle with a broad or specific contact surface, and move the limb passively. There are a few variations:

1. Apply static compression to the area, and passively shorten the limb. Remove the pressure, return the body part to the starting position, reapply pressure, and repeat. This is effective for trigger points and muscle spasms.
2. Shorten the limb, and then apply static pressure and lengthen the tissue. Repeat this shortening, compressing, and lengthening cycle; move pressure around the body part being treated.
3. Shorten the limb and perform deep parallel stripping along the muscle as the limb is passively lengthened (Fig. 3-11). This can be repeated in strips over the entire area.

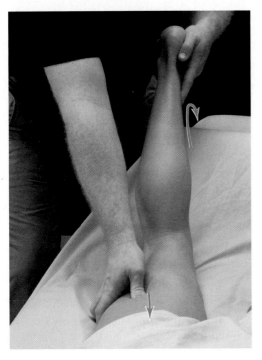

Figure 3-11 Deep parallel stripping with passive movement. Shorten the muscle and perform the stroke as the limb is passively lengthened.

Active Movement with Compression

This stroke uses the client's active movement while the therapist applies pressure or strokes to effect change. There are several variations:

1. Apply static compression to the hypertonic area or trigger point. Direct the client to perform an isotonic contraction of the muscle and return it to the original starting position. Repeat this several times until a change is noticed. This is effective for treating trigger points and adhesions.
2. This technique requires communication and timing between the therapist and client: Place the treatment area in a lengthened position. Perform a perpendicular compressive effleurage stroke while the client concentrically contracts the muscle (Fig. 3-12). The stroke should begin when the client starts to move and should end when the muscle is fully contracted.
3. This technique is typically the most intense and is used primarily during the late stages of healing and for chronic conditions: Place the area in a shortened position. Begin deep parallel stripping at the distal end of the muscle as the client actively lengthens the muscle (Fig. 3-13). You will travel a short distance, and the client will shorten the muscle and begin to lengthen it again. Move along the muscle during the lengthening phase, and repeat this process until the entire muscle is covered.

These techniques can be intensified through the use of manual resistance or resistance with weights, exercise bands, and the like. The greater

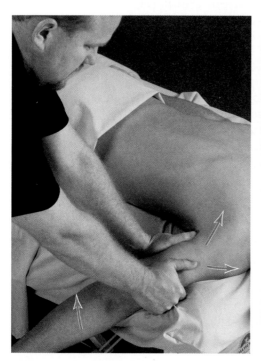

Figure 3-12 Perpendicular compressive effleurage with active movement. The stroke should begin when the client starts to move and should end when the muscle is fully contracted.

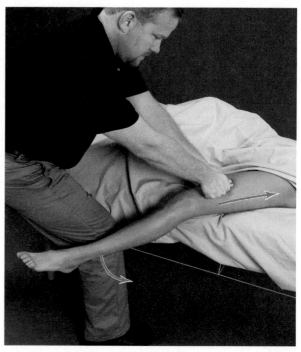

Figure 3-13 Deep parallel stripping with active movement. Move along the muscle during the lengthening phase, and repeat this process until the entire muscle is covered.

the resistance, the more motor units that are recruited, thereby increasing the pressure and number of fibers affected.

FLEXIBILITY TRAINING

Just as massage therapy has been around for centuries, the origins of stretching can be traced back to the Greeks who used flexibility training to prepare themselves for wrestling, acrobatics, and other sports. **Flexibility** is the ability of a joint to move through a normal range of motion without creating an excessive amount of stress to the muscle-tendon unit (Zakas, 2002).

This is influenced by the associated bones and bony structures and the characteristics of the surrounding soft tissues. The human body is a complex system that needs movement to function properly. Restrictions to normal motion negatively affect function and can lead to compensational behavior and subsequent dysfunction.

flexibility The ability of a joint to move through a normal range of motion without creating an excessive amount of stress to the muscle-tendon unit.

Benefits

Stretching increases flexibility and decreases stiffness, thereby reducing injury and restoring normal functioning. "Flexibility and proper stretching have played a very important role for enhancing performance, rehabilitation, and wellness" (Mattes, 2000). The goal of any effective stretching program should be to improve the range of motion at a joint by changing the ability of the musculotendinous units at that joint to lengthen. These effects are derived from two mechanisms:

1. *Neurophysiologic:* Muscles that are exposed to stretching are more inhibited to the activity of the contractile component of the muscle. This inhibition results in an increased extensibility of the muscle, leading to an increase in range of motion at the joint.
2. *Biomechanical:* This mechanism is a result of the viscoelastic property of the muscle tissue. When force is applied through the stretch, the elastic component of the muscle causes it to elongate. When a muscle is repeatedly stretched to a certain tension, the acting force at that length will decrease over time.

Through these mechanisms, the length of the muscle is gradually changed over time and will result in a variety of benefits, including:

1. *Improved preparation for activity:* Stretching will increase tissue temperature, reduce muscle tension, and improve tissue pliability.
2. *Improved tissue nutrition:* The increase in circulation to the area will facilitate the removal of metabolic waste products and the oxygenation and nutrition of the tissues.
3. *Reduced soft tissue injury:* Flexible tissue is able to absorb more energy and move through its range without restriction.
4. *Improved lymph flow:* Stretching manually compresses the tissue through lengthening and encourages the movement of lymph.
5. *Improved posture:* A release of fascial tissue allows the body to properly accommodate the effects of gravity.

Obstacles

Despite the multiple benefits of stretching, it is not uncommon for people to avoid stretching because of the following reasons:

- *Time constraints:* When incorporated into a fitness or rehabilitation program, stretching can be viewed as time-consuming.
- *Boredom:* Some techniques can be boring because of the length of time the stretches are held.
- *Pain:* It is a common misconception that stretching is beneficial only when it is painful; hence, it is avoided.
- *Complexity:* Some types of stretching involve complicated positions and sequences that can be hard to remember.

Other obstacles to achieving optimal flexibility through stretching include:

1. *Medical or physical conditions:* Trauma, inflammation, injury, and other conditions can change the soft tissue and restrict flexibility.
2. *Chronic improper posture:* Connective tissue adapts to shortened positions over time and exerts tremendous force, locking the body into posture patterns. Until the fascia is released, it will inhibit flexibility of the surrounding joints.
3. *Aging:* Aging causes increases in connective tissue concentration within the muscle and decreases in its elastic component.
4. *Rapid growth:* Changes in height or weight place stress on muscles and soft tissue as they try to keep up with the growth of the skeletal system.

Research Findings

While the use of stretching is widespread, there is conflicting scientific evidence over whether flexibility training reduces injury and enhances performance. Still, anecdotal and experiential evidence has supported the use of stretching throughout the ages, citing its benefits for improved posture, ease of movement, increased efficiency of tissue nutrition, and more.

Epidemiological evidence has cited reduced flexibility as an etiological factor in acute muscle-strain injuries, suggesting that increased flexibility reduces injury. "Tissue level research has established the fact that there is a positive relationship between duration of tensile loading and elongation of soft tissue structures" (Ford, 2005). However, the link between increased tissue length and reduced injury has not been positively made. In fact, several studies show that stretching, especially immediately prior to activity, will actually decrease the muscle's ability to produce force and increase the chance of injury. This concept is based on the mechanical changes in muscle stiffness and alterations in the viscoelastic properties of the musculotendinous unit, specifically the length-tension relationship and the plastic deformation of the connective tissues such that the maximal force-producing capabilities of the musculotendinous unit could be limited. It has also been hypothesized that neural factors such as decreased motor-unit activation and decreased reflex sensitivity will affect force production. These factors result in the creation of several theories about why there is a decrease in performance and an increase in injury potential:

1. *Increased flexibility around a joint can reduce its stability.* A certain amount of tone is needed around a joint to provide structural integrity. An increase in the range of motion at a joint can compromise its ability to remain stable.

2. *Creating hypermobility can affect the muscle's ability to control the body part that is moving.* In considering the level of flexibility needed during movement, a balance must be established between dynamic control and range of motion. One can have a tremendous amount of flexibility in a joint, but if the joint cannot be controlled during motion, the added range of motion is useless. There must be a synergistic combination of motion and stability. An optimal range of motion for one activity may be detrimental for a different activity.

3. *Most muscle strains occur when the muscle is active and functioning in an eccentric manner wherein flexibility is not an issue.* The ability of a muscle to absorb energy is a combination of both active and passive components. In an active capacity, it is more a function of contractile strength than tissue compliance. It is unclear whether passive-tissue flexibility affects active-tissue compliance.

Although the conflicting research may cast doubt on the validity of stretching and flexibility training, it is clear that there are two distinct categories when it comes to stretching:

- Stretching to improve motion and relieve pain
- Stretching to reduce injury and improve performance

Before implementing a flexibility program, contemplate the following questions:

1. *What is the intent of the added flexibility?* We must look at the individual person to determine his or her goals. The goals of an elderly person will be vastly different from those of an elite athlete.

2. *Where is the flexibility needed?* Flexibility is personal and can vary from one person to another. It can even vary from one side of the body to the other. With each person, flexibility is not a general trait—it is specific to each joint in the body; therefore, the type and intensity of the activity will help determine the best game plan for designing a flexibility program.

3. *To what extent is flexibility determined by body structure?* A person can be flexible if his or her muscles have a high level of compliance or his or her joint structure allows for hypermobility.

4. *What is the best time to develop flexibility?* Just as performing specific massage techniques at certain times can affect muscle function, research shows that stretching at the wrong time can disrupt normal neuromuscular patterns in the muscle. The time to improve flexibility is not immediately before competition. Stretching to improve range of motion should be included as part of the preparation for competition, while a warm-up, active type of gentle stretching should be used immediately prior to activity.

5. *What are the flexibility requirements?* When it comes to athletes and people engaged in performance-based activities, not every sport requires the

same level of flexibility. Establish a baseline according to the needs of the individual, and then customize the routine to fit the demands of the activity. Each person requires a certain level of flexibility for normal functioning, and the level can be additionally modified to fit each situation.

Despite the lack of conclusive research, it is generally accepted that flexibility training is beneficial as a regular part of an overall wellness program. When recommending a flexibility program to a client, remember to take into consideration all the factors involved.

Methods of Stretching

Before employing any method of stretching, it is necessary to understand some common neuromuscular principles.

1. *Myotatic stretch reflex:* There are two types of muscle receptors responsible for a protective mechanism known as the *stretch reflex.* Muscle spindle fibers are located within the muscle itself and monitor both the magnitude and the velocity of a stretch. If a muscle is lengthened too far or too fast, the reflex is engaged, causing a contraction of that muscle. Golgi tendon organs are located in the muscle tendons and monitor the force of the contraction. If a stretch is sustained or creates excessive force, the Golgi tendon organs respond by causing reflexive relaxation of the muscle, which allows it to stretch and avoid injury. Several factors can affect the stretch reflex, including pain, the type of muscle contraction, precontraction tension levels, and imposed motor tasks.

2. *Postisometric relaxation:* A latency period occurs immediately following an isometric contraction; this prevents the muscle from contracting again too rapidly. The latency period is attributed to the repolarization of the muscle fibers and can be utilized to enhance the stretching process.

3. *Reciprocal inhibition:* Reciprocal inhibition is created by a reflex loop between opposing pairs of muscles. As one muscle contracts, there is simultaneous inhibition of the opposing muscle on the other side of the joint.

Ballistic Stretching

Also known as *dynamic, kinetic,* or *body-momentum stretching, ballistic stretching* involves bouncing or bobbing in the direction of desired length increase. Ballistic stretching has fallen out of favor in recent years for several reasons:

- Its rapid movements can engage the stretch reflex and increase the chances of tissue damage.
- It can irritate the tissue because of the inability to determine the stretch tolerance of the tissue.
- It can result in the formation of scar tissue, which is less flexible than muscle, by causing micro-traumas in the tissue.

Because the method has been deemed unsafe in many instances, therapists are encouraged to use other, more beneficial forms of stretching.

Static Stretching

This popular method of flexibility training has been around for centuries in various applications, including yoga. It can be performed by a client on his or her own or with the help of the therapist. When working in pairs, communication between the client and the therapist is essential to avoid overstretching.

1. The static stretching routine begins with a warm-up exercise to increase the core temperature.
2. The desired muscle group is stretched to a point of mild tension that causes slight discomfort but not pain and is held for between 15 and 60 seconds.

Research shows that a minimum of a 15-second hold can change length but a longer duration does not necessarily yield greater results. Most studies agree that a 30-second hold is optimal for gains in flexibility. Static stretching can be performed after activity. In fact, some believe that this is the optimal time to improve one's flexibility due to the increased pliability of the tissue. Static stretching is usually the easiest to teach and remember.

Proprioceptive Neuromuscular Facilitation

The *Proprioceptive Neuromuscular Facilitation (PNF)* system of stretching was developed in the 1940s by Maggie Knott, Dorothy Voss, and Herman Kabat. Its goal is to promote functioning through the use of the neuromuscular principles mentioned earlier in this section. There are typically two types of PNF stretches:

1. *Hold/relax:* The therapist stretches the muscle to its end range of motion. The client holds a submaximal (10%) isometric contraction of the target muscle for 5 to 10 seconds while the therapist resists the motion. The therapist allows the postisometric relaxation of the muscle and then gently stretches the muscle to its new end range of motion. The process is repeated several times.
2. *Contract/relax:* The therapist stretches the muscle to its end range of motion. The client holds a submaximal (10%) isometric contraction of the target muscle for 5 to 10 seconds while the therapist resists the motion. After a few seconds, the client is instructed to engage the antagonistic muscle to the one being stretched, while the therapist assists the muscle into its new end range of motion. Not only does this method utilize postisometric relaxation by engaging the opposite side of the target muscle, but it also employs reciprocal inhibition.

While this method of stretching is highly effective, it is also complex and physically demanding; hence, it is best utilized under the guidance of an experienced therapist. The technique also requires a sustained amount of coordination between the client and the therapist.

Active Isolated Stretching

Active Isolated Stretching (AIS) was developed by Aaron Mattes and incorporates the key concept that only relaxed structures will allow themselves to be optimally stretched (Mattes, 2000). Mattes holds a bachelor's degree in physical education and a master's degree in kinesiology. He is both a massage therapist and a kinesiotherapist and has lectured all over the world as well as written several books. He is a consultant for various sports teams and has been integral in organizing massage therapy at the Olympics.

This method of stretching has several advantages and can be adapted to fit any situation. There are three main principles of the AIS technique:

1. *Contract the muscle opposite to the one being stretched.* This incorporates the principle of reciprocal inhibition.
2. *Hold the stretch for 1.5 to 2 seconds, performing 10 to 15 repetitions.* The short duration of the stretch phase decreases the chance of engaging the myotatic stretch reflex.
3. *Breathe.* Breathing ensures that the tissues will be supplied with oxygen.

Several benefits of Active Isolated Stretching are listed in Table 3-3.

Table 3-3   Benefits of Active Isolated Stretching

The positions isolate the muscles that need to be stretched.

The use of repetitive isotonic contractions ensures increased blood flow and tissue nutrition more efficiently than other methods.

Repeated contractions warm up the muscle tissue as it is stretched.

The focus on breathing decreases fatigue and lactic acid buildup by ensuring the presence of oxygen.

The stretch is held for no more than 2 seconds, which ensures safety and comfort because the stretch reflex is not engaged; irritation is kept to a minimum.

The opposite side to that being stretched is strengthened through motion.

The active nature of the stretches ensures improved neuromuscular coordination.

Active Isolated Stretching can be applied by a client on his or her own or with the help of a therapist. Steps for the therapist to follow include:

1. Determine the muscle to be stretched.
2. Have the client take a deep breath. On the exhale, the client moves the joint to its end range through the contraction of the muscle opposite the one being stretched.
3. After the client has reached the end range, gently assist with the stretch (Fig. 3-14). The pressure should be gentle and not cause discomfort. Additionally, the client should continue to engage the muscle involved in the movement, as this ensures reciprocal inhibition.
4. Have the client return the limb to the starting position and repeat the movement for the desired amount of repetitions.

When stretching alone, clients can use a rope to replace the assistance of the therapist.

Practical Tip

Make sure that the client moves the limb to the end range and that you assist only at the end.

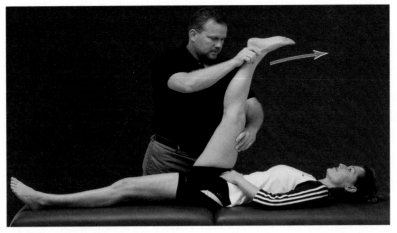

Figure 3-14 Example of Active Isolated Stretching to the hamstrings.

While several different methods of stretching are beneficial, therapists must find those that best fit their needs. Active Isolated Stretching is further discussed in the treatment section of this text.

SUMMARY

This chapter dealt with the advanced techniques that are used in treating a condition with clinical massage therapy. The components of connective tissue were discussed, along with how this unique tissue fits into the overall treatment plan. A review of four connective tissue treatment theories, their history, and their application gave a good look at the different treatment styles of each. The next section provided an in-depth discussion on the myofascial trigger point, the history of its diagnosis, and the pathophysiology involved in its treatment. Using the principles discussed in the previous chapter, the next section focused on the application of advanced strokes, when to apply them, and their benefits. The last portion of the chapter reviewed the major philosophies of stretching and discussed the benefits of and major research on the subject.

REVIEW QUESTIONS

1. What are the three types of fibers in connective tissue?
2. What is ground substance?
3. What are the two types of fibrous connective tissue, and how do they differ?
4. How does the fascia respond to stresses placed on it?
5. Who devised Bindegewebsmassage, and what is it based on?
6. What were Ida Rolf's two central ideas for Structural Integration?
7. What are the three phases of Rolfing?
8. What is the main concept of myofascial release?

9. What is Kinesis Myofascial Integration based on?
10. What is tensegrity?
11. What are the principles of application of connective tissue therapy?
12. What are the key components of a muscle contraction?
13. What are the different types of trigger points?
14. What are the three causes of trigger points?
15. What are the signs and symptoms of a trigger point?
16. How is a trigger point palpated?
17. List the steps in the formation of a trigger point.
18. List the benefits of stretching.
19. List the neurologic principles involved in stretching.
20. Describe the four stretching methods discussed in the chapter.

CRITICAL-THINKING QUESTIONS

1. Why is treating connective tissue important in clinical massage?
2. Why do people develop connective tissue problems?
3. What are the underlying philosophies of the different types of connective tissue work?
4. Why does static compression work when treating a trigger point? How does movement contribute to the treatment?
5. Why is it effective to apply strokes that incorporate movement?

part II

Regional Approach to Treatment

Formulating a Treatment Plan

chapter outline

chapter objectives

At the conclusion of this chapter, the reader will understand:

- why treating more than just the primary complaint is important
- three phases of injury and key points of each
- five forces on the body
- four roles of a muscle
- three types of contractions
- four basic muscle shapes
- three degrees of muscle tissue and ligament injury
- difference between tendonitis and tenosynovitis
- two methods of gathering information during an assessment
- importance of obtaining a client history
- correct posture alignment of the structures
- phases of the gait cycle
- principles in assessing active and passive ranges of motion and administering isometric strength tests
- six levels of learning
- five steps of the clinical massage treatment framework

key terms

active range of motion

acute injury

anisotropic

chronic injury

force

gait cycle

passive range of motion

primary curves

secondary curves

signs

sprain

strain

symptoms

tendonitis

tendonosis

tenosynovitis

Introduction   In utilizing clinical massage, it is imperative that therapists maintain structured treatment sessions. This chapter looks at creating a treatment plan, including how and where to start, the properties of the involved structures, the components of a treatment plan, how to systematically work through the information gathered, and how to apply that information to a treatment framework.

TREATMENT PHILOSOPHY

As massage therapists, we are trained to focus on the fact that the body is an integrated organism and that in order to treat a person effectively, we must look at the whole picture. This includes not only the physical symptoms but also the way other factors such as lifestyle, diet, and activity level relate back to the changes we are seeing in the body.

When deciding how to treat a client, therapists must focus on restoring balance to the system. By gathering as much information as possible, we can see how the body has changed its functioning and work to correct the system.

Focused Approach vs. Global Approach

Most anatomy courses, regardless of the discipline, break the body into individual systems and parts; however, this is not a true reflection of how the body functions. All the body systems are interdependent on each other, and when something happens to one system, all the other systems are affected as well. Traditionally, modern medicine treats dysfunction in the body by focusing solely on the area of complaint. It seldom considers the possible involvement of other body systems.

The first step in developing a treatment plan is to identify the primary area of complaint and begin treatment in this area. While it is not necessary to spend the entire session on the primary complaint, there is a psychological component to acknowledging the client's source of pain or dysfunction. If a therapist begins treatment on a different part of the body, even if doing so will ultimately benefit the client, the therapist risks jeopardizing the relationship with the client, who may subsequently question the therapist's skill level. Once the primary area has been treated, the therapist can treat other global areas of involvement.

A stone thrown into a still pond causes ripples to radiate from the center (Fig. 4-1). The size of the ripples and the distance they travel is determined by two factors. The first factor is the size of the stone, which relates to the impact on the pond. The larger the stone (or, in this case, the client's complaint), the bigger the impact and the farther the ripples travel. The other factor is the length of time from when the stone was thrown to when the ripples were measured. The longer the window of time, the farther the ripples radiate. In other words, there is a link between how much time has elapsed from the onset of the complaint to the start of treatment. The length of time that has passed since the onset of the complaint will

> **Practical Tip**
> Addressing the primary complaint lets the client know you acknowledge his or her pain.

Figure 4-1 Just as ripples in a pond radiate out farther over time, the longer a client has had a condition, the greater the compensation that has occurred.

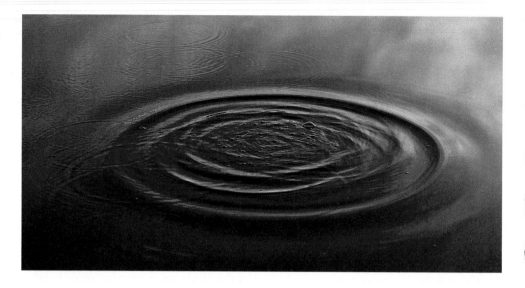

determine how far out the therapist must go to address all the related areas. As the regional issues are resolved, the therapist can then return to the initial area and complete any work there. This stone-in-the-pond concept relates to how the body compensates for dysfunction. The larger the initial trauma to the body, the greater the compensation and the more structures will likely be affected.

Compensation

The body is susceptible to injury from a variety of sources ranging from severe physical trauma to emotional abuse. Regardless of the source, however, the body reacts to injury the same way: through compensation. The human body is an amazing organism capable of adapting to just about any situation in order to accomplish any task. When it comes to the musculo-skeletal system, damage results in one of two ways:

- The efforts of other muscles are modified to make up for the damaged ones in order to complete the same task.
- Movement is modified into another motion that naturally results in a smaller load being placed on the damaged tissue(s).

While compensation makes sense in the short term, the long-term effects of improper mechanics can be as damaging as the original injury.

Muscles are classified into one of two groups based on their functional tasks. *Stabilizers* typically have a postural role. They are associated with the eccentric resistance of momentum and control through a wide range of motion. *Mobilizers* tend to have a role in generating movement and will concentrically accelerate body segments to produce motion. The balance of efficient dynamic movement is much more complex than the simple production of force by the muscles. There is a precisely coordinated inter-action between synergistic groups of muscles, as well as interaction with antagonistic groups. This creates a delicate dance between systems of the body. Some components involved in the movement process include sensory and biomechanical elements, movement strategies, and learned responses.

Movement dysfunction can be a local or global problem. Locally, it can present as a motor-recruitment deficiency, which results in poor control

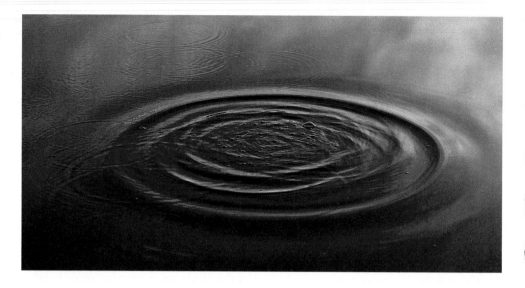

Practical Tip

Consider the length of time a complaint has existed to determine the extent of compensation.

of the area. Globally, it may occur as an imbalance between the stabilizers and the mobilizers. This imbalance alters the normal resting length of the muscles involved, whether they are chronically lengthened or shortened, and results in abnormal force. Through the use of associated muscles, force patterns on muscles, connective tissues, bones, and joints are changed, and this leads to the breakdown of the system. When dealing with this phenomenon, therapists need to consider the effect of the deactivated injured tissues on the biomechanics of the whole system to avoid additional problems, as well as to know how much additional training is needed by the other muscles to compensate.

While injury is the most common method of starting this breakdown in the kinetic chain, repetitive behavior can also play a major role. Overusing one particular muscle or movement pattern can result in muscle imbalances or connective tissue restrictions that can start a cascade of dysfunction. Pain can lead to decreased proprioceptive input, which can affect movement patterns, and decreased force production by a muscle, which can result in alterations of the functional length of the muscle. Although pain and dysfunction are often related, improper movement patterns created as the result of pathology can remain after the pain is gone. The results of these patterns can include increased recurrence, possible degenerative changes, and the perpetuation of the global imbalances.

Therapists must follow the kinetic chain from the area of complaint to the related areas of the body. Understanding the process of compensation will help therapists view the body as a whole entity and address all the areas involved.

Deciding to Treat

From a clinical standpoint, the safe and effective treatment of specific musculoskeletal conditions begins with knowing when *not* to treat. One major purpose of having a systematic way to gather information is to determine whether massage therapy will truly benefit the client. As health care practitioners, therapists have a duty to provide proper care, even if that means referring clients to other health care providers.

There are several reasons that a therapist may decline to treat a client. The first is contraindications, of which there are two types: absolute and local. *Absolute contraindications* are typically chronic ailments or conditions brought about through contagious viral or bacterial pathologies. It is wise to obtain a physician's clearance before working on a client with this type of contraindication. Some examples are kidney stones, fever, lupus (during a flare-up), and chickenpox.

In the case of *local contraindications,* massage is applied using modified or adapted techniques, or the area in question is simply avoided. Consider each situation on its own merit, and consult a physician if necessary. Always use common sense to avoid a negative outcome. Some examples of local contraindications are poison ivy, decubitus ulcers, shingles (absolute contraindication when acute), and acute injuries.

Another reason to avoid working with a client is the presence of a condition that falls outside the scope of practice for massage therapy. Depending on the massage regulations in individual states, some techniques are prohibited and massage therapists cannot treat clients who have certain conditions. In this case, it is best to refer the client to an outside health care provider. Since skill level and experience with certain conditions will vary among therapists, a therapist may choose not to treat a client whose condition falls outside his or her comfort level. During the assessment process, if a therapist becomes uncomfortable with a situation, he or she should refer the client to someone with more experience. It is always best to err on the side of caution.

COMPONENTS OF A TREATMENT PLAN

When gathering information to create a treatment plan, the therapist must first determine the phase of the injury. Soft tissue heals through a series of three interrelated physical and chemical phases. Since these phases are regular and predictable, a knowledgeable therapist can monitor the healing process to determine what type of treatment should be applied or whether a referral is necessary. Keep in mind that while this text discusses the phases as individual stages, there is an overlap of the phases during the healing process.

Phases of Injury

Phase I: Inflammatory Phase

The *inflammatory phase* of the healing process results from a variety of causes, including injury, which is the focus of this section. This first phase of the healing process can last up to 6 days and has familiar signs and symptoms, including heat, redness, swelling, pain, and loss of function. Depending on the cause of the injury, inflammation can be acute or chronic. *Acute inflammation* is usually brief in duration and generates swelling called *exudate,* which comprises plasma, protein, and white blood cells. *Chronic inflammation* is prolonged in duration and characterized by the presence of white blood cells and scar tissue.

While most therapists view the inflammatory process as negative, it is a necessary process to initiate healing. The initial job of the inflammatory phase is to stop the loss of blood from the wound. This occurs through three mechanisms:

1. Local vasoconstriction occurs as a result of chemical mediators causing an increase in blood viscosity. This can last for a few seconds or up to 10 minutes, and it reduces blood flow and loss. Vasospasm of large and small vessels results in increased viscosity of the blood, which further reduces loss.
2. Platelets stick to each other and combine with fibrin to occlude the defect in the vessel, creating a mechanical plug that blocks the opening.
3. A heightened physiologic response occurs. This consists of several interrelated components known as a *coagulation cascade,* which converts fibrinogen to fibrin, resulting in the formation of a clot.

Once the vasoconstriction phase is over and the blood loss is under control, a period of vasodilation transpires. This process occurs in order to bring white blood cells to the area for infection control and to rid the injury site of dead and damaged tissue through phagocytosis. Along with vasodilation, there is an increase in the permeability of the vessels, which contributes to the formation of exudate. The change in permeability can last a few minutes or longer depending on the severity of the injury. In some cases, if the trauma is extensive, the change in permeability will not occur for some time after the injury. The exudate that is created is important to the overall healing process. In addition to diluting toxins in the area, it provides the cells necessary to remove damaged tissue and enable reconstruction. These two factors cause swelling in the area and, in conjunction with the damaged and necrotic tissue, form what is known as the *zone of primary injury.*

While this swelling process is beneficial to the overall healing process, it also can be detrimental to the area. If excess fluids, damaged tissues, chemical mediators, and white blood cells remain in the area for too long, the environment may become hypoxic. The inability of the surrounding tissues to access oxygen and nutrients, and remove waste products due to the congestion created by the swelling, will result in the expanded death of those tissues and create the *zone of secondary injury.* This area will continue to expand through this process until the initial inflammation is under control and the tissue returns to its normal metabolism.

Phase II: Proliferative Phase

The next phase in the healing process is called the *proliferative phase,* sometimes referred to as the *repair and regeneration phase.* This phase can overlap the latter part of the inflammatory phase and last up to 21 days. It includes the development of new blood vessels, fibrous tissues, and epithelial tissues. The process of new tissue formation begins when the hematoma created by the inflammation reduces in size enough to allow new growth. The accumulated fluid, containing a high level of protein and cellular materials, will form the foundation for the fibroblasts, which will generate the collagen. The formation of connective tissue and blood vessels is an interdependent process. The fibroblasts are fueled by nutrients brought in by the blood vessels, and the vessels are supported and protected by the connective tissue matrix. This highly vascularized mass is transformed into the necessary structures in the third and final phase of healing.

Phase III: Maturation Phase

The *maturation phase* is the final phase of healing and is sometimes known as the *remodeling phase.* It involves the maturation of the newly formed mass from the repair phase into scar tissue. It can last over a year depending on the severity of the initial injury and whether any interventions occur. The maturation process includes decreased fibroblast activity, increased organization in the matrix, reduced vascularity, and a return to normal histochemical activity. While the tissue has been regenerated by this time, its tensile strength is only 25% of normal. This is thought to occur because of the orientation of the collagen fibers, which are more vertical than they are in normal tissue, where orientation is horizontal. This deficit can last for several months depending on what is done to support the process. Scar tissue is less elastic, more fibrous, and less vascular than the original tissue. This creates weakness within the tissue and decreases flexibility in the area, leaving it vulnerable for re-injury. As the scar matures, the fibers align themselves along the lines of tension. This process of creating a more "functional" scar can be enhanced through soft tissue work, flexibility training, and strength training.

Damaged muscle tissue develops an adhesion—a type of scarring—within the muscle fibers that glues them together, decreasing their ability to function normally. This can result in a muscle regaining only 50% of its preinjury strength. This process can occur even slower in tissues that have a limited blood supply, such as tendons, ligaments, and other inert tissues. Through soft tissue work to the damaged areas, healing rates can be improved as a result of an increase in circulation.

Knowledge of Anatomy

A critical component of clinical massage is a thorough working knowledge of anatomy and physiology. It is the basis for the formulation of any treatment plan and leads to all other steps of therapy. Because their composition varies, different types of tissues are damaged differently, heal differently, and respond to treatment differently. (The chapters that follow review the regional anatomical structures before considering individual conditions.)

Before discussing the different types of tissues and their pathologies, it is necessary to address some of the basic forces that can cause damage to them. One of the first steps in treating an injury is to understand the different ways that force can act on the body. In addition to understanding force, knowing the structural properties of the different tissues and how they respond to force is valuable in developing a treatment plan.

force A push or a pull that acts on the body.

A **force** is a push or pull acting on the body. This action can have two different effects: a change in direction or velocity and a change in shape. Both of these can damage the tissues, but the amount of damage will depend on the magnitude of the force and the properties of the tissue on which the force is applied.

All tissues have an elastic region and a plastic region. As long as the force remains within the elastic region, the tissue will return to its original shape once the force is removed. When a tissue moves beyond the elastic region into the plastic region, it no longer has the ability to return to its original shape: The deformation of the structure will remain even after the force is removed. However, regardless of tissue type, if the force is too great, it will exceed the ultimate failure point and rupture the tissue.

anisotropic Able to resist force better from one direction than another.

The physical properties of the tissues factor into the effects of force because many tissues are **anisotropic**. This means that the structure resists force better from some directions than others. One example of this occurs in ankle injuries. The lateral ligaments are damaged much easier than the medial ones because the laterals do not have as much support and are not as strong.

Types of Force

Force is generally described on the basis of the direction in which it is applied. An important factor, regardless of direction, is the magnitude of the stress applied. Another factor is the surface area: The larger the surface area on which the force is applied, the more the force is dispersed, allowing the tissue to handle a greater load. The opposite is also true: The smaller the surface area on which the force is applied, the less it is dispersed, decreasing the amount of load the tissue can handle. There are five categories of force that can act on the body:

1. *Compression:* Force that is directed along the long axis of a structure and squeezes the structure together.
2. *Tension:* A pulling force that is directed along the long axis and stretches the structure.
3. *Shear:* Force that acts parallel to a plane and causes the tissues to slide past each other in opposite directions.
4. *Bending:* The result of the combination of compression and tension that is applied perpendicular to the long axis. The side of the structure where the force is applied is compressed, while the opposite side is loaded under tension.
5. *Torsion:* The application of torque about the long axis of a structure, which creates a shear stress throughout the structure.

Soft Tissue Properties

Muscle Although there are three types of muscle tissue (cardiac, smooth, and skeletal), this chapter focuses only on skeletal muscle. *Skeletal muscle* is the main contractile tissue and has a myriad of functions: providing movement, maintaining posture, communicating with other muscle tissue, and providing feedback about the body's position in space.

The structure and function of skeletal muscle classify it as *viscoelastic* tissue. This means it has elastic properties, which enable the muscle to return to its original length and extensibility or affect its ability to stretch. When working with muscle injuries, the therapist has several factors to consider in determining the severity of damage and the type of treatment needed.

The first factor is the role that the muscle was playing when it was injured. A muscle can assume one of four roles:

1. *Agonist:* This muscle provides the desired movement. If more than one muscle performs the same movement, the one that contributes to movement the most is called the *prime mover;* the others are called *synergists.* Agonist muscles can switch roles depending on the position of the body.
2. *Antagonist:* This muscle performs the motion opposite that of the agonist.
3. *Stabilizer:* This muscle fixates or supports a body part so that other muscles can perform a particular function.
4. *Neutralizer:* Muscles typically have more than one function at a particular joint. The neutralizer cancels out unwanted movement so that only the desired action is performed.

The second factor is determining the type of contraction that occurred during the activity. There are three main types of contractions:

1. *Concentric:* This contraction occurs when the two ends of the muscle move closer together and shorten during the contraction. The angle at the joint is decreased during this type of contraction.

2. *Eccentric:* This contraction generates more force on the muscle than does the concentric contraction, and it lengthens the muscle as it is contracting. An outside force is acting on the muscle that is greater than the stimulus to contract, so lengthening takes place. This can also occur if there is controlled lengthening of a muscle: a biceps curl, for example. Once the muscle is fully shortened, the weight is slowly lowered to the starting position.

3. *Isometric:* During this contraction, no movement takes place at the joint. The force of the muscle contraction equals the outside force, or the simultaneous contraction of the agonist and antagonist causes no movement.

The third factor is the shape of the muscle. The strength and direction of a muscle's pull are determined partly by the orientation of the fibers. Some muscles are more easily injured than others, so this becomes relevant during the assessment. There are four basic shapes that a muscle can assume (Fig. 4-2):

1. *Fusiform:* These muscles are thick in the middle and taper at the end. An example is the biceps brachii.

2. *Parallel:* These are long muscles with uniform width. They cover great distances and can shorten more than any other muscle type. Examples are the rectus abdominus and the sartorius.

3. *Convergent:* These are strong, fan-shaped muscles that are wide at their origin and narrow at their insertion. The pectoralis major is one example.

4. *Pennate:* These are feather-shaped muscles; their fibers insert obliquely along a central tendon that runs the length of the muscle. They are classified by how their fibers attach to the central tendon. This classification has three subclasses:

   - *Unipennate* muscle fibers all approach the tendon from the same side, such as the semimembranosis.
   - *Bipennate* muscle fibers approach from both sides, such as the rectus femoris.
   - *Multipennate* fibers approach from multiple tendons that converge on a single point, such as the deltoids.

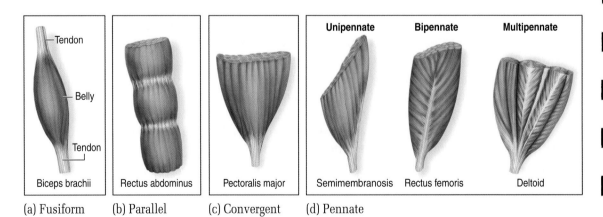

(a) Fusiform   (b) Parallel   (c) Convergent   (d) Pennate

Figure 4-2 The four basic muscle shapes.

Muscle Injuries When discussing injuries to muscle tissue, it is necessary to determine whether the injury was acute or chronic. An **acute injury** occurs when a single force produces the injury; its severity is determined by the magnitude of the force. Regardless of the severity, the force that causes the injury is termed a *macro-trauma.* A **chronic injury** occurs as the result of the repeated loading of a muscle over a period of time. This is termed a *micro-trauma* because of the level of individual force that is applied over time. An injury can exist in limbo between the acute and chronic stages, moving in and out of each, depending on activity levels. This is referred to as the *subacute phase.*

One type of muscle injury is a **strain**. A strain, or "pulled muscle," typically occurs due to an excessive tensile force. Muscle strains can result from force that causes the muscle to stretch past its elastic region or, more commonly, from an excessive eccentric load. When force exceeds the ability of a muscle, it causes the muscle to work eccentrically and often results in injury. When a muscle strain occurs, it is graded into one of three degrees depending on its severity and the extent of damage:

1. *First degree:* A first-degree strain is the mildest type, characterized by only a few torn muscle fibers. Symptoms include mild weakness and spasm, which results in some loss of function. There is mild swelling but no palpable defect in the muscle. Pain occurs on both contraction and stretching, and range of motion is decreased.

2. *Second degree:* A second-degree strain is a moderate injury with nearly half of the muscle fibers torn, resulting in bruising or ecchymosis. Significant weakness occurs due to a reflexive inhibition in the area caused by pain. Spasm, swelling, and loss of function are moderate to severe, but there is still no palpable defect. Pain is worse with contraction and stretching, and there is decreased range of motion.

3. *Third degree:* A third-degree strain is the most severe and results from the total rupture of the muscle. Swelling, weakness, and spasm are severe, and some bruising may occur. Loss of function is significant, and there is a palpable defect in the muscle. Despite being the most severe type of strain, the pain level is mild to nonexistent due to the rupture of the nerves in the area.

Tendon Tendons are also classified as contractile tissue even though they contain no contractile fibers. Their purpose is to transmit the force of the muscular contraction to the bones so that movement of the skeleton can occur. Tendons are composed of dense fibrous connective tissue, which is arranged in parallel patterns. This structure is well suited to their function and allows them to withstand high longitudinal tensile force.

Tendon Injuries The mechanisms of tendon injuries are different from those of muscle tissue. Instead of an excessive tensile force, there is either a sudden maximum loading of the tendon or a repeated submaximal loading. This load usually results in damage close to the musculotendinous junction on the muscle side because the tendon portion is much stronger than the muscle portion. Actual damage to the tendon occurs after the tendon is stretched about 5% to 8% past its normal resting length.

acute injury An injury caused by a single force.

chronic injury An injury caused by a repetitive load placed on an area.

strain An injury to a muscle or tendon.

Three of the most common injuries to the tendon are due to chronic repetitive micro-traumas to the area:

1. **Tendonitis** is the inflammation of the tendon. Its symptoms include a history of chronic onset, repetitive mechanism, pain throughout the tendon, swelling, and pain during active motion.
2. **Tenosynovitis** involves the sheath around certain tendons. The purpose of the sheaths is to reduce friction to the tendon. Overuse and chronic irritation can cause an inflammatory reaction resulting in the formation of connective tissue cross-bridges between the tendon and the sheath and in the roughening of the tendon surface. Symptoms are similar to those of tendonitis except for a few differences. Tenosynovitis occurs only in tendons that have a sheath, and there is a distinct crepitus sound with movement. If the condition becomes chronic, a nodule may develop within the sheath that can further restrict the motion of the tendon.
3. **Tendonosis** is a degeneration of the collagen matrix within the tendon, causing an overall breakdown of the tissue. It can arise from a single incident but is more likely caused by repeated insults to the tendon. It has been described as a failed healing response in that there is a repeated cycle of insults and partial healing that, over time, leads to the degeneration of the tissue.

Ligament Ligaments are included in a category known as *noncontractile* or *inert tissues.* Their job is to connect adjacent bones to each other. Ligaments are made up of the same fibrous connective tissue that tendons are, with a few exceptions. Ligaments contain a higher percentage of elastin fibers, and some of these fibers are oriented in nonlongitudinal planes. This gives the ligament more flexibility and strength to resist force that originates from different directions. While tendons need to resist force only in one direction, ligaments act around joints; most joints are exposed to force from multiple directions.

Ligament Injuries Ligaments are most often damaged from excessive tensile force on the fibers. Depending on the magnitude of the force, the ligament may or may not be able to return to its original length. Once the tissue moves beyond its elastic limits, the result is permanent deformation, which decreases joint stability. If the force is large enough to cause the ligament fibers to fail, the resulting injury is a **sprain.** Sprains are classified into three degrees:

1. *First degree:* A few of the fibers are torn, with no recognizable joint instability; a firm end-feel is present. Symptoms include mild weakness and loss of function, as well as mild swelling and decreased range of motion.
2. *Second degree:* In this more severe sprain, almost half of the fibers tear. Some joint laxity occurs, and there is a definite end point with mild to moderate weakness. Symptoms include loss of function, swelling, and decreased range of motion.
3. *Third degree:* This degree is the most severe and results in the total rupture of the ligament. There is gross joint instability, which results

in an absent end point with moderate weakness. Due to the instability, symptoms include severe loss of function and marked swelling. Range of motion may increase due to instability or decrease due to swelling. Typically, because of the magnitude of the force, other structures will be involved.

Joint Capsule The tissue that makes up the capsule is similar to that which makes up the ligaments. It is designed to contain the joint and produce synovial fluid to lubricate it. Depending on the joint's location and necessary motion, the capsule can be very elastic or stiff. To accommodate the different demands placed on it, the capsule can change its level of tension, as it moves through its range of motion. It can be tight in some positions and lax in others. Injuries to the capsule usually accompany injuries to the ligaments. Since the capsule varies in its levels of tension, its injuries, unlike those of muscles and ligaments, are not graded. Another type of injury evolves from adhesions in the capsule, which limits range of motion in certain directions. This injury is discussed in more detail in Chapter 7.

Cartilage There are two types of cartilage: hyaline and fibrous. Both have poor blood supply and are slow or unable to heal if damaged. *Hyaline cartilage* covers the ends of the bones and provides a smooth articular surface. *Fibrocartilage* is located between the bones in certain joints and acts to provide extra cushioning against compressive force. The intervertebral disks and the meniscus in the knees are examples of fibrocartilage. Described below are general cartilage injuries; individual types of cartilage injuries are discussed in later chapters.

Cartilage Injuries Compressive force is the most common cause of cartilage injury. Injuries to the hyaline cartilage are generally irreversible without surgical intervention and may result in chronic joint pain and dysfunction. Compressive force can cause ruptures in the disks or splitting and cracking in the menisci. When compressive force is coupled with other force, such as shear and torsion, the chance of injury greatly increases. A therapist's role in treating such injuries is more supportive in nature (this topic is covered in greater detail in Chapter 11).

Nerve Nerves carry information via electrical and chemical means. They are the lifeblood of the body and control every activity. Any type of nerve injury can be detrimental to the proper functioning of the body. The two types of force to which nerves are susceptible are tension and compression. Tensile injuries usually result from a high-speed accident and are graded on three levels:

1. *Grade I:* This is referred to as *neurapraxia* and is the mildest lesion. The nerve, epineurium, and myelin sheath are stretched but still intact. There is a localized conduction block, which causes a temporary loss of sensation and motor function. This usually lasts a few days to a few weeks.
2. *Grade II:* This is more severe and is known as an *axonotmesis* injury. This type of injury disrupts the axon and myelin sheath but

leaves the connective tissue covering, the epineurium, intact. Sensory and motor deficits last for at least 2 weeks, and full function is usually restored.

3. *Grade III:* This is the most severe lesion and is known as a *neurotmesis* injury. The entire nerve is disrupted and may never recover. Surgical intervention is usually necessary to aid in the recovery process, which can last up to a year.

In addition to tension injuries, compression force can lead to dysfunction in the nerves. This type of injury is much more complicated than tension injuries and depends on several factors such as the size of the force, the length of time the force was applied, and whether the pressure of the force was direct or indirect.

With compression injuries, damage to the vascular supply can result in nerve damage because of the dependency of the nerves on oxygen and nutrients supplied by the vessels. Regardless of the cause, the symptoms of nerve damage range from severe pain to loss of sensation. Changes in sensation can be placed in one of three categories:

1. *Hypoesthesia:* A reduction in sensation
2. *Hyperesthesia:* An increase in sensation
3. *Paresthesia:* A sense of numbness, prickling, or tingling

ASSESSMENT PROTOCOL

signs Objective, measurable findings obtained during an assessment.

symptoms Information obtained from the client during an assessment.

Performing assessments is nothing more than searching for dysfunctional anatomy, physiology, or biomechanics. This involves identifying **signs**, which are objective, measurable physical findings, and **symptoms**, which consist of information provided by the client. The purpose of identifying signs and symptoms is to gather as much information as possible about the condition from the perspectives of both the client and the therapist. Having a systematic and sequential method of gathering information is an important element of assessment. This ensures that nothing is overlooked and that information is obtained properly.

There are two methods of gathering information during an assessment. The first is the *HOPS method.* The acronym stands for:

- *H:* History
- *O:* Observation
- *P:* Palpation
- *S:* Special tests

The second is the *SOAP method.* The acronym stands for:

- *S:* Subjective
- *O:* Objective
- *A:* Assessment
- *P:* Plan

Both methods gather the same information, but the SOAP method applies the information gathered during the HOPS evaluation to the assessment section and formulates a treatment plan. Regardless of the method used, several key components are common to both, as listed in Table 4-1.

Table 4-1 Key Components to Gathering Information

History of the injury

Observation and inspection

Palpation

Functional tests

Special stress test

Neurologic tests

A vital step in the assessment process is taking care to test the uninvolved side or limb first. This provides an immediate reference to the affected side, as well as a means for the client to demonstrate the mechanism of injury. The uninvolved side plays a role in all aspects of the assessment, including:

- *History:* Helps determine the mechanism of injury and whether the uninvolved side has a preexisting injury.
- *Observation:* Provides a reference for appearance, symmetry, and obvious deformity.
- *Palpation:* Provides a baseline for the normal feel of the tissues.
- *Functional tests:* Provide a frame of reference for range of motion, strength, and painful arcs.
- *Special tests:* Help determine the end-feel and normal joint laxity.

There are two schools of thought when it comes to testing the uninvolved side. One says that testing the uninvolved side first reduces a client's apprehension by showing him or her the process. The other perspective states that letting the client experience the test on the uninvolved side first will cause more apprehension and guarding in anticipation of the test. The therapist should use the method that best fits the individual situation.

Client History

The client history is the most important component of the assessment and provides much more information than that related to the primary complaint: "80% of the information needed to clarify the cause of symptoms is contained within the subjective assessment" (Goodman et al., 1990). The history gives insight into the client's personality, lifestyle, stress levels, work patterns, and recreational pursuits, as well as other treatment the client has received and how the injury has manifested.

To take a client's history, begin by building a rapport with the client in a professional and comfortable atmosphere. This will ensure that the client feels validated and listened to. Maintain eye contact and ask easy, open-ended questions; however, closed-ended questions may be used if

Practical Tip

It is important to test the uninvolved side first.

Practical Tip

Building a rapport with a client will help the therapist obtain the desired information more quickly and easily.

Table 4-2 Examples of Questions for the Client

Open Ended	Closed Ended
1. Why are you here?	1. Can you lie on your back?
2. Where is it bothering you the most?	2. Is it pain or numbness?
3. What caused your problem?	3. Do you have x-rays?

the client is not divulging the necessary information. Questions should be asked one at a time and should not lead the client in any particular direction; Table 4-2 shows some examples. Other relevant information to gather during the history includes:

1. *The primary complaint:* Asking about the primary complaint elicits information in the client's own words about the reason for the visit.
2. *The mechanism of injury:* Discussing the mechanism of injury provides the most important information that comes from the history—the client's description of what happened to cause the injury. Questions that can help expand on this information include:

   - Was there any trauma?
   - If it was a fall, in what position did you land?
   - Did the problem arise suddenly or occur over time?
   - What was the position of your body when you first noticed the pain?
   - Did you feel or hear anything?
   - Have you performed any new activities or movements?
   - Have you changed any of your exercise equipment?

   Determining the mechanism of injury provides clues to the direction and magnitude of the force, the type of muscle contraction occurring at the time, and the type of force that was applied. If no discernable mechanism or memorable incident occurred when the complaint was noticed, then peripheral information, including signs and symptoms, areas of pain, and dysfunction patterns, can be useful in coming to a reasonable conclusion.

3. *Symptoms:* Acquiring information about the client's symptoms requires investigating the primary complaint. There are two categories of pain: somatic and visceral. Both have unique descriptive characteristics:

   - *Somatic pain* occurs from structures other than organs; it can be deep or superficial pain.
   - *Deep somatic pain* lasts longer than superficial somatic pain and is diffuse and nagging; it also feels as if there is pressure on the structures. This type of pain usually indicates more significant damage.
   - *Superficial somatic pain* affects the superficial structures; it is sharp, prickly pain that is brief in duration.
   - *Visceral pain* results from injury to organs. It is similar to deep somatic pain but includes nausea and vomiting. It is important to obtain as specific a location of the pain as possible. Asking the cli-

ent to place one finger on the area of complaint will help narrow down the structures that could possibly be involved.

For the most part, the location and the characteristics of the pain indicate which tissues are involved; however, do not rule out referred pain. The therapist must be knowledgeable in common referral areas to ensure an accurate assessment. Certain questions can help in obtaining information about the pain:

- Where was the pain originally, and has it moved?
- What situations make the pain worse or better?
- How long has the problem lasted?
- When do the symptoms occur?
- Are there any unusual sensations?
- Does the pain stay in one spot or radiate into other areas?
- Does it prevent you from sleeping?
- Does a joint lock, give way, or feel unstable?
- Has this problem occurred before?
- Is the pain constant or occasional?
- What type of pain is it?
  - Nerve pain is sharp and burning, and it tends to follow patterns.
  - Bone pain is very deep and localized.
  - Muscle pain, which is harder to localize, is dull and aching and can be referred.

When questioning about pain, have the client put the information in measurable terms by using a pain scale. This rates the client's pain on a scale of 1 to 10, with 1 being minimal and 10 being unbearable, and provides an objective baseline to use later. Keep in mind that each client will have a different interpretation of the pain scale.

Additional information to obtain includes whether the client has experienced any disabilities as a result of the injury and whether there is a previous medical history that relates to the injured area.

> **Practical Tip**
> Remember that each client will have a different interpretation of the pain scale.

Observation

Observation begins the moment the client walks in the door. It includes a visual analysis of the client's overall appearance, posture, and dynamic movement and of the symmetry of his or her body. In addition to observing the client, inspect the injury site for factors such as redness, bruising, swelling, deformities, and other marks in the area. Once the client has disrobed to the appropriate level, scan the body's symmetry and appearance from the anterior and posterior, as well as both sides. While observing the client from different views, consider these specific questions:

- Is there any obvious deformity?
- Does the client possess normal balance?
- Are the bony and soft tissue contours symmetrical?
- Are limb positions equal and symmetric?
- Are there any scars or other signs that indicate recent injury?
- Is the color of the skin normal?

Once the general scan is complete, assess the client in static and dynamic phases.

Posture

According to the Posture Committee of the American Academy of Orthopedic Surgeons:

> Posture is usually defined as the relative arrangement of the parts of the body. Good posture is that state of muscular and skeletal balance which protects the supporting structures of the body against injury or progressive deformity, irrespective of the attitude (erect, lying, squatting, or stooping) in which these structures are working or resting. Under such conditions the muscles will function most efficiently and the optimum positions are afforded for the thoracic and abdominal organs. Poor posture is a faulty relationship of the various parts of the body which produces increased strain on the supporting structures and in which there is less efficient balance of the body over its base of support (Kendall et al., 2005).

If the posture is such that joints become hyper- or hypomobile or the muscles become weak or shortened, pathology can develop. This pathology may arise from the repetitive effect of small stresses over time, which causes the body to alter its structure to accommodate repeated stresses.

In an assessment of posture, it is important to review the normal curves of the spine. Humans are born with two curves, and two additional curves develop over time. The curves present at birth, or **primary curves**, are the thoracic spine and sacral curves; they are concave in shape anteriorly and convex in shape posteriorly. **Secondary curves**, located in the cervical and lumbar spine, develop as the body accommodates for the effects of gravity; they are convex in shape anteriorly and concave in shape posteriorly.

It is necessary to use a straight line as a reference for testing. This is accomplished easiest by hanging a plumb line, which is nothing more than a plumb bob suspended by a string from the ceiling, and having the client stand in front of it. When assessing from the front or back, have the client stand with feet equidistant from the line. When the client is standing sideways, line up the plumb just in front of the lateral malleolus. Deviations are described as slight, moderate, or marked.

Anterior

Use the following guidelines when assessing posture from the anterior side (Fig. 4-3):

- The head should sit squarely on the shoulders. Check for tilts or rotations, and try to establish their causes.
- The tip of the nose should be in alignment with the manubrium, xiphoid process, and umbilicus. This is known as the *anterior line of reference.*
- The contour of the trapezius should appear equal bilaterally. Check for unusually prominent bony areas.
- The shoulders, clavicles, and acromioclavicular joints should appear to be equal. Deviations may indicate joint pathology.
- The tops of the iliac crests should appear level. Deviations may indicate the presence of scoliosis.
- The arms should face the same direction.

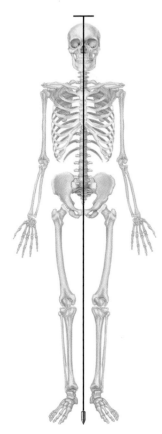

primary curves The curves of the spinal column that are present at birth.

secondary curves The curves in the spinal column that develop as a result of adapting to the forces of gravity.

Figure 4-3 Correct posture from the anterior view.

- The anterior superior iliac spine (ASIS) should appear level bilaterally. Dysfunction may indicate leg-length discrepancies or pelvic rotation.
- The pubic bones should appear level.
- The patella should face forward. An outward-facing patella is known as "frog eyes." A patella facing inward is called a "squinting" patella.
- The knees should appear straight.
- The malleoli should appear to be equal.
- The arches on both sides of the feet should be checked, noting any pes planus or cavus.

Lateral

Use the following guidelines when assessing posture from the lateral side (Fig. 4-4):

- Check the lateral line of assessment, which is the line from the earlobe to the tip of the shoulder. It continues through the highest point on the iliac crest, slightly anterior to the axis of the knee joint and slightly anterior to the lateral malleolus.
- Determine whether the back has excessive curvature. Look at each spinal segment in relation to the sacrum.
- Check the musculatures of the back, abdominal, and chest regions. They should have good tone with no obvious deformity.
- Check the pelvis. It should appear level.
- Look for visible trunk rotation.
- Examine the position of the knees. Determine whether they are flexed, straight, or in recurvatum (hyperextended).

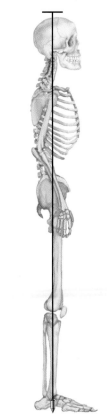

Figure 4-4 Correct posture from the lateral view.

Posterior

Use the following guidelines when assessing posture from the posterior side (Fig. 4-5):

- Check the head and neck. They should sit squarely on the shoulders, matching the anterior view.
- Determine whether the scapulae are positioned similarly on both sides. Note the rotation and tilt, levels of the superior and inferior angles, and whether they sit flat on the rib cage.
- Look for lateral curves on the spine.
- Look for atrophy of the posterior musculature.
- Look for equal space between the elbows and trunk.
- Determine whether the ribs are symmetrical.
- Check the posterior superior iliac spine (PSIS). It should appear level bilaterally.
- Check the tops of the iliac crests and gluteal folds. They should appear equal.
- Determine whether the backs of the knees appear level.
- Check the Achilles. They should run vertical on both sides.
- Determine whether the heels are straight. Check for valgus or varus positioning.

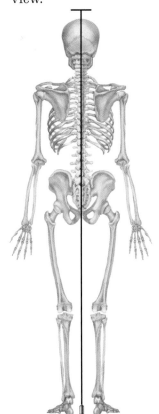

Figure 4-5 Correct posture from the posterior view.

Gait

The last phase of observation is the assessment of gait. As the main source of the body's locomotion, improper gait can be a major source of dysfunction. This section provides a general overview of the phases related to gait and explains what happens during each phase.

The Gait Cycle The gait cycle includes the cooperative functioning of the lower extremities, pelvis, and spinal column. This dance of articulations is composed of a kinetic chain through which motion occurs. The position and function of one joint affects the position and function of the others. During the gait cycle, there are times when the chain is closed and times when it is open. The weight-bearing portion of the cycle is a closed kinetic chain in which the distal joints influence the proximal ones. The other half of the cycle is a non-weight-bearing, or open, kinetic chain in which the proximal joints influence the distal ones.

The process of walking can be described as the act of falling forward and catching oneself. One foot is always in contact with the ground, and there are two periods of single-leg and two periods of double-leg support. The term **gait cycle** is the sequence of motions that occur between two consecutive initial contacts of the same foot (Magee, 1997). The gait cycle of one foot is 180° opposite that of the other and consists of two phases: stance and swing.

Stance The stance phase makes up 60% to 65% of the gait cycle and occurs when the foot is in contact with the ground (Fig. 4-6). This is the

📖 **gait cycle** The sequence of motions that occur between two initial contacts of the same foot.

Figure 4-6 The stance phase of gait and its five stages.

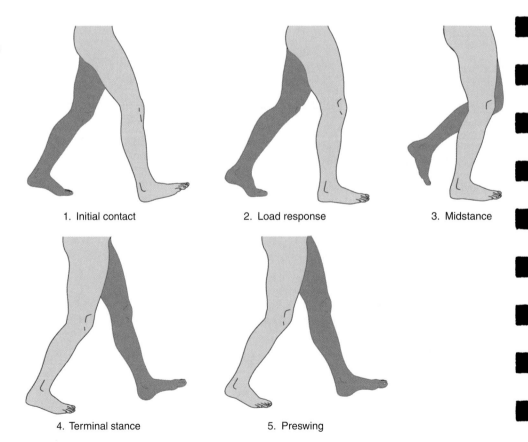

1. Initial contact

2. Load response

3. Midstance

4. Terminal stance

5. Preswing

Part II Regional Approach to Treatment

weight-bearing portion of the cycle and enables forward movements. There are five stages of this phase:

1. *Initial contact:* This is also known as *heel strike* and occurs when the heel of one foot contacts the ground and begins to accept the weight of the body, while the opposite foot is simultaneously ending its stance phase and coming off the ground.
2. *Load response:* As the foot begins to bear weight, this stage lasts until the opposite foot leaves the ground.
3. *Midstance:* This phase occurs when only one leg bears the entire weight of the body. During the midstance of one leg, the other leg is going through the swing phase.
4. *Terminal stance:* This phase is also known as the *weight-unloading period* and occurs when the stance leg is shifting the weight to the contralateral side to prepare to enter the swing phase.
5. *Preswing:* This is the last period of the stance phase; it begins with the initial contact of the opposite foot and ends with the toe-off of the stance foot.

Swing The swing phase constitutes 35% to 40% of the gait cycle and occurs when the foot is suspended in the air. The swing phase of gait is the non-weight-bearing period when the leg moves forward (Fig. 4-7). There are three parts to this phase:

1. *Initial swing:* This begins with the toe leaving the ground and ends with the knee reaching the maximum amount of flexion needed for the foot to clear the ground, which is about 60°.
2. *Midswing:* This occurs when the swing leg is next to the stance leg, which is in midstance, and begins to straighten so that the tibia is vertical.
3. *Terminal swing:* This is the last period of the swing phase; it begins with the deceleration of the leg and ends with the initial contact or heel strike.

Parameters of Gait Before discussing observation of gait, it is important to define some normal baseline parameters related to gait, which will assist in determining the presence of dysfunction. These parameters are

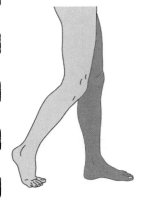
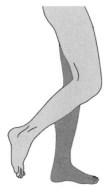
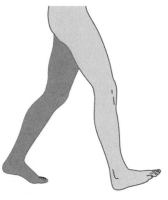

1. Initial swing   2. Midswing   3. Terminal swing

Figure 4-7 The swing phase of gait and its three stages.

standard for the population between 8 and 45 years old; however, there are variations among genders and ages and within the same gender.

1. *Center of gravity:* This is an important component of gait and posture. The normal center of gravity in standing is 2 inches anterior to the second sacral vertebra; this can be lower in women.
2. *Base width:* This is defined as the distance between the feet and is normally 2 to 4 inches.
3. *Step length:* This is the distance between successive contact points on opposite feet. While it should be the same for both legs, normally 14 to 16 inches, there are various factors that can alter it: Children take smaller steps than adults; women take smaller steps than men; and taller people take longer steps than shorter people. There are other factors that affect step length regardless of age or gender, including fatigue, pain, and disease.
4. *Stride length:* While step length is the distance between opposite feet, stride length is the distance between successive points of contact on the same foot. This distance is normally 27 to 32 inches. The factors that affect stride length are the same as those that alter step length.
5. *Lateral pelvic shift:* Also known as *pelvic list,* this is the lateral side-to-side movement of the pelvis during walking. The purpose of the shift is to center the body's weight over the stance leg. The normal amount of shift is 1 to 2 inches and, if varied, can affect balance.
6. *Vertical pelvic shift:* A vertical shift during gait keeps the center of gravity moving up and down about 2 inches. The highest point occurs during midstance; the lowest, during heel strike.
7. *Pelvic rotation:* Rotation takes place on both sides of the pelvis, and this lengthens the femur. In order to maintain balance, the trunk rotates in the opposite direction.
8. *Cadence:* This is the pace of gait and is normally 90 to 120 steps per minute in men. Factors such as gender, age, and injury can alter normal cadence.

Observation of Gait Once the static assessment of posture is complete, observe the body during motion. When assessing gait, watch all the components involved, including the lumbar spine, pelvis, hips, knees, feet, and ankles. Ensure that the client is dressed appropriately, and observe movement from the anterior, posterior, and lateral sides.

- *Anterior view:* When observing from the anterior, pay attention to the motions of the pelvis. Watch for lateral tilt to determine whether the pelvis rotates on a horizontal plane. Does the trunk shift sideways and rotate in the opposite direction of the pelvis? Note the movements at the other joints. Check for hip and knee rotation; ankle and foot plantar or dorsiflexion; and pronation and supination. These are best noted during the weight-loading period.
- *Lateral view:* Examine trunk rotation, reciprocal arm swing, hip and knee flexion, ankle movement, step length, stride length, and cadence on the lateral side.
- *Posterior view:* Observing the same structures as in the anterior view, watch heel rise and stance width, as well as movement of the lumbar spine, musculature of the back, and posterior hips and legs.

To help facilitate a treatment plan, use the information from the observation of posture and gait to determine the specific musculature that may be shortened or lengthened, as well as joints that may be restricted.

Palpation

Palpation is the next component in developing a treatment plan, and it is an extension of observation because the hands are used to "see" the structures. Specific structures that should be palpated are discussed in later chapters based on the regions of the body; however, some general principles and characteristics are addressed here.

Just as the entire assessment process is systematic, so too is palpation. Start at a point away from the injury site, and move toward the point of greatest pain last. Pressure should be light at first and increased as the deeper structures are felt. Depending on the type of information desired, use the corresponding body part. For example, to determine tissue temperature, use the entire ventral surface of the hand. To obtain more specific information, use the sensitive parts of the hand, such as the fingertips. As the areas are palpated, gather information about the physical findings, including:

1. *Tissue temperature:* Determine tissue temperature using a larger surface of the hand or fingertips; this can provide information about the phase of the injury. Warmth in the area can mean an increase in circulation.
2. *Obvious deformity:* Take care to identify obvious changes in the structures or the presence of abnormal structures.
3. *Swelling:* Depending on where swelling is located, the tissue will feel different. *Edema* is excess fluid in the interstitial spaces and can leave indentations when pressure is applied (pitting edema). Swelling can be general or localized, such as within a joint or bursa. Acute swelling is softer and more mobile, whereas fluid that has been in an area for a period of time has a thicker feel and is more gel-like.
4. *Tissue tone:* Note muscle tone and whether the muscle is in spasm or flaccid. Assess the presence of tight bands within the muscle and tension in other structures such as the ligaments, tendons, and fascia. Note the presence of spasms, tremors, fasciculation, or abnormal structures.
5. *Point tenderness:* Note the area with the highest level of pain, which is graded on four levels:
   - *Grade 1:* The client complains of pain.
   - *Grade 2:* The client complains and winces.
   - *Grade 3:* The client winces and withdraws the limb.
   - *Grade 4:* The client will not allow the area to be palpated.
6. *Crepitus:* A creaking or cracking sensation during palpation indicates damage to the bony or soft tissue structures. If this occurs over the bone, it may indicate a fracture. If this occurs over soft tissue, inflammation can cause the sensation in tendons, bursas, and joint capsules.
7. *Abnormal sensation:* Changes in sensation such as dysesthesia (decreased), hyperesthesia (increased), or anesthesia (absence) may indicate

nerve damage. This is assessed by running a finger along both sides of the area and asking the client if there are any differences between the sides.

8. *Pulses:* Check for changes in the major pulses in the area of palpation.

Functional Testing

This next component of assessment consists of several steps and tests muscle, nerve, and other noncontractile tissues. Specific functional testing for each region is included in correlating chapters. This section covers the principles in the application of the tests.

There are several rules of thumb to follow when you are performing functional testing:

- If it is appropriate for the situation, test the uninvolved side first unless bilateral movement is required. This lets the client know what to expect and establishes what is normal for the individual.
- Perform active motion before passive motion; this will prevent moving the limb past the client's ability. It will also help determine the structures, contractile or inert, that are involved.
- Perform painful movements last; this prevents pain from affecting future tests during the assessment.
- Apply overpressure gently to determine end-feel of the tissues.
- Hold or repeat movement to obtain accurate information. Clients will present with conditions that are aggravated by repetitive movements, so re-creating the conditions will provide a truer picture of the problem.
- Perform resisted muscle tests with the joint in a resting position to cancel out force on inert tissues; this allows for the isolation of contractile tissues.
- After completing the testing, inform the client that symptoms may worsen due to the assessment.

These principles are summarized in Table 4-3.

Table 4-3   Principles in Application of Functional Testing

If it is appropriate for the situation, test the uninvolved side first unless bilateral movement is required.

Perform active motion before passive motion.

Perform painful movements last.

Apply overpressure gently to determine end-feel of the tissues.

Hold or repeat movement to obtain accurate information.

Perform resisted muscle tests with the joint in a resting position.

Inform the client that symptoms may worsen due to the assessment.

Active Range of Motion

Active range of motion is motion performed by the client with no help from the therapist. Objective measurements of active range can be obtained through the use of a goniometer; however, this text discusses how a therapist can approximate the ranges of both sides and compare the differences.

Active motion tests the range of motion, the client's willingness to move through the range, and the control the client has over the body part that is being assessed. Active motions primarily test contractile tissue and are generally performed a few times in each direction while the therapist makes notes. The movements are usually standard and follow the cardinal planes. If the client experiences pain outside the planes or from a combination of the planes, instruct the client to re-create those movements; while the client is doing so, observe:

- The client's reaction to the pain
- The movement pattern
- The quality of the movement
- The location of the restrictions and when they occur
- The location of the pain and when it occurs
- Any compensatory movements

Passive Range of Motion

Passive range of motion is motion performed on the client by the therapist while the client remains totally relaxed. To perform a passive-range-of-motion test, place the area in a position wherein the joint is in a relaxed state. Instruct the client to refrain from contracting the area during the test because passive range of motion tests noncontractile, or inert, tissues and a contraction can affect the results. The movement should be as complete as possible and in the same direction as movements that were tested actively. During testing, note:

- The location of pain and when it occurs
- Whether the movement changes the pain
- Any patterns of restriction
- The end-feel
- Any compensatory movement

As discussed earlier, determining end-feel during passive motion is accomplished when the therapist gently applies overpressure to the client. The end-feel can help determine which structures are responsible for the dysfunction. There are four types of end-feel:

1. *Soft:* This occurs as a result of soft tissue approximation, such as when the calf touches the thigh during knee flexion, for example. Some abnormal causes would result from swelling or a ligamentous tear.
2. *Firm:* This feels as though there is a rising sense of tension and creates a feeling of springy or elastic resistance. It can occur as a result of

active range of motion Motion performed by the client with no help from the therapist.

passive range of motion Motion performed on the client by the therapist while the client remains totally relaxed.

muscle tightness or capsular or ligamentous stretching. Abnormally, the stretch is felt before the normal end range.

3. *Hard:* This occurs from two bones' coming in contact with one another, such as the ulna and humerus in elbow extension. If dysfunction is present, it will occur before reaching normal range for a joint; it can result from bony abnormalities.

4. *Empty:* This occurs when there is no end-feel because the full range is never reached due to pain; it occurs only if dysfunction is present.

Resisted Isometric Motion

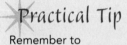
Practical Tip

Remember to create an isometric contraction by placing an eccentric load on the muscle.

Resisted isometric motion gauges the strength of the contractile tissues and their ability to facilitate movement, stability, and support. It is important to create an isometric contraction through the application of an eccentric load so that only the contractile tissues are tested. This will determine whether they are at fault. If the joint moves, the inert tissues will also move and subsequently skew the results.

It takes a lot of practice to become proficient at muscle testing, including understanding the intricacies of positioning, the resistance used in testing small or weak muscles, and the anatomical details, all of which ensure accuracy. The results of testing expose areas of weakness and muscle imbalance that can lead to undue stress and strain on the system, and these areas are graded on a scale depending on how much force the muscles can resist. There are several basic principles related to performing the tests:

- Place the client in a position that offers the most stability. If necessary, stabilize additional regions of the client's body to prevent compensation.
- Stabilize the body part proximal to the one being tested.
- Apply pressure directly opposite the line of pull to the muscle being tested using as long a lever as possible. As a general rule, apply the pressure near the distal end of the bone in which the muscle is inserted, unless it does not allow adequate leverage.
- Tell the client to prevent you from moving him or her. Apply pressure gradually, and maintain it for at least 5 seconds; repeat throughout the joint's range of motion. This allows a better overall assessment of weakness and will establish the presence of a painful arc.

There are five numerical grades for gauging a client's strength, several of which have a plus and minus system. The scale is based on the pull of gravity; a 3 represents a fair score. Table 4-4 summarizes the testing scale.

Damage to the muscle-tendon unit is not the only cause of muscle weakness. Pain, injury to the nerve root or peripheral nerve, pathology to the tendon, fractures, and psychological reasons can also produce weakness.

Orthopedic Tests

Just as testing the contractile tissues of the body is important, assessing the noncontractile structures is equally important. Orthopedic tests are specific to each region of the body and are designed to expose pathology in the area. As with the other tests, these tests should be performed bilaterally to obtain baseline results. Throughout the book, specific tests are addressed for different pathologies in the appropriate chapter for the region.

Table 4-4 Manual Muscle Testing Scale

5	Normal	The muscle can move through the full range of motion against gravity and hold the maximum pressure a therapist applies for what might be the "full strength" of the muscle.
4+	Good [+]	The muscle moves through the complete range of motion against gravity and resists moderate to strong pressure.
4	Good	The muscle can move through the complete range of motion against gravity and resist moderate pressure.
4-	Good [-]	The muscle can move through the complete range of motion against gravity and resist slight to moderate pressure.
3+	Fair [+]	The muscle can move through the complete range of motion and resist minimal pressure.
3	Fair	This is the middle ground. The muscle has the ability to move through the entire range of motion against gravity but with no pressure.
3-	Fair [-]	The muscle can move through some of the range of motion against gravity.
2+	Poor [+]	The muscle can start the movement through the range but cannot continue it.
2	Poor	The muscle can move through the range with some gravity-eliminating assistance.
2-	Poor [-]	The muscle will initiate movement if gravity is eliminated.
1	Trace	A contraction is felt in the muscle, but no motion occurs.
0	Zero	There is no evidence of contraction.

Neurologic Tests

The functioning of the nerves in the area is an important component to assess when dealing with injuries. The portion of the nerve that originates from the spinal cord is referred to as the *nerve root*. Most nerves have two components:

- *Motor component:* This innervates various skeletal muscles and provides sensory information from the skin, connective tissue, joints, and muscles.

- *Visceral component:* This is part of the autonomic nervous system and innervates structures such as the dura mater, blood vessels, periosteum, and intervertebral disks.

The motor component of a segmental nerve is assessed using a myotome, and the sensory component is tested using a dermatome. Most roots form a plexus as they exit the spinal cord and become peripheral nerves. Because of this, injuries to a segment often affect more than one peripheral nerve and demonstrate a different neurologic presentation than would occur if just one nerve was affected. These tests are used to determine the integrity of the central nervous system.

Dermatomes

A *dermatome* is the area of skin innervated by a single nerve root. Slight differences occur between individuals, and there is a great deal of overlap between dermatomes. The sensitivity of these nerves is usually tested using light touch discrimination. This can be accomplished using items such as a paper clip, a cotton ball, fingernails, or the pads of the fingers. The areas innervated by the nerves are touched lightly bilaterally, and then the client is asked if the sensations were equal. It is important to stay in the middle of the dermatome to avoid any overlap into adjacent dermatomes. Variations between the sides can indicate pathology.

Myotomes

Myotomes are defined as adjacent muscles that receive their innervation from one or two nerve roots. Testing the motion of certain muscles by using resistive tests can assess the condition of the nerve root. These tests should be held for at least 5 seconds; deviations between the sides may indicate pathology in the nerve root.

Designing a Treatment Plan

Treating a condition through clinical massage is a very involved process that requires a significant time investment. Each client should receive a customized plan based on his or her unique situation. This requires a high level of clinical reasoning on the part of the therapist. Before addressing clinical reasoning, it is necessary to expand on the concepts from *Bloom's Taxonomy of Educational Objectives*, introduced in Chapter 1.

As discussed in Chapter 1, there are six levels of learning. Each level builds on the previous one and increases in difficulty:

- *Knowledge:* This level involves basic memorization regardless of the information. As this level evolves, information is placed into trends and sequences, or classifications and categories, and moves from specific and concrete knowledge to more abstract ideas.
- *Comprehension:* This level is where the process of understanding and perceiving begins; it involves insight and the processing of information, including transforming the information into a more useful form.

- *Application:* This level involves using the information in a very specific manner; it requires an element of creativity since the information can be applied to a new situation for which no specified solution exists.
- *Analysis:* This phase involves higher-level objectives and the breakdown of the whole into its parts. It can include simply listing the elements or determining the relationship between the elements.
- *Synthesis:* This level involves creating a whole from parts using deductive logic; it requires a heavy dose of thinking and creativity.
- *Evaluation:* This is the highest level of learning. It is a combination of the five previous levels and is concerned with value judgments.

Clinical Reasoning

Clinical reasoning is an important part of the clinical treatment process. It "provides a safeguard against the risk of having the popular theory and clinical techniques of the day adopted without question and hence thwarting alternative theories and clinical practice" (Jones, 1995).

The process of clinical reasoning always begins with gathering initial information. This information generally causes a wide range of impressions and interpretations, leading to the formulation of an initial general hypothesis; however, most therapists usually have an established assessment routine, which develops through experience, although it will vary among practitioners. Despite having a general routine in place, therapists should view each client as a unique individual whose symptoms require a tailored assessment. The process of formulating a hypothesis and assessing on the basis of the individual continues until enough information is gathered to make a treatment and management decision.

The more experience a therapist has with these techniques, the better he or she will be at recognizing common patterns associated with specific conditions. Although no two situations are exactly the same, similarities do exist. The process of recognizing patterns without the need for hypothesis testing is called *forward reasoning.* While this ability is linked to experience and typically employed by experts, therapists at any skill level who are faced with an unfamiliar situation employ what is known as *backward reasoning.* This is the process of formulating and testing a hypothesis to obtain information.

Factors That Influence Clinical Reasoning A variety of internal and external factors affect clinical reasoning. Externally, the client's needs, expectations, values, beliefs, and available resources are influential. Internally, the therapist's knowledge base, reasoning strategies, and personal beliefs can have tremendous influence.

Errors can occur and are typically related to data analysis and hypothesis testing. Examples include overemphasizing information that supports a popular theory or misinterpreting unimportant information. The most common error, however, occurs when a therapist is biased toward a favorite hypothesis. It is important for therapists to continually add to their skill sets to avoid becoming preoccupied with a single theory.

One consistent clinical-reasoning research finding shows that the more knowledge a therapist has in a particular area, the more accurate he or she is at assessing.

Treatment Framework

Regardless of the condition, the sequence of treatment techniques should not change. Certain techniques may be used more than others, along with different styles; however, the order of application should always stay the same:

1. *Connective tissue restrictions:* Connective tissue has a wonderful symbiotic relationship with every other tissue in the body; therefore, it must be addressed first if any subsequent treatment techniques are to be effective.
2. *Trigger points:* Trigger points are key components of dysfunction and can affect the entire body.
3. *Muscle tissue:* Once the connective tissue and trigger points have been handled, the inconsistencies in the muscle due to hypertonicity or adhesions must be addressed.
4. *Flexibility restrictions:* To prevent the same conditions from recurring, the muscles must be in proper balance; this requires restoring the proper length to the tissue.
5. *Strength training:* Though not addressed in this text, strength training is the final component necessary for restoring balance to the tissues.

SUMMARY

"For a treatment to work, it must be specific" (Kraft, 2003). Formulating a treatment plan is an ongoing process for each client. It involves a constant sequence of assessing, treating, reassessing, and either continuing with the same treatments or trying something different. This requires that therapists continually use all of their resources to provide the most effective therapy possible. This chapter has discussed the components of gathering information to create a treatment plan. In order to know how to heal, the therapist must first understand the types of tissue involved, the ways injuries can occur, and the injury process itself. Information must be gathered from the client that will contribute to the overall picture of the problem. This information is gathered in several different ways, ranging from verbal questioning to manual assessment techniques. When an injury occurs, other structures may be affected far away from the injury site. The methods of assessing the kinetic chain and determining the level of compensation were discussed in this chapter. Once the necessary information is obtained, various methods presented in the chapter help assemble it into useful patterns and an overall treatment plan.

REVIEW QUESTIONS

1. What are the characteristics of the three phases of injury?
2. What are the three types of contractions that a muscle can perform?
3. What are the five types of force that can affect the body?
4. What are the four basic muscle shapes?
5. What is the difference between tendonitis and tenosynovitis?
6. What are the characteristics of the three degrees of injury to muscles and ligaments?
7. What is the proper alignment of the body in the anterior, posterior, and side views?
8. What are the two phases of the gait cycle?
9. What are the six levels of learning?
10. What are the five steps in the treatment framework of clinical massage?

CRITICAL-THINKING QUESTIONS

1. Why is it important to look beyond the direct source of the complaint for underlying causes of dysfunction?
2. Why is it important to obtain as detailed a client history as possible?
3. Explain the difference between testing active and testing passive ranges of motion as they relate to the tissues being tested.
4. Discuss the importance of having a referral network of outside health care providers.
5. Why is it important to know what type of contraction the muscle was performing at the time of an injury?
6. What is the importance of testing the uninvolved side first?
7. What is the importance of grading a client's pain levels?
8. Why is it important to continually reassess a client's treatment?

chapter **5**

Conditions of the Head and Neck

chapter outline

I. Introduction

II. Anatomical Review
 a. Bony Structures of the Head and Face
 b. Soft Tissue Structures of the Head and Face
 c. Bony Structures of the Cervical Spine
 d. Soft Tissue Structures of the Cervical Spine
 e. Associated Bony Structures
 f. Muscles of the Head and Neck

III. Movements and Manual Muscle Testing of the Region
 a. Movements of the Region
 b. Manual Muscle Testing for the Region

IV. Dermatomes for the Head and Neck

V. Trigger-Point Referral Patterns for Muscles of the Region

VI. Specific Conditions
 a. Whiplash
 b. Temporomandibular Joint Dysfunction
 c. Torticollis
 d. Cervical Disk Injuries
 e. Thoracic Outlet Syndrome

VII. Summary

VIII. Review Questions

IX. Critical-Thinking Questions

X. Quick Reference Tables
 a. Bony Surface Anatomy of the Skull
 b. Soft Tissue Surface Anatomy of the Skull
 c. Bony Surface Anatomy of the Neck
 d. Soft Tissue Surface Anatomy of the Neck
 e. Bony Surface Anatomy of the Shoulder
 f. Muscles of the Head and Face
 g. Muscles of the Posterior Neck
 h. Muscles of the Anterior Neck
 i. Trigger Points for the Head and Neck Muscles
 j. Orthopedic Tests for the Head and Neck

chapter objectives

At the conclusion of this chapter, the reader will understand:

- bony anatomy of the region
- how to locate the bony landmarks and soft tissue structures of the region
- where to find the muscles and the origins, insertions, and actions of the region
- how to assess the movement and determine the range of motion for the region
- how to perform manual muscle testing to the region
- how to recognize dermatome patterns for the region
- trigger-point locations and referral patterns for the region
- the following elements of each condition discussed:
  - background and characteristics
  - specific questions to ask
  - what orthopedic tests should be performed
  - how to treat connective tissue, trigger points, and muscles
  - flexibility concerns

key terms

congenital muscular torticollis
muscular cervical dystonia
neurologic cervical dystonia
release phenomenon
temporomandibular disorder (TMD)
thoracic outlet syndrome (TOS)
torticollis
whiplash

94

Introduction
The head, neck, cervical, and thoracic regions of the body are extremely susceptible to injury and are a common area of complaint in the massage therapy profession. Injuries to these areas can develop from both chronic conditions and acute trauma. Although traumatic mechanisms of injury, such as automobile accidents, falls, or sports-related activities, are more common, chronic conditions such as repetitive motion injuries and postural misalignments can be just as debilitating. In order to understand how to treat dysfunction in these areas, it is necessary to first understand the anatomy of the region and how it interacts with the rest of the body in a normal capacity.

This chapter reviews the skeletal anatomy of the head and neck and discusses the unique bumps, projections, holes, hills, and valleys of the skeletal structures, all of which perform various functions. In addition, this chapter covers:

- Specific bony landmarks that identify important areas for palpation
- Soft tissue structures, including the muscles of the region
- The movements of the region
- Manual muscle tests for the head and neck
- Dermatome and trigger-point referral patterns for the involved muscles

ANATOMICAL REVIEW

Bony Structures of the Head and Face

The head is divided into two parts: the skull and the face. The skull is the most complex part of the skeleton and forms the cranial vault; this area houses the brain. The *cranium,* which refers to the head and not the face, consists of eight bones joined by a synarthritic joint called a *suture.* The sutures of the cranium are not fused at birth as this allows for the shifting of the cranial bones during the passage of the head through the birth canal. The cranial bones typically fuse around the age of 2 and are generally considered immovable by the medical community (Fig. 5-1). Table 5-1 lists the bones of the cranium.

The face comprises 14 bones and is more delicate than the cranium (see Fig. 5-1). Its bones develop more slowly than the cranium and give the face its shape and unique characteristics. The facial bones perform many important functions such as holding the upper and lower teeth intact and enabling movement of the mouth. Table 5-2 lists the major bones in the face.

All the bones in the skull and face are listed in Table 5-3.

Bony Landmarks and Surface Anatomy

In order to accurately treat the head and neck region, massage therapists must be able to identify and locate relevant landmarks. The following sections describe how to find the landmarks in this region.

The Anterior Structures (See Fig. 5-1) The *frontal bone* is located on the forehead. Locate the *supraciliary arch* by tracing the frontal bone inferiorly at the top of the orbit of the eye just above the bony ridge around the eyebrow area. The *supraorbital foramen* and *frontal sinus* are located at the medial corner of the eyebrow and are found by following medially

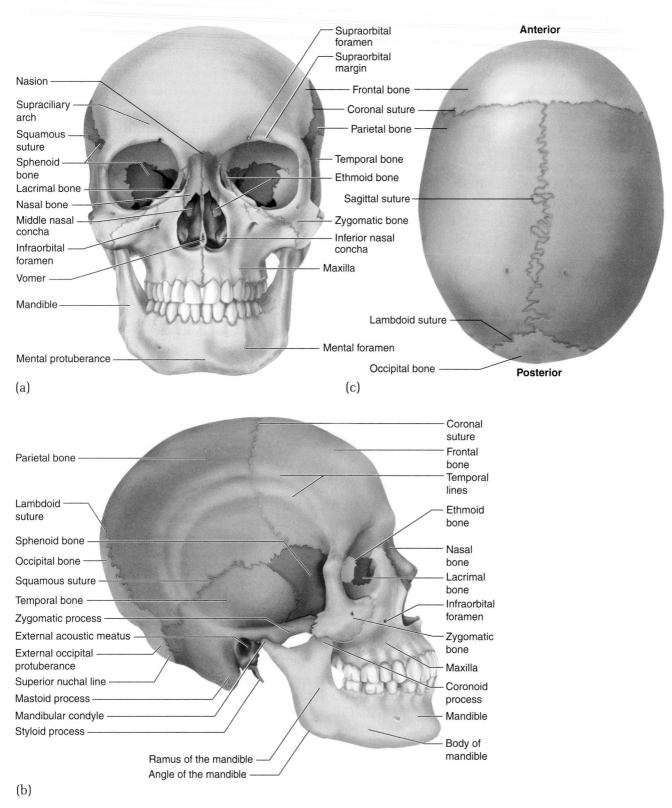

Figure 5-1 The skull.
(a) Anterior view. *(b)* Lateral view. *(c)* Superior view.

Table 5-1 The Bones of the Cranium

Bone	Location
Frontal bone	Comprises the front of the skull, the roof of the cranial cavity, and the upper portion of the orbits of the eyes; also contains the frontal sinus.
Parietal bones (2—one on either side of midline)	Form the top and posterior lateral portions of the skull.
Temporal bones (2)	Encompass the ears. They are the weakest cranial bones.
Occipital bone	Forms the posterior skull and articulates with the 1st cervical vertebra at the occipital condyles, which are on the inferior surface of the bone. It is the strongest cranial bone.
Ethmoid and sphenoid bones	Form the floor of the skull.

Table 5-2 Major Facial Bones

Bones	Function
Maxilla	Holds the upper teeth intact. It is the largest facial bone.
Zygomatic bones	Form the inferior border of the orbits of the eyes and the prominence of the cheek.
Nasal bones	Form the bridge of the nose and support the nasal cartilage.
Mandible	Holds the lower teeth intact. It is the only movable bone in the face.

Table 5-3 Bones of the Skull and Face

Cranium	Facial
Frontal (1)	Maxilla (2)
Parietal (2)	Zygomatic (2)
Occipital (1)	Nasal (2)
Temporal (2)	Inferior nasal conchae (2)
Sphenoid (1)	Mandible (1)
Ethmoid (1)	Palatine (2)
	Lacrimal (2)
	Vomer (1)

along the supraorbital arch to a rounded and flat area. The supraorbital nerve exits the foramen here, and the frontal sinus lies deep to it. This area is a common source of pain and pressure associated with allergies and sinus problems.

On the inferior side of the orbits are the *infraorbital foramens*, which are just lateral to the inferior portion of the nose at the inferior medial orbit of the eye. They are home to the infraorbital nerves, and the maxillary sinuses lie deep to them.

At the junction between the nasal bone and the frontal bone is the *nasion*. A horizontal ridge that designates the suture can be felt by palpating in a vertical direction. Just below the nasion on each side is a *nasal bone*. Moving in an inferior direction yields the junction between the bone and the cartilage at the tip of the nose.

The *maxilla* comprises the center of the face, the area around the nose, the inferior portion of the orbit of the eye, and the front portion of the cheek. The maxilla also holds the upper teeth intact. Starting at the inferior lateral corner of the eye and tracing laterally to either side of the maxilla yields the *zygomatic bone*. Continuing laterally yields an arch, or the cheekbone.

The mandible, or jaw, is the only movable bone in the face. The *mandibular condyle* is located just anterior to the external auditory meatus, or ear canal, and forms the temporomandibular joint (TMJ) with the temporal bone. Tracing the zygomatic arch to the ear and moving inferiorly is an alternate method of locating this structure. To feel the condyle move forward and down, have the client open and close his or her mouth. Anterior to the condyle is the *coronoid process*, which is the insertion point for the temporalis muscle. Using the mandibular condyle as a starting place, move about an inch anteriorly and roll under the zygomatic arch. Have the client open his or her mouth fully; the process should move into your finger. To find the location using an alternate method, have the client open his or her mouth fully while you trace along under the zygomatic arch in the hollow part of the cheek until you feel the process.

The *ramus of the mandible* is located inferior to the TMJ. This is the vertical portion of the mandible, running down from the mandibular condyle to the corner of the jaw. At the end of the ramus is the *angle of the mandible*. From the angle, moving toward the chin is the *body of the mandible*, the long horizontal portion of the jaw that holds the lower teeth intact. At the junction between the two bodies of the mandible is the *mental protuberance*, which is the very front midline of the jaw and can be felt when palpating in a transverse direction.

The Posterior Structures (See Fig. 5-1) The *occipital bone* is located at the inferior and posterior part of the skull, which is the back of the head. In the center of the occipital bone is a bump at the midline known as the *external occipital protuberance*, or inion. The *superior nuchal lines* are located laterally in either direction from the external occipital protuberance. These lines run horizontally and should be palpated vertically. They are the insertion points for the upper trapezius and the splenius capitis.

Located at the side of the head, the *temporal bone* encompasses the ear; it is the weakest bone of the skull. The *mastoid process* is located on the temporal bone and is the large, fairly prominent bump behind the ear. It is the insertion point for the sternocleidomastoid muscle (SCM). On the top of the skull, the *sagittal suture* runs between the parietal bones. It is oriented in a vertical direction, so it should be palpated in a transverse direction. The last bony landmark of the skull is the *coronal suture,* which is located between the frontal and parietal bones. It runs in a horizontal direction, so it must be palpated in a vertical direction. The intersection of the two sutures forms the frontal fontanel in an infant.

Soft Tissue Structures of the Head and Face

To ensure the most effective treatment of the area possible, it is necessary to know the location of some important soft tissue structures (Fig. 5-2).

The *glabella* is located on the midfrontal bone; it is the area of skin between the eyebrows. Find the *superficial temporal artery/pulse* by moving under the eye along the orbit and tracing the zygomatic arch to just in front of the ear. Move just superior to the arch, and use light pressure since the artery is very superficial.

Move inferiorly from the arch to locate the *parotid gland,* a salivary gland located superficially over the posterior portion of the masseter muscle; it envelops the angle of the mandible. Palpate over the angle in a circular motion with the fingertips; the gland should feel like a small cluster of nodules. The duct for the parotid gland, the *parotid duct*, runs horizontally from the gland into the mouth. To find it, locate the anterior border of the masseter muscle by having the client clench his or her teeth. Palpate just below the zygomatic arch at the anterior border of the masseter in an up-and-down fashion; the duct should feel like a small tube running horizontally.

The *submandibular gland* is a salivary gland located up and under the mandible. It sits about halfway between the angle of the mandible and the mental protuberance, and it feels like a round nodule. Have the client press his or her tongue to the roof of the mouth to make the gland more prominent. The *submandibular lymph nodes* are located in the same area as the submandibular salivary gland. They are smaller and rounded and are responsible for draining the forehead and anterior face region, as well as the lateral upper lip and chin.

The *facial artery/pulse* lies on the body of the mandible at the anterior border of the masseter muscle. Locate the anterior border of the masseter by having the client bite down. At the most anterior border of the muscle, trace down to the body of the mandible and palpate using very light pressure while feeling for a pulse. Trace the body of the mandible distally to the chin at the mental protuberance to find the *submental lymph nodes* up and under the jaw; these drain the central portion of the lower lip and chin.

Figure 5-2 Soft tissue structures of the head and face.

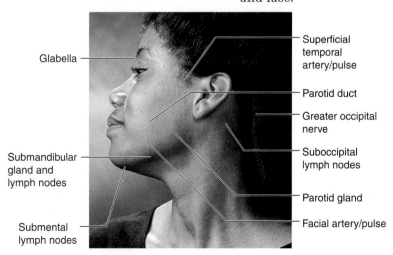

Glabella

Submandibular gland and lymph nodes

Submental lymph nodes

Superficial temporal artery/pulse

Parotid duct

Greater occipital nerve

Suboccipital lymph nodes

Parotid gland

Facial artery/pulse

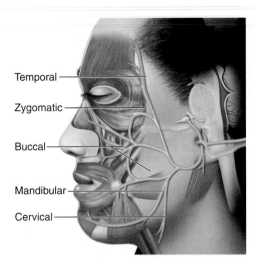

Temporal
Zygomatic
Buccal
Mandibular
Cervical

Figure 5-3 The branches of the facial nerve.

The *facial nerve* is responsible for the face and neck (Fig. 5-3). To identify its branches, stand behind the client and place an open hand on the side of his or her face so that the ear is under your palm. Place your thumb and fingers as described below to locate the branches:

- *Temporal branch:* Thumb just above the orbit of the eye
- *Zygomatic branch:* Index finger over the zygomatic arch
- *Buccal branch:* Middle finger between the nose and the upper lip
- *Mandibular branch:* Ring finger under the bottom lip above the chin
- *Cervical branch:* Little finger down and anterior across the neck

There are numerous structures relative to the ear (Fig. 5-4):

- *Auricle:* The cartilaginous outer portion of the ear
- *Helix:* The outer ring of the auricle
- *Antihelix:* The inner smaller ring of the auricle running parallel to the helix
- *Triangular fossa:* An anterior/superior fossa dividing the helix and antihelix
- *External auditory meatus:* The external opening of the ear canal
- *Tragus:* A posterior-facing projection that partially covers the external auditory meatus
- *Antitragus:* The projection that sits opposite and inferior to the tragus
- *Lobule:* The earlobe

Located just in front of the ear canal and just behind the ears, the *pre- and postauricular lymph nodes* are very small and difficult to palpate. Use

Figure 5-4 The surface anatomy structures of the ear.

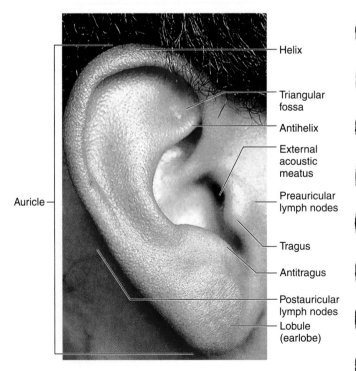

Auricle

Helix
Triangular fossa
Antihelix
External acoustic meatus
Preauricular lymph nodes
Tragus
Antitragus
Postauricular lymph nodes
Lobule (earlobe)

very light pressure in a circular fashion to find them, keeping in mind that they are often not palpated in healthy individuals.

On the posterior head (see Fig. 5-2), the *suboccipital lymph nodes* are located at the base of the occiput on either side. They are posterior to the mastoid process but not all the way to the midline. Have the client tuck his or her chin slightly to help in locating them.

Lastly, the *greater occipital nerve* is located at the midpoint between the mastoid process and the external occipital protuberance along the occiput. This nerve runs vertically, so it should be palpated in a transverse direction. It is easiest to locate while the client is in the prone position with relaxed muscles, but it can also be located with the client in the sitting position.

Bony Structures of the Cervical Spine

The cervical spine comprises seven vertebrae, which are interlocked and shaped to allow a generous range of motion; however, the region is also vulnerable to injury. The cervical spine is divided into two parts:

- *Upper:* The occiput and the first two vertebrae
- *Lower:* The 3rd through 7th vertebrae

A secondary lordotic curve develops as we grow and the spine begins compensating for the weight of the head and bipedal locomotion. How the head sits on the cervical spine is similar to how a basketball balances on a broomstick. Each vertebra has similar features and is divided into anterior and posterior portions.

Anterior Vertebra Components

- *Body:* Supports the weight of the vertebra above it, except for C1, and provides an attachment point for the disks
- *Intervertebral disks:* Consist of concentric rings of fibrous connective tissue (annulus fibrosis) and a gel-like substance (nucleus pulposis) in the center of the disk. This gel provides cushioning and shock absorption and shifts depending on the force placed on the spine

The disks in the cervical region make up 25% of the height of the cervical spine, and they are wedge-shaped to help facilitate the normal lordotic curve in the area.

Posterior Vertebra Components

- *Spinous process:* Allows various muscle and ligament attachments
- *Two transverse processes connected by arches:* Allow various muscle and ligament attachments while the arches define the borders of the vertebral foramen, giving the spinal cord a protective column in which to rest
- *Two pairs of facet joints (superior and inferior):* Enable mobility
- *Vertebral foramen:* Allows passage of the spinal cord

The vertebrae are locked into one another through two sets of facet joints, one on the superior surface and one on the inferior surface. These joints enable mobility, rather than weight bearing. When the facets articulate with one another, they create a space known as the *intervertebral foramen,* which allows for the exit of the cervical spinal nerves.

Table 5-4 lists the cervical spinal nerves.

Table 5-4 Cervical Spinal Nerves

Level	Innervation
C1	None
C2	Longus coli, sternocleidomastoid, rectus capitis
C3	Trapezius, splenius capitis
C4	Trapezius, levator scapulae
C5	Supraspinatus, infraspinatus, deltoid, biceps
C6	Biceps, supinator, wrist extensors
C7	Triceps, wrist flexors
C8	Ulnar deviators, thumb extensors, thumb adductors

The following ligaments add stability to the vertebral column:

- *Anterior longitudinal ligament (ALL):* Prevents excessive extension of the spine and increases its thickness as it moves from the cervical to the lumbar region
- *Posterior longitudinal ligament (PLL):* Prevents excessive flexion of the spine and decreases its thickness as it moves into the lumbar region
- *Supraspinous ligament:* Connects the spinous processes of the vertebrae to prevent excessive flexion

In the cervical spine, there are two atypical vertebrae, neither of which has disks, that have special names (Fig. 5-5). The 1st cervical vertebra (C1) is known as "the atlas," after the Greek god Atlas, who held the weight of the world on his shoulders. C1 is little more than a bony ring, lacking both transverse and spinous processes. On each side is a lateral mass, which forms the superior articular facet and acts like a "washer" as it articulates with the occipital bone of the skull at the occipital condyles. C1 also does not have a true body. Its body is actually formed by the 2nd cervical vertebra (C2), known as "the axis" (named for the odontoid process); it forms the body of C1 when the two come together. The process is held in place by a transverse ligament, and it is this process that enables rotation of the head.

Collectively, the cervical vertebrae are unique because each has a distinct tunnel known as the *transverse foramen* in each transverse process. This foramen allows a protective passageway for the vertebral arteries that supply blood to the brain.

Bony Landmarks and Surface Anatomy

Many therapists are hesitant to work on the anterior neck because of its delicate structures; however, understanding the structures and how to palpate them should help alleviate this fear.

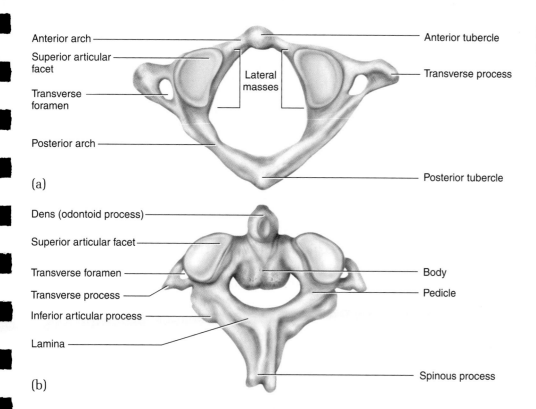

Anterior arch

Superior articular facet

Transverse foramen

Posterior arch

Lateral masses

Anterior tubercle

Transverse process

Posterior tubercle

(a)

Dens (odontoid process)

Superior articular facet

Transverse foramen

Transverse process

Inferior articular process

Lamina

Body

Pedicle

Spinous process

(b)

Figure 5-5 The 1st and 2nd vertebrae of the cervical spine. *(a)* Atlas. *(b)* Axis.

Depending on one's body type, the *posterior tubercle of C1* (see Fig. 5-5) is usually too small to palpate; however, it lies midline directly inferior to the external occipital protuberance in the soft tissue space. This is palpated easier in the supine position, which facilitates the relaxation of the neck musculature and allows you to passively flex and extend the client's head. From the posterior neck, the *C1 transverse process* is located by picking a point midway between the angle of the mandible and the mastoid process. Very gently palpate behind the ear, anterior to the SCM, looking for a bony prominence. You may laterally flex the client's neck passively to help with palpation. The *C1 posterior arch* is located between the tubercle and the transverse process. To find the location, move laterally from the posterior tubercle on either side; the arch is halfway between the tubercle and the mastoid processes lateral to the paraspinal musculature. The arch, which is palpated easier in the supine position, is the bony landmark for the greater occipital nerve and lymph nodes.

The *C2 spinous process* is usually the first palpable spinous process and is directly inferior from the external occipital protuberance; it is almost always bifurcated. It is the largest and longest spinous process in the cervical region until C7. From the C2 spinous process, the *C2 cervical facet joints* are found by moving out lateral to the paraspinal musculature. This is the superior facet of C2. To find the C2 and C3 joints, move inferiorly less than a finger's width. Use caution, as this is typically a tender area.

The *C7 spinous process* is also known as the *vertebral prominens;* it is the most prominent and easiest cervical vertebra to palpate. To distinguish between C7 and C6 or T1, locate what you think is the C7 spinous process. Have the client extend his or her neck to see whether it disappears. If the spinous process disappears, move down and repeat the movement until finding one that does not disappear; this is C7. If the starting spinous process does not disappear, move up until finding one that does. The last spinous process before the one that disappeared is C7.

Chapter 5 Conditions of the Head and Neck

103

At the front of the neck, the *hyoid bone* lies under the chin above the voice box. Place your thumb and first finger on either side of the anterior neck just below the mandible and above the trachea. Gently squeeze, and move your thumb and finger back and forth to feel the bone move. Once you think you have it, have the client swallow to feel it elevate. It lies at the level of C3 and can be used as a landmark for that vertebra.

Soft Tissue Structures of the Cervical Spine

Known as the "Adam's apple," the *thyroid cartilage* lies on the anterior neck just below the hyoid bone; it is at the C4-C5 level. It should be midline and can be gently moved from side to side using the fingers. Figure 5-6 shows the soft tissue structures of the cervical spine.

The *1st cricoid ring* lies below the thyroid cartilage at C6 anteriorly. Using the thyroid cartilage as a starting point, move inferiorly until finding an indentation. The next structure down is the cricoid ring, followed by the rest of the trachea.

Using the 1st cricoid ring, move lateral to the trachea but stay medial to the sternocleidomastoid muscle. Palpate posteriorly until you feel a bony prominence. This is the *anterior tubercle of the C6 transverse process*, just anterior to the C6 nerve root exit. The structure is in a delicate area, so use caution. Pathology or pressure in this area may reproduce radicular symptoms in the upper extremity, or what is termed a "positive doorbell sign"; that is, by pressing on the nerve (the buzzer), you reproduce the symptoms (ring the doorbell).

The *posterior cervical triangle* is bound by three structures:

- *Anteriorly:* Sternocleidomastoid muscle
- *Posteriorly:* Upper trapezius
- *Inferiorly:* Near the clavicle

There are several structures within this triangle. The 1st rib makes up a bony portion of the floor where the scalenes are also located. The *brachial plexus* (Fig. 5-7) emerges from the cervical spine in this region as it passes into the shoulder and arm. It consists of the nerve roots of C5 through T1.

Figure 5-6 Soft tissue structures of the cervical spine.

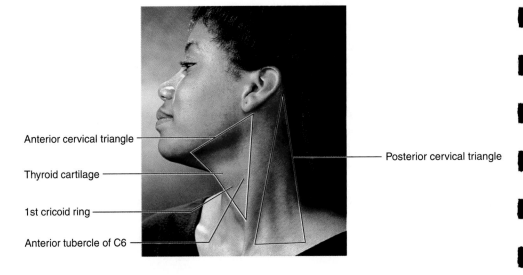

Anterior cervical triangle

Thyroid cartilage

1st cricoid ring

Anterior tubercle of C6

Posterior cervical triangle

Part II Regional Approach to Treatment

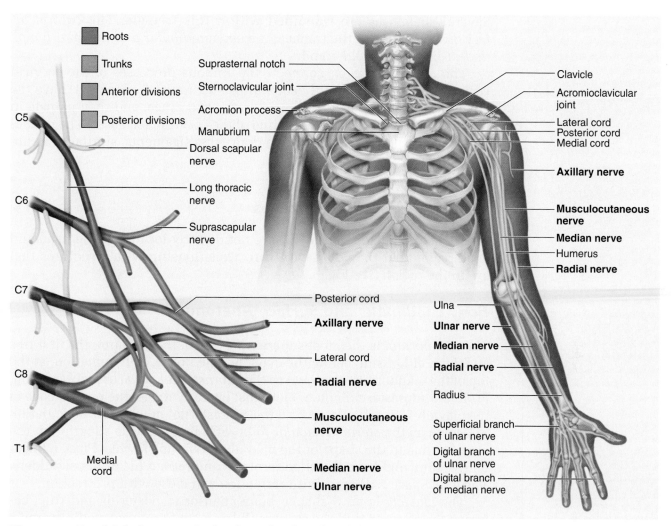

Figure 5-7 Brachial plexus and other bony landmarks of the neck and upper shoulder.

The brachial plexus starts as separate nerves as it leaves the foramen and then converges into three trunks: The upper trunk is formed by C5 and C6; the middle trunk consists of C7; and the lower trunk consists of C8 and T1. As the plexus continues distally, it splits into anterior and posterior divisions. The posterior divisions branch off to form the posterior cord, while the anterior divisions of the upper and middle trunks form the lateral cord. The anterior division of the lower trunk creates the medial cord, which branches to form the nerves that enter the arm. The posterior cord branches into the radial and axillary nerves; the lateral half of the medial cord converges with the medial half of the lateral cord to form the median nerve; and the rest of the medial cord becomes the ulnar nerve. The remaining part of the lateral cord becomes the musculocutaneous nerve. There are minor branches off the plexus at different levels that innervate surrounding structures.

The *anterior cervical triangle* is another general region of the neck. This triangle is bound by three structures:

- *Anteriorly:* Midline of the neck
- *Superiorly:* Inferior border of the body of the mandible
- *Posteriorly:* Sternocleidomastoid muscle

Several structures are contained within this triangle: The *carotid artery* on either side of the trachea; the *submandibular and tonsillar lymph nodes;* and the thyroid gland.

The *nuchal ligament* connects the spinous processes of the cervical vertebrae with the external occipital protuberance. To locate it, have the client flex his or her head and neck to the end range, and then palpate in a transverse direction at the midline of the cervical vertebrae. The nuchal ligament should feel more flexible than other ligaments, similar to a rubber cord.

Associated Bony Structures

The structures discussed below are not directly located in the head and neck region, but they do have a direct relationship with structures that are in the region (see Fig. 5-7).

Bony Landmarks and Surface Anatomy

The *manubrium* is the most superior portion of the sternum; the first ribs attach on either side below the clavicle. The notch, or indentation, at the top of the manubrium is known as the *suprasternal notch* or jugular notch. From the suprasternal notch, move just laterally to feel the medial edge of the clavicle as it articulates with the suprasternal notch. This articulation is known as the *sternoclavicular joint (SC)*. It sits a little superior on the sternum due to the shape of the medial end of the clavicle. Place a finger on the joint, and have the client protract and retract his or her shoulders. The joint space will open with retraction and close with protraction.

The *clavicle* is an S-shaped bone anterior to posterior and runs between the sternum and the scapula. It has a convex curve medially and a concave curve laterally. The lateral end is larger and flatter; it forms a joint with the acromion process of the scapula called the *acromioclavicular joint (AC)*. This can be a difficult structure to find on some people. Trace the clavicle to its lateral edge. You should feel a space where it meets the acromion process. You can also locate this joint by finding the acromion process and working medially until finding a "step" up to the clavicle. The space before the step is the joint. Have the client protract and retract his or her shoulders to feel the joint open and close.

The *acromion process* is the L-shaped lateral end of the spine of the scapula. It is flat and forms the acromioclavicular joint with the clavicle. To palpate, place the palm of your hand on the lateral tip of the shoulder and move it in a circular fashion. You will feel a flat, bony surface and can use your fingertips to trace the borders. If you are uncertain, have the client move his or her shoulder. If you are on the process, it should not move. If it moves, you are probably on the AC joint or the head of the humerus.

Muscles of the Head and Neck

These muscles either are directly part of the head and neck or have an attachment there (Fig. 5-8). Refer to the Quick Reference Table "Muscles of the Head and Neck" at the end of this chapter.

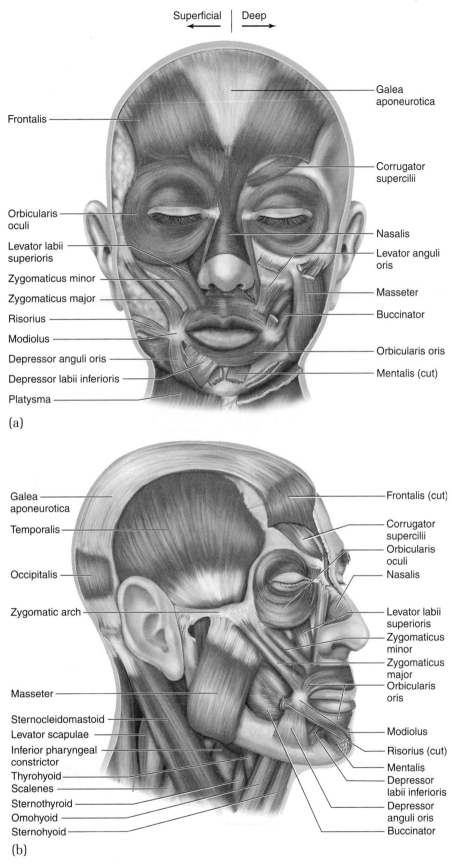

Superficial | Deep

Galea aponeurotica

Frontalis

Corrugator supercilii

Orbicularis oculi

Nasalis

Levator labii superioris

Levator anguli oris

Zygomaticus minor

Masseter

Zygomaticus major

Buccinator

Risorius

Modiolus

Orbicularis oris

Depressor anguli oris

Mentalis (cut)

Depressor labii inferioris

Platysma

(a)

Galea aponeurotica

Frontalis (cut)

Temporalis

Corrugator supercilii

Orbicularis oculi

Occipitalis

Nasalis

Zygomatic arch

Levator labii superioris

Zygomaticus minor

Zygomaticus major

Orbicularis oris

Masseter

Modiolus

Sternocleidomastoid

Risorius (cut)

Levator scapulae

Mentalis

Inferior pharyngeal constrictor

Depressor labii inferioris

Thyrohyoid

Scalenes

Depressor anguli oris

Sternothyroid

Omohyoid

Buccinator

Sternohyoid

(b)

Figure 5-8 Muscles of the head and neck.
(a) Anterior view. *(b)* Lateral view. *(continued)*

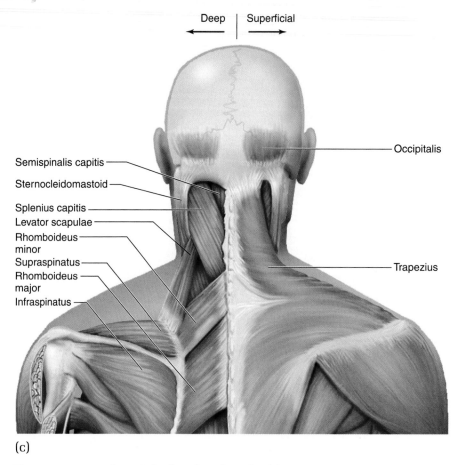

Deep | Superficial

Semispinalis capitis

Sternocleidomastoid

Splenius capitis

Levator scapulae

Rhomboideus minor

Supraspinatus

Rhomboideus major

Infraspinatus

Occipitalis

Trapezius

(c)

Figure 5-8 Muscles of the head and neck. *(c)* Posterior view

MOVEMENTS AND MANUAL MUSCLE TESTING OF THE REGION

There are some general assessment tools that can help therapists establish a baseline for more specific assessments regardless of the dysfunction.

Movements of the Region

The cervical spine has six basic movements:

- Flexion
- Extension
- Left and right lateral flexion
- Left and right rotation

When you are looking at normal ranges of motion, it is a good idea to assess both passive and active movements. They are typically within a few degrees of each other, but comparing the two can be a valuable tool for determining the tissues involved in the restrictions. The client is tested in the seated or standing position, and the normal ranges of motion for the neck are as follows:

- *Flexion:* Have the client bring the chin to the chest; the average range is 80°.
- *Extension:* Have the client look up at the ceiling; the average range is 70°.
- *Left and right lateral flexion:* Have the client bring the ear to the shoulder; the average range is 45°.
- *Left and right rotation:* Have the client look over the shoulder; the average range is 80°.

The temporomandibular joint (TMJ) is unique. When the mouth opens, the mandible moves down and forward. TMJ movements are listed below, along with the normal range of movement for each:

- *Depression:* Opening the mouth—40 millimeters (mm)
- *Elevation:* Closing the mouth from depression until the teeth meet
- *Protrusion:* Jutting the jaw forward—4 mm
- *Retrusion:* Pulling the jaw backward—3 mm
- *Lateral deviation:* Moving the jaw side to side—12 mm

Manual Muscle Testing for the Region

The client stays seated for all manual muscle tests. Figure 5-9 shows how the following tests should be performed:

- *Neck flexion:* Stand at the client's side, and place one hand around C7 to T1 to support the trunk. Place the other hand on the forehead of the client. Press into the forehead while the client resists the movement.
- *Extension:* Stand at the client's side, and place one hand at the top of the sternum to support the trunk. Place the other hand on the occipital bone of the client. Press into the back of the head while the client resists the movement.
- *Lateral flexion:* Stand behind the client, and place your hand on the shoulder of the opposite side that you are testing to support it. Place your other hand on the side of the head that you are testing. Press into the side of the head while the client resists the movement. Repeat for the opposite side.
- *Rotation:* Stand in front of the client, and place both hands on the client's head, one on each side of the face. Rotate the head in one direction while your client resists the movement. Repeat for the other side.

> **Practical Tip**
> Make sure to apply an eccentric load to produce an isometric contraction when testing muscle strength.

There are additional manual muscle tests that will help indicate whether a specific nerve root is experiencing dysfunction. These tests to the myotomes evaluate the dorsal (motor) nerve root and are performed having the client resist the movement:

- *C1-C2:* With the client seated, have the client slightly flex his or her neck. Stand to the side of the client, and place one hand between the scapulas to stabilize the trunk. Press into the forehead while the client resists the movement.
- *C3:* Stand behind the client, and place one hand on the shoulder opposite the side of the neck being tested to stabilize it. Place the other hand on the side of the client's head, and have him or her resist lateral flexion.

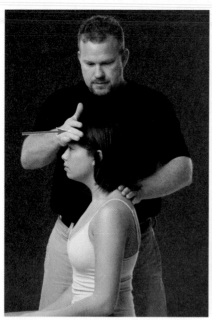

(a)

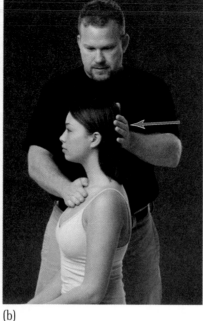

(b)

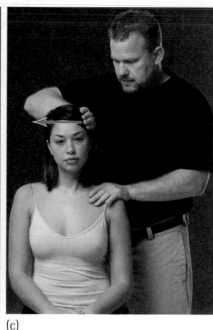

(c)

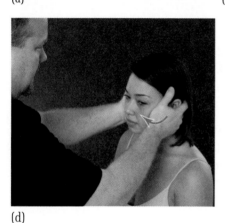

(d)

Figure 5-9 Manual muscle tests for the neck.
(a) Flexion.
(b) Extension.
(c) Lateral flexion.
(d) Rotation.

- *C4:* Stand in front of the client, and have him or her shrug the shoulders. Place your hands on the shoulders, and have the client resist your attempt to depress the shoulders.
- *C5:* Abduct the client's arms to about 70°. Place your hands on the middle of the client's arms, and apply a downward force while he or she resists.
- *C6 and C7:* Standing in front of the client, have the client put his or her arms at the side and flex the elbows to 90°. For C6, supinate the forearm, and place your hands on the client's wrists. Have the client resist downward pressure to test the elbow and forearm flexors. For C7, pronate the forearm. Place your hands under the client's forearm, and have the client resist an upward force to test the elbow extensors; move your hands to the dorsal wrist, and have the client resist a downward force to test the wrist extensors.
- *C8:* Have the client extend the thumb to its end range. Have the client resist as you move his or her thumb into flexion.
- *T1:* Have your client spread his or her fingers and resist while you adduct them.

DERMATOMES FOR THE HEAD AND NECK

Just as there is weakness associated with dysfunction in the motor nerve root, there are sensory changes with dysfunction in the sensory nerve root. These sensations can differ from person to person. Figure 5-10 shows the dermatomes of the area, which are listed below:

- *C1-C2:* Top of the head
- *C2:* Back of the head, temple, and forehead
- *C3:* Entire neck and posterior cheek
- *C4:* Shoulder area and upper clavicle
- *C5:* Deltoid area, radial side of the humerus, and forearm to the thumb
- *C6:* Anterior arm, radial side of the hand to the thumb, and lateral index finger
- *C7:* Lateral arm and forearm, lateral index finger, entire long and ring fingers
- *C8:* Medial arm and forearm, ulnar side of the hand, and last two fingers
- *T1:* Ulnar side of the forearm

TRIGGER-POINT REFERRAL PATTERNS FOR MUSCLES OF THE REGION

Trigger points in the head and neck region have been the source of many misdiagnosed conditions. They are prevalent in all parts of the body and can arise from chronic postural issues, poor body mechanics during activity, repetitive motion syndromes, and acute trauma to the area. There

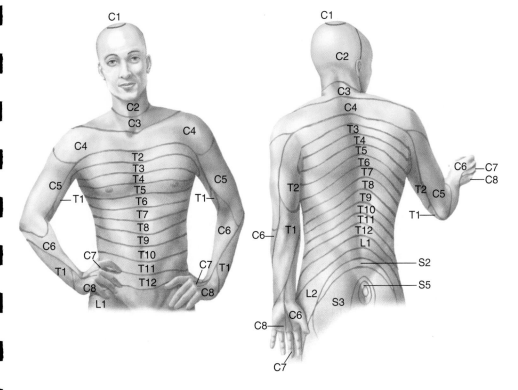

Figure 5-10 Dermatomes of the cervical region.

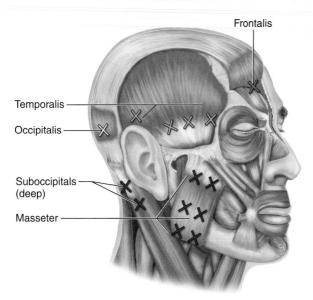

Figure 5-11 Trigger-point locations for the temporalis, frontalis, occipitalis, suboccipitals, and masseter.

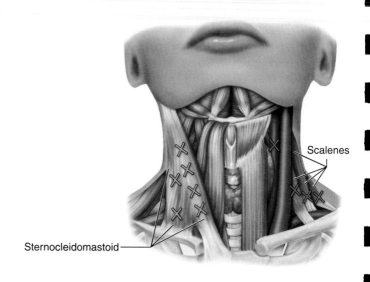

Figure 5-12 Trigger-point locations for the sternocleidomastoid, and scalenes.

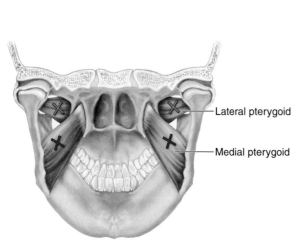

Figure 5-13 Trigger-point locations for the medial and lateral pterygoids.

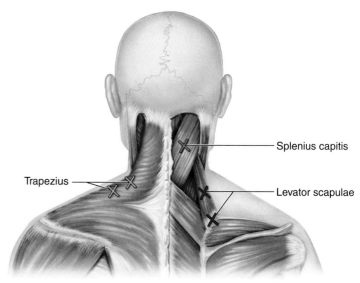

Figure 5-14 Trigger-point locations for the trapezius, splenius capitis, and levator scapulae.

are many common active-trigger-point locations for several muscles in the head and neck, all of which have referral patterns and symptoms.

The *frontalis* (see Figs. 5-11 and 5-18) has an active trigger point just superior to the eye and refers pain up and over the forehead on the same side. Its antagonist partner, the occipitalis, has an active trigger point in the belly of the muscle at the back of the head. It refers pain diffusely over the back of the head and deep into the orbit. While the chief symptom for both of these muscles is pain, people with trigger points in the occipitalis typically complain that they cannot bear the weight of the back of their head on a pillow and must lie on their side.

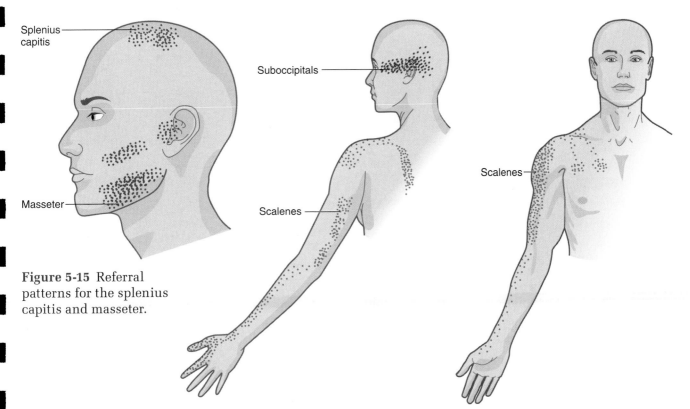

Figure 5-15 Referral patterns for the splenius capitis and masseter.

Figure 5-16 Referral patterns for the suboccipitals and the posterior pattern for the scalenes.

Figure 5-17 Referral patterns for the anterior pattern for the scalenes.

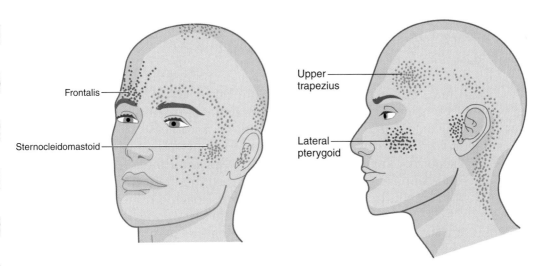

Figure 5-18 Referral patterns for the frontalis and sternocleidomastoid.

Figure 5-19 Referral patterns for the upper trapezius and lateral pterygoid.

The *temporalis* (see Figs. 5-11 and 5-20) is located in the temporal fossa above the ear but can refer pain into the eyebrow, upper teeth, temple, and temporomandibular joint (TMJ). There are four active trigger points in the temporalis. The first lies in the anterior portion of the muscle above and in front of the ear. The second and third are in the middle of the muscle; the fourth is toward the posterior aspect of the muscle. Based on their locations, they will have different referral patterns. The chief symptom

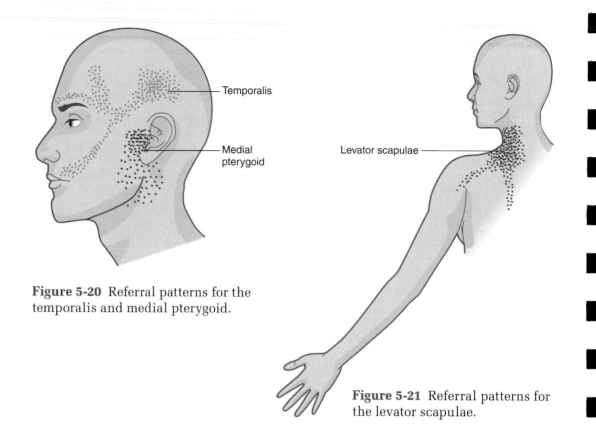

Figure 5-20 Referral patterns for the temporalis and medial pterygoid.

Figure 5-21 Referral patterns for the levator scapulae.

of temporalis trigger points is head pain in different locations; they are commonly involved in TMJ disorders.

The *masseter* shares its function with the temporalis but has a different pain presentation. (See Figs. 5-11 and 5-15.) Clients with masseter trigger points can have problems with their TMJ as well as restricted jaw movement and unilateral tinnitus. Trigger points in the superficial layer of the muscle can be in three different locations. The points in the musculotendinous junction refer to the upper molars and maxilla. The midbelly points refer to the lower molars and the mandible. The lowest points at the angle refer to the mandible and up and over the eyebrow. The deep layer has only one point, which refers to the anterior ear.

On the opposite side of the mandible are the *medial and lateral pterygoids*. The medial pterygoid trigger point is located midbelly of the muscle and refers to the ear, the back of the mouth, and the TMJ. Chewing, opening the mouth too wide, and clenching the teeth exacerbate the pain caused by this muscle. The lateral pterygoid is more difficult to access; its trigger point lies on the muscle adjacent to the medial surface of the coronoid process. (See Fig. 5-13.) It is strongly associated with TMJ dysfunction and refers deep into the joint and the maxillary sinus. Intraoral palpation is more effective with this muscle, but access to the muscle is limited (see Figs. 5-13, 5-19, and 5-20).

Down the anterior neck is the *sternocleidomastoid (SCM)*, shown in Figs. 5-12 and 5-18. This muscle has two heads, and trigger points can develop in both. Surprisingly, there is no neck pain or stiffness associated with these trigger points. The sternal head has several points and can refer downward into the upper sternum or across and up into the cheek, maxilla, occipital ridge, and top of the head. The clavicular head also has several points and refers to the frontal bone and deep into the ear.

Medial to the SCM are the *scalenes,* as seen in Figs. 5-12, 5-16, and 5-17. They reside in the posterior triangle and are a common source of scapular, shoulder, back, and arm pain. Each of the three muscles develops trigger points. The anterior scalene refers pain to the upper border of the scapula and the posterior shoulder, as well as down the front and back of the arm to the radial side of the forearm, thumb, and index finger in conjunction with the medial scalene. The posterior scalene can refer pain into the anterior chest, and if the trigger point is activated on the left side, the pain referral can be mistaken for a heart attack.

The *supra- and infrahyoid* muscles also have myriad referral patterns. Complaints range from difficulty swallowing or the feeling of something stuck in the throat to referred pain to the lower teeth or up the SCM.

Moving around to the posterior head and neck, the *suboccipital* muscles are the deepest muscles at the base of the skull (see Figs. 5-11 and 5-16). Their referral pattern is more general than the patterns of most trigger points and can be a source of frustration for clients. Because of their size and location, these muscles rarely develop trigger points without the involvement of other larger cervical muscles.

Splenius capitis trigger points (see Figs. 5-14 and 5-15) limit neck range of motion and cause pain in the area. They can also cause pain behind the eye, and splenius capitis refers pain to the top of the head.

The *levator scapula* is a unique muscle because of its spiral twist that moves from the scapula to the neck. It has two main trigger points (see Figs. 5-14 and 5-21), one at the superior angle of the scapula and one about halfway up the muscle. Typical symptoms include pain and stiffness in the neck, with limited range of motion; The trigger points refer into the angle of the neck and posterior shoulder.

The *trapezius* (see Figs. 5-14 and 5-19) is the muscle most often affected by trigger points. There are two points in the upper fibers at approximately the same level, one anterior and one posterior. The anterior point refers behind, up, and over the ear in a ram's horn pattern, while the posterior point refers up the back of the neck to the area behind the ear. Both of these points are major contributors to tension headaches. Refer to the Quick Reference Table "Trigger Points for the Head and Neck Muscles" at the end of this chapter (page 153).

SPECIFIC CONDITIONS

When it comes to the head and neck, the same structures can be involved in more than one condition; thus, treatment overlaps may occur. The structures involved will vary from person to person and with the severity of the condition. The area of involvement may be localized or large and move into other regions, depending on how long the client has had the condition.

Whiplash

Background

"Whiplash injuries, although not associated with a high fatality rate, present a risk for permanent disability and are a significant cost to society"

(Winkelstein et al., 2000). Approximately 4 in every 1000 people suffer from whiplash injuries. Between the cost of treatment, lost work time and productivity, chronic pain issues, and psychological concerns, the total financial impact on society can be in the billions.

Whiplash, or hyperextension-hyperflexion injury, seems to be a common traumatic injury to the soft tissue structures around the cervical spine (Childs, 2004). Physician Harold Crowe first introduced the term *whiplash* in 1928 to describe a neck injury caused by a motor vehicle crash; however, when the term first appeared in the medical literature in 1945, the condition was not based on scientific evidence.

Any therapist who has treated a client with whiplash knows how complicated it can be. In fact, whiplash has been such an enigma that a task force called the Quebec Task Force on Whiplash-Associated Disorders (WAD) was created in 1995 in Canada to develop a grading scale for whiplash-related disorders. The grading system consists of a scale from 0 to IV:

- *Grade 0:* No complaints about the neck and no physical signs
- *Grade I:* A complaint of pain or tenderness and stiffness but no physical signs
- *Grade II:* A neck complaint with physical signs that is musculoskeletal in nature (point tenderness and loss of range of motion)
- *Grade III:* Symptoms of grade II plus neurologic involvement such as decreased reflexes, weakness, and sensory deficits
- *Grade IV:* Neck complaints accompanied by a fracture or dislocation of the vertebra; the most serious grade

The most common classifications among clients are grade I and grade II, which make up 80% of whiplash injury claims (Ferrari, 2003). While motor vehicle collisions are the most common mechanism, there are numerous other types of trauma that can cause whiplash. Falls that cause axial loading (landing on the head), sports collisions, and even a push from behind can cause whiplash. The involvement of several structures has been identified in relation to whiplash, but the involvement of the cervical facet joints has been supported by numerous clinical observations. Both mechanoreceptors and nociceptors play a part in the facet capsule and are involved in pain sensation and proprioception through neural input from the facets (Winkelstein et al., 2000).

There are two common classifications of whiplash: acute and chronic. While the majority of people will recover within a few weeks or months, it is estimated that between 12% and 40% will go on to have persistent problems (Treleaven et al., 2003). Both acute whiplash and chronic whiplash cause several common symptoms:

Acute Phase (symptoms usually develop within the first 24 hours)
- Headache
- Neck pain
- Stiffness
- Interscapular pain
- Arm and hand paresthesia
- Dizziness
- TMJ symptoms
- Emotional and psychological disturbances

Chronic Phase
- Pain (most prevalent symptom)
- Increased TMJ complaints

whiplash
An acceleration-deceleration mechanism of energy transfer to the neck resulting in a hyperextension-hyperflexion injury.

- Loss of neck mobility
- Increased muscle tension
- Increased neurologic symptoms such as sensory disturbances, brachial plexus irritation, weakness, and radiculopathy

While the existence of acute whiplash, and the ability to diagnose it, seems universal, chronic whiplash-related disorders have been linked to psychosocial factors and the injured party's cultural background. Several studies have described a phenomenon termed an "expectation of symptoms" wherein society reinforces the anticipation, symptom amplification, and other behaviors that foster chronic pain (Virani, 2001). A 1996 study found that Lithuanians who had little or no knowledge of whiplash-related chronic pain did not have as high an incidence rate of whiplash-related injuries as Americans did, suggesting that knowledge and expectation play a key role in whiplash injuries.

A study in 2000 surveyed physicians and nonphysicians who had been in automobile accidents and received whiplash injuries. Of the respondents, 71% were physicians and 60% were nonphysicians. Only 31% of physicians compared to 46% of nonphysicians reported acute symptoms, and only 9% of physicians recalled chronic problems, whereas 32% of nonphysicians reported lasting symptoms.

Assessment

Throughout the assessment phase, it is important for therapists to consider their ability to treat the condition, taking care to refer clients to outside health care providers if treatment appears to be contraindicated.

Condition History Since whiplash can be multifactorial, taking a detailed history of the injury is critical in creating an appropriate treatment plan. In addition, there are some specific questions to ask in relation to whiplash. These questions can be modified to fit any mechanism of injury, whether it was a fall, sports collision, or automobile accident. Here are some questions that are relevant to automobile accidents:

Question	Significance
What was the vehicle's speed at the moment of impact, or was the vehicle stationary at the time of collision?	Helps determine the severity of the injury.
Were you aware of the impending collision?	Awareness causes a person to tense up, increasing injury severity.
Were you wearing a seat belt?	Gives indications of overall trauma.
Did you hit any other surfaces?	Indicates other possible areas of trauma.
What were your symptoms?	Helps determine if other structures are involved.
Were/are you intact from a neurovascular standpoint?	Helps determine severity and whether physician referral is warranted.
What was the size of the other vehicle or structure involved?	The bigger the vehicle/structure, the greater the force.
In what position was your head at the time of impact?	Helps isolate the muscles involved.

On which side were you hit?	Helps determine the mechanism.
What was your condition immediately after the collision?	Gives indication of severity.
Did you lose consciousness?	Gives indication of severity.

If the client indicates that he or she experienced any loss of consciousness or neurologic symptoms, ask for a physician's clearance prior to treating.

Visual Assessment After taking the condition history, the therapist should conduct a visual examination based on the observation criteria discussed earlier. Generally, the easiest and first observation includes noting the position of the neck, followed by observing the overall posture of the upper body. Next, observe the client during motion. Assess active range of motion first, followed by passive range of motion.

Practical Tip

It is best to observe the client when he or she is not aware of being watched, such as when the client is walking through your office.

Palpation The first step in palpation is to notice any obvious changes in the tissue, such as swelling, bruising, abrasions, or deformities. Palpate the structures in a systematic order, starting with the head and face; then palpate the structures that would be involved based on the mechanism of injury. Note areas of tenderness and the client's facial expressions during palpation.

Move on to the neck, and adjust pressure based on the severity of the injury and the client's pain level. Use the information obtained from the history to guide the treatment. Pay special attention to the structures on the side opposite that of impact; these structures are typically more involved due to the initial eccentric load placed on them. In many injuries, the side that experiences the most pain is not the side that is injured more.

Orthopedic Tests There are no specific orthopedic assessments for whiplash; however, tests are typically administered to rule out other conditions. This includes performing manual muscle testing, dermatome and myotome assessment, and other tests such as cervical compression and Spurling's test, both of which identify nerve involvement. Treatment is largely based on the mechanism, history, observations, and findings during palpation.

Soft Tissue Treatment

Treatment for whiplash will vary based on the severity of the injury and the stage of healing it is in. If the injury is in the acute phase, treatments such as rest and ice should be implemented to reduce discomfort and facilitate healing. Once the condition moves out of the acute phase (usually after 24 to 72 hours), active therapies tend to produce better results. The use of a soft collar to immobilize the neck can lead to additional problems; a collar should be used as a means of decreasing activity rather than preventing it. Determine which structures to treat based on the findings from the assessment. The treatment protocol should be modified to fit the situation.

Connective Tissue Many techniques are available for treating whiplash. The following are some approaches to treatment.

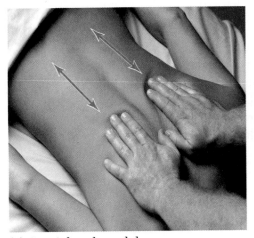 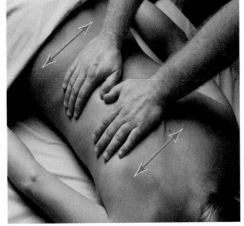

Figure 5-22 Assessment of superficial connective tissue. *(a)* Cranial and caudal. *(b)* Medial and lateral.

(a) Cranial and caudal

(b) Medial and lateral

Prone Position Start with the general assessment of the connective tissue from a cranial and caudal direction and a medial and lateral direction (Fig. 5-22). Move into the restriction, paying special attention to the tissue from the base of the skull through the upper trapezius. Change the angle to address the oblique restrictions as well. Once the superficial fascia has been released, move to the deeper tissues and address the restrictions in each muscle involved. Apply these techniques to the muscles that you have identified through your assessments.

This is a good position in which to unwind the upper trapezius: Squat down at the head of the table, facing the client. Hook into the muscle at the bend in the neck, and press up and then inferiorly as the hands come over the shoulder. This can also be done standing at the shoulder of the client and facing his or her head. Reach across to the opposite side; take hold of the muscle and "unwind" it using a pulling motion. Stripping out local restrictions to the upper trapezius works well in this position, starting at the bend of the neck and defining the anterior edge of the muscle, working laterally toward the acromion.

Supine Position Start superficially with the fascia of the neck and upper chest, assessing it and moving into any restrictions until they have released. Releasing the sternoclavicular joint by tracing the inferior and superior borders of the clavicle from medial to lateral and removing restrictions between the clavicle and 1st rib are beneficial in improving symptoms. This is the optimal position for working on the scalenes and sternocleidomastoid muscles.

To work the scalenes, cradle the head and work in the posterior cervical triangle from superior to inferior, tracing three lines medial to lateral, sinking in behind the clavicle toward the 1st rib. Incorporating rotation of the head, if tolerable, into and away from the restrictions increases this technique's effectiveness.

For the SCM, continue cradling the head, and grasp the muscle between your thumb and first finger. Rub the muscle back and forth, or hold pressure while rotating the client's head, if tolerable, to the opposite side within his or her comfort level.

Another technique that addresses both muscles is performed by standing at the head of the client at the side of the table. Using a loose back of the hand with your fingers pointing into the table, hook into the tissue just lateral to the trachea. Move the tissue in a posterior direction, conforming the back of your hand to the neck during the stroke.

The supra- and infrahyoids are also typically involved and can be difficult to access. To access the suprahyoids, find the hyoid and perform a stroke from the superior aspect of the bone up to the mandible. Repeat while moving laterally until reaching the angle of the mandible. For the infrahyoids, move the thyroid cartilage laterally, and use the other hand to perform a stroke from the hyoid bone to the sternum. Repeat this while moving laterally to the clavicular head of the SCM.

Addressing posterior structures from a supine position can be very effective. Pulling your hands up the back of the neck, using the weight of the head to apply the pressure, prevents you from using too much force.

Side-Lying Position In treating whiplash, the side-lying position can be useful for performing a broadening stroke to the upper trapezius. Standing at the front of the table facing the feet, put the heels of your hands on the upper trapezius; spread your hands apart and define the anterior border of the upper trapezius using the thumbs or fingertips. A nice depression stroke to the shoulder can be performed by standing behind the client at the shoulder, facing the head of the table. Use the same arm as the side of the table where you are standing, and place your forearm at the base of the skull. Use the other hand to help pull your forearm along the muscle, up and over the trapezius and deltoids, while you depress the shoulder girdle at the same time.

Tissue Inconsistencies As you free restrictions in the connective tissue, you will come across trigger points in the various muscles that you will need to release. On the basis of your assessments, address muscles that may be restricting movement or causing pain. Some of the common neck muscles involved in whiplash are:

- Suboccipitals
- Trapezius
- Sternocleidomastoid
- Scalenes
- Suprahyoids
- Infrahyoids
- Levator scapulae
- Splenius capitis

Other muscles may be involved depending on the severity of the injury.

Muscle Concerns

Muscle tension and adhesions can inhibit the healing process and must be addressed. After determining which muscles are involved, use the various strokes discussed in earlier chapters to treat these concerns. Since active therapies have been shown to produce the best results in rehabilitation, using strokes that incorporate movement is very effective.

Prone Position Stand at the head of the table, facing inferiorly to either side of the client's head. Using the loose fist of the same side where you are standing, start at the bend of the neck and lean on the client as you slide your fist laterally to the acromion, being careful not to slide over the bone. Brace your elbow in your hip if you need to apply more pressure.

Another stroke is applied by squatting at the head of the table and running your forearm up and over the bend in the neck. This is also an effective position for stripping out the upper trapezius using either of two methods:

1. Run your thumb or finger from the base of the skull out laterally.
2. Approach from the opposite side, and pull your fingers medially along the anterior border of the muscle from the acromion.

Supine Position The supine position is excellent for working on the anterior neck structures. An effective stroke is performed by cradling the head and rotating it to the opposite side. Using a loose fist, apply the stroke starting at the occipital ridge and working down to the acromion and back, staying toward the posterior aspect of the neck. Incorporating both active and passive movement with the strokes in this position is easy to do.

Side-Lying Position The entire upper trapezius is easily accessed in this position. Be careful not to apply too much downward pressure toward the table on the lateral side of the neck.

Stretching

Active Isolated Stretching is beneficial for whiplash, although any of the stretching methods mentioned earlier in the text can be used as well.

Neck Extensors Place the client in the seated position. Stretch the extensors of the neck, ensuring that the client is sitting up straight. Have the client tuck and retract the chin as close to the neck as possible and contract the neck flexors. Make sure the client keeps his or her mouth closed and exhales during the movement.

Once the client has moved through the entire range, provide a gentle assist in the same direction (Fig. 5-23). This stretch addresses the deep neck extensors. Repeat 10 to 15 times, using two sets if necessary.

Neck Flexors Place the client in the seated position. Place your hand just below C7 to stabilize the trunk, and have the client lean forward about 45°. Have the client engage the neck extensors by looking up toward the ceiling. When he or she reaches the end range of motion, assist in the same direction by pressing on the client's forehead with a slight traction component (Fig. 5-24). Perform 10 repetitions. This stretch concentrates deep and superficial flexors of the neck. In severe cases of injury, performing this stretch in the seated position is contraindicated and should be modified (this is discussed later).

Lateral Flexors of the Neck Stretching the lateral flexors of the neck, such as the scalenes, SCM, and splenius capitis, begins with the client in the seated position, sitting up straight. Stand on the opposite side from the one being stretched, and

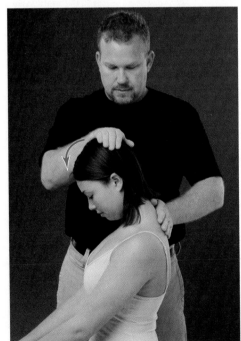

Figure 5-23 Neck extensor stretch.

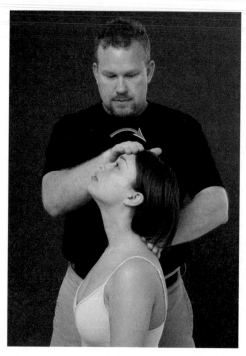

Figure 5-24 Neck flexor stretch.

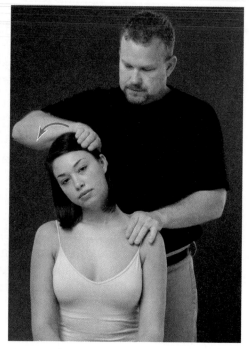

Figure 5-25 Stretching the lateral flexors of the neck.

place your hand on the shoulder of the side you are stretching to stabilize it. Have the client bring the ear to the shoulder, exhaling during the motion. At the end of the movement, provide a gentle assist in the same direction (Fig. 5-25). Perform one to two sets of 10 depending on the need.

Neck Rotators Rotation can be performed in the same position as that used for the previous stretches. This stretch targets the neck rotators. Stand at the client's side, on the side opposite the one being stretched. Place one hand on the ramus of the mandible on the side opposite the one where you are standing. Place the other hand behind the ear of the side where you are standing. Have the client turn the head toward you while exhaling. Once the client has reached the end range of motion, gently assist in the motion (Fig. 5-26). Have the client perform 10 repetitions.

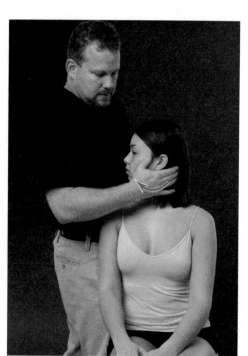

Figure 5-26 Stretching the rotators of the neck.

Posterior Neck, Oblique Aspect Stretch the posterior oblique muscles by having the client turn the head 45° to the same side you are stretching. Have the client exhale and bend the head down toward the opposite knee. Once he or she reaches the end range of motion, assist in the movement (Fig. 5-27). Support the client's opposite shoulder to prevent it from elevating. Have the client perform 10 repetitions.

Anterior Neck, Oblique Aspect Stretch the anterior muscles by having the client turn the head 45° to the side opposite the one being stretched. Have the client bend his or her head over the shoulder while exhaling. Gently assist the client at the end range of active motion (Fig. 5-28). These stretches can be

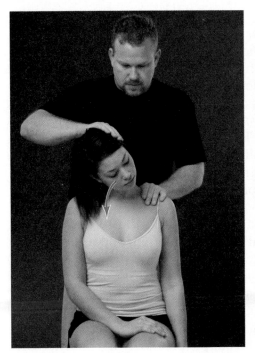

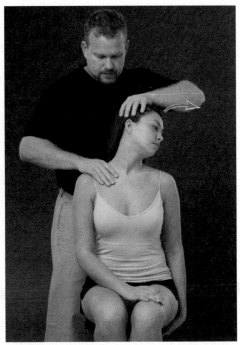

Figure 5-27 Stretching the posterior oblique aspect of the neck.

Figure 5-28 Stretching the anterior oblique aspect of the neck.

modified for postsurgical clients or for those suffering from disk involvement or severe whiplash.

Temporomandibular Joint Dysfunction

Background

The jaw forms important bilateral joints, the *temporomandibular joints (TMJs)*, between the condyloid process of the mandible and the mandibular fossa of the temporal bones. These synovial joints are two of the most frequently used joints and can be a source of dysfunction in the body. They combine the movements of a hinge, gliding, and condyloid joint. Movements include depression, elevation, protrusion, retrusion, and lateral and medial deviation. The TMJ is surrounded by a loose joint capsule and is separated into a superior and inferior chamber by an articular disk.

It is not surprising that problems with this joint affect millions of individuals in the United States, with the problems ranging from minor discomfort to disabling chronic pain (Gremillion, 2003). Although a large percentage of the general population displays signs of dysfunction, only 5% seek medical or dental treatment (Cleland and Palmer, 2004).

While anyone can develop TMJ dysfunction, it often affects women more than men. A study by Johansson et al. showed that "pain from the TMJ was almost twice as prevalent in women than in men" (2003). **Temporomandibular disorder (TMD)** is defined by the International Association for the Study of Pain as aching in the muscles of mastication, sometimes with occasional brief, severe pain on chewing, often associated with restricted jaw movement and clicking or popping sounds (Cleland and Palmer, 2004).

This disorder encompasses both the muscles and the joint. The muscle pain is a diffuse, dull pain in and around the jaw muscle area, while the

temporomandibular disorder (TMD)
An aching in the muscles of mastication, sometimes with occasional brief, severe pain on chewing, often associated with restricted jaw movement and clicking or popping sounds.

most common joint issue is internal derangement (Vazquez-Delgado et al., 2004). The derangement is a disorder in which the articular disk is in an abnormal position, resulting in restriction of normal mandibular function (Cleland and Palmer, 2004). This dysfunction can be described as "an achy, sharp pain, localized in the preauricular area, accompanied by clicking, crepitation, and catching or locking of the TMJ" (Vazquez-Delgado et al., 2004). The joint is formed by the condyle of the mandible and the mandibular fossa of the temporal bone. The presence of an articular disk on the condyle divides the joint into a superior and an inferior compartment. During normal motion, the disk will translate to accommodate the condyle, rotating up and down and gliding forward and backward. When there is dysfunction in the joint, the condyle is not seated correctly on the disk or can slip off the disk anteriorly or posteriorly. This can cause various clicking or popping sounds, limit the joint's range of motion, and cause the jaw to lock in an open or closed position.

Even with our technology in the new millennium, the etiology of TMD has been a very controversial issue and the knowledge of what causes it is still limited (Johansson et al., 2003). Contributing factors that seem to be consistent are bruxism (clenching the teeth), trauma, stress, malocclusion, and muscle imbalance. While the pain is primarily in the jaw, many patients have also reported a variety of related musculoskeletal problems, including neck and shoulder pain, upper- and lower-back pain, and tension headaches (DeBar et al., 2003).

Assessment

Because TMJ dysfunction can arise from trauma to other areas of the head and neck, therapists must always be prepared to expand the assessment to include these areas, keeping in mind potential contraindications. The most obvious contraindication includes neurologic involvement either from the joint itself or from associated trauma.

Condition History Here are some questions that are relevant to TMJ dysfunction:

Question	Significance
Do you experience pain when opening or closing your mouth?	Helps determine the involved structures.
	• Extra-articular pain, like muscle pain, is likely to be involved if there is pain while opening.
	• Intra-articular problems are indicated by pain while biting.
Do you experience pain while chewing?	Muscle imbalances can occur as a result of chewing on one side.
Does the client chew equally on both sides?	Muscle imbalances can occur as a result of chewing on one side.
What movements or actions cause pain?	If biting, yawning, chewing, swallowing, or speaking cause discomfort, determine exactly where it hurts.

Is there any clicking sound in the jaw?	If so, determine how many clicks and when they occur (on opening or closing, etc.).
Has your jaw ever locked?	Locking is a symptom of a displaced articular disk.
	• Locking in the open position: The disk has displaced posteriorly.
	• Locking in the closed position: The disk has moved anteriorly.
Do you grind your teeth?	If so, or if the client is missing any teeth, a muscle imbalance could develop because of the malocclusion. This could lead to TMD.

Visual Assessment Balance between the two TMJ joints is very important. Check the face for symmetry both horizontally and vertically. This can be a quick check for structural as well as neurologic involvement. Check for overbite, underbite, and malocclusion. Note whether the client demonstrates normal bony and soft tissue contours at rest and during motion.

Do not forget to observe the surrounding structures, such as the cervical spine, to check their involvement. Additionally, observe the mouth during opening and closing to determine whether motion is smooth and continuous and occurs in a straight line. If the chin deviates toward the affected side, there may be a muscular cause. Early deviation typically involves the soft tissue, whereas late deviation is articular.

> **Practical Tip**
> Early chin deviation toward the affected side may indicate a muscular cause, while late deviation is articular.

Palpation When palpating the TMJ, look for symmetry, noting obvious swelling, bruising, or deformity. To feel the TMJ, place your fingers in or just in front of the client's external auditory canals. Have the client open and close the mouth while you determine whether both sides are moving simultaneously and whether the movement is smooth. Include the neck structures in the palpation.

Orthopedic Tests There are no specific tests for TMD. The joint can be auscultated during movement to help determine when the joint makes noise and what it sounds like. "'Soft' or 'popping' clicks that are sometimes heard in normal joints are caused by ligament movement, articular surface separation, or sucking of loose tissue behind the condyle as it moves forward. 'Hard' or 'cracking' clicks are more likely to indicate joint pathology or joint surface defects" (Magee, 1997). Perform a functional opening test by having the client put two flexed proximal interphalangeal joints sideways in his or her mouth. This will determine whether the jaw can open wide enough for everyday activity (25 mm to 35 mm). The dermatomes of the head and neck identified earlier should be assessed in addition to performing manual muscle tests to the area.

For each movement, have the client seated, and place one hand on the client at the base of the occiput for stability.

- *Depression:* Have the client open his or her mouth. Place your free hand under the chin, and press up while the client resists the movement.
- *Elevation:* Have the client close his or her mouth and hold it closed while you place your hand just under the mouth, on the chin, and press down.
- *Protrusion and retrusion:* Do not test for these.
- *Lateral deviation:* Place your hand along the body of the mandible, and push to one side while the client resists the movement.

Soft Tissue Treatment

Regardless of the etiology of the client's TMD, addressing the soft tissue is beneficial. If, however, on the basis of the assessment, you suspect that the cause is articular, refer the client to an appropriate health care provider. The actual size of the treatment area is relatively small when dealing with the joint. You will primarily deal with the four muscles of mastication (masseter, temporalis, and medial and lateral pterygoids) and the supra- and infrahyoids; however, do not neglect other areas if it is necessary to treat them.

This section discusses only TMJ-specific treatment, but the methods used for other parts of the region can be applied for TMJ dysfunction as well (see pages 118–123). It is easiest to work on a client in the supine position.

Connective Tissue Address the superficial fascia of the neck and face first. Assess the restriction in multiple directions, and move into it. Typically, because of posture, restrictions tend to be into the clavicle and chest and up into the mandible and face. After treating the neck and face, address each muscle and separate it out using the methods described earlier. Perform these techniques extraorally.

Tissue Inconsistencies The trigger points in TMD are:

- Temporalis
- Masseter
- Suprahyoids
- Infrahyoids
- Medial pterygoids
- Lateral pterygoids

When addressing the trigger points in the involved muscles of TMD, treat them both intraorally and extraorally using the methods described earlier. Use a nonpowdered, nonlatex-gloved finger, and discuss which techniques you are going to perform with the client prior to starting. Be sure to check any local and state guidelines before treating intraorally, and always gain the consent of the client.

The easiest muscles to access are the temporalis and masseter. The supra- and infrahyoids are a little more difficult because of their proximity to other delicate structures in the area. The most difficult muscles to access are the medial and lateral pterygoids. Externally, the lateral pterygoids can be accessed between the mandibular condyle and the coronoid process. Locate this point, and roll just under the zygomatic arch; compress in different directions, stopping to release tender points. Make sure that you have released the masseter's trigger points first.

Intraorally, access the muscles by sliding the finger with the pad facing medially between the maxilla and the coronoid process. Reach all the way to the superior border of the cheek where it meets the maxilla. Press in toward the pterygoid plate to access the inferior division of the muscle. The medial pterygoids can also be accessed externally, but they are best treated internally. To access their trigger points intraorally, slide a gloved finger, with the pad facing outward, along the inside of the mandible to the last molar. Slide off the last molar on the medial side of the mandible toward the angle. The trigger point will be in the belly of the muscle.

Muscle Concerns

Since muscle imbalance is a big contributor to TMD, thorough treatment of the involved muscles is beneficial. The goal should be to remove the imbalance and restore equal motion to both sides. Treatments that incorporate movement are especially effective for this condition.

Manual Muscle Treatment Suggestions Start by treating the muscles that are directly involved, the muscles of mastication and the supra- and infrahyoids, and then move into the neck and other areas as necessary. For the masseter and temporalis, use parallel and cross-fiber strokes, incorporating movement. These muscles can also be accessed intraorally.

Temporalis Have the client open the mouth fully. For the temporalis, place a gloved finger between the last upper molar and the cheek, with the pad facing laterally. If you press laterally, you should feel the medial aspect of the coronoid process and the tendon of the temporalis. Apply pressure, being careful to stay within the client's level of tolerance. Treat the lateral aspect of the tendon by moving to the outside aspect of the coronoid process.

Masseter Treat the masseter intraorally by placing the client in the supine position with the mouth open and using a gloved finger facing laterally. Apply pressure just lateral to the last inferior molar. You can also use the first finger to pinch the muscle between your finger and thumb. Have the client clench his or her teeth, as this will verify your finger placement and incorporate movement into the treatment.

Suprahyoids For the suprahyoids, find the hyoid bone, and perform a stroke from the superior aspect of the bone up to the mandible. Repeat as you move laterally until you reach the angle of the mandible.

Infrahyoids For the infrahyoids, move the thyroid cartilage laterally, and use the other hand to perform a stroke from the clavicle to the hyoid bone. Repeat this while moving laterally to the clavicular head of the SCM.

Medial Pterygoid For the medial pterygoid, place your fingers under the mandible, just anterior to the angle. Press up and into the bone to access the muscle. Intraorally, use the same technique as you did for the trigger points.

Lateral Pterygoids The lateral pterygoids are treated externally between the mandibular condyle and the coronoid process. The same method is used for treating trigger points internally.

Stretching

The only direct stretch used for this condition is depressing the mandible. While the client is seated, place a hand on his or her forehead for support. Have the client open the mouth fully. When the client has reached his or her end range of motion, gently assist the motion by pressing the chin down. Perform 10 repetitions. Stretching the neck as described previously is important since those structures can contribute to the TMD.

Torticollis

Background

"**Torticollis** is a diagnosis used for a variety of muscular, bony, and neurologic conditions" (Luther, 2002). It is essentially a dystonia, which is an extended muscle contraction. Dystonia can occur in any voluntary muscle; however, it is called *cervical dystonia (CD)* when it involves neck muscles. Torticollis can arise from three sources: congenital, neurologic, and muscular.

"**Congenital muscular torticollis** is a painless condition usually presenting during infancy with a tight sternocleidomastoid muscle causing the child's head to be tilted to the tightened side" (Luther, 2002). This is commonly referred to as the "cocked robin" deformity. The incidence of congenital torticollis is rather common and believed to be caused by one of three factors:

1. A hematoma in the sternocleidomastoid
2. Intrauterine positioning of the head
3. Trauma to the SCM during a vaginal birth

A study in 2001 subdivided congenital torticollis into three groups:

1. *Sternomastoid tumor:* Characterized by the palpable presence of a tumor and muscle tightness
2. *Muscular torticollis:* Has tightness but no tumor
3. *Postural torticollis:* Has clinical features but no tumor or tightness

Although this condition is painless, it can cause permanent deformity if it is not addressed.

Neurologic cervical dystonia is sometimes known as *spasmodic torticollis.* It typically occurs in adults between the ages of 25 and 60 and can be secondary to a known neuropathological process such as trauma, brain tumor, stroke, or neurodegenerative disease. It can

torticollis A type of dystonia that affects the cervical region in which the head is tilted toward one side and the chin is elevated and turned toward the opposite side.

congenital muscular torticollis A painless condition usually presenting during infancy with a tight sternocleidomastoid muscle causing the child's head to be tilted to the tightened side.

neurologic cervical dystonia A type of dystonia that typically occurs in adults between the ages of 25 and 60 and can be secondary to a known neuropathological process such as trauma, brain tumor, stroke, or neurodegenerative disease. It can also occur as a primary disorder, with no abnormality found.

also occur as a primary disorder, with no abnormality found (Gilman, 1999). One theory suggests that it is the result of either dysfunction in the spinal accessory nerve (11th cranial nerve), which innervates the sternocleidomastoid and trapezius muscles, or abnormal functioning of the basal ganglia, which are involved with the control of movement. The course of CD varies from one individual to another, and the symptoms of a particular patient may vary throughout the course of the illness.

Muscular cervical dystonia is often referred to as *wryneck*. This type of torticollis arises from the body's protective mechanism for safeguarding the neck. Its causes can vary and include:

- Trauma to the area
- A sleeping position that is wrong for the neck
- Repetitive motion of the head for extended periods of time

More often than not, the cause is muscular; however, other causes include infection, postural problems, ear conditions, and malocclusions of the teeth. The root of the problem seems to come from the facet joints. As a result of the trauma or other causes, the facet joints lock down and restrict motion, resulting in a painful, protective spasm. This spasm causes the neck to become "stuck" in one position with the head tilted to the side of the spasm and rotated to the opposite side.

muscular cervical dystonia A type of torticollis that arises from the body's protective mechanism for safeguarding the neck; its causes include trauma to the area, a sleeping position wrong for the neck, or repetitive motion of the head for extended periods of time. Also referred to as *wryneck*.

Assessment

Since the condition can arise from several different causes, it is necessary to rule out more serious origins. Generally, congenital CD is evident in infants and small children. Taking a thorough history will be helpful in determining if the origins are neurologic or muscular. Once again, it is important to be aware of possible contraindications and make the appropriate referral when necessary.

Condition History Here are some questions that are relevant to torticollis:

Question	Significance
How long have you had the condition?	While muscular wryneck can be a lengthy disorder, neurologic cervical dystonia usually has a longer history of symptoms.
Was there any associated trauma or mechanism with the injury?	Mechanisms can range from a car accident to turning of the head too fast to a neurologic cause. Unexpected occurrences indicate a possible muscular origin.
Are there symptoms other than neck pain and stiffness?	Other symptoms, including ticks, tremors, and migrations of pain and stiffness to other parts of the body, occur in neurologic-based dystonia.

Visual Assessment The most obvious observation involves the position of the client's head. With torticollis, the head is tilted to the affected side and rotated away from it. Checking symmetry in the face and malocclusions in the mouth can help determine whether other structures are involved. Active and passive ranges of motion should be assessed at this point as well.

Palpation Regardless of the origin of the torticollis, the muscles in the cervical area will be hypertonic. Palpation for this condition should include the head and face, as it is common for structures outside the cervical spine to be involved.

Starting with the face, investigate any abnormalities or deformities. Depending on the length of the symptoms, facial structures can become deformed due to the pull of the soft tissue. Palpate the TMJ as described previously. Move on to the neck, checking for any obvious swelling, bruising, or deformity, and include all the structures mentioned at the beginning of the chapter. Torticollis can arise from infection, so the lymph nodes in the area may be involved. The muscles that are hypertonic should be noted to guide the treatment.

Orthopedic Tests There are no specific orthopedic tests for torticollis. Assess both the TMJ and the cervical spine to determine whether they are involved, as well as dermatomes and myotomes to ensure there is no neurologic involvement. Manual muscle testing of the area can be included if the therapist feels it is necessary.

Soft Tissue Treatment

Regardless of the cause of the hypertonicity, soft tissue treatment is beneficial. While the primary muscles involved are the trapezius and the sternocleidomastoid, various layers of muscles of the cervical spine can all contribute to the client's reported pain and restricted movement; they should be addressed in order to achieve comprehensive and lasting therapeutic resolution (Vaughn, 2003).

Working with infants and small children can be challenging, and treatments may need modification depending on the situation. The therapist should incorporate the help of the parent or caregiver to facilitate the treatment.

Treatment should be as comfortable as possible because the structures involved are already irritated and inflamed; therefore, it is important to remain within the client's comfort zone. Modifications to client positioning or stroke technique can help facilitate comfort as well. In the early stages of treatment, the supine and side-lying positions will probably be of more use because of the tilting of the head. Once the muscles are sufficiently released to allow prone positioning, it should be utilized.

Connective Tissue Depending on the length of the symptoms, there may be significant connective tissue involvement. If the origin is congenital, the SCM tumor will become fibrotic as it heals.

Supine Position Start superficially with the neck, working into the restrictions until they have released. Pay special attention to the upper trapezius, the SCM, and the scalenes. Staying within the client's comfort zone, work the scalenes by cradling the head and tracing three lines medial to lateral in the posterior cervical triangle, sinking in behind the clavicle toward the 1st rib. Rotate the head, if tolerable for the client, into and away from the restrictions; this increases the technique's effectiveness. For the SCM, incorporating active movement gives the client more control over the treatment and keeps it tolerable. The same techniques used to treat whiplash can be applied here:

- Stand at the head of the client at the side of the table.
- Hook into the tissue just lateral to the trachea.
- Move the tissue in a posterior direction.

Address the smaller muscles of the neck with the same methods as those used for whiplash. The deep suboccipitals can be addressed here very effectively by tracing along their fiber direction.

Side-Lying Position The client may not be able to lie on the affected side, so use caution. If the client lies on the unaffected side, perform a depression stroke to the shoulder; the weight of the head will create a stretch of the tissue in the opposite direction. Stand behind the client's shoulder, and face the head of the table. Use the same arm as the side of the table where you are standing, and place your forearm at the base of the skull. Use the other hand to help pull your forearm along the muscle, up and over the deltoids and upper trapezius, while you depress the shoulder girdle at the same time.

Tissue Inconsistencies Address trigger points in the following muscles when treating torticollis:

- Trapezius
- SCM
- Scalenes
- Suboccipitals
- Any other muscles that contribute to cervical movement

Muscle Concerns

Massage techniques that incorporate simultaneous movement of the head and neck will stimulate both the motor nerve system and the myofascial system (Vaughn, 2003). Use the techniques discussed earlier to treat the involved muscles, adapting the techniques to each individual situation (see pages 120–121).

Stretching

"Manual stretching still is the most common form of treatment for muscular torticollis" (Luther, 2002). Active Isolated Stretching is very effective for this condition because of its incorporation of reciprocal inhibition. For infants and small children, enlist the help of a toy or the parent to have the child perform the motion. Passive stretching for this population may be more appropriate if the children are young. Stretching should be focused on the affected side until a more normal head positioning is achieved. Use the modified neck stretches described below for flexion and lateral flexion before using the seated stretches.

Neck Extensors—Modified To modify stretching the neck extensors, place the client in the supine position, keeping his or her shoulder and upper back on the table. Position one of your hands just above the occiput and the other on the client's chin. Have the client tuck the chin in while lifting the head off the table, looking toward the feet. At the end range of motion, gently assist the client with tucking the chin and lifting the head (Fig. 5-29). Perform 5 to 8 repetitions, increasing to 15 when ready. Using the same position, perform lateral flexion by having the client bend his or her ear toward the shoulder. At the end range of motion, assist the motion with your hands on either side of the client's head (Fig. 5-30).

As the client's range improves, you can further modify this stretch by placing the client in a side-lying position with his or her neck beyond the end of the table and the bottom arm hanging off the front of the table. Stand behind with one hand on the top shoulder to stabilize it. Guide the ear to the shoulder to prevent unwanted movement, and assist at the end range of motion. Start with 5 to 8 repetitions, increasing them as necessary.

For flexion, rotation, and oblique stretches, start with the seated version and move to the modified positions.

Neck Flexors—Modified To modify the neck flexors stretch, place the client in the prone position with his or her neck beyond the edge of the table and the arms hanging down and holding the table. Stand to the side, and place one hand on C7 to stabilize the trunk. Have the client extend his or her head to the end range of motion, and with your hand

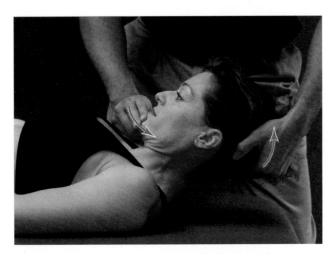

Figure 5-29 Modified neck extensor stretch.

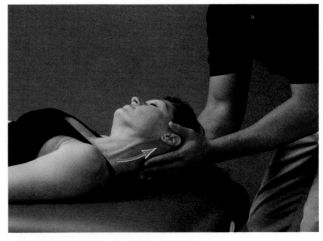

Figure 5-30 Modified stretch of the lateral flexors of the neck.

on the client's forehead gently assist with the motion (Fig. 5-31). Start with 5 to 8 repetitions, working up to 15.

Anterior Neck, Oblique Aspect—Modified For the anterior oblique stretch, start from the position used for modified neck flexion, and have the client rotate his or her head 45° to the unaffected side. The client should extend the head to look over the shoulder on the same side. With your hands on the temporal bone, assist at the client's end range in the same direction as the motion. Start with 5 to 10 repetitions, increasing to 15.

Neck Rotation—Modified Perform modified cervical rotation with the client in the same position as that for lateral flexion. With your hands on the forehead and occiput, help support the client's head parallel to the ground, and have him or her rotate toward the ceiling and floor. Assist at the end of each direction, making sure to prevent unwanted movements (Fig. 5-32).

Posterior Neck, Oblique Aspect—Modified The last modified stretch is for the posterior oblique muscles. Place the client in the supine position, and have him or her rotate the head 45° toward the affected side. Your hand should be on the temporal bone on the bottom side. Have the client flex up at the 45° angle. Assist the motion at the end of the client's range, performing 5 to 10 repetitions (Fig. 5-33).

Cervical Disk Injuries

Background

Various structures of the spine that emanate pain are a major cause of chronic problems (Manchikanti

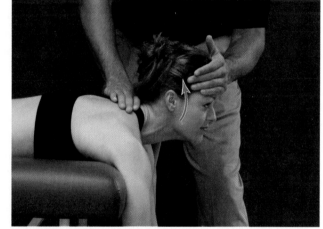

Figure 5-31 Modified neck flexors stretch.

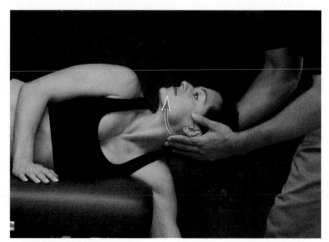

Figure 5.32 Modified stretch of the rotators of the neck.

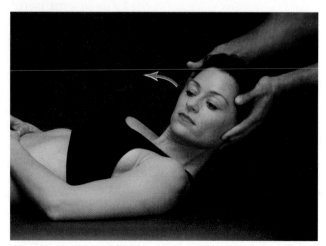

Figure 5.33 Modified stretch of the posterior oblique aspect of the neck.

et al., 2004). Among the causes of pain, injuries to the cervical disk are a significant contributor. The stability of a cervical segment is derived mainly from the anterior spinal elements, while compression to the spinal column is resisted primarily by the vertebral bodies and intervertebral disks. Shear forces on the spine are opposed by the paraspinal musculature and ligamentous support. The orientation of the facets prevents forward vertebral motion, while the ligamentous structures and the annulus fibrosis are the primary restraints to distraction of the spine (Banerjee et al., 2004).

Traumatic forces are the most common mechanism of disk injuries. Motor vehicle accidents are the most prevalent cause of injury, followed by violence, falls, and sports-related activities. Injury occurs when the force is greater than the stability of the structures. Chronic conditions such as posture, repetitive mechanical loading of the spine, hydration levels, and age can also cause injury. Repeated micro-traumas and forces on the disk, combined with age and decreased disk pliability, cause cracks and allow for the migration of the nucleus.

The degree of disk injuries varies. Micro-tears to the annulus and rim lesions (tears away from the body) are considered minor injuries, while major injuries include avulsions of the disk away from the body, annular longitudinal ligament tears, and herniated disks. Disk herniation has a wide range of presentations and clinical significance and is considered a common spine disorder (McLain, 2005).

There are varying degrees of herniations, ranging from a slight bulge to a complete rupture and loss of nucleus pulposis. Tears usually occur in the posterior lateral portion of the disk because that is where the annulus is thinnest. Anterior bulges are often asymptomatic because the spinal nerves exit posteriorly.

When a tear in the annulus fibrosis occurs, the nucleus is allowed to migrate abnormally as a result of the forces on the disk. As the annular tear gets larger, the nucleus migrates more and more until it bulges. If the disk ruptures, the nucleus, which is caustic to the surrounding structures, leaks out. This changes the height of the disk, resulting in decreased disk space. Despite the degree of herniation, the end result is the same: a reduction in space for the spinal nerve roots and cord.

When the spinal nerves are compressed due to contact with the disk, pain and neurologic symptoms occur. The degree of herniation that produces symptoms varies from person to person and is based on the preexisting stenosis that is normal for the individual. Contributing factors such as posture, muscle tension, and age can cause some people to be symptomatic when others are not. Other dysfunctions that can mimic disk problems are brachial plexus injuries, facet joint irritation or misalignment, and muscular tension. These conditions can also compress the spinal nerves but occur at locations other than the disks.

Symptoms from disk injuries will not occur until the surrounding tissue has been contacted; they include sharp pain in the area of the bulge, weakness and paresthesia, diminished reflexes, and limited range of motion. Therapists can determine the level that is involved by using the dermatomes and myotomes discussed earlier to map out the spinal nerve that is affected.

Assessment

When dealing with potential nerve involvement, use extra caution and awareness in order to determine contraindications. Cervical disk injuries can have a variety of etiologies; thus, a thorough assessment is advised.

Condition History

Here are some questions that are relevant to cervical disk injuries:

Questions	Significance
How severe are your symptoms?	More severe symptoms may indicate a higher level of involvement.
What was the mechanism of injury?	Obvious trauma, such as an automobile accident, may help identify the type of injury and the structures involved.
Where is the pain or other symptoms (such as radiation and paresthesia)?	Helps identify the level of disk involvement.
Does the pain change as the day progresses?	Morning pain and stiffness that dissipates might indicate muscle versus disk involvement. Pain that develops after activity or after standing could be a stenosis without disk involvement.

Visual Assessment Because symptoms vary depending on the severity, observing the client both at rest and in motion is an important part of the assessment process. Head and neck position is a key factor in cervical disk injuries. Look for any obvious muscular spasm or deformity. Facial expressions on movement will give clues as to severity as well. Noting the posture of the rest of the body can determine the extent of compensation. Passive and active ranges of motion should be assessed here using previously described methods.

Palpation Palpation should include all the structures that are involved. Typically this involves only the neck, but it can include the face if the symptoms have migrated due to compensation. Check for swelling, bruising, and obvious deformity in the area. Palpate bony structures as well as soft tissue and muscles using the techniques described earlier; be aware of the client's pain threshold and adjust pressure accordingly. Note any areas that cause discomfort.

Orthopedic Tests There are specific orthopedic tests for assessing cervical disk injuries. To begin, make sure you have performed manual muscle tests to the area and have checked the dermatomes and myotomes. Once the results have been recorded, begin the specific tests. Table 5-5 lists some orthopedic tests and explains how to perform them.

Soft Tissue Treatment

The focus in treating cervical disk injuries should be the decompression of the spine. When space is created, theoretically, pressure will be alleviated

Table 5-5   Orthopedic Tests for Cervical Disk Injuries

Orthopedic Test	How to Perform
Cervical compression test 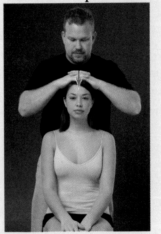	Client is in seated position. Stand behind client with head and neck in a neutral position. Interlace your fingers, and place them on top of the client's head. Gently press straight down, being careful not to create any movement but compression. Any pain or increase in neurologic symptoms is considered a positive sign. If a positive sign is obtained from cervical compression, or the client is in constant pain, move on to the cervical distraction test.
Cervical distraction 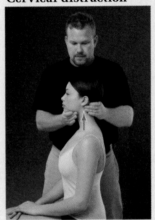	Client is in seated position. Stand to the side of client. Cradle the occiput, using the hand that is furthest from the client; with the hand nearest to the client, cradle the mandible. Gently lift up on the head. A decrease in pain or associated symptoms in this position indicates a positive sign because the pressure on the nerve root has been lifted. If the pain increases in this position, this is an indication of a possible ligamentous injury.
Spurling's test 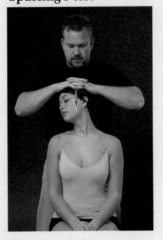	Client is in seated position. Stand behind client. Have client laterally flex and rotate the head to the side of the complaint. Interlace your fingers, and press down on the head. An increase in pain and symptoms indicates a positive sign. This test will significantly close down the foramen on the tested side, so other conditions such as stenosis, bone spurs, and facet problems can elicit a positive sign even if there is no disk involvement.

and symptoms will improve. Make sure to address the condition appropriately based on its phase (acute or chronic). The treatment area can be local or regional depending on how long the client has had to compensate for the discomfort.

★ Practical Tip
The focus in treating cervical disk injuries should be the decompression of the spine.

Connective Tissue Typically, there are underlying postural issues that have contributed to the condition. Since most postural dysfunction is chronic, addressing the connective tissue in the area will be of significant benefit.

Prone Position Start with the general assessment of the connective tissue from cranial to caudal and medial to lateral. Move into the restriction, paying special attention to the tissue from the base of the skull through the upper trapezius. Once the superficial fascia has been released, remove the restrictions in each muscle involved based on the assessments. Unwind the upper trapezius using the method described for whiplash. Stripping out local restrictions works well for the upper trapezius, starting at the bend of the neck and working laterally toward the acromion.

Supine Position Start superficially by releasing the fascia of the neck and upper chest. If indicated, you can release the sternoclavicular joint using the same method as used for whiplash. Spend a significant amount of time working on the scalenes and sternocleidomastoid muscles. Incorporating rotation of the head, if tolerable for the client, into and away from the restrictions increases the effectiveness of the work.

The supra- and infrahyoids are also typically involved and should be addressed. To access the suprahyoids, find the hyoid and perform a stroke from the superior aspect of the bone up to the mandible. Repeat while moving laterally until reaching the angle of the mandible. For the infrahyoids, move the thyroid cartilage laterally with one hand, and use the other hand to perform a stroke up to the hyoid bone. Repeat this while moving laterally to the clavicular head of the SCM. The suboccipitals should be a posterior structure you address here. Pulling your hands up the back of the neck into the base of the skull can be an effective technique.

Side-Lying Position Use caution when working on clients in this position. Be careful not to compress directly into the spine or press the neck into extension. This can close down the foramen and re-create the symptoms. Access to the upper trapezius is convenient here. A broadening stroke while depressing the shoulder is very effective.

Tissue Inconsistencies Trigger points for cervical disk injuries are similar to those involved in whiplash. Use the assessment information to determine which muscles are involved, and release them using the methods described earlier. Some neck muscles that are commonly involved include:

- Suboccipitals
- Trapezius
- SCM
- Scalenes
- Suprahyoids
- Infrahyoids

- Levator scapulae
- Splenius capitis

Other muscles may be involved depending on the severity of the injury.

Muscle Concerns

Focus on spinal decompression when choosing stroke direction. Incorporating movement can be effective as long as it is not too aggressive. Techniques used to treat whiplash can also be used for this condition (see pages 120–121).

Stretching

When stretching the neck, be careful of the amount of pressure used in assisting. If any symptoms are reproduced, use the modified position. If they continue, a referral to a physician or other health care provider may be indicated.

Neck Extensors To stretch the neck extensors, make sure the client is sitting up straight. Have the client tuck and retract the chin as close to the neck as possible, and contract the neck flexors. Advise the client to keep the mouth closed and exhale during the movement.

Once the client has moved through the entire range, gently assist in the same direction (see Fig. 5-23); this stretch addresses the deep neck extensors. Repeat 10 to 15 times, in two sets if necessary.

Neck Flexors—Modified For the flexors, place your client in the prone position with the neck beyond the edge of the table and the arms hanging down and holding the table. Stand to the side, and place one hand on C7 to stabilize the trunk. Have the client extend to the end of the range; place your hand on the forehead, and gently assist in the motion (see Fig. 5-31). Start with 5 to 8 repetitions, working up to 15.

Lateral Neck Flexors Stretch the lateral flexors of the neck with the client sitting up straight. Stand on the side opposite the one being stretched. Place your hand on the shoulder of the side you are stretching to stabilize it. Have the client bring the ear to the shoulder, exhaling during the motion. At the end of the movement, gently assist in the same direction (see Fig. 5-25). Perform one to two sets of 10 depending on the need.

Neck Rotators Rotation can be performed in the same position as that for the previous stretches. This stretch targets the neck rotators. Stand at the client's side on the opposite side to that being stretched. Place one hand on the ramus of the mandible of the side opposite the one where you are standing. Place the other hand behind the ear of the side where you are standing. Have the client turn his or her head toward you while exhaling. Once the client has reached the end range, gently assist in the motion (see Fig. 5-26). Have the client complete 10 repetitions.

Posterior Neck, Oblique Aspect Stretch the posterior oblique muscles by having the client turn his or her head 45° to the side you are stretching. Have the client exhale and bend the head down toward the opposite knee. Once the client has reached the end range, assist with the movement (see

Fig. 5-27). Support the client's opposite shoulder to prevent it from elevating. Perform 10 repetitions.

Anterior Neck, Oblique Aspect   Stretch the anterior muscles by having the client turn the head 45° to the side opposite the one being stretched. Have the client bend the head backward, looking over the shoulder, while exhaling. At the end range of active motion, gently assist the client. Perform 5 to 10 repetitions (see Fig. 5-28).

Thoracic Outlet Syndrome

Thoracic outlet syndrome involves structures in the shoulder girdle as well as the neck. This section focuses primarily on the neck; however, the techniques discussed in Chapter 7, on the shoulder, can be applied here as necessary.

Background

"Thoracic outlet syndrome has been reported since antiquity" (Casbas et al., 2005). Peet introduced the term *thoracic outlet syndrome* in 1956 to describe all cervical brachial pain and numbness syndromes of the upper extremity (Atasoy, 1996). It is a condition included in a larger classification known as *nerve entrapments.* While nerve entrapment is not a primary disease, it is caused by pathologic changes in the tissues through which nerves pass (Schoen, 2002). Nerve entrapments are usually chronic, characterized by pain and paresthesia with or without sensory or motor loss. As the nerve travels its course, it passes through many narrow anatomical passages. Since the nerve is the softest structure, entrapment occurs at these vulnerable passages.

The term **thoracic outlet syndrome (TOS)** describes symptoms related to compression or tension of the brachial plexus and/or subclavian vessels in the region of the thoracic outlet (Brismee et al., 2004). Due to the lack of objective diagnostic criteria and the danger associated with operative management, both skeptics about its existence and voices of conservatism regarding its management have evolved (Rayan, 1998). "The brachial plexus lies posterior, lateral, and superior to the subclavian artery, and its lower roots (C8 and T1) have a close relationship with the artery" (Atasoy, 1996). (See Fig. 5-7).

A variety of symptoms may occur as a result of the compression, including:

- Pain
- Numbness
- Tingling
- Paresthesia
- Weakness in the thenar, hypothenar, and interossei muscles

The neurogenic symptoms are primarily along the ulnar nerve distribution but can be along the medial or radial nerves as well; they are dependent on the frequency, duration, and degree of compression. Vascular compromise is much less common (only 2% of cases) and can involve the subclavian artery, resulting in coldness, pallor, and arm fatigue, or the subclavian vein, resulting in edema, cyanosis, and pain.

The thoracic outlet is created by the area leaving the thorax superiorly into the neck and laterally to the axilla. It is bordered by the anterior and

thoracic outlet syndrome (TOS)
A compression or tension of the brachial plexus and/or subclavian vessels in the region of the thoracic outlet.

middle scalenes and the 1st rib. Associated structures that can also be related to dysfunction in this area are:

- Clavicle
- Subclavius
- Pectoralis minor
- Omohyoid
- Cervical rib
- Transverse process of C7

These structures form four gates that the neurovascular structures pass through. These gates, from medial to lateral, are:

- *Gate 1:* Anterior scalenic triangle
- *Gate 2:* Posterior scalenic triangle
- *Gate 3:* Costoclavicular space
- *Gate 4:* Coracothoracopectoral space (Brismee et al., 2004)

As these neurovascular structures pass through the gates, they can be entrapped at any location. The three most common are the costoclavicular space (Gate 3); the interscalene triangle (Gates 1 and 2); and the space between the coracoid process and the pectoralis minor insertion (Gate 4) (Ritter et al., 1999). Compression of the brachial plexus as it passes through the gates is usually caused by a band of taut tissue, whether it is congenital or fibrotic, pressing on the lower trunk. More often than not, clients with TOS have underlying congenital anomalies that predispose them to developing space problems (Brantigan and Roos, 2004). When compression occurs, the pressure diminishes capillary perfusion and results in ischemia. The ischemic portion of the nerve does not repolarize normally and causes a conduction delay. This produces the vague aching in the general region of the compression that is reported.

Thoracic outlet syndrome can arise from a variety of sources. The most common age range affected is 25 to 40, with women four times as likely to develop symptoms as men (Brismee et al., 2004). Trauma is a common cause, whether it is major, such as whiplash, or minor, such as repeated micro-traumas that form fibrotic bands as the tissue heals. Whiplash injuries are the most common mechanism of neurogenic TOS, with up to 30% of motor vehicle accident victims developing symptoms. At least 60% to 70% of people who present with symptoms have had an injury to the neck or shoulder girdle area (Atasoy, 1996). Repetitive stress also accounts for a large number of TOS injuries. Repeated small neck traumas from frequent head turning or improper body mechanics can lead to symptoms over time. Chronic improper postures and positions of the head and spine are also common mechanisms for TOS. These postures have three major influences:

- Direct pressure on nerves and vessels at various entrapment sites
- A shortening adaptation that causes muscles to become painful when stretched or overused
- Muscular imbalance wherein some muscles are underused and weak, while others are overused

A forward head position, drooping shoulders, and lowering of the anterior chest wall all produce shortened muscle positions, which result in strength imbalances that will adapt over time (Ritter et al., 1999).

Assessment

Diagnosis of thoracic outlet syndrome is challenging and controversial because of the subjectivity of patient complaints and the difficulty in objectively quantifying those complaints (Ritter et al., 1999). Moreover, "there is no universally reliable and accurate diagnostic test for TOS" (Rayan, 1998). Clinicians typically rely on a combination of a thorough history, a comprehensive physical examination, and a variety of specific tests to assess TOS (Brismee et al., 2004). This combination prevents misdiagnoses from occurring.

When assessing thoracic outlet syndrome, therapists must include the cervical spine, shoulder, elbow, and hand to determine whether neural compression is causing or contributing to the symptoms. This section addresses cervical concerns.

Condition History Here are some questions that are relevant to thoracic outlet syndrome:

Question	Significance
Was there an injury?	A large majority of clients who display thoracic outlet syndrome recall some type of trauma.
What does the pain feel like?	Disk pain is typically sharper and more severe. It follows a dermatomal pattern. TOS often involves the whole limb with no distinguishable dermatomal patterns.
When does pain occur?	TOS usually surfaces after exercise or exertion, which separates it from orthopedic problems that produce discomfort during exercise.
Where are the neurologic symptoms?	TOS presents along the ulnar nerve distribution. Cervical disk dysfunction presents along the radial nerve distribution. Carpal tunnel syndrome strictly presents along the median nerve distribution.

Visual Assessment There can be many different levels of involvement in thoracic outlet syndrome. Observe the head, neck, and upper shoulder, noting their positions in relation to each other. Note other observations based on the criteria discussed in previous sections. Since whiplash can be a mechanism for this condition, include the same observations as those for whiplash assessment. Be sure to include active and passive movements to check ranges of motion.

Palpation Since TOS can involve more than one part of the body, make sure palpation includes the neck, shoulder, elbow, and wrist. Muscular dysfunction is common, so pay special attention to hypertonicity in the area. Check for obvious signs of swelling, discoloration, or deformity.

Orthopedic Tests Several tests for vascular and neurologic symptoms help provide objective results in assessing thoracic outlet syndrome; however, these tests should not be used as a definitive assessment of TOS.

Rather, factor the results of the tests into the overall picture created by the different components of the evaluation. Since the majority of patients have symptoms relating to compression of the brachial plexus, the reproduction of their symptoms may be a more accurate assessment criterion than the changing of their pulse (Novak and Mackinnon, 1996).

To begin, make sure to perform the appropriate manual muscle tests, as described earlier, and assess the dermatomes and myotomes (see Fig. 5-10). The Roos test, the most reliable test for thoracic outlet syndrome (Brantigan and Roos, 2004); Adson maneuver; and Allen test are performed to reproduce a client's symptoms. Table 5-6 lists some orthopedic tests and explains how to perform them.

Table 5-6 Orthopedic Tests for Thoracic Outlet Syndrome

Orthopedic Test	How to Perform
Roos test 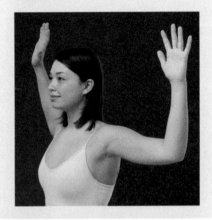	Client is in standing position. Have the client abduct the shoulder to 90° and flex the elbows to 90°. Slightly externally rotate the client's shoulders and horizontally abduct the shoulders so that he or she is just behind the frontal plane. Have the client slowly open and close the hands for 3 minutes. A positive sign is ischemic pain, profound weakness in the arm, or numbness or tingling in the hand. Minor symptom reproduction is considered a negative sign.
Adson maneuver 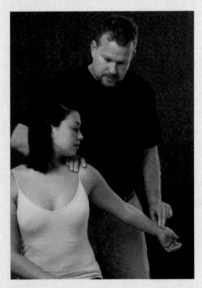 *Note:* This is the most common test performed, but it has also been proved unreliable.	Client is in seated position. Locate the radial pulse on the side you are testing. Extend and externally rotate the arm, keeping it below horizontal. Have the client rotate the head and look at the hand being tested. Instruct the client to take a deep breath and hold it. Any diminishing or disappearance of the pulse indicates a positive sign.

Table 5-6 Orthopedic Tests for Thoracic Outlet Syndrome *(Continued)*

Orthopedic Test	How to Perform
Allen test 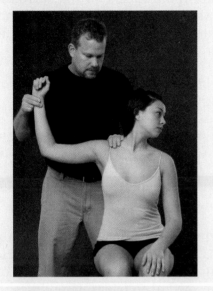	Client is in seated position. Locate the radial pulse of the client on the test side. Flex the elbow and shoulder to 90°. Horizontally abduct and laterally rotate the arm. Have the client rotate the head and look away from the side being tested. Any change or disappearance of the pulse is an indication of a positive test.
Cyriax release test 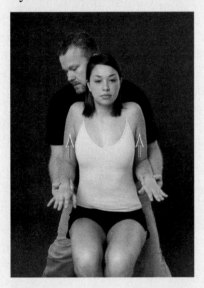 *Note:* This is also known as the *passive shoulder girdle elevation test* and involves the **release phenomenon.** That is, neurovascular symptoms that present as a result of compression will change if the structures causing the compression are moved.	Client is in seated position. Stand behind the client, and hold the elbows in 90° of flexion and the forearms and wrists in a neutral position. Lean the client back about 15°, and passively elevate the shoulders just shy of the end range. Hold the position for 1 to 3 minutes. A positive result can take one of two forms: • If the client has active symptoms, a reduction or relief of those symptoms indicates a positive test. • One interpretation of the release phenomenon is that compressed nerve trunks will initially display symptoms but will return to normal; hence, a reproduction of the client's symptoms also indicates a positive test. 📖 release phenomenon The principle that neurovascular symptoms that present as a result of compression will change if the structures causing the compression are moved.

Soft Tissue Treatment

Whether the condition is caused by a congenital abnormality or results from trauma, soft tissue work can be extremely beneficial. Although it is not possible to address the presence of a cervical rib or enlarged C7 transverse process, it is possible to counteract their effects on the surrounding structures. Pay special attention to the anterior and middle scalenes, since they can create potential entrapment sites. Many of the techniques discussed previously can be applied here.

Connective Tissue Since there are typically underlying postural concerns with TOS, addressing the connective tissue will be beneficial.

Prone Position Assess the superficial connective tissue from superior to inferior and medial to lateral. Move into the restrictions until they are sufficiently released. Use the techniques used for treating whiplash in the upper trapezius, and separate each muscle in the area (see page 119).

Supine Position After releasing the superficial connective tissue, move into the individual muscles of the area. Releasing the sternoclavicular joint and 1st rib is beneficial in reducing the symptoms of this condition. Trace the underside of the clavicle from medial to lateral to address the subclavius. Tightness in this area can restrict SC joint motion.

While the SCM does not directly entrap any structures, its effect on cervical lordosis and the clavicle makes it a prime candidate for work. Strip out the scalenes, especially the anterior and median, to open up that gate. Use caution, as excessive movement may aggravate the symptoms. Working the supra- and infrahyoids will help take pressure off the general area.

Side-Lying Position This position is beneficial in treating the associated involved structures in the shoulder. Although this position can be used to treat the neck, it is most effective for treating the shoulder.

Tissue Inconsistencies The same trigger points may be involved, in the same muscles, as those described earlier for other conditions. Focus initially on the anterior muscles of the neck and into the chest.

Muscle Concerns

Fibrotic adhesions from acute or chronic trauma are key players in thoracic outlet syndrome. Once the area can tolerate it, incorporate movement into the strokes to help break them up. Use the same techniques in the same positions here as those described for treating whiplash (see pages 120–121). The focus should be to remove pressure on the structures that are involved, as discovered during the assessment.

Stretching

Active Isolated Stretching techniques are very effective in lengthening the tissues without irritating the entrapped structures. The anterior stretches should be emphasized first because the postural predispositions and entrapment sites are on the anterior side. Therapists may use the stretches that were used for the neck, adapting them to each situation (see Figs. 5-23 to 5-28). The stretches for the chest and shoulder are discussed in Chapter 7 and can be used for this condition, as well (see pages 249–252).

SUMMARY

This chapter began with a review of the anatomy of the head and neck region and gave detailed directions on how to locate various bony landmarks and structures. The range of motion and manual muscle tests for the region were covered so that any abnormalities can be noted. Next, the chapter discussed the last piece of general information for the region: the trigger-point locations for the various muscles in the area. Once the baseline information for the region is obtained, the therapist can begin treatment. Thus, the chapter concluded with a detailed explanation of specific conditions and how to assess and treat them.

REVIEW QUESTIONS

1. What are the bones of the skull and face?
2. What are the anterior and posterior components of the cervical vertebrae?
3. What are the structures that create the boundaries for the anterior and posterior cervical triangles?
4. Which nerve roots make up the brachial plexus?
5. What are the movements of the cervical region?
6. What are the dermatomes for the cervical region?
7. What is the grading system for whiplash, and what does each grade mean?
8. What causes the clicking noises in TMJ?
9. What are the three causes of torticollis? Describe them.
10. What is the difference between a bulging disk and a ruptured disk?
11. What are the neurologic and vascular symptoms of thoracic outlet syndrome?
12. What are the four gates that the neurovascular structures pass through in the neck?

CRITICAL-THINKING QUESTIONS

1. How does the position of the head at the time of impact influence assessing and treating whiplash?
2. Why is it important to limit but not prevent motion during the initial phases of whiplash?
3. Why is it important to determine the classification of torticollis?

4. How is connective tissue massage beneficial in treating cervical disk injuries?

5. What is the reason for performing cervical distraction if the test for cervical compression is positive?

6. How can breathing patterns affect thoracic outlet syndrome?

7. Why is thoracic outlet syndrome sometimes misdiagnosed as an elbow or wrist condition?

8. How does posture contribute to thoracic outlet syndrome?

Bony Surface Anatomy of the Skull

Frontal bone	Bone that is located at the front of the skull and constitutes the forehead.
Supraciliary arch	Arch at the top of the orbit at the approximate location of the eyebrows.
Supraorbital foramen/ frontal sinus	Follow medially along the arch until feeling a rounded, flat area at the medial corner of the eyebrow. This is where the supraorbital nerve exits; the frontal sinus is deep to it.
Infraorbital foramen	This is just lateral to the inferior portion of the nose at the inferior medial orbit of the eye. It is home to the infraorbital nerve; the maxillary sinus is deep to it.
Nasion	Junction between the nasal and frontal bones. A horizontal suture designates the spot and can be felt by palpating in a vertical direction.
Nasal bone	Just below the nasion on either side.
Maxilla	This bone makes up the center of the face, the area around the nose, the inferior portion of the orbit of the eye, and the front portion of the cheek. It holds the upper teeth intact.
Zygomatic bone and arch	Follow the inferior orbit of the eye and continue laterally to find the arch, which constitutes the cheekbone.
Mandibular condyle	Located just anterior to the external auditory meatus. Open and close the mouth to feel it move forward and down. This forms the TMJ with the temporal bone.
Coronoid process	Use the mandibular condyle as a starting place, and move about 1 inch anteriorly and under the zygomatic arch. Have the client open his or her mouth fully to feel the process.
Ramus of the mandible	The vertical portion from the mandibular condyle to the corner of the jaw.
Angle of the mandible	The corner of the jaw.
Body of the mandible	The long horizontal portion of the mandible from the angle to the front of the jaw. It holds the lower teeth intact.
Mental protuberance	The very front midline of the jaw.
Occipital bone	Located at the inferior and posterior positions of the skull, it constitutes the back of the head.
External occipital protuberance or inion	Bump located midline and at the center of the occiput.
Superior nuchal line	Located laterally in either direction from the external occipital protuberance.
Temporal bone	Located at the side of the head; it encompasses the ear.
Mastoid process	Located on the temporal bone, this is the "bump" behind the ear.
Sagittal suture	The suture between the parietal bones.
Coronal suture	The suture between the frontal and parietal bones.

Soft Tissue Surface Anatomy of the Skull

Glabella	The area of skin between the eyebrows.
Superficial temporal artery/ pulse	Trace the zygomatic arch to the ear. Move just superior, and use very light pressure.
Parotid gland	Located superficially over the posterior portion of the masseter muscle, this gland envelops the angle of the mandible. It feels like a small cluster of nodules.
Parotid duct	This duct runs horizontally from the gland into the mouth. Locate the anterior border of the masseter muscle. Palpate just below the zygomatic arch at the anterior border of the masseter in an up-and-down fashion.
Submandibular gland	Located up and under the body of the mandible. It sits about halfway between the angle of the mandible and the mental protuberance.
Submandibular lymph nodes	These nodes are located in the same area as the submandibular salivary gland. They are smaller and more rounded in feel.
Facial artery/ pulse	This structure lies on the body of the mandible at the anterior border of the masseter muscle. Locate the anterior border of the masseter. Go to the most anterior border of the muscle on the body of the mandible, and palpate for a pulse.
Submental lymph nodes	Located under the chin at the mental protuberance.
Facial nerve	Stand behind the client, and place an open hand on the side of his or her face so that the ear is under your palm and your thumb is aimed just above the orbit (temporal branch); index finger is over the zygomatic arch (zygomatic branch); middle finger is aimed between the nose and upper lip (buccal branch); ring finger is aimed under the bottom lip above the chin (mandibular branch); and little finger is facing down and anterior across the neck (cervical branch).
Auricle	The cartilaginous outer portion of the ear.
External auditory meatus	The external opening of the ear canal.
Helix	The outer ring of the auricle.
Antihelix	The inner smaller ring, which runs parallel to the helix.
Triangular fossa	Superior fossa dividing the antihelix.
Tragus	The projection or flap that lies on the anterior part of the external auditory meatus. It faces posterior and partially covers the ear canal.
Antitragus	The projection that sits opposite and inferior to the tragus.
Lobule	The earlobe.
Pre- and postauricular lymph nodes	Located just in front of the ear canal and just behind the ears.
Suboccipital lymph nodes	Located at the base of the occiput on either side, posterior to the mastoid process but not all the way to the midline.
Greater occipital nerve	Located midpoint between the mastoid process and the external occipital protuberance along the occiput. This nerve runs in a vertical direction, so palpate in a transverse direction.

Bony Surface Anatomy of the Neck

Posterior tubercle of C1	Usually too small to palpate. It lies midline directly inferior to the external occipital protuberance in the soft tissue space. This is palpated easier in the supine position.
Transverse process of C1	Pick a point midway between the angle of the mandible and the mastoid process. Palpate behind the ear, anterior to the SCM, going deep but gently.
Posterior arch of C1	Move lateral to the tubercle on either side. The arch is halfway between the tubercle and the mastoid process. Move from the tubercle lateral to the paraspinal musculature, and palpate vertically for a bony ridge.
Spinous process of C2 (axis)	Usually the first palpable spinous process. It is inferior from the external occipital protuberance. It is almost always bifurcated.
Cervical facet joints of C2	From the C2 spinous process, move out laterally until you are off the erector spinae and other musculature. This is the superior facet of C2.
C7 spinous process	The most prominent and easiest cervical vertebra to palpate. To distinguish between C7 and C6 or T1, locate what you think is C7. Have the client extend the neck. If the spinous process disappears, move down until finding one that does not disappear. This is C7. If the spinous process does not disappear, move up until finding one that does. The last spinous process before the one that disappeared is C7.
Hyoid bone	This bone lies under the chin above the voice box. Place your thumb and first finger on either side of the anterior neck just below the mandible. Gently squeeze and move your thumb and finger back and forth.

Soft Tissue Surface Anatomy of the Neck

Thyroid cartilage	Known as the "Adam's apple." This structure lies on the anterior neck, just below the hyoid bone.
1st cricoid ring	Using the thyroid cartilage, move inferiorly until finding an indentation. The next structure down is the cricoid ring.
C6 transverse process (anterior tubercle)	Using the 1st cricoid ring, move lateral but stay medial to the sternocleidomastoid muscle. Palpate posteriorly until feeling a bony prominence.
Posterior cervical triangle	This triangle is bound by several structures: anteriorly by the sternocleidomastoid muscle, posteriorly by the upper trapezius, and inferiorly by the clavicle
Anterior cervical triangle	This triangle is bound anteriorly by the midline of the neck, the inferior border of the mandible, and the sternocleidomastoid muscle.
Nuchal ligament	Have the client flex the head and neck to the end range; then palpate in a transverse direction at the midline of the cervical vertebrae.

Bony Surface Anatomy of the Shoulder

Manubrium	Most superior portion of the sternum.
Suprasternal notch	This is the notch or indentation at the top of the sternum.
Sternoclavicular joint	Using the suprasternal notch, move just lateral and you will feel the medial edge of the clavicle.
Clavicle	An S-shaped bone anterior to posterior that runs between the sternum and the scapula. Trace the bone from the sternum to the scapula.
Acromion process	The L-shaped lateral end of the spine of the scapula. Place the palm of your hand on the lateral tip of the shoulder, and move it in a circular fashion. You will feel a flat, bony surface. Use your fingertips to trace the borders.
Acromioclavicular joint	Trace the clavicle to its lateral edge. You should feel a space where it meets the acromion process.

Muscles of the Head and Face

Muscle	Origin	Insertion	Action	How to Palpate
Frontalis	Galea aponeurotica	Skin over eyebrows	Raises eyebrows; wrinkles forehead	Supine position; wrinkle forehead
Occipitalis	Galea aponeurotica	Superior nuchal line	Retracts the galea	Slide superior to nuchal line
Temporalis	Temporal fossa	Coronoid process of the mandible	Elevates the mandible	Clench teeth and palpate over ear
Obicularis occuli	Skin around eyes	Skin around eyes	Squeezes eyes closed	Squeeze eyes closed and palpate around them
Obicularis oris	Skin around lips	Skin around lips	Puckers lips	Pucker lips and palpate around them
Masseter	Zygomatic arch	Angle and ramus of the mandible	Closes, protracts, and laterally shifts jaw	Clench teeth and palpate over jaw in front of ear
Medial pterygoid	Pterygoid plate	Medial surface of the ramus of the mandible	Closes, protracts, and laterally shifts jaw	Intraorally or extraorally
Lateral pterygoid	Pterygoid plate	TMJ	Closes, protracts, and laterally shifts jaw	Intraorally or extraorally

Muscles of the Posterior Neck

Muscle	Origin	Insertion	Action	How to Palpate
Erector spinae group	Thoracolumbar aponeurosis; posterior sacrum; iliac crest; lumbar vertebra	Posterior ribs; thoracic and cervical vertebrae; mastoid process; nuchal line	Extends vertebral column; laterally flexes vertebral column to same side	Prone position; extend legs and trunk
Levator scapulae	Transverse processes of C1-C4	Superior angle of the scapula	Elevates, endorotates the scapula; laterally flexes head and neck; extends head and neck	Prone position; find superior angle and shrug shoulder
Splenius capitis	C7-T3 spinous processes; ligamentum nuchae	Lateral nuchal line; mastoid process	Laterally flexes and rotates neck to same side; extends head	Prone position; extend and rotate head; palpate between upper trapezius and SCM
Suboccipitals	Spinous process of C2; transverse process and tubercle of C1	Nuchal line; transverse process of C1	Extends head; rotates head to same side	Outlined by triangle between C2 spinous process, C1 transverse process; nuchal line
Trapezius	External occipital protuberance; nuchal ligament; C7-T12 spinous processes	Lateral third of clavicle; spine; acromion process of scapula	Elevates, depresses, retracts, endorotates, exorotates scapula; laterally rotates head to opposite side; extends head	Prone or standing position; resist shoulder elevation, retraction, or depression

Muscles of the Anterior Neck

Muscle	Origin	Insertion	Action	How to Palpate
Scalenes	Transverse processes of C2-C7	1st and 2nd ribs	Laterally flexes head to same side; rotates head to opposite side; flexes neck; elevates ribs during forced inhalation	Supine position; rotate head to opposite side and palpate in posterior cervical triangle
Sternocleidomastoid	Medial third of clavicle; manubrium of sternum	Mastoid process	Laterally flexes to same side, rotates to opposite side; flexes neck	Supine position; rotate head to opposite side, prominent muscle running from mastoid process to sternum
Suprahyoids (mylohyoids, digastrics, stylohyoids, geniohyoids)	Underside of mandible; styloid process; mastoid process	Hyoid bone; inferior border of the mandible	Elevates hyoid and tongue; depresses mandible	Supine position; superior to hyoid bone running to mandible
Infrahyoids (thyrohyoid, sternohyoid, sternothyroid, omohyoid)	Manubrium; superior border of scapula	Hyoid bone; thyroid cartilage	Depresses hyoid bone and thyroid cartilage	Supine position; inferior to hyoid running to sternum

Trigger Points for the Head and Neck Muscles

Muscle	Trigger-Point Location	Referral Pattern	Chief Symptom
Frontalis	Just superior to eye	Up and over forehead on same side	Pain
Occipitalis	Belly of muscle at back of head	Diffusely over back of head; deep into orbit of eye	Pain; cannot rest head on pillow; must lie on side
Temporalis	1. Anterior portion of muscle above and in front of ear 2. Middle of muscle 3. Middle of muscle 4. Posterior aspect of muscle	Eyebrow; upper teeth; temple; TMJ	Pain in the different locations; commonly involved in TMJ dysfunction
Masseter	1. Musculotendinous junction 2. Midbelly 3. Angle 4. Deep layer	Upper molars; maxilla; lower molars; mandible; up and over eyebrow; anterior ear	TMJ dysfunction; restricts jaw opening; tinnitus
Medial pterygoid	Midbelly of muscle	Ear; back of mouth; TMJ	Exacerbated by chewing, opening mouth too wide, clenching teeth
Lateral pterygoid	On the muscle adjacent to medial surface of coracoid process	Deep into TMJ; maxillary sinus	TMJ dysfunction
Sternocleidomastoid	1. Sternal head 2. Clavicular head	Sternum; cheek; maxilla; occipital ridge; top of head; frontal bone; deep into ear	No neck pain or stiffness associated with these points
Scalenes	1. Anterior 2. Posterior 3. Middle	Upper border of scapula; posterior shoulder; front and back of arm; radial sides of forearm, thumb and index finger; anterior chest	Scapular, shoulder, back, and arm pain
Supra- and infrahyoids	Various points in the muscles	Lower incisor teeth; tongue; head and neck	Difficulty swallowing; something stuck in throat
Suboccipitals	Base of skull	Deep into skull; diffuse pain in back of head	Often involves larger cervical muscles

Trigger Points for the Head and Neck Muscles *(Continued)*

Splenius capitis/cervicis	Upper portion of muscle where upper trapezius crosses, midmuscle	Pain behind eye, top of head, base of neck	Limited neck ROM; pain
Levator scapulae	Superior angle of the scapula, halfway up muscle	Angle of neck; posterior shoulder	Pain, stiffness; limited neck ROM
Upper trapezius	In angle of neck on anterior and posterior side of muscle	Up and over ear in ram's horn pattern; back of the neck behind ear	Tension headaches

Orthopedic Tests for the Head and Neck

Condition	Orthopedic Test	How to Perform	Positive Sign
Whiplash	None	Various tests are performed to rule out other conditions.	NA
TMJ dysfunction	None	Joint can be auscultated to determine sounds.	NA
Torticollis	None	Assess TMJ and cervical spine for involvement.	NA
Cervical disk injuries	Cervical compression test	Client seated. Stand behind client with head and neck in a neutral position. Interlace fingers and place on top of client's head. Gently press straight down.	Any pain or increase in neurologic symptoms
	Cervical distraction	Client seated. Stand to side of client. Cradle occiput using one hand; cradle the mandible with the other. Gently lift up on the head.	A decrease in pain or associated symptoms (increase in pain indicates possible ligamentous injury)
	Spurling's test	Client seated. Stand behind client. Have client laterally flex and rotate the head to the side of the complaint. Interlace your fingers and press down on the head.	An increase in pain and symptoms

Orthopedic Tests for the Head and Neck

Condition	Orthopedic Test	How to Perform	Positive Sign
Thoracic Outlet Syndrome	Roos Test	Client in standing position. Have client abduct the shoulder to 90° and flex the elbows to 90°. Slightly externally rotate and horizontally abduct shoulders so that they are just behind the frontal plane. Have the client slowly open and close the hands for 3 minutes.	Ischemic pain, profound weakness in the arm, or numbness or tingling in the hand. Minor symptom reproduction is considered a negative sign.
	Adson maneuver *Note:* This is the most common test performed, but it has also been proved unreliable.	Client seated. Locate the radial pulse on side you are testing. Extend and externally rotate the arm, keeping it below horizontal. Have client rotate head and look at hand being tested. Instruct the client to take a deep breath	Any diminishing or disappearance of the pulse indicates a positive sign.
	Allen test	Client in seated position. Locate the radial pulse of the client on the test side. Flex the elbow and shoulder to 90°. Horizontally abduct and laterally rotate the arm. Have the client rotate the head and look away from the side being tested.	Any change or disappearance of the pulse is an indication of a positive test.
	Cyriax release test *Note:* This is also known as the *passive shoulder girdle elevation test* and involves the release phenomenon. That is, neurovascular symptoms that present as a result of compression will change if the structures causing the compression are moved.	Client in seated position. Stand behind the client, and hold the elbows in 90° of flexion and the forearms and wrists in a neutral position. Lean the client back about 15°, and passively elevate the shoulders just shy of the end range. Hold the position for 1 to 3 minutes.	A positive result can take one of two forms: If the client has active symptoms, a reduction or relief of those symptoms indicates a positive test. One interpretation of the release phenomenon is that compressed nerve trunks will initially display symptoms but will return to normal; hence, a reproduction of the client's symptoms also indicates a positive test.

chapter 6

Conditions of the Lumbar Spine and Sacrum

chapter outline

chapter objectives

At the conclusion of this chapter, the reader will understand:

- bony anatomy of the region
- how to locate the bony landmarks and soft tissue structures of the region
- where to find the muscles, and the origins, insertions, and actions of the region
- how to assess the movement and determine the range of motion for the region
- how to perform manual muscle testing to the region
- how to recognize dermatome patterns for the region
- trigger-point location and referral patterns for the region
- the following elements of each condition discussed:
  - background and characteristics
  - specific questions to ask
  - what orthopedic tests should be performed
  - how to treat connective tissue, trigger points, and muscles
  - flexibility concerns

key terms

congenital spondylolysis

contranutation

developmental spondylolysis

facet joint syndrome

nutation

sacroiliac joint (SIJ) dysfunction

spondylolisthesis

spondylolysis

Introduction The lumbar spine and the sacrum can be significant sources of dysfunction. Studies have estimated that up to 70% of adults have experienced low-back pain during their lifetime, with 50% reporting it every year (Jackson and Browning, 2005). Compared to pain in the cervical spine, low-back pain more often originates from chronic behavior than from acute trauma. "Back pain has been identified as the leading cause of disability among persons under the age of 45 years and the third leading cause of disability among those 45 years of age or older" (McGeary et al., 2003). Back pain accounts for 200,000 office visits per year—1.8% of the total medical visits in the United States (Jackson and Browning, 2005). Despite its high percentage of occurrence, only 25% of people with physical symptoms seek medical attention. Most back injuries are relatively minor and will resolve within a month; however, a minority of people—around 10%—develop chronic conditions that make up 80% of the cost associated with the disorder.

Management of low-back pain continues to be challenging (Maluf et al., 2000), especially because there are many different variables and sources from which the pain can originate. Despite having knowledge of the structures involved, a large percentage (up to 85%) of cases are classified as "nonspecific" because a definitive diagnosis cannot be made with current methods (O'Sullivan, 2005). A nonspecific diagnosis is sometimes referred to as "lumbago," but the cause of pain is usually narrowed down through a process of elimination to ensure that the correct treatment is administered.

This chapter seeks to clarify some of the major causes of lumbar spine and sacral dysfunction. In addition to reviewing the structures, this chapter discusses:

- Specific bony landmarks for palpation
- Soft tissue structures, including the muscles of the region
- The movements of the region, and basic biomechanics of the lumbar spine and sacrum
- Manual muscle tests for the lumbar spine
- Dermatome and trigger-point referral patterns for the involved muscles
- Some common causes of dysfunction and how to assess and treat them using soft tissue therapy

ANATOMICAL REVIEW

Bony Anatomy of the Lumbar Spine

Each region of the spine—cervical, thoracic, and lumbar—has its own vertebrae. The shape of each individual vertebra changes from region to region, enabling function or restricting movement in the area. Moving in an inferior direction, you'll notice a progressive increase in the size of each vertebra in order to support the weight of each vertebra above it. The lumbar vertebrae are the largest and densest because they furnish support to the upper body and transmit that weight to the pelvis and lower limbs.

Of the total vertebrae, there are five segments that create the *lumbar spine.* They are shaped very differently and have characteristic thick, stout bodies with squared spinous processes (Fig. 6-1). This lumbar spine is the location of one of the secondary curves in the spine that develops as a result of supporting the weight of the torso and upright locomotion; the other secondary curve is the *cervical spine.*

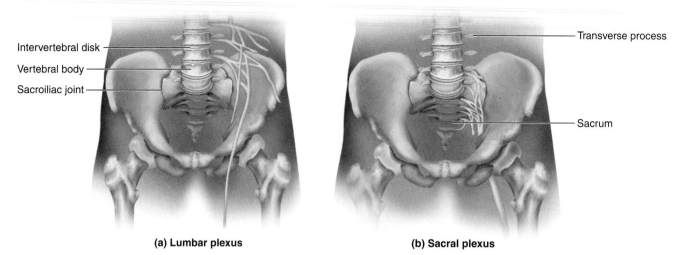

Intervertebral disk
Vertebral body
Sacroiliac joint
Transverse process
Sacrum

(a) Lumbar plexus　　　　**(b) Sacral plexus**

Figure 6-1 Structures of the lumbar spine and sacrum. *(a)* Lumbar plexus. *(b)* Sacral plexus.

> **Practical Tip**
>
> The two locations of the secondary curves are the lumbar and cervical spines.

Continuing from the other vertebrae in the spine, the lumbar spine has a vertebral foramen that allows for the passage of the spinal cord. The transverse processes of the lumbar vertebrae lie directly lateral to the corresponding spinous processes. When the vertebrae are stacked, an intervertebral foramen is created to allow the lumbar spinal nerves to exit. These nerve roots create the lumbar plexus (see Fig. 6-1). The posterior branches of the 2nd through 4th nerve roots form the femoral nerve that supplies the quadriceps, while its anterior branches form the obturator nerve, innervating a majority of the adductors. The lumbar plexus is summarized in Table 6-1.

The orientation of the lumbar facets contributes to their function. There are five pairs of facets (superior and inferior) that are oriented in a vertical fashion, which limits rotation but allows side bending, flexion, and extension at the segment (see Fig. 6-2). The primary job of the facets is to allow movement; they should not function as weight-bearing structures.

The *intervertebral disks* function as weight-bearing structures; their main functions are to absorb shock, allow movement, and hold the vertebrae apart in conjunction with the facets to allow the free passage of the nerve roots out of the spinal cord to the body. It is the last function—creating a space for the nerve root to exit—that is so important. The disks create 20% to 25% of the height of the spinal column. As we age, the disks lose

Table 6-1　Nerves and Motor Innervations of the Lumbar Plexus

Level	Innervation
L1	Internal and external obliques, transverse abdominus
L2	Iliopsoas, anterior thigh muscles
L3	Quadriceps, pectineus, sartorius
L4	Adductor longus, brevis, magnus, gracilis

their height as a result of degeneration and the loss of hydrophilic action. The loss of height within the spinal column leads to less space for the nerve to exit and can result in problems with nerve entrapments.

The same three ligaments that support the cervical spine support the lumbar spine region as well:

- *Anterior longitudinal ligament (ALL):* Prevents excessive extension of the spine and increases its thickness as it moves from the cervical to the lumbar region
- *Posterior longitudinal ligament (PLL):* Prevents excessive flexion of the spine and decreases its thickness as it moves into the lumbar region
- *Supraspinous ligament:* Connects the spinous processes of the vertebra to prevent excessive flexion

Despite this support, there are certain positions that can place more stress on the lumbar spine than others can. Constant excessive extension in the spine can cause a lot of stress through the facet joints. Rotation in the spine can lead to wear and tear on the disks. Repetition of these postures can lead to dysfunction in the area.

Bony Structures and Surface Anatomy of the Lumbar Spine

Palpation in the lumbar spine region is not easy. While there are fewer delicate structures in this region than in the anterior neck, the therapist must take care to avoid causing injury. There is generally more tissue in this area to palpate, and the structures are typically deeper (Fig. 6-2).

Posterior Lumbar Spine

The *lamina groove* is continuous through all the regions of the spine. It runs on either side of the spinous processes from the cervical region to the sacral region. Using this groove, it is possible to identify the spinous processes of the lumbar spine. First, find the junction between the thoracic and lumbar divisions. The last thoracic vertebra (T12) should be in line with the 12th rib. With the client in the prone position, place

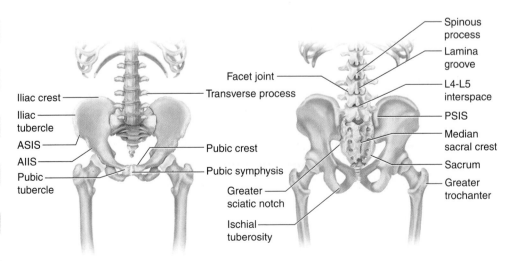

Iliac crest
Iliac tubercle
ASIS
AIIS
Pubic tubercle

Facet joint
Transverse process

Pubic crest
Pubic symphysis

Greater sciatic notch

Ischial tuberosity

Spinous process
Lamina groove
L4-L5 interspace
PSIS
Median sacral crest
Sacrum
Greater trochanter

Figure 6-2 Bony structures and surface anatomy of the lumbar spine.

your hands in the soft flank, and press up and in. Trace the rib back to the spine, and you will be on T12. Using that spinous process as a starting point, move in an inferior direction, locating each lumbar spinous process. There are some quick reference landmarks you can use to check yourself. The *umbilicus* is generally opposite L3-L4. The *L4-L5 interspace* should line up with the top of the iliac crest. To locate the interspace, stand behind the client, and place the palms of your hands in the flank area just below the ribs. Press down and in; you should feel the top of the *iliac crests*, using your fingertips to trace the edges. With your hands on the top of the crests, touch your thumbs together and place them on the client. They should fall into the L4-L5 interspace. If you move up, you will be on the spinous process of L4; if you move down, you will be on the spinous process of L5.

Once you have located the spinous processes, the *transverse processes of L1-L5* are directly lateral. Start on the corresponding spinous process of the transverse process you want to locate. Move laterally so that you are lateral to the musculature. Press in toward the spine; you should feel a projection, which is the transverse process. The longest and easiest to find is L3. L1 and L5 are more difficult to locate as they are partially covered by other structures—the 12th rib and the iliac crest, respectively.

Anterior Lumbar Spine and Pelvis

Moving around to the front, identify structures on the pelvis to help define the region (see Fig. 6-2). From the iliac crest, move anteriorly to find the widest points on the crests: the *iliac tubercles*. Continuing around the front of the ilium, the *anterior superior iliac spine (ASIS)* is the most anterior part of the crest and should be obvious.

An alternate method of finding this landmark is to have the client lie in the supine position and place the palms of your hands on the front of the client's hips. You should feel two bony prominences, which might be sensitive to the touch. From the ASIS, move inferiorly about one-half inch where the thigh blends into the trunk to locate the *anterior inferior iliac spine (AIIS)*. Because of its depth and the fact that it is the origin of the rectus femoris, you won't be able to directly palpate this structure.

The *pubic crest* is palpated by placing your fingertips in the umbilicus and resting your hand in an inferior direction on the abdomen. Slowly press down and in; the heel of your hand will hit a bony ledge. This is the crest. Use your fingertips to trace its edges and the other landmarks in the area. The *pubic symphysis* is the joint directly in the middle of the crest; it joins the two pelvic bones anteriorly. The *pubic tubercles* lie on either edge of the pubic crest and are palpated by moving laterally to either side of the crest.

The last bony structures are the *anterior transverse processes of the lumbar spine* (see Fig. 6-2). These structures are deep and need to be palpated carefully. Have the client lie in the supine position and flex the knees to soften the abdomen. Use the umbilicus and ASIS as reference points. Starting at the ASIS, slide into the tissue until you reach the lateral edge of the rectus abdominus. Once there, direct pressure downward while the client relaxes and continues to breathe normally. As you sink into the abdomen, you should feel the firmness of the lumbar vertebrae. The iliopsoas muscle lies over the top of these. Verify your hand placement by having the client gently flex the hip to feel the psoas contract into your fingers.

Soft Tissue Structures of the Lumbar Spine

Identifying the lumbar spine soft tissue structures, though they are not necessarily treated through soft tissue manipulation, will help the overall treatment plan (Fig. 6-3). The *inguinal ligament* is located on a line between the ASIS of the ilium and the pubic tubercles; it is the inferior edge of the oblique abdominal muscles. The *costal margin* is the border formed by the inferior aspect of the rib cage separating it from the upper abdomen. The *umbilicus*, or the belly button, lies at the level of L3-L4. It is an important reference point for finding other landmarks.

To find the *abdominal aorta*, pick a point between the xiphoid process and the umbilicus, just left of midline. Use your fingertips, and press in gently as the client relaxes. It is an easily palpated strong pulse in most people, but you may have to move up or down to find it. The *spleen* is found by placing one hand on the left back around T10-T11 and lifting up. Place the other hand at the left costal margin, and gently press up and in. Have the client take a deep breath; you should feel the edge of the spleen move into your fingers.

The *liver* is found in much the same way. Place one hand on the right side of the back around T10-T11, and lift up gently. Using the fingers of the other hand, press up and in at the right costal margin with moderate pressure. Have the client take a deep breath; you should feel the edge of the liver move into your fingers. Don't be surprised if you cannot feel the liver or the spleen. Depending on the health and size of the person, you will feel them only if there is a problem in the area. On the posterior side, the *cluneal nerves* are located along the iliac crest. Locate the posterior superior iliac spine (PSIS) and the iliac tubercles. Find the midpoint along the iliac crest, and palpate these vertically oriented nerves in a transverse direction.

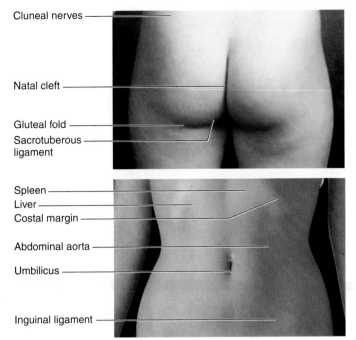

Cluneal nerves
Natal cleft
Gluteal fold
Sacrotuberous ligament
Spleen
Liver
Costal margin
Abdominal aorta
Umbilicus
Inguinal ligament

Figure 6-3 Soft tissue structures of the lumbar spine region.

Bony Anatomy of the Sacrum

The *sacrum* is an important structure that can affect the hips, pelvis, and lumbar spine (see Fig. 6-2). It is essentially a bony plate that forms the back of the pelvic girdle, which comprises the two ilium bones and the sacrum. This locks the two pelvic bones together and acts as the "keystone" of the pelvis the same way the central, wedge-shaped stone of an arch locks its parts together. The sacrum is the link between the axial and lower appendicular skeletons. The sacrum comprises five vertebrae that begin to fuse around the age of 16 and are fully fused by the age of 26. In some cases, the first sacral section does not fuse and will essentially function as a 6th lumbar vertebra. This condition is referred to as a *lumbarization of S1,* and it may or may not cause problems. Additionally, there is a condition in which the 5th lumbar vertebra can become fused to the sacrum, resulting in what is known as a *sacrilization of L5* and leaving only four mobile lumbar vertebrae. In a normal spine, the angle between the lumbar spine and the sacrum is 140°, and the sacrum is positioned at an angle of 30°. Any deviation in these angles can be a predisposition to dysfunction.

The anterior surface of the sacrum is concave and relatively smooth. It has four large holes on either side called *sacral foramina,* which allow the passage of nerves and vessels to the pelvic organs. The posterior surface, in contrast, is very rough as a result of the various soft tissue attachments to it. As the spinous processes fused, they formed a ridge down the center known as the *median sacral crest.* The transverse processes also fused into a less prominent structure called the *lateral sacral crest.* As with the anterior side, four posterior sacral foramina allow the passage of nerves that supply the gluteals and lower limbs.

These anterior nerve roots make up what is known as the *sacral plexus* (see Fig. 6-1). The upper portion of the plexus is actually formed by the lower part of the lumbar plexus (L4-L5); the lower portion of the plexus forms the sciatic nerve, which comprises two distinct nerves. The tibial nerve is formed by the anterior branches of the five upper roots and supplies the posterior leg. The common peroneal nerve is formed by the posterior branches of the four upper roots and supplies the short head of the biceps femoris before splitting behind the knee to form the deep and superficial peroneal nerves, which innervate the anterior and lateral compartments of the lower leg. Table 6-2 summarizes the sacral plexus.

Table 6-2 Nerves and Motor Innervations of the Sacral Plexus

Level	Innervation
L4-L5	Gluteus medius, gluteus minimus, tensor fascia latae
S1	Gluteus maximus
S2	Piriformis, deep lateral rotators, extensor hallucis longus, extensor digitorum longus
S3	Hamstrings, gastrocnemius, soleus, flexor digitorum longus, tibialis posterior, flexor hallucis longus
S4	Muscles of perineum

On either side of the sacrum are articular surfaces that form the sacroiliac joints with the iliums of the pelvis. Through these joints, the weight of the upper body is transferred to the lower limbs, lessening the bumps and jars received by the lower extremities.

The joints are both synovial and syndesmotic. The *synovial* portion of the joint is formed by the articulation of the C-shaped convex surface of the ilium with the concave surface of the sacrum. Both surfaces are covered with hyaline cartilage, but the cartilage is three times thicker on the sacral surface. These surfaces start out smooth in children and roughen through age due to the stresses placed on the joint. As a result, the joint becomes less mobile and more stable. The *syndesmotic* portion of the joint comes from the numerous strong ligaments that bind the joint together and fill in the spaces between the sacrum and the ilium. The ligaments in the area are:

- *Interosseous sacroiliac ligaments:* Bind the anterior and posterior portions of the sacrum, thereby filling in gaps between the sacrum and ilium
- *Dorsal sacroiliac ligament:* Binds the posterior ilium to the upper portion of the sacrum, and binds the lower sacrum to the PSIS
- *Ventral sacroiliac ligament:* Lines the anterior sacrum
- *Sacrotuberous ligament:* Arises from ischial tuberosity and merges with the dorsal sacroiliac ligament
- *Sacrospinous ligament:* Indirectly supports the sacrum through its attachment from the ischial spine to the coccyx

Injury to these structures or imbalances in the muscles can lead to dysfunction in the joint and cause pain.

Bony and Soft Tissue Structures and Surface Anatomy of the Sacrum

Since there are so few soft tissue structures associated with the sacrum, they are included in this section with the bony landmarks (see Figs. 6-2 and 6-3).

The *posterior superior iliac spines (PSISs)* are located on the most posterior aspect of the iliac crest. Using the crest, trace in a posterior direction until you are at the most posterior part. The PSIS prominences are commonly referred to as the "dimples" in the low back and are located at the level of the S2 spinous process. From the PSIS, fall medially onto the *sacrum*, which consists of four to five fused vertebrae and sits inferior to the lumbar spine. Once on the sacrum, use your fingertips to trace the *median sacral crest* down the center and its *lateral edge* in an inferior direction. The inferior end of the sacrum is generally at the top of the *natal cleft*, which is the area of tissue on the medial side between each buttock.

The *greater trochanter* of the femur is used as a reference to identify several other landmarks and lies on the proximal lateral thigh. Have the client lie in the prone position, and place the palm of your hand over his or her lateral hip. Bend the knee to 90°, press in on the hip, and rotate the leg medially and laterally. You should feel a large bony structure rotating under your hand. Use your fingertips to trace its borders, noting that the *trochanteric bursa* lies posterior to its lateral edge.

The *gluteal fold* is formed by the thigh as it meets the hip. Have the client lie in the prone position, and locate the fold at the base of the gluteus maximus muscle and the top of the hamstrings. Once you have located the fold, the *ischial tuberosity* is easy to locate. This structure is on the inferior ischium and is the common origin for the hamstrings. Using the gluteal fold, place the webspace of your hand with the thumb pointing medially along the fold. Press in; your thumb should be on the tuberosity.

The *sacrotuberous ligament* runs between the ischial tuberosity and the inferior lateral angle of the sacrum. Using the ischial tuberosity, roll a little superior and medial, and then press in. To make sure you are on the ligament, have the client cough; the ligament will tighten.

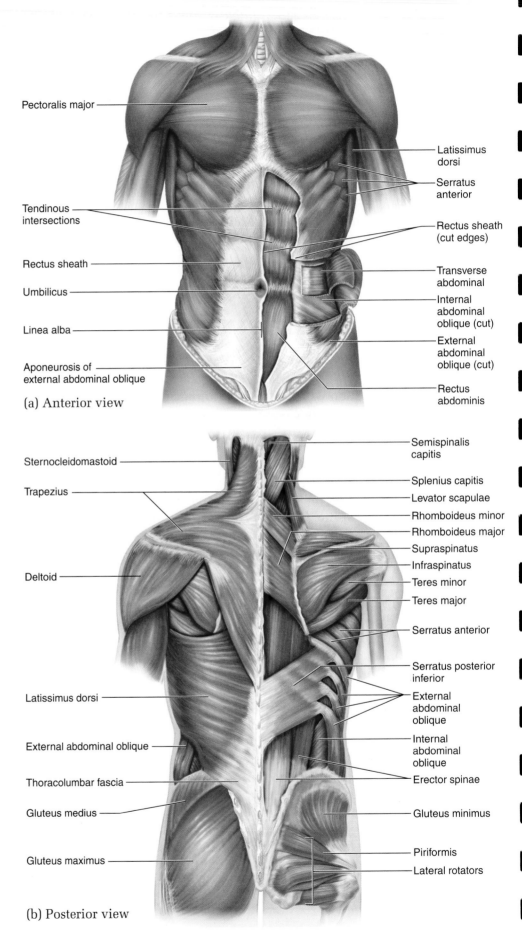

Figure 6-4 Muscles of the lumbar spine region. *(a)* Anterior view. *(b)* Posterior view.

Pectoralis major

Latissimus dorsi

Serratus anterior

Tendinous intersections

Rectus sheath (cut edges)

Rectus sheath

Transverse abdominal

Umbilicus

Internal abdominal oblique (cut)

Linea alba

External abdominal oblique (cut)

Aponeurosis of external abdominal oblique

Rectus abdominis

(a) Anterior view

Semispinalis capitis

Sternocleidomastoid

Splenius capitis

Trapezius

Levator scapulae

Rhomboideus minor

Rhomboideus major

Supraspinatus

Deltoid

Infraspinatus

Teres minor

Teres major

Serratus anterior

Serratus posterior inferior

Latissimus dorsi

External abdominal oblique

External abdominal oblique

Internal abdominal oblique

Thoracolumbar fascia

Erector spinae

Gluteus medius

Gluteus minimus

Gluteus maximus

Piriformis

Lateral rotators

(b) Posterior view

Part II Regional Approach to Treatment

The *greater sciatic notch* lies approximately in the middle of the hip and is the passageway of the sciatic nerve from the sacrum into the hip and leg. To find the notch, draw a line between the posterior superior iliac spine on the opposite side of the notch you are trying to locate and the greater trochanter on the same side of the notch you are trying to locate. Press in at the midpoint; you should be in a depression, which is the notch.

Muscles of the Lumbar Spine and Sacrum

The muscles of the lumbar spine and sacrum either are directly attached to or have an affect on the region (Fig. 6-4). Refer to the Quick Reference Table "Muscles of the Lumbar Spine and Sacrum" at the end of this chapter (page 206).

MOVEMENT AND MANUAL MUSCLE TESTING OF THE REGION

In order to assess specific conditions of the region, it is necessary to establish a baseline from which to work. This baseline is obtained using the tools discussed below.

Movements of the Region

Lumbar Spine

As is the case with the other regions of the spine, movement is generated through the coupling of movements in the individual segments. These movements are governed by the anatomical constraints of the region. For the lumbar spine, there are six basic movements:

- Flexion
- Extension
- Left and right rotation
- Left and right lateral flexion

No muscles directly control the movement of the sacrum; therefore, the contraction of other muscles affects the position of the sacrum. There are only two true movements that do not arise from a dysfunction. These occur in a nodding fashion and are referred to as:

1. **Nutation:** The posterior rotation of the ilium on the sacrum
2. **Contranutation:** The anterior rotation of the ilium on the sacrum

If these movements occur on one side and not the other, this will lead to dysfunction in the sacroiliac joint, which is discussed later in the chapter.

To begin gathering baseline information, it is necessary to determine both the active and the passive movements that are available at the joints. Chapter 4 discussed key points to look for when assessing ranges of motion; however, for the lumbar region, the normal ranges of motion are assessed differently. All assessments are done with the client in the standing position. The therapist should look for symmetry of movement

nutation The posterior rotation of the ilium on the sacrum.

contranutation The anterior rotation of the ilium on the sacrum.

between the sides and the willingness of the client to move, performing the most painful motions last. The greatest amount of movement occurs at L4-L5 and L5-S1.

- *Flexion:* Have the client bend forward with the arms hanging down. The client should be able to bend between 40° and 60°. Make sure that the motion is not arising from the hips or other parts of the spine. To check this, verify that the normal lordotic curve becomes flat or slightly reversed. If it does not, this can indicate hypomobility in the area.
- *Extension:* Extension is more limited due to the shape of the vertebra. Typically, extension is only about 20° to 35°. Have the client place his or her hands in the small of the back and bend backward.
- *Lateral flexion:* Have the client run his or her hand down the side of the thigh. Compare how far down he or she can go bilaterally. Flexion should be about 15° to 20°. The curve in the spine should be smooth with no obvious angles, which could indicate hypomobility at a segment. Make sure the client does not combine any other movement with lateral flexion.
- *Rotation:* This is the most limited movement due to the orientation of the facets; it occurs as a result of a shearing movement of the vertebra. Pelvic and hip movement must be canceled out either manually or by testing in a seated position. The normal range is 3° to 18°.

For the sacrum, since there is very little motion at the sacroiliac joint, look for unequal movement or a loss or increase in movement as other associated joints are moved.

Combined Movements

In assessing active ranges of motion in the lumbar spine, it is necessary to combine movements. Injuries in this area rarely occur from a "pure" movement such as flexion or extension. There are four combined movements that should be assessed. They are performed with the client in the standing position and should be done bilaterally.

- *Flexion with lateral flexion:* With the hands on the hips, the client bends forward and leans over to the side at the same time.
- *Extension with lateral flexion:* With the hands on the hips, the client bends backward and leans to the side at the same time.
- *Rotation with flexion:* From the same starting position, the client bends forward and twists at the same time.
- *Rotation with extension:* The client bends backward and twists at the same time.

Passive Range of Motion

Passive range of motion is difficult to test due to the size of the trunk and how it would have to be handled. Assess passive range of motion by applying gentle overpressure during active testing or by checking the end-feel of each vertebra during joint-play assessment.

Manual Muscle Testing

Once the range of motion in the region is determined, assess the overall strength of the region and individual muscles that pertain to conditions in the region. To handle issues of compensation, test the client in a seated position (Fig. 6-5).

- *Flexion:* Stand in front of or on the side of the client. Have the client resist while you push him or her into extension. Make sure the contraction is isometric by advising the client, "Don't let me move you."
- *Extension:* Stand behind or on the side of the client. Have the client resist while you push him or her into flexion.

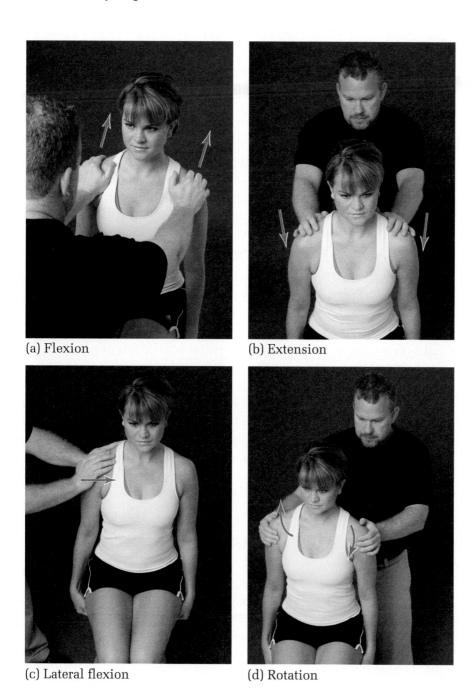

(a) Flexion

(b) Extension

(c) Lateral flexion

(d) Rotation

Figure 6-5 Manual muscle tests for the lumbar spine. *(a)* Flexion. *(b)* Extension. *(c)* Lateral flexion. *(d)* Rotation.

- *Lateral flexion:* Stand on the side of the client. Have the client resist while you push him or her into lateral flexion to the opposite side. Repeat for the other side.
- *Rotation:* Stand behind the client. Place your hands on the client's shoulders, and have the client resist while you rotate him or her in either direction.

In addition to tests for the general strength of the region, there are specific tests to determine whether individual nerve roots are involved. They test the myotomes of the region and are performed the same way as are other resisted-muscle tests:

- *L1-L2—hip flexion:* Have the client lie in the supine position. Flex the thigh to 40° while supporting the lower leg off the table with your bottom hand. Place your other hand just proximal to the client's knee. While the client resists, try to move him or her into hip extension. Make sure the client does not increase his or her lumbar lordosis during this test.
- *L3—knee extension:* This can be performed with the client's leg hanging off the table. Flex the client's knee to 30°, and apply a force with the other hand at the midshaft of the tibia while the client resists.
- *L4—ankle dorsiflexion:* Have the client lie in the supine position. Place his or her feet at 90° relative to the leg. Place your hands on the tops of the feet, and push them into plantar flexion while the client resists.
- *L5—great-toe extension:* Place the client in the supine position, and have him or her hold the great toes in a neutral position. Apply force to the tops of the toes while the client resists.
- *S1—ankle plantar flexion, ankle eversion, hip extension:*
  - *Ankle plantar flexion:* Have the client lie in the supine position, and hold his or her feet in a neutral position. Have the client resist while you apply force on the bottom of the feet and push him or her into dorsiflexion.
  - *Ankle eversion:* Have the client resist while you apply force to the outside of the foot and move it into inversion.
  - *Hip extension:* This test is done only if the client is unable to perform the other two. Have the client lie in the prone position, and flex his or her knee to 90°. Lift the client's thigh off the table, and instruct the client to hold it there while you apply a downward force to the thigh.
- *S1-S2—knee flexion:* Keep the client in the prone position, and flex the knee to 90°. Place your hand just proximal to the ankle, and apply a force into extension while the client resists.

DERMATOMES FOR THE LUMBAR SPINE AND SACRUM

Along with the motor nerves, sensory nerves indicate dysfunction in an area. To assess the areas innervated by the nerves, touch the areas lightly bilaterally and ask the client whether the sensations are equal. It is important to stay in the middle of the dermatome to avoid any overlap into adjacent dermatomes. Any variation between the sides can indicate pathology, which can vary from person to person (Fig. 6-6). The dermatomes of the lumbar spine and sacrum are listed in Table 6-3.

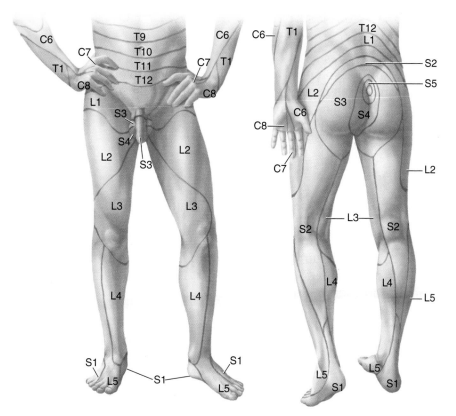

Figure 6-6 Dermatomes of the lumbar spine.

Table 6-3 Dermatomes of the Lumbar and Sacral Region

L1: Side of the hip over the trochanter; front of the hip into the groin

L2: Back, just over the PSIS running toward the trochanter; front of the thigh to the knee

L3: Back, upper gluteal along the iliac crest; front of the thigh, knee, and medial lower leg

L4: Inner gluteal; lateral thigh, running to the medial lower leg below the knee; top of the foot on the great-toe side, including toes

L5: Gluteal; back and side of the thigh; lateral aspect of the lower leg; top of the foot on the lateral side, including toes; distal medial sole of the foot including the first three toes

S1: Gluteal; back of the thigh and lateral lower leg; distal lateral sole of the foot, including the last two toes

S2: Same as S1

S3: Groin; inner thigh to knee

S4: Perineum; genitals; lower sacrum

TRIGGER-POINT REFERRAL PATTERNS FOR MUSCLES OF THE REGION

This section examines some of the common muscles involved in back pain and the location and symptoms of the corresponding myofascial trigger points, which can arise as a result of postural issues, acute trauma, poor body mechanics, and repetitive stress.

Erector Spinae

This discussion focuses only on the two main muscles of the erector spinae group that can cause pain and dysfunction in the low back: the iliocostalis lumborum and the longissimus thoracis (see Figs. 6-8, 6-12, and 6-13).

The trigger point for the *iliocostalis lumborum* is located in the belly of the muscle just under the last rib. Its referral pattern is strongly downward to the midbuttock region; its chief symptom is unilateral posterior hip pain and can be an underlying factor in lumbago.

The *longissimus thoracis* has two points. The first point is located at the lower thoracic region around T10 or T11, just over the transverse process. It refers pain down to the lower part of the buttock almost to the ischial tuberosity; its chief symptom is buttock pain. The other point in the thoracis is located at the level of L1 just lateral to the spinous process. Its chief symptom is diffuse, nonspecific pain along with difficulty rising from a chair or climbing stairs; it refers inferiorly several lumbar segments to the posterior iliac crest.

Serratus Posterior Inferior

The referral of the *serratus posterior inferior* muscle (see Figs. 6-9 and 6-12) stays local to the trigger point, which is located about the middle of the muscle around the 10th rib. Clients will complain of an annoying but not serious ache in the lower thoracic area.

Quadratus Lumborum

Among the deeper muscles in the lumbar area, the *quadratus lumborum* (see Figs. 6-8 and 6-12) is a major player in low-back pain. "The quadratus lumborum is one of the most commonly overlooked muscular sources of low back pain and is often responsible, through satellite gluteus minimus trigger points, for the 'pseudo-disc syndrome' and the 'failed surgical back syndrome'" (Travell and Simons, 1999). There are four active trigger points located throughout the muscle. The chief symptoms include low-back pain, difficulty turning over in bed or standing upright, and pain when coughing or sneezing.

Two of the points are superficial and located laterally on the muscle, one superior to the other. The first point located on the lateral edge of the muscle just under the last rib refers pain along the crest of the ilium and anteriorly to the adjacent quadrant of the lower abdomen. The second superficial point is located laterally at the inferior edge of the muscle just above the iliac crest. This point refers to the greater trochanter, and the pain can be so intense that the client cannot tolerate lying on his or her side. The other two points are located deep and medial on the muscle. The superior point is located just lateral to the transverse process of L3 and refers strongly into the sacroiliac joint on the same side. The inferior deep point is located between the transverse processes of the 4th and 5th lumbar vertebrae and refers to the lower buttock.

Multifidus and Rotatores

The deepest muscles of the lumbar spine are the deep paraspinal muscles *multifidi and rotatores* (see Figs. 6-8 and 6-13). The chief complaint from a trigger point in these muscles is a persistent, worrisome bone pain from either of the two muscles. Multifidus trigger points tend to refer to the area around the spinous process of the adjacent vertebra but can also refer anteriorly and be mistaken for visceral pain. Trigger points in the rotatores refer midline and cause tenderness in the spinous process.

Gluteus Maximus

On the pelvis, the gluteals can develop trigger points that affect both the lumbar spine and the sacrum. Three points in the *gluteus maximus* (see Figs. 6-9 and 6-11) can refer pain. Symptoms include pain and restlessness after long periods of sitting and pain while walking uphill and swimming

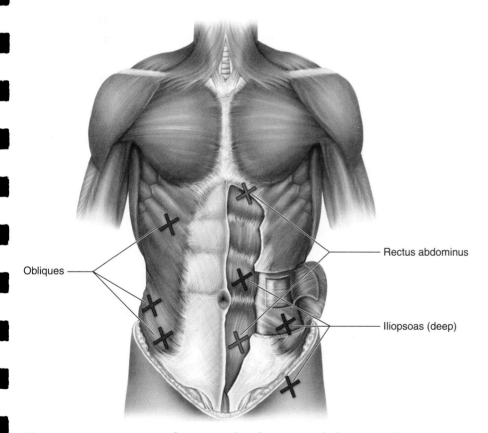

Figure 6-7 Trigger-point locations for the rectus abdominus, iliopsoas, and obliques.

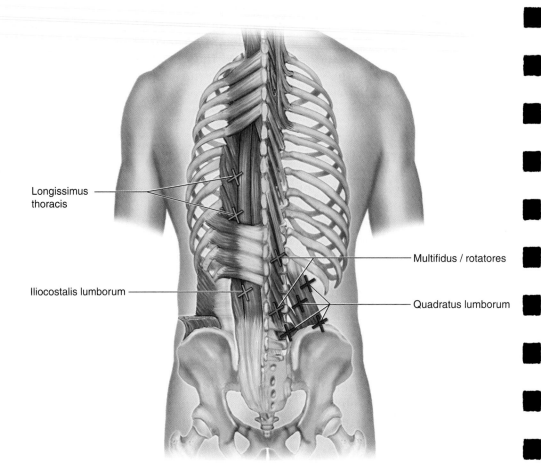

Figure 6-8 Trigger-point locations for the longissimus thoracis, iliocostalis lumborum, multifidus/rotatores, and quadratus lumborum.

Longissimus thoracis

Iliocostalis lumborum

Multifidus / rotatores

Quadratus lumborum

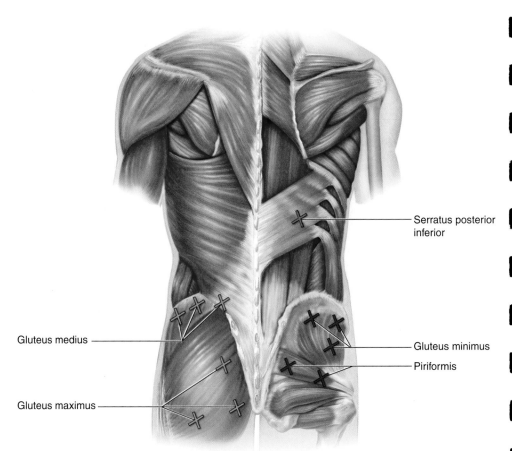

Figure 6-9 Trigger-point locations for the serratus posterior inferior, gluteus maximus, gluteus medius, gluteus minimus, and piriformis.

Serratus posterior inferior

Gluteus medius

Gluteus maximus

Gluteus minimus

Piriformis

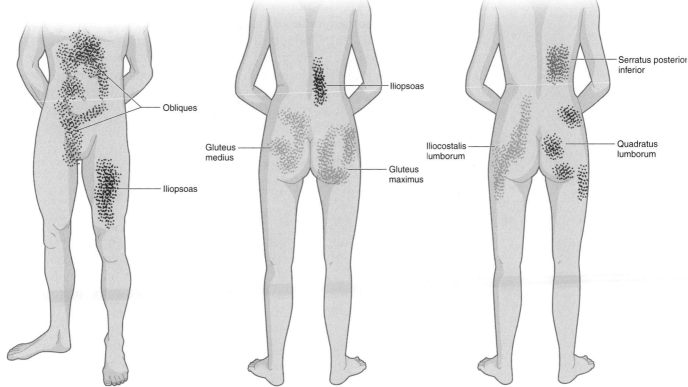

Figure 6-10 Trigger-point referrals for the obliques and the anterior pattern for the iliopsoas.

Figure 6-11 Trigger-point referrals for the gluteus medius, the posterior pattern for the iliopsoas, and the gluteus maximus.

Figure 6-12 Trigger-point referrals for the serratus posterior inferior, quadratus lumborum, and iliocostalis lumborum.

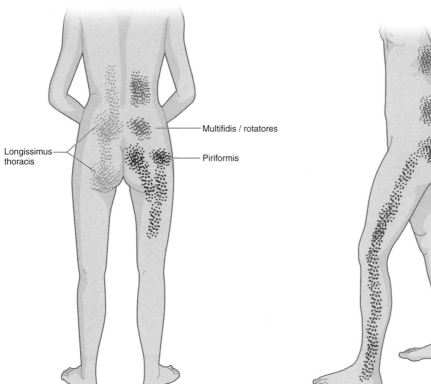

Figure 6-13 Trigger-point referrals for the multifidus/rotatores, piriformis, and longissimus thoracis.

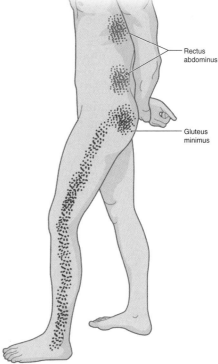

Figure 6-14 Trigger-point referrals for the rectus abdominus and the gluteus minimus.

the crawl stroke. All the points refer to the general gluteal region and do not travel any considerable distance. The first trigger point is along the lateral edge of the sacrum about halfway down. It refers in a semicircle pattern up along the sacrum and natal cleft to the sacroiliac joint and down along the gluteal fold. The second trigger point is located just superior to the ischial tuberosity and is the most common location for this muscle. This point refers to the entire buttock both superficially and deep; it encompasses the entire sacrum and moves laterally just under the iliac crest. The last point is located medial to the ischial tuberosity and refers to the coccyx; pain at this point is often mistaken for problems with the coccyx.

Gluteus Medius

The *gluteus medius* (see Figs. 6-9 and 6-11) also has three points that can cause problems. Clients with active trigger points in this muscle will complain of pain on walking and sitting in a slumped position, as well as difficulty sleeping on the affected side. The first point is located just inferior to the posterior iliac crest near the sacroiliac joint. It refers along the crest and up into the sacroiliac joint and lumbar spine. It also refers over the sacrum and can extend over much of the buttock. The second point is also located just inferior to the iliac crest but is midway along its length. Its referral is more lateral and to the midgluteal region and may extend into the upper lateral thigh. The last point is located near the anterior superior iliac spine just inferior to the crest. Referral pain from this point travels along the crest and encompasses the lower lumbar and sacral region.

Gluteus Minimus

The last gluteal muscle, *gluteus minimus* (see Figs. 6-9 and 6-14), has several trigger points in both the anterior and the posterior portions of the muscle. Common symptoms include hip pain that can affect gait, difficulty lying on the affected side, and difficulty standing after prolonged sitting. Active trigger points in the gluteus minimus can be misdiagnosed as sciatica. The two points in the anterior portion of the muscle are located one below the other, inferior to the anterior iliac crest. They refer pain to the lower lateral buttock and down the lateral thigh, along the peroneals sometimes as far as the ankle. The points in the posterior portion of the muscle lie along the superior edge of the muscle. They refer to most of the buttock and down the back of the thigh and into the calf.

Piriformis

Deep to the gluteals is the *piriformis* (see Figs. 6-9 and 6-13). It is another muscle that can lead to the misdiagnosis of sciatica because of its relationship with the nerve. Symptoms from trigger points in this muscle include pain and numbness in the low back, groin, buttock, hip, and posterior thigh and leg. They can be aggravated by prolonged sitting or through activity. There are two points located along the length of the muscle, one just lateral to the sacrum and the other just before the greater trochanter. The referral is over the sacroiliac region for the medial point and over the posterior hip joint for the lateral point.

Rectus Abdominus

On the anterior side of the trunk, several muscles can cause low-back pain. The four abdominal muscles contain trigger points that refer to other areas of the body, and pain from the points can be commonly mistaken for visceral or other somatic conditions. The *rectus abdominus* (see Figs. 6-7 and 6-14) contains multiple points, and symptoms will vary depending on where the point is located. In the upper portion of the muscle, symptoms can include heartburn, indigestion, and back pain along the same level as the point. Referral patterns for these points include the midback bilaterally and the xiphoid process.

The next area in the rectus abdominus is the periumbilical region. The points in this region refer to the area directly around the trigger point and can cause symptoms such as abdominal cramping, colic, and diffuse pain that is exacerbated by movement. The lower points can refer to the lower back and sacrum and can cause dysmenorrheal or pseudo-appendicitis pain.

Obliques and Transverse Abdominus

The obliques have multiple referral patterns that can extend up into the chest, across the abdomen, or down into the groin. Trigger points located in the upper portion of the *internal and external obliques* (see Figs. 6-7 and 6-10) can produce deep epigastric pain and mimic heartburn symptoms. Active trigger points in the lower portion of the muscle along the inguinal ligament can cause groin pain. The last abdominal, the *transverse abdominus*, refers pain laterally in a band out from the points.

Iliopsoas

The *iliopsoas* (see Figs. 6-7 and 6-10) is often overlooked as a source of low-back pain. Symptoms from active points in the muscle include pain during weight-bearing activities with relief through hip flexion. Pain is described as running up and down the spine and can include the front of the thigh. The three main trigger points within the muscle have a common referral pattern. There is a distinct ipsilateral vertical pattern along the lumbar spine. It may extend into the sacroiliac area and include the groin and anteromedial thigh on the same side. Points in the belly of the psoas or iliacus refer primarily to the back, whereas the point near the insertion of the muscle refers into both the thigh and the back. The three points are located just lateral to the umbilicus, just medial to the anterior iliac crest on the fossa, and on the anterior thigh just inferior to the inguinal ligament, respectively. Refer to the Quick Reference Table "Trigger Points for the Lumbar Spine and Sacrum" at the end of this chapter (page 209).

SPECIFIC CONDITIONS

Dysfunction in the lumbar spine, sacrum, pelvis, and hips overlaps and involves the same structures, and this results in a crossover of the treatments. As with all conditions, each client will present with his or her unique set of symptoms and must be looked at individually.

Lumbar Spine Conditions

Background

Injuries to the structures in the lumbar spine are common and have a wide range of presentations and clinical significance (McLain, 2005). Despite the different presentations, the end result is the same: a decrease in the space of the intervertebral foramen. This results in an eventual compression or entrapment of the neural elements in the area, leading to myriad dysfunctions (Chen and Spivak, 2003). Two of the more common disorders in the area are degenerative lumbar spinal stenosis and lumbar disk injuries.

Degenerative lumbar spinal stenosis can result from congenital conditions and degenerative conditions. Table 6-4 lists the results of these two conditions.

Table 6-4   Etiology of Degenerative Lumbar Spinal Stenosis

Etiology	Result
Congenital	Narrow spinal canal dimensions
	Bone dysplasias
	Dwarfism
Degenerative	Spinal disease
	Instability
	Scoliosis
	Chronic improper posture and movement patterns

Source: (Chen and Spivak, 2003)

The disorder typically presents in people over the age of 60, with males reporting a higher percentage of problems. Stenosis can be localized to one segment or can span several, and the process typically begins with the breakdown of the disk. This results in altered biomechanics at the segment and causes a chain reaction. As the mechanics change, the anatomical structures morph to accommodate the new movement and a decrease in foraminal space occurs. Essentially, this is the "wearing out" of the disk and the surrounding joint; however, the degeneration of the disk and the narrowing of the intervertebral space do not mean that pain is imminent. Underlying anatomical, congenital, and pathologic factors complete the puzzle of dysfunction and result in a symptomatic spine.

In the lumbar spine, the disks create 20% to 25% of the height of the region and function to absorb shock, create movement between vertebrae, and create a space for the spinal nerve root to exit. The disk comprises the annulus fibrosis, which is concentric rings of fibrocartilage, and the nucleus pulposus, which is a hydrophilic gelatinous tissue that initially contains about 90% water and that decreases with age. The nucleus pulposus lies slightly posterior in the lumbar spine because of the lordotic curve in the region. When different forces on the disk are applied, the nucleus shifts to accommodate the pressure. As the disk loses its ability to reabsorb and hold water, the space between adjacent vertebrae lessens, resulting in a narrowing of the foramen from which the spinal nerve exits.

While acute injuries can occur in the lumbar spine, chronic stresses as a cause of dysfunction are more common. Prolonged submaximal loading can lead to micro-tears in the annulus fibrosis and result in one of four conditions:

1. *Protrusion:* The disk protrudes in a posterior direction but does not rupture the annulus.
2. *Prolapse:* The annulus is not ruptured, but its outermost fibers contain the nucleus.
3. *Extrusion:* The annulus is perforated, and the nucleus material moves into the epidural space.
4. *Sequestrated:* Fragments from the annulus and nucleus move outside the disk. This is the most severe condition.

Lumbar disk injuries are most prevalent in men between the ages of 35 and 45. Herniations most commonly occur at the L4-L5 level, followed by L5-S1, and are generally posterior or posterolateral in direction due to the positioning of the disk. Just as in other areas of the spine, injuries to the disk can exist without any clinical symptoms. When the severity of the injury is such that the disk causes a stenosis of the foramen and contacts the nerve, the symptoms can range from a mild discomfort to severe pain and neurologic dysfunction.

Some symptoms include:

- Sharp pain
- Spasm at the site of the injury
- Radiating pain down the sciatic nerve
- Compensation, such as walking in a crouched position, leaning away from the injury site

Since both disk injuries and disk degeneration can cause stenosis of the foramen, which may impinge the nerve, the symptoms of each are similar. Often, additional tests are required to differentiate between the two conditions. Based on the referral patterns of the dermatomes and myotomes for the area, a better understanding of which disk is possibly involved can be achieved. There are other conditions that can mimic both degenerative spine and disk injuries, including:

- Sacroiliac joint dysfunction
- Facet joint dysfunction
- Vertebral fractures
- Visceral conditions

Assessment

Because different conditions can present with the same symptoms, a thorough assessment is recommended. It is important for therapists to consider their ability to treat the condition, taking care to refer the client to another health care provider if treatment appears to be contraindicated.

Condition History Here are some questions that are relevant to lumbar spine conditions:

Question	Significance
What is the client's occupation?	Occupations that are more strenuous have higher rates of injury.
What was the mechanism of injury?	Involved structures can be narrowed down if the mechanism is known.
Where is the pain located?	The more specific the location, the easier it is to determine the structures involved.
Does the pain radiate?	Helps determine whether the pain has a neurologic origin.
What type of pain is it (deep, superficial, burning, sharp)?	Helps identify the source of pain.
Are there any positions, postures, or activities that change the pain?	Pain resulting from the degeneration of the disk usually increases with activity and decreases with rest. Pain from a disk injury tends to increase if a single posture is held for an extended period of time.
Does the pain get worse or better as the day progresses?	Helps identify the source structures. Facet joint conditions are typically stiff in the morning and improve with activity.
Are there any changes in sensations?	Identifies whether there is pressure on a nerve root.

Forces on the disk are greater in certain postures or positions, and this can help determine whether the cause of the discomfort is disk-related. If the pressure on the disks while standing is the baseline norm, the following are the increases in pressure in the disks in various postures:

- Coughing or straining   5% to 35%
- Walking   15%
- Side bending   25%
- Bending forward   150%
- Lifting a weight with the back and knees straight   169%
- Lifting a weight with the knees bent   73%

Visual Assessment As with the cervical spine, observe the client in static and dynamic capacities. Before beginning a formal assessment, simply watching the client enter and maneuver around your facility can reveal a plethora of information. Notice the position and gait of the client's body, whether he or she is guarding any areas, and any facial expressions during movement that can lend information about pain levels. Have the client disrobe to the appropriate level, and scan the area for obvious deformity or muscle spasm. Move into a systematic assessment of posture, movement, and gait as described earlier in the text. Include associated areas if necessary.

Palpation When palpating the region, remember to include the related structures on the anterior side of the body. Begin with the structures listed earlier in the chapter, and expand to other regions as necessary. Note areas of bruising, swelling, and obvious deformity such as step-offs between vertebrae.

Orthopedic Tests Administer specific tests after you have performed the assessments for the ranges of motion, dermatomes, and myotomes. Table 6-5 lists some orthopedic tests and explains how to perform them.

Soft Tissue Treatment

Since the resulting anatomical change in the spine is a stenosis of the intervertebral foramen, the focus of the treatment should be to create an increase in that space. The body's soft tissues create a tremendous force on the vertebrae, adding to the stenosis by compressing the segments together. Relieving tension in the tissues will, in theory, remove pressure

> **Practical Tip**
> Don't confuse tight hamstrings for a disk injury. Use all the information gathered to help make your decision.

Table 6-5 Orthopedic Tests for Lumbar Spine Conditions

Orthopedic Test	How to Perform
Lasegue's (straight-leg-raise) test 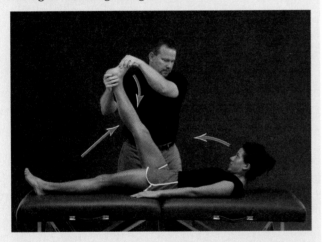 *Note:* This test asserts that moving the lower limb will increase tension on the nerve, which will subsequently pull on the root and cause symptoms. It tests for irritation to the sciatic nerve from a variety of underlying causes, including disk injuries.	Client is in the supine position with both legs straight and the tested leg internally rotated at the hip. Client should be completely relaxed and lift the leg slowly until he or she complains of pain or tightness. Then have the client lower the leg until the pain or tightness is relieved. Have the client dorsiflex the foot as far as possible or until symptoms return. If this does not cause any pain or tightness, ask the client to flex his or her head off the table as far as possible. If either movement does not cause the pain to return, the source is not disk-related and is most likely tight hamstrings. If the client is able to flex the leg past 70°, the cause is most likely facet or sacroiliac in origin, since the sciatic nerve is fully stretched at that range. Pain that moves from the back down into the leg along the sciatic nerve distribution during one of the movements is a positive sign. Pain in the lumbar spine on the side opposite the lifted leg can indicate a space-occupying lesion, such as a herniation.

Table 6-5 Orthopedic Tests for Lumbar Spine Conditions
(Continued)

Orthopedic Test	How to Perform
Slump test 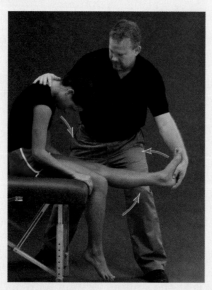 *Note:* This is the most common neurologic test for the lower limb and is an indicator of impingement of the dura and spinal cord or nerve roots.	Client is seated on the edge of the table with the legs hanging over and the hands behind the back. Have the client "slump" so that he or she flexes the spine and rolls the shoulders forward but keeps the head in a neutral position. If this does not produce any symptoms, have the client flex the head down and hold the shoulders slumped forward. If there are still no symptoms, passively extend the client's lower leg and dorsiflex the foot while he or she maintains the slumped position. The reproduction of pain down the sciatic nerve at any stage of the test is a positive sign.

Practical Tip

To rule out hamstring tightness, perform more than one orthopedic test.

from the involved structures. Be sure to address the condition appropriately based on the phase of the injury, and include any compensatory areas as needed.

Connective Tissue Since a majority of problems stem from chronic stress placed on the area, underlying postural issues play an important role. Addressing the connective tissue restrictions will dramatically improve the posture in the area.

Prone Position Start with a general assessment of the superficial fascia, from superior to inferior, from medial to lateral, and at various oblique angles. Apply pressure to the restrictions, including the gluteals. Change the angle to address restriction in an oblique direction; then move into the deeper tissues by separating them out and clearing any restrictions within each muscle involved. Working from the side of the table can be very effective and is a good position for addressing the paraspinal tissue:

1. While applying pressure with the heel of your hand to the opposite-side musculature, apply counterpressure to the opposite-side paraspinals or secure the sacrum, depending on the level at which you are working.
2. Reach across and around the front to the abdominals and iliac crest. While pulling the tissue at the iliac crest toward the back, apply coun-

180   **Part II** Regional Approach to Treatment

terpressure to the sacrum. The anterior iliac crest is defined very effectively using this method.

Another specific technique involves tracing around the posterior iliac crests with the thumbs or fingertips to free the fascia around the joint. Be careful not to apply too much downward pressure to the spine or increase lumbar extension as this may exacerbate symptoms.

Supine Position Include the abdominals, lower thoracic area, and anterior hip in the assessment and treatment of the superficial fascia. Begin by assessing these areas in different directions, and treat them by moving into the restrictions superficially and separating out each muscle as you move deeper. The abdominal area may be difficult to release due to the pliability of the tissue. The lateral edge of the rectus abdominus can be stripped out by securing the tissue either at the superior border and working down along its lateral edge or at its inferior border and working up along the lateral edge. Because of its influence on the position of the pelvis, an effective area to release is the area along the inguinal ligament and the iliac crest, working into the iliacus. Trace on both the superior and inferior edges of the ligament, releasing any restrictions as you work. Move into the iliacus by sliding into the "bowl" of the ilium at the ASIS. Work into the restrictions as they are encountered.

Side-Lying Position This is the most effective position for addressing the gluteals and hip rotators. When standing behind the client, place your fingertips on the client's greater trochanter and radiate out. You can also access the anterior pelvis and iliopsoas from this position. Start at the ASIS and sink into the tissue, pressing back into the client when you find a restriction.

Tissue Inconsistencies While you are releasing the connective tissue in the area, trigger points will become evident in various muscles. Depending on the muscle, decide whether the flat or pincer palpation technique would be more appropriate. Use the methods described in Chapter 3 to address the points, and be sure to keep the pain levels no higher than 7 out of 10. Utilizing passive and active movements will improve the effectiveness of the direct pressure techniques. Involved muscles may include:

- Paraspinals
- Quadratus lumborum
- Gluteals
- Iliopsoas
- Abdominals

However, do not neglect any compensatory areas that may be involved.

Muscle Concerns

Pressure from tension and adhesions in the muscle tissue can exacerbate the symptoms associated with spinal conditions. Once you've identified the involved muscles, you can apply various strokes, including advanced techniques that incorporate movement (described in Chapter 3).

Prone Position The prone position is the most common position for addressing conditions of the lumbar spine and sacrum. Stripping out the paraspinals and quadratus lumborum is very effective in this position. Due to the density of the area, forearm and elbow strokes are extremely useful here. Facing either the head or feet, place the elbow of your arm closest to the table on the border or the belly of the muscle. Move slowly up or down the muscle, being careful not to cross over the spine.

The gluteals can also be effectively treated in this position; using a loose fist ensures that the appropriate depth is obtained:

1. Stand on the side of the client, and place the back of your fist just lateral to the sacrum. Use the other hand to apply counterpressure on the sacrum; then slowly slide your hand toward you, being careful not to pinch the tissue into the table.
2. Defining the sacrum and its lateral edge removes a lot of the restrictions in the gluteus maximus. From the PSIS, move medially onto the sacrum and find its lateral edge. Run your fingertips or thumb inferiorly along its border.

The thoracolumbar fascia and muscle tissue are thick in this area. Removing any muscular restrictions along the iliac crest is effective at improving movement.

Supine Position Addressing the iliopsoas is a key factor in effectively treating conditions of the lumbar spine (Fig. 6-15).

1. Have the client bend the knees to about 45°.
2. Place the client's feet on the table, and have him or her take a deep breath. Starting at the anterior superior iliac spine, slide your fingertips in along the inside of the "bowl" of the pelvis as the client exhales; stay lateral to the edge of the rectus abdominus muscle.
3. Once you locate a restriction, direct your pressure down toward the table.
4. Have the client slowly extend the leg, keeping the heel on the table as he or she slides it as far as possible and brings it back up.
5. While you continue to hold the restriction, have the client repeat this process several times or until you feel the tissue release. Slowly remove your hand and repeat the process, changing the location and angle that you slide in.

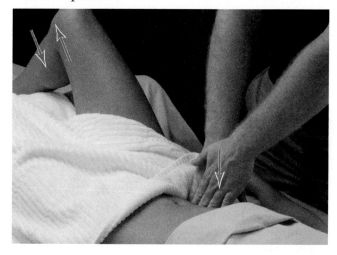

Figure 6-15 Massage using active engagement to the iliopsoas.

The more inferior you move along the bowl of the pelvis, the greater the focus on the iliacus. Moving superiorly toward the umbilicus will focus more on the psoas. Generally, avoid going any higher than the level of the umbilicus because you may encounter solid organs.

Side-Lying Position This position is most effective for treating the gluteals and lateral hip rotators. Radiating strokes using a loose fist from the greater trochanter out to the iliac crest and sacrum are very effective for the area. The iliopsoas can also be accessed from the side. The process is the same as far as the stroke progression except that gravity assists in moving internal organs out of the way. Have the client take a deep breath. As he or she exhales, slide your fingertips around the front of the pelvis. Once you find a restriction, have the client straighten the leg as far as possible and bring it back up. Repeat this process until you remove all the restrictions. The paraspinal muscles can also be accessed here; however, use care when pressing down toward the table. Pressure directly into the transverse processes can be painful.

Stretching

Flexibility in this region of the body is essential in treating and preventing dysfunction. In addition to the lumbar spine, hip range of motion is an integral part in the overall functioning of the region; therefore, it is important to incorporate several hip stretches. This section discusses Active Isolated Stretching as it relates to the lumbar spine and the anterior muscles.

Lumbar Spine and Hip Extensors To stretch the lower spine and hips, have the client lie in the supine position and bring the leg of the side you are stretching up toward the armpit by contracting the hip flexors and the abdominal muscles (Fig. 6-16). Once the client reaches the full range, assist in the same direction by placing the client's hand either behind his or her knee or under the foot and holding for 1½ to 2 seconds while the client exhales. Release to the starting position, which is the thigh in a vertical position. Repeat for one to two sets of 10 repetitions.

Lumbar Spine To stretch the lower spine, have the client sit on the table with the legs bent to about 30° (Fig. 6-17). Stand in front of the client, and have him or her tuck the chin, contract the abdomen, and curl forward on the exhale. Once the client has reached the end range, assist him or her in the same direction by placing your hands on the client's midback and providing downward traction for 2 seconds. Perform 10 to 15 repetitions, being careful to apply traction, not a vertical force downward.

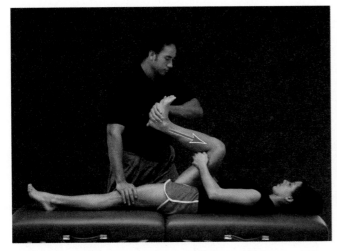

Figure 6-16 Lumbar spine and hip extensor stretch.

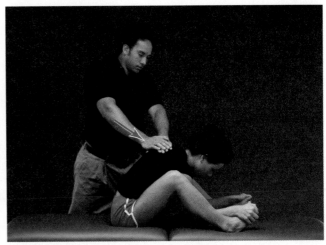

Figure 6-17 Lumbar spine stretch.

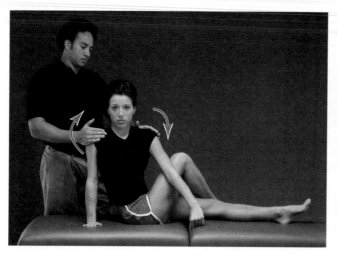

Figure 6-18 Trunk rotation stretch.

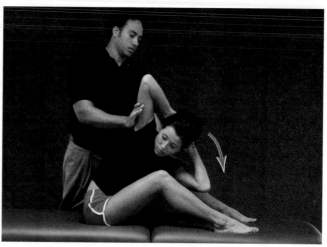

Figure 6-19 Seated lateral trunk stretch.

Trunk Rotators To stretch the trunk rotators, have the client sit on the table with one leg straight and the other one bent to 90°, crossing the foot over the straight leg (Fig. 6-18). Have the client rotate the trunk toward the bent knee and place the elbow on the outside of the bent knee if possible. Once the client has reached his or her end range, assist by standing on the side and placing your hands on the client's shoulders. Rotate the shoulders and hold for 2 seconds as the client exhales. Repeat for one to two sets of 10 repetitions.

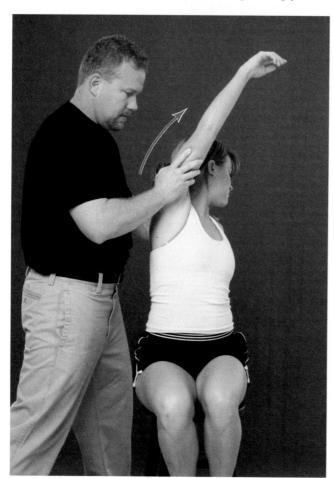

Figure 6-20 Anterior trunk stretch.

Lateral Spine and Abdominals To stretch the lateral spine and abdominal muscles, place the client in a seated position on the table with the knees bent to a 45° angle and the legs spread wider than the shoulders (Fig. 6-19). Standing at the side of the table, have the client fully rotate the trunk away from the side where you are standing and then bend the trunk between the knees. Once the client has reached the end range, place your hands on the client's shoulders and assist in flexing the trunk while keeping the client rotated. Hold the stretch for 2 seconds while the client exhales. Perform 10 repetitions.

Anterior Trunk Stretching the anterior trunk is important as well. Have the client, from the seated position, rotate the trunk to 45° (Fig. 6-20). Have the client lean backward at a 45° angle while lifting the front arm over the head. Assist the client in the motion to the end range for 2 seconds while he or she exhales. Repeat for two sets of 10 repetitions.

Posterior Hips To stretch the posterior hips, place the client in the supine position, move

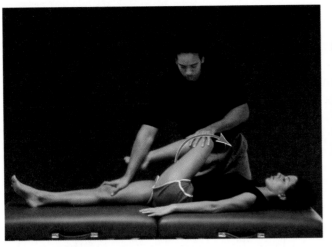

Figure 6-21 Posterior hip stretch.

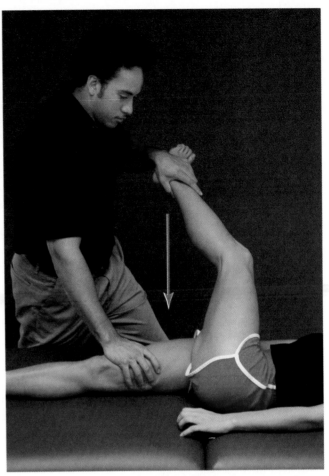

Figure 6-22 Stretch to the lateral rotators.

the leg opposite to that being stretched across the midline, and medially rotate it (Fig. 6-21). Have the client flex the thigh toward the opposite shoulder while exhaling. Stand on the side opposite that being stretched. Assist the leg as it is flexed while stabilizing the leg on the table with the other hand. Return to the starting position, and repeat for two sets of 10 repetitions. In the same position, have the client lift the leg as far as possible, but not more than 90°, while keeping a slight bend in the knee (Fig. 6-22). While you maintain internal rotation on the leg that is on the table, have the client move the leg across his or her body as far as possible. Gently assist the client at the end range for one to two sets of 10 repetitions.

Iliopsoas To stretch the iliopsoas, have the client lie on his or her side and pull the bottom leg up to the chest and hold it (Fig. 6-23). Place your hand that is closest to the client's head on the client's hip to keep it from rolling backward. The client's bottom hand will support the thigh at the knee, keeping the knee at a greater-than-90° angle. Instruct your client to extend the thigh back as far as possible, and assist him or her in the same direction at the end range. Repeat for two sets of 10 repetitions.

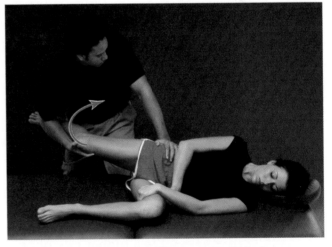

Figure 6-23 Side-lying iliopsoas stretch.

Spondylolysis and Spondylolisthesis

Background

Spondylolysis and spondylolisthesis, although different in their presentations, involve related structures and frequently occur simultaneously.

Chapter 6 Conditions of the Lumbar Spine and Sacrum

These conditions create a lot of controversy in their etiology and treatment because of poor correlations between clinical symptoms and radiographic evidence (McNeely et al., 2003).

Spondylolysis stems from the Greek words *spondylos*, which means "vertebra," and *lysis*, which means "break." It is a defect or break in an area of the vertebra between the superior and inferior facets of the vertebral arch known as the *pars interarticularis.* It occurs in 6% of the population and affects twice as many boys as girls (McNeely et al., 2003). In addition, higher rates of occurrence were found in certain ethnic populations, such as some Alaskan natives and individuals who had a family history of the condition (Wong, 2004).

There are two theories that seek to explain the causes of spondylolysis:

1. **Congenital spondylolysis** occurs when there is a predisposed weakness in the pars interarticularis. This theory is supported through the study of family histories.

2. **Developmental spondylolysis** occurs as the result of a fracture in the pars due to continued micro-traumas, which weaken the structure. The micro-traumas can occur from a variety of sources, including postural conditions, various activities, and repetitive movement patterns.

There is a higher rate of occurrence in the adolescent population, caused by micro-traumas placed on immature spines (Cook et al., 2004). There is also a high rate of occurrence in young athletes. Up to 40% of sports-related back pain can be attributed to pars damage, which is common in sports that combine extension with rotation (McNeely et al., 2003). The most common site of fracture is L5, but defects can occur at L4 and above. Some common symptoms associated with spondylolysis include:

- Pain
- Loss of mobility
- Paraspinal muscle spasm
- Flattening of the lumbar curve
- Changes in gait

The pain is usually localized over the spine, gluteals, and posterior thigh.

Spondylolisthesis is a similar condition characterized by the forward slippage of one vertebra on another and the spine's inability to resist the shear force associated with this shifting. It was first described in the late 1700s by obstetricians who noted that it caused a barrier to the passage of the infant through the birth canal (Dickson, 1998). The reported incidence of occurrence is estimated to be between 2% and 6%, with L5-S1 most commonly affected (McNeely et al., 2003). There is a higher rate of occurrence in the adolescent population, particularly girls, which is due to the increased mobility of the adolescent spine and the fact that facets in adolescents are more horizontal in orientation than they are in adults.

Spondylolysis and spondylolisthesis frequently occur together. Radiographic studies have reported that 50% to 81% of cases of spondylolisthesis also contain a fracture of the pars interarticularis (McNeely et al.,

---

spondylolysis A defect or break in an area of the vertebra between the superior and inferior facets of the vertebral arch known as the *pars interarticularis.*

congenital spondylolysis A type of defect that occurs when there is a predisposed weakness in the pars interarticularis.

developmental spondylolysis A type of defect that occurs as the result of a fracture in the pars due to continued micro-traumas, which weaken the structure. The micro-traumas can occur from a variety of sources, including postural conditions, various activities, and repetitive movement patterns.

spondylolisthesis The forward slippage of one vertebra on another and the spine's inability to resist the shear force associated with this shifting.

2003). This shows that one condition will typically lead to the other. The classifications of spondylolisthesis are:

- Dysplastic or congenital
- Isthmus
- Degenerative
- Traumatic
- Pathological

The International Society for the Study of the Lumbar Spine (ISSLS) has created five classifications of spondylolisthesis:

Classification I—dysplastic or congenital spondylolisthesis: Affects the posterior facets of L5-S1 and occurs only at that level. The problem is twice as common in women as in men (Dickson, 1998). Elongation of the pars interarticularis allows for significant slippage—up to 100% if bilateral fractures occur.

Classification II—isthmus spondylolisthesis: Occurs secondarily to a defect in the pars and may be attributed to hormonal influences, since the slippage can progress during adolescence along with postural and gravitational forces (Wong, 2004).

Classification III—degenerative spondylolisthesis: Occurs as a result of the degeneration of the posterior facet joints and is more likely to occur at the L4-L5 level. Because of its etiology, it does not present in the population under the age of 50, and the degree of slippage does not exceed 30°.

Classification IV—traumatic spondylolisthesis: Occurs as a result of fractures that are on other parts of the vertebrae, such as the body and pedicles, and are not discrete entities within the pars region of the vertebrae.

Classification V—pathological spondylolisthesis: Occurs as a result of an overall process and does not result from isolated defects in the pars.

A disease process will affect the entire segment and indirectly affect the pars and cause slippage. Clinical presentation can vary depending on the type of deformity. Common symptoms include:

- Chronic midline ache at the lumbosacral junction that is exacerbated with extension
- Hamstring tightness
- Abnormal gait
- Cramping in the legs

Depending on the degree of slippage, neurologic symptoms may occur along the L5 nerve root. There is also a feeling of "giving way" when moving from flexion into extension. A high incidence of disk herniation, up to 25%, is associated with spondylolisthesis; therefore, take care to investigate all possible causes of dysfunction (Dickson, 1998).

Assessment

Since other conditions are associated with spondylolysis and spondylolisthesis, make sure the assessment reflects that possibility. Ruling out contraindications is a priority when there are neurologic symptoms.

Condition History Here are some questions that are relevant to spondylolysis and spondylolisthesis:

Question	Significance
What is the client's age?	While these conditions are more prevalent in certain age groups, age also lends information on the category of the dysfunction.
What is the client's gender?	The occurrence rate of these conditions can be more frequent in one gender than another.
Where is the pain?	These conditions tend to have specific pain patterns.
Which movements hurt?	These conditions are aggravated by hyperextension, especially when coupled with rotation or lateral flexion.
What activities does the client perform on a regular basis?	Certain movement patterns lend themselves to the development of these conditions.
Are there any postures that cause pain or discomfort?	Prolonged extension will cause pain if this condition is present.
Does the pain radiate? Is there any numbness or change in sensation?	This is an indicator of neurologic involvement.

Visual Assessment While dysfunction may be present in the absence of symptoms, there are some visual observations that may occur with this condition. The client may present with an increased lordotic or scoliotic curve. The significance of the deviated posture lies in whether the posture will increase the pressure on the pars interarticularis.

Tilts in the pelvis, changes in the lumbar curve, and avoidance of certain movements or postures in sitting or standing can also indicate dysfunction. Check for obvious deformities or spasm in the lumbar region. Assess both active and passive ranges of motion for any limitations.

Palpation Regardless of the origin of the defect in the vertebra, the surrounding musculature will be hypertonic and will try to compensate for the instability in the area. Check for swelling or bruising, including on the gluteals and posterior thighs. With spondylolisthesis, there may be a palpable step-off at the spinous process of the involved level. Take care not to apply too much force down toward the table—it is contraindicated and will put the spine into hyperextension. Focus on the structures mentioned earlier, beginning with the spine, and expand the area as necessary.

Orthopedic Tests Diagnosis of either spondylolysis or spondylolisthesis is achieved primarily through imaging techniques. One specific test can help with the assessment. Table 6-6 lists that orthopedic test and explains how to perform it.

Table 6-6   Orthopedic Test for Spondylolysis and
                Spondylolisthesis

Practical Tip

For accurate results, be sure the client performs a true extension and does not combine movements.

Orthopedic Test	How to Perform
Stork (single-leg) standing test 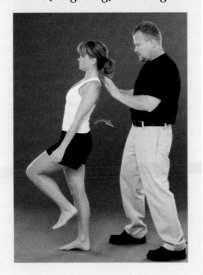	Have the client stand on one leg. Stand behind the client to prevent him or her from falling. Have the client extend the spine. Repeat on the other leg. A positive test is pain in the low back, which is associated with a fracture of the pars. *Note:* If the fracture is only on one side, standing on the ipsilateral leg will cause more pain. Have the client perform true extension; combining movements will not give an accurate result.

Soft Tissue Treatment

The primary structure involved with these two conditions cannot directly be treated with massage; however, massage therapy can support the normal healing process of the skeletal system by affecting the surrounding tissue directly. Muscle spasm, congestion in the tissues, and pain in the area are all treated effectively through massage. The focus of soft tissue treatment is on relieving pressure at the site of the fracture, caused by tight tissues, and assisting with correcting posture, which will reduce the force causing the slippage of the vertebra. Be careful not to cause hyperextension of the spine, which can exacerbate the condition. Place a pillow or cushion across the front of the hips when the client is in the prone position or under the knees when in the supine position to add to the client's comfort if necessary.

Connective Tissue The inherent instability that arises from these conditions results in an extreme guarding of the area; therefore, the tissues can be extremely tight.

Prone Position Begin with a general assessment of the area, from superior to inferior, from medial to lateral, and at various oblique angles. Since an anterior tilt of the pelvis can be present, working around the front of the pelvis and tracing the anterior iliac crest is effective for these conditions. Working deeper and stripping out and removing restrictions within the muscles in the region is also beneficial, especially to the paraspinals. One effective technique is static pressure in an inferior direction to the sacrum. An increased lumbosacral angle will increase the pressure on the posterior structures of the vertebra. Distracting the sacrum will change the lumbosacral angle and take pressure off the area.

1. Stand on the side of the client, and place your hand on the sacrum with the heel at its apex.
2. Apply gentle pressure in an inferior direction to create a distraction of the sacrum. Be careful not to press straight down into the table.
3. Place the other hand on top to generate more force if needed. Hold for 10 to 30 seconds and release.

A result of chronic pain in the area is an increase in connective tissue over the sacroiliac joint. Tracing the posterior iliac crest and clearing the restrictions is beneficial and will improve mobility in the area. Remember to address the gluteals, as they can affect the pull on the pelvis. The instability of the spine will cause the gluteals to assume a stabilizing role and result in chronic hypertonicity in the muscles.

Supine Position The main focus when working in this position should be to reduce the anterior tilt of the pelvis and restore the normal curve to the lumbar spine. After releasing the superficial connective tissue, work along the superior and inferior borders of the inguinal ligament and anterior hip with the fingertips to remove any restrictions. Along with stripping out the iliac crest, focus on the iliopsoas by sliding into the restriction from the ASIS. Because of the path it takes as it passes over the pelvis from the lumbar spine, the iliopsoas has an enormous effect on the tilt of the pelvis and the curve in the lumbar spine.

Side-Lying Position Utilize this position to access the gluteals with strokes radiating out from the trochanter. It is also important to use this position if the client cannot lie prone. You can treat the same tissues in this position as those treated in the prone position. Have the client assume a fetal position, and place a pillow or bolster between the legs for comfort.

Tissue Inconsistencies Releasing trigger points of the involved muscles can provide relief to the client. Pay special attention to the anterior muscles and the muscles that control the tilt of the pelvis. Use the methods described in Chapter 3, and apply them to the appropriate muscles.

Muscle Concerns

Focus on restoring the normal curves in the lumbar spine so that the forces are distributed evenly. If the client cannot lie in the prone position, treat the muscles in the side-lying position.

Prone Position This position is effective for stripping out the paraspinals and quadratus lumborum. When using forearm and elbow strokes, be careful to avoid applying too much pressure down toward the table. Facing toward the head or feet, move slowly up or down the muscle, being careful not to cross over the spine. Treat the gluteals using a loose fist to ensure that the appropriate depth is obtained:

1. Stand on the side of the client, and place the back of your fist just lateral to the sacrum. Use the other hand to apply counterpressure on the sacrum; then slowly slide your hand toward you, being careful not to pinch the tissue into the table.
2. Defining the sacrum and its lateral edge removes a lot of the restrictions in the gluteus maximus. From the PSIS, move medially onto the

sacrum and find its lateral edge. Run your fingertips or thumb inferiorly along its border.

Supine Position Addressing the iliopsoas is a key factor in effectively restoring the curve in the lumbar spine (see Fig. 6-15):

1. Have the client bend the knees to about 45°.
2. Place the client's feet on the table and have him or her take a deep breath. Starting at the anterior superior iliac spine, slide your fingertips in along the inside of the "bowl" of the pelvis as the client exhales; stay lateral to the edge of the rectus abdominus muscle.
3. Once you locate a restriction, direct your pressure down toward the table.
4. Have the client slowly extend the leg, keeping the heel on the table as he or she slides it as far as possible and brings it back up.

While you continue to hold the restriction, have the client repeat this process several times or until you feel the tissue release. Slowly remove your hand and repeat the process, changing the location and angle that you slide in. The more inferior you move along the bowl of the pelvis, the greater the focus on the iliacus; moving superiorly toward the umbilicus will focus more on the psoas. Generally, avoid going any higher than the level of the umbilicus because you may encounter solid organs.

Side-Lying Position This position is the most effective for treating the gluteals and lateral hip rotators. Using radiating strokes with a loose fist from the greater trochanter out to the iliac crest and sacrum is effective for the area. You can access the iliopsoas from this position using the same stroke progression, and gravity assists in moving internal organs out of the way. Have the client take a deep breath and as he or she exhales, slide your fingertips around the front of the pelvis. Once you find a restriction, have the client straighten the leg as far as possible and bring it back up. Repeat this process until all the restrictions are removed.

Stretching

Tightness from the muscles can place a great amount of stress on the surrounding structures; therefore, improving flexibility will dramatically improve this condition. The stretches that were utilized for lumbar disk conditions can be utilized here with a few exceptions (see pages 183–185). Avoid stretches requiring that the client move into spinal extension, or administer them with extreme caution. Take care when using stretches that involve lateral flexion or rotation of the spine.

Quadriceps with Emphasis on the Rectus Femoris One stretch that helps reduce the anterior tilt of the pelvis is a quadriceps stretch with special emphasis on the rectus femoris (Fig. 6-24). Have the client, in the side-lying position, bring the bottom leg to the chest and hold it.

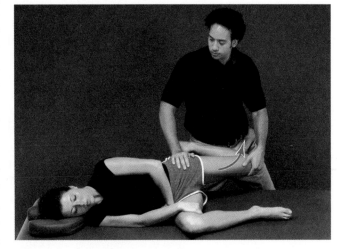

Figure 6-24 Side-lying quadriceps stretch.

This prevents the spine from hyperextending. Support the top leg, and keep the knee bent to at least 90°. Use the other hand to support the hip so that it does not roll backward. Have the client exhale and extend the thigh as far as possible. Assist at the end of the range of motion for 2 seconds. Repeat for 8 to 10 repetitions, and perform additional sets with the knee flexed greater than 90°.

Facet Joint Syndrome

Background

Also known as *zygapophysial joints,* facet joints are paired synovial joints that join one vertebra to another. In each region of the spine, the orientation of the facets changes based on the anatomical demands of the area. In the lumbar spine, the plane of orientation of the facets is vertical, which severely restricts motion, particularly rotation. As with other synovial joints, the facets are surrounded by a capsule, lined with a synovial membrane, and contain a meniscoid structure on the inside.

The existence of **facet joint syndrome** has been controversial. Ghormley first used the term around 1933, stating that arthritic changes on the facets could lead to sciatica (Wong, 1984). In 1994, Schwarzer et al. showed that the facet joint can be the source of back pain in a percentage of patients. This finding was based on a study in which anesthesia was injected directly into the facet joint and subsequently relieved symptoms (Cavanaugh et al., 1996).

The facets are highly innervated. Anatomical studies by Wyke confirmed that the medial branch of the posterior primary rami supplies the joint, which is densely innervated with pain receptors (Wong, 1984). So what causes joint dysfunction? One theory holds that biomechanical stresses can predispose the area to pain. During normal motion and at rest, the facets can be exposed to numerous forces. These forces, which can arise from different sources, can cause damage to the joint capsule or the surrounding muscle tissue. Shear force produced during normal movement or trauma to the spine can stress the facets and initiate degenerative changes. Compression from persistent faulty posture or the approximation of the facets as a result of degenerative conditions can also generate a pain response. With disk narrowing from compression, as much as 70% of the force will be transmitted across the facets. Normally, pain fibers have a high mechanical threshold and are stimulated only when the stress is noxious. The forces placed on the facets may be enough to cause the capsule to stretch and initiate the firing of pain nerves, but this still does not explain the ongoing pain. When tissue is damaged, however, chemical mediators are released that sensitize nerve endings and reduce their firing threshold, allowing lower levels of stress and strain to initiate the pain response. If the force through the facet is great enough to damage the capsule or other tissues, the ensuing inflammatory response will result in continued pain.

Another potential source of facet joint irritation is the "locking" of the joint. This occurs when a person has performed a movement, typically returning to extension from deep flexion, and is unable to achieve a fully

facet joint syndrome Low-back pain that is caused from a dysfunction in the facet joints of the spine.

upright position. When deep movement in any direction is performed, a small gap is created between the facet joints. This gap can entrap soft tissue on the return of the joint to its normal position. The entrapped tissue can be the synovial capsule, loose bodies, or the meniscoid structure in the joint. Pain is usually unilateral, and very sharp and localized, causing significant muscle spasm that reinforces the locking. Manual therapy and mobilization of the joint are extremely effective methods of treatment for facet joint irritation, especially joint locking.

Assessment

There is no gold standard for determining whether irritation of the facets is the source of back pain. Perform as thorough an assessment as possible to rule out referral or contraindications.

Condition History Here are some questions that are relevant to facet joint syndrome:

Question	Significance
What was the mechanism of injury?	Irritation to the facet often has no memorable mechanism. The locking of the joint can occur as the client moves from deep flexion to extension.
Where is the pain?	Pain from facet joints is specific, localized, and unilateral.
Does the pain radiate?	Facet pain rarely radiates.
What movement hurts?	Movements that compress the facets will typically generate pain.

Visual Assessment Facet joint irritation often presents in a client who is unable to stand erect. The client may have shifted to one side and have an antalgic gait. There may be muscle spasm over the lumbar area. Check for bruising or swelling, and assess passive and active ranges of motion to determine any limitations.

Palpation In addition to feeling for swelling and deformities, assess muscle tone over the lumbar area. Begin with the structures listed earlier in the chapter, and expand to include compensatory areas as needed.

Orthopedic Tests After assessing the dermatomes and myotomes using the touch discrimination and manual muscle testing methods described earlier, you may perform the quadrant test, which is the only test for this condition. Table 6-7 lists that orthopedic test and explains how to perform it.

Soft Tissue Treatment

Since the underlying cause of pain is pressure through the facets or the locking of the joint, the focus of treatment should be on distracting the joint to reduce pressure and remove derangement. Focus on the muscles

Table 6-7 Orthopedic Test for Facet Joint Syndrome

Orthopedic Test	How to Perform
Quadrant test 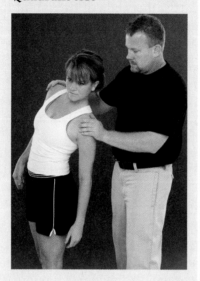	Stand behind the client, and place your hands on the shoulders. Have the client extend the spine while you control the movement by holding the shoulders. Move the client into lateral flexion and rotation to the side of pain while the client is in extension. Continue the movement until you reach the end range or reproduce the pain. This will cause the maximum narrowing of the foramen and put the most stress on the facets. A positive test occurs if pain is produced.

surrounding the site of pain that can cause compression in the area; expand the treatment area if necessary.

Connective Tissue Chronic forces through the facets can be a factor in this condition. Most of these forces are caused by faulty postural positions. Since restricted connective tissue plays a major role in posture, addressing it can be beneficial.

Prone Position Begin with a general assessment of the area, from superior to inferior, from medial to lateral, and at various oblique angles. Move into the deeper layers, and strip out the involved muscle, paying special attention to the paraspinals and quadratus lumborum. Working from the side of the table is a good position for addressing the paraspinal tissue. Apply pressure with the heel of your hand to the opposite-side musculature while either using counterpressure to the same side paraspinals or securing the sacrum.

Supine Position The abdominals, lower thoracic area, and anterior hip should be included in the assessment and treatment of the superficial fascia. Begin by assessing these areas in different directions, and treat them by moving into the restrictions superficially and separating out each muscle as you move deeper. When moving deeper, focus on the muscles that control the curvature of the lumbar spine, namely, the iliopsoas.

Side-Lying Position This position is helpful in addressing the associated areas such as the gluteal region. Standing behind the client, place your fingertips on the client's greater trochanter and radiate out.

Tissue Inconsistencies The same trigger points addressed in earlier conditions may present here. The involved muscles may include:

- Paraspinals
- Quadratus lumborum
- Gluteals
- Iliopsoas
- Abdominals

Pay special attention to the multifidus and rotatores. Because of their influences on the position of the joint, releasing them can significantly benefit the client. The flat palpation technique will be most effective in releasing any restrictions.

Muscle Concerns

Depending on the acuteness of the condition, other modalities such as ice may be used to help the client tolerate manual techniques. Focus on creating mobility in the segment responsible for the dysfunction.

Prone Position This condition is most commonly addressed in the prone position. Stripping out the paraspinals and quadratus lumborum is effective in relieving tension in the area. Use forearm and elbow strokes because of the depth of the tissue. Facing either the head or feet, place the elbow of the arm closest to the table on the border or belly of the muscle. Move slowly up or down the muscle, being careful not to cross over the spine.

Supine Position Addressing the iliopsoas is a key factor in treating facet joint problems:

1. Have the client bend the knees to about 45°.
2. Place the client's feet on the table, and have him or her take a deep breath. Starting at the anterior superior iliac spine, slide your fingertips in along the inside of the "bowl" of the pelvis as the client exhales; stay lateral to the edge of the rectus abdominus muscle.
3. Once you locate a restriction, direct your pressure down toward the table.
4. Have the client slowly extend the leg, keeping the heel on the table as he or she slides it as far as possible and brings it back up.

While you continue to hold the restriction, have the client repeat this process several times or until you feel the tissue release. Slowly remove your hand and repeat the process, changing the location and angle that you slide in. The more inferior you move along the bowl of the pelvis, the greater the focus on the iliacus. Moving superiorly toward the umbilicus will focus more on the psoas. Generally, avoid going any higher than the level of the umbilicus because you may encounter solid organs.

Side-Lying Position Treat the paraspinal muscles in this position, taking care when pressing down toward the table. Direct pressure into the transverse processes can be painful. Since the gluteals can be indirectly related to this condition, treating them can be beneficial. Using radiating strokes with a loose fist from the greater trochanter out to the iliac crest and sacrum is effective for the area.

Stretching

Muscle tightness can exacerbate the locking of the facets. Once the muscles have been relaxed, improving the flexibility in the area can prevent the recurrence of this condition. The stretches for the low back, hips, and anterior trunk can be applied to this condition (see Figs. 6-16 through 6-19 and 6-21 through 6-23). As with spondylolisthesis, take care with the stretches that cause hyperextension of the spine.

Sacroiliac Joint Dysfunction

Background

"The sacroiliac joint continues to be one of the most misunderstood joints in the body" (Cibulka, 2002). It is classified as a *synchondrosis,* which by definition is an immovable joint, yet it is subject to the same inflammatory and infectious conditions that affect synovial joints. As more information is gathered about its true function, it is routinely being described as a synovial articulation with motion as a characterizing feature (McGrath, 2004). "There are 35 muscles that attach directly to the sacrum and/or the innominate bones" (Thompson et al., 2001). The sacroiliac joint primarily functions as a shock absorber, but it also serves to complete the pelvic ring and dissipates the load from the upper body to the lower extremities. It is estimated that 15% to 30% of clients with low-back pain have **sacroiliac joint (SIJ) dysfunction**. Repetitive or high-force loads can result in bony, ligamentous, or muscle overuse syndromes. Several anatomical, biomechanical, and neurophysiologic studies have shown that the loss of stability in the lumbopelvic region, more specifically, the SIJ, can be crucial in the etiology of nonspecific back pain (Pool-Goudzwaard, et al., 2003). The main conclusions from these studies are:

- In loading conditions, muscle forces are necessary for stability.
- Mechanoreceptors present in the massive ligaments of the area are important in the activation of the muscles for posture control.
- Restriction of the range of motion by the ligaments plays an important role in stability.

The motions at the SIJ have been described as upslips, downslips, torsions, outflares, inflares, rotations, and side bending (Cibulka, 2002). Since the movements at a joint are dictated to a large extent by their anatomical structure, all of these different motions cannot occur at the sacroiliac joint. According to Cibulka, the only two motions possible at that joint are a nodding movement of the sacrum and an anterior or posterior tilt (2002). This motion will change over time as a result of the changes in the anatomical structure of the joint. As the mobility in the joint decreases, compensatory motion in the lumbar spine increases. This also works in reverse; that is, decreased mobility in the lumbar spine leads to increased motion in the SIJ. This motion is not always biomechanically desirable

sacroiliac joint (SIJ) dysfunction Misalignment of the sacroiliac joint, which can result in damage to the joint and thus cause pain.

and can lead to dysfunction in the joint. There are two common hypotheses for SIJ involvement in low-back pain:

1. Asymmetry in the pelvic ring results in an increase in stress on a particular structure.
2. The lack of mobility results in tissue stress and pain.

Despite the lack of evidence of the involvement of the SIJ in low-back pain, the presentation of clients who have SIJ dysfunction has been consistent. Ipsilateral gluteal pain, typically around the posterior superior iliac spine, is the most common complaint and is often accompanied by a palpable soft tissue nodule over the PSIS. In addition to pain in the gluteal region, the pain and discomfort can radiate into the groin and lower extremities and can cause numbness, clicking, or popping in the posterior pelvis.

Assessment

While many diagnostic tests have been developed to identify dysfunction at the sacroiliac joint, there is no gold standard to confirm its presence (Riddle et al., 2002). Traditionally, the tests used in manual medicine to identify SIJ involvement have poor inter- and intraexaminer reliability when it comes to assessing landmarks. The two basic types of assessments are:

• Motion tests
• Pain provocation tests

There are challenges with each type of test, and it is important to consider other clinical findings along with the test results. Motion tests for the SIJ are still up for debate. Pain provocation tests for the SIJ are unlikely to load the targeted structures alone; therefore, the challenge is to determine whether the pathology is in the joint or in a nearby structure (Laslett, 2005). Motion and pain provocation tests, the asymmetry of bony landmarks, and soft tissue texture change should all be combined to create the most accurate assessment of the condition (Peace and Fryer, 2004).

Condition History Since this condition can develop from a variety of sources, it is important to perform a thorough history. Here are some questions that are relevant to SIJ dysfunction:

Question	Significance
What was the mechanism of injury?	The SIJ can be injured from sudden jarring as the result of a fall or intense extreme movement at the joint or from lift and twist action.
Where is the pain? Does it radiate?	SIJ pain tends to be focused over and around the PSIS and can radiate down the leg.
When does the pain occur?	Pain can be constant or occur primarily during extension from a flexed position or stepping up with the affected leg.

Question	Significance
Is there a habitual posture?	Certain postures can stress the joint.
Is there any weakness?	Dysfunction in the joint can cause neurologic weakness.
Was there a recent pregnancy?	The increase in the laxity of the ligaments due to hormonal changes during pregnancy can lead to dysfunction in the area.

Visual Assessment Have the client disrobe to the appropriate level. In addition to noting any obvious discoloration, swelling, or deformity, check on the following:

- Is there an anterior or posterior tilt to the pelvis? This will indicate a nutation or contranutation position.
- Does the client favor one side when standing? Unequal distribution of weight on both feet can indicate pathology.
- Are the contours of the gluteals and the gluteal folds normal?
- Are the iliac crests level?
- Are the ASIS and PSIS level? The ASIS will tend to be higher and slightly forward on the affected side. If the ASIS and PSIS are higher on one side than the other, this indicates a shift on the high side. This may result in a short leg or muscle spasm on the affected side. If the ASIS is higher and the PSIS is lower on the same side, this indicates an anterior torsion of the sacrum on that side.
- Are the pubic bones level at the symphysis?
- Are the ischial tuberosities level?
- Are the ASISs of equal distance from the midline?

Palpation When palpating the area, check for obvious deformity or swelling. Palpate the structures discussed at the beginning of the chapter to check for any asymmetry. Be sure to include the hip rotators, gluteal muscles, iliolumbar ligament, and other areas of compensation. Check for palpable nodules over the PSIS, as they are common in this condition.

Orthopedic Tests In addition to assessing the dermatomes and myotomes and conducting other active and passive range-of-motion tests, look for asymmetrical movements, hypo- or hypermobility, and tissue restrictions.

1. Kneel behind the client. Start by noting the position of the static bony landmarks such as the PSIS, ASIS, ischial tuberosities, sacrum, and iliac crests.
2. Place one thumb over the PSIS and the other over the spinous process of S2. Have the client flex the hip as high as possible. In normal motion, the PSIS of the flexed hip will drop while hypomobility causes the PSIS to move up. Repeat on both sides and compare. Move the thumb that was on the PSIS to the ischial tuberosity of the same side; have the client flex the hip again. In normal motion the ischial tuberosity moves laterally, while a hypomobile joint causes the ischial tuberosity to move in a superior direction.

Table 6-8 lists some orthopedic tests and explains how to perform them.

Table 6-8   Orthopedic Tests for SIJ Dysfunction

Orthopedic Test	How to Perform
Gillet's (sacral fixation) test 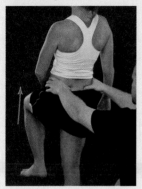 (This is a mobility test.)	Have the client stand directly in front of you, facing away. Place your thumbs on the PSIS on both sides, and have the client fully flex one thigh to the chest while standing on one leg. The PSIS on the flexed side should move in an inferior direction. If it does not move or moves in a superior direction, it indicates a hypomobile joint or a "blocked" joint; this is a positive test.
Sacroiliac compression (gapping) test 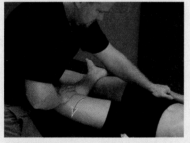 (This is a pain provocation test.)	Client is in the supine position. Place your hands cross-armed on the ASIS, and repeatedly apply a downward and outward pressure to the ASIS as if you were trying to spread the two iliums apart. Unilateral pain in the posterior leg, the PSIS, or the gluteals may indicate an anterior sprain to the SIJ. Pain elsewhere may indicate the involvement of other structures.
Patrick's (Faber's) test 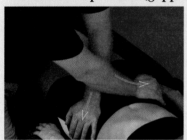 (This is a pain provocation test.)	Client is in a supine position. Place the outside of the foot and ankle of the involved leg on the knee of the contralateral leg, and let it fall out to the side. Place one hand on the knee of the involved leg and the other hand on the ASIS of the uninvolved leg. Stabilize the ASIS, and apply pressure to the bent knee. Pain in the SIJ of the involved side may indicate pathology and is considered a positive test.
Gaenslen's test 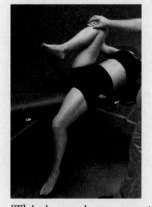 (This is a pain provocation test.)	Client is in the supine position close enough to the edge of the table that the hip extends beyond the edge. Have the client draw both legs up to the chest and slowly lower one into extension. Pain in the SIJ of the extended leg is considered a positive test and may indicate pathology. *Note:* If the client cannot lie in the supine position, place him or her on the side and draw the bottom leg up to the chest; have the client hold the position. Bring the top leg into hyperextension while stabilizing the pelvis. Pain in the SIJ is considered a positive test.

Soft Tissue Treatment

Since SIJ dysfunction stems from a lack of motion at the joint, the primary intent of the treatment should be to restore normal motion to the joint. The iliopsoas and gluteal muscles can be major contributors to this condition and should be a principal area of concentration.

Connective Tissue The loss of motion associated with this condition can be chronic, developing over time and involving adaptive layers of connective tissue restrictions. Releasing these tissues is beneficial in restoring normal functioning in the area.

Prone Position After releasing the superficial restrictions in all directions in both the lumbar and the gluteal regions, move into the deeper layers and strip out the borders of the involved muscles. An important area to release is the border between the gluteus maximus and the gluteus minimus. Start at the PSIS, and work in a line toward the greater trochanter. Another effective area to address is around the greater trochanter itself. Trace around its borders to release the lateral rotators. Tracing along the inferior border of the iliac crest will help release the rest of the gluteals.

Supine Position Once the superficial layers have been addressed, remove the restriction along the abdominal muscles, especially at the inguinal ligament attachments. It is important to address the anterior hip because it has a great deal of influence on anterior pelvic tilt. Release the muscles that attach in that area. Along with the anterior hip, the iliopsoas, particularly the iliacus division, can dramatically affect motion at the SIJ. Be sure to spend ample time on this muscle.

Side-Lying Position This position is the most efficient and effective for accessing the gluteals and lateral hip rotators.

Tissue Inconsistencies Trigger points are involved in several different conditions of this region. Some of the muscles that may be involved are:

- Paraspinals
- Quadratus lumborum
- Gluteals
- Iliopsoas
- Abdominals

The same muscles can cause dysfunction in the SIJ and should be addressed using digital compression techniques and active and passive movement.

Muscle Concerns

More often than not, this condition is the result of a muscle imbalance in the area. Effective treatment can benefit the client. Focus on the restoration of normal motion in the joint.

Prone Position With the client in this position, treat the muscles that attach to the iliac crest and sacrum. Treat the gluteals using a loose fist to obtain the appropriate depth.

1. Standing on the side of the client, place the back of your fist just lateral to the sacrum. Use the other hand to apply counterpressure on the sacrum; then slowly slide your hand toward you, being careful not to pinch the tissue into the table.
2. Defining the sacrum and its lateral edge removes a lot of the restrictions in the gluteus maximus. From the PSIS, move medially onto the sacrum and find its lateral edge. Run your fingertips or thumb inferiorly along its border.

Forearm strokes to the paraspinals and the quadratus lumborum can dramatically affect movement at the SIJ.

Supine Position The iliopsoas has a powerful effect on the mobility of the SIJ; therefore, spending ample time on this muscle is important (see Fig. 6-15).

1. Have the client bend the knees to about 45°.
2. Place the client's feet on the table, and have him or her take a deep breath. Starting at the anterior superior iliac spine, slide your fingertips in along the inside of the "bowl" of the pelvis as the client exhales; stay lateral to the edge of the rectus abdominus muscle.
3. Once you locate a restriction, direct your pressure down toward the table.
4. Have the client slowly extend the leg, keeping the heel on the table as he or she slides it as far as possible and brings it back up.

While you continue to hold the restriction, have the client repeat this process several times or until you feel the tissue release. Slowly remove your hand and repeat the process, changing the location and angle that you slide in. The more inferior you move along the bowl of the pelvis, the greater the focus on the iliacus. Moving superiorly toward the umbilicus will focus more on the psoas. Generally, avoid going any higher than the level of the umbilicus because you may encounter solid organs.

Side-Lying Position This is the best position for addressing the gluteals and hip rotators. Along with radiating strokes out from the greater trochanter, a forearm stroke to the gluteals is effective in this position.

Stretching

Lack of motion in a joint has a direct relationship with the flexibility of the tissue in the area. Using the stretches for the iliopsoas, hip flexors, and gluteals can dramatically improve this condition. (See Figs. 6-21, 6-23, and 6-24).

SUMMARY

A review of the regional anatomy and a detailed description of how to locate various bony landmarks and structures began the first section of this chapter. The next section discussed how to gather information to create a physiologic baseline of the lumbar spine and trunk. This included the various ranges of motion, dermatomes, trigger-point locations, and manual muscle tests. Numerous conditions that affect the lumbar spine and sacral area were discussed, including their presentation characteristics. For each condition mentioned, assessment and treatment techniques were given so that the therapist can effectively work on the condition.

REVIEW QUESTIONS

1. What bones make up the lumbosacral region?
2. Which three spinal ligaments support the region?
3. Which nerve roots make up the lumbar and sacral plexuses?
4. What are the movements of the lumbar and sacral region?
5. What are the dermatomes for the lumbar and sacral region?
6. What are the four degrees of injury that can occur to the vertebral disks?
7. What is the end result of the degeneration of or injury to a disk?
8. What is the difference between spondylolysis and spondylolisthesis?
9. What are the five classifications of spondylolisthesis?
10. What are the two mechanisms for facet joint irritation?
11. What are the two types of assessments for sacroiliac joint dysfunction?
12. What are the mechanisms of injury for SIJ dysfunction?

CRITICAL-THINKING QUESTIONS

1. How do the special tests for lumbar disk injuries indicate an injury?
2. Why is it important to differentiate between hamstring tightness and nerve involvement for a low-back injury?
3. How does posture contribute to lumbar spine and sacral problems?
4. Why is preventing hyperextension important in spondylolysis and spondylolisthesis?
5. How does releasing the iliopsoas benefit the conditions discussed in the chapter?
6. How does the quadrant test indicate a facet joint problem?

Bony Structures of the Lumbar Spine

Lamina groove	Groove on either side of the spinous processes from the cervical region to the sacral region.
Umbilicus	Known as the belly button and lies at the level of L3-L4.
L4-L5 interspace	L4-L5 interspace should line up with the top of the iliac crest.
Iliac crest	Place the palms of your hands in the flank area just below the ribs, and press down and in. You should feel the top of the crests.
Transverse processes L1-L5	Directly lateral to their spinous processes. Make sure you are lateral to the musculature. The longest and easiest to find is L3. Use the L4-L5 interspace to locate L4 and the rest of the segments. L1 is more difficult to locate as it is partially covered by the 12th rib. L5 is also difficult, as it is covered by the iliac crest.
Iliac tubercle	From the top of the crests, move anteriorly to find this tubercle. It is the widest point on the crests.
Anterior superior iliac spine (ASIS)	Most anterior part of the crest. Have the client lie supine, and place the palms of your hands on the front of his or her hips.
Anterior inferior iliac spine (AIIS)	From ASIS, move inferiorly about ½ inch. You won't be able to directly palpate this structure.
Pubic crest	Place your fingertips in the umbilicus. Rest your hand in an inferior direction on the abdomen. Slowly press down and in; the heel of your hand will hit a bony ledge.
Pubic symphysis	Once you find the crest, there is a joint directly in the middle.
Pubic tubercles	On either edge of the pubic crest are small bumps.
Anterior transverse processes of lumbar spine	Have the client flex the knees to soften the abdomen. Use the umbilicus and ASIS as reference points. Starting at the ASIS, slide into the tissue until you reach the lateral edge of the rectus abdominus. Once there, direct pressure downward.

Soft Tissue Structures of the Lumbar Spine

Inguinal ligament	Located on a line between the ASIS of the ilium and the pubic tubercles. It is the inferior edge of the oblique abdominal muscles.
Abdominal aorta	Pick a point between the xiphoid process and the umbilicus, just left of midline. Use your fingertips, and press in gently as the client relaxes. The aorta is easily palpated in most; you may have to move up and down the line to find it.
Spleen	Place one hand on the left back around T10-T11, and lift up. Place the other hand at the left costal margin, and gently press up and in. Have the client take a deep breath; you should feel the edge of the spleen move into your fingers.
Liver	Place one hand on the right side of the back around T10-T11, and lift up gently. Using the fingers of the other hand, press up and in at the right costal margin with moderate pressure. Have the client take a deep breath; you should feel the edge of the liver move into your fingers.
Cluneal nerves	Locate the PSIS and the iliac tubercles. Find the midpoint along the iliac crest, and palpate these vertically oriented nerves in a transverse direction.

Bony and Soft Tissue Structures and Surface Anatomy of the Sacrum

Posterior superior iliac spine (PSIS)	These are the most posterior aspects of the iliac crest. They are commonly referred to as the "dimples" in the low back. They are located at the level of S2.
Sacrum	Using the PSIS, move medially onto the sacrum. Once you are on the bone, use your fingertips to trace its lateral edge in an inferior direction.
Medial sacral crest	The fused spinous processes of the sacral vertebra.
Natal cleft	The area between the buttocks.
Greater trochanter of femur	Have the client lie in the prone position, and place the palm of your hand over his or her lateral hip. Bend the client's knee to 90°, press in on the hip, and rotate the leg medially and laterally. You should feel a large bony structure rotating under your hand.
Trochanteric bursa	This bursa is generally not palpable. Using the greater trochanter, palpate just posterior to and behind the trochanter.
Gluteal fold	This fold is formed by the thigh as it meets the hip. Have the client lie in the prone position, and locate the fold at the base of the gluteus maximus muscle and the top of the hamstrings.
Ischial tuberosity	This structure is on the inferior ischium and is the common origin for the hamstrings. Using the gluteal fold, place the webspace of your hand with the thumb pointing medially along the fold. Press in; your thumb should be on the tuberosity.
Sacrotuberous ligament	Using the ischial tuberosity, move superior and medial and press in. To make sure you are on the ligament, have the client cough; the ligament will tighten.
Greater sciatic notch	Draw a line between the posterior superior iliac spine on the side opposite the notch you are trying to locate and the greater trochanter on the same side as the notch you are trying to locate to find the midpoint. Press in, and you should be in a depression, which is the notch.

Muscles of the Lumbar Spine and Sacrum

Muscle	Origin	Insertion	Action	How to Palpate
Posterior Lumbar Spine				
Erector spinae group	Thoracolumbar aponeurosis; posterior sacrum; iliac crest; lumbar vertebra	Posterior ribs; thoracic and cervical vertebra; mastoid process; nuchal line	Extends vertebral column; laterally flexes vertebral column to same side	Prone position; extend legs and trunk
Quadratus lumborum	Posterior iliac crest	12th rib; transverse processes of L1-L4	Laterally flexes trunk to same side; elevates hip (hip hiker)	Prone position; palpate between the last rib and the iliac crest lateral and deep to erector spinae
Multifidus	Sacrum; iliac crest; transverse processes of C4-L5	Spinous processes of vertebra above origin	Extends and rotates spinal column to opposite side	Not directly palpable. Press deep along attachment line
Rotatores	Transverse processes of lumbar through cervical vertebrae	Spinous processes of vertebra above origin (one span)	Extends and rotates spinal column to opposite side	Not directly palpable. Press deep along attachment line
Serratus posterior inferior	Spinous processes of T11-L3	Ribs 9-12	Depresses rib cage	Prone position; palpate along muscle fibers during exhalation
Posterior Hip				
Gluteus maximus	Posterior iliac crest; sacrum; sacrotuberous and sacroiliac ligaments	Gluteal tuberosity of femur; Gerty's tubercle by way of the iliotibial tract	Extends thigh at hip; laterally rotates thigh at hip; extends leg at knee while standing; extends trunk at hip when standing; abducts thigh at hip	Prone position; palpate during hyperextension of thigh at the hip
Gluteus medius	Iliac crest and lateral surface of the ilium	Greater trochanter of the femur	Abducts, flexes, medially rotates the hip; stabilizes the pelvis on the hip during gait	Side-lying position; palpate between greater trochanter and iliac crest during abduction of thigh

Muscle	Origin	Insertion	Action	How to Palpate
Posterior Hip (Continued)				
Gluteus minimus	Posterior ilium between the middle and inferior gluteal lines	Anterior aspect of the greater trochanter	Abducts, medially rotates, flexes hip	Side-lying position; palpate between greater trochanter and 1 inch inferior to the iliac crest during abduction at the hip
Piriformis	Greater sciatic notch and the anterior surface of the sacrum	Greater trochanter of the femur (medial aspect)	Laterally rotates, abducts thigh at hip	Side-lying position; palpate between greater trochanter and sacrum during lateral rotation of thigh
Anterior Trunk				
Rectus abdominus	Pubic symphysis	Costal cartilages of ribs 5, 6, 7; xiphoid process	Supports compression of abdominal contents; flexes trunk	Supine position; palpate anterior surface of abdomen during trunk flexion
External oblique	Ribs 5-12	Abdominal aponeurosis and linea alba; iliac crest	Bilateral: flexes trunk; compresses abdominal contents. Unilateral: laterally flexes trunk to same side; rotates trunk to opposite side	Supine position; palpate lateral sides of abdomen during trunk rotation to the opposite side
Internal oblique	Inguinal ligament; iliac crest; thoracolumbar aponeurosis	Costal cartilages of ribs 9-12; abdominal aponeurosis and linea alba	Bilateral: flexes trunk and compresses abdominal contents. Unilateral: laterally flexes, rotates trunk to same side	Supine position; can be felt between the ribs and pelvis during rotation of the trunk to the same side
Transverse abdominus	Inguinal ligament; iliac crest; thoracolumbar aponeurosis; costal cartilages of ribs 7-12	Abdominal aponeurosis; linea alba	Compresses abdominal contents	Supine position; difficult to palpate and differentiate from overlying structures. More palpable toward the pubic crest on either side of the rectus abdominus

Chapter 6 Conditions of the Lumbar Spine and Sacrum

Iliopsoas	Iliac crest and fossa; anterior vertebral bodies T12-L5	Lesser trochanter of femur	Flexes hip	Supine position; on a line between ASIS and umbilicus. Press down into iliac fossa for iliacus; press down and in at lateral edge of rectus abdominus for psoas

Trigger Points for the Lumbar Spine and Sacrum

Muscle	Trigger-Point Location	Referral Pattern	Chief Symptom
Iliocostalis lumborum	Belly of muscle just under the last rib	Strongly downward to midbuttock region	Unilateral posterior hip pain
Longissimus thoracis	1. Lower thoracic region (T10 or T11) over transverse process 2. L1 just lateral to spinous process	1. Down to lower part of buttock to ischial tuberosity 2. Inferiorly several segments to posterior iliac crest	Buttock pain; lumbago-type symptoms
Serratus posterior inferior	Middle of muscle around 10th rib	Local to trigger point	Annoying ache in lower thoracic area
Quadratus lumborum	1. Lateral edge of muscle just under the last rib 2. Inferior edge of muscle just above iliac crest 3. Lateral to transverse process of L3 4. Between transverse processes of L4-L5	1. Along crest of ilium and adjacent quadrant of abdomen 2. Greater trochanter 3. Sacroiliac joint 4. Lower buttock	Low-back pain; difficulty turning over in bed or standing upright; pain when coughing or sneezing
Multifidi/rotatores	Within the bellies	Area around the spinous process; midline to spinous process	Persistent, worrisome, bone pain
Gluteus maximus	1. Lateral edge of the sacrum halfway down 2. Just superior to ischial tuberosity 3. Medial to ischial tuberosity	1. Semicircle up along sacrum and natal cleft to SIJ; down along gluteal fold 2. Entire buttock, both superficially and deep; just under iliac crest 3. Coccyx	Pain and restlessness after long periods of sitting; pain while walking uphill and swimming the crawl stroke
Gluteus medius	1. Inferior to posterior iliac crest near SIJ 2. Inferior to iliac crest midway along length 3. ASIS inferior to crest	1. Along crest up into SIJ and lumbar spine 2. Midgluteal region; may extend to upper lateral thigh 3. Along crest; encompasses lower lumbar and sacral region	Pain on walking and sitting in a slumped position; difficulty sleeping on the affected side

Chapter 6 Conditions of the Lumbar Spine and Sacrum

Trigger Points for the Lumbar Spine and Sacrum *(Continued)*

Muscle	Trigger-Point Location	Referral Pattern	Chief Symptom
Gluteus minimus	1. One below the other, inferior to the anterior iliac crest 2. Superior edge of the muscle	1. Lower lateral buttock down lateral thigh, along the peroneals sometimes to ankle 2. Most of buttock down back of thigh into calf	Hip pain that can affect gait; difficulty lying on affected side and standing after prolonged sitting
Piriformis	1. Just lateral to the sacrum 2. Just before the greater trochanter	1. Sacroiliac region 2. Posterior hip joint	Pain and numbness in the low back, groin, buttock, hip, and posterior thigh and leg
Rectus abdominus	1. Upper portion of muscle 2. Periumbilical region 3. Lower portion of muscle	1. Midback bilaterally; xiphoid process 2. Area around point 3. Lower back and sacrum	Heartburn; indigestion; back pain; abdominal cramping; colic; diffuse pain; dysmenorrheal or pseudo-appendicitis pain
Obliques	Within the belly	Up into chest; across the abdomen; down into the groin	Deep epigastric pain; mimics heartburn symptoms; groin pain
Iliopsoas	1. Just lateral to the umbilicus 2. Just medial to the anterior iliac crest on the fossa 3. Anterior thigh just inferior to the inguinal ligament	Ipsilateral vertical pattern along the lumbar spine, sacroiliac area, groin, and anteromedial thigh on the same side	Pain during weight-bearing activities with relief through hip flexion

Orthopedic Tests for the Lumbar Spine and Sacrum

Condition	Orthopedic Test	How to Perform	Positive Sign
Lumbar disk injuries	Lasegue's (straight-leg-raise) test	Client is in the supine position with both legs straight and the tested leg internally rotated at the hip. Client should be completely relaxed and lift the leg slowly until he or she complains of pain or tightness. Lower leg until pain or tightness is relieved. Have client dorsiflex foot as far as possible or until symptoms return. If this does not cause any pain or tightness, ask client to flex the head off the table as far as possible. If either movement does not cause the pain to return, the source is not disk-related and is most likely tight hamstrings. If the client is able to flex the leg past 70°, the cause is most likely facet or sacroiliac in origin, since the sciatic nerve is fully stretched at that range.	Pain that moves from the back down into the leg along the sciatic nerve distribution during one of the movements is a positive sign. Pain in the lumbar spine on the side opposite the lifted leg can indicate a space-occupying lesion such as a herniation.
	Slump test (This is the most common neurologic test for the lower limb and is an indicator of impingement of the dura and spinal cord or nerve roots.)	Client is seated on the edge of the table with the legs hanging over and the hands behind the back. Have the client "slump" so that he or she flexes the spine and rolls the shoulders forward but keeps the head in a neutral position. If this does not produce any symptoms, have the client flex the head down and hold the shoulders slumped forward. If there are still no symptoms, passively extend the client's lower leg and dorsiflex the foot while he or she maintains the slumped position.	The reproduction of pain down the sciatic nerve at any stage of the test is a positive sign.
Spondylolysis or spondylolisthesis	Stork (single-leg) standing test	Have the client stand on one leg. Stand behind the client to prevent him or her from falling. Have the client extend the spine. Repeat on the other leg. *Note:* If the fracture is only on one side, standing on the ipsilateral leg will cause more pain. Have the client perform true extension because combining movements will not give an accurate result.	A positive test is pain in the low back, which is associated with a fracture of the pars.

Orthopedic Tests for the Lumbar Spine and Sacrum *(Continued)*

Muscle	Trigger-Point Location	Referral Pattern	Chief Symptom
Facet joint syndrome	Quadrant test	Stand behind the client, and place your hands on the shoulders. Have the client extend the spine while you control the movement by holding the shoulders. Move the client into lateral flexion and rotation to the side of pain while the client is in extension. Continue the movement until you reach the end range or reproduce the pain. This will cause the maximum narrowing of the foramen and put the most stress on the facets.	A positive test occurs if pain is produced.
Sacroiliac joint dysfunction	Gillet's (sacral fixation) test (This is a mobility test.)	Have the client stand directly in front of you, facing away. Place your thumbs on the PSIS on both sides, and have the client fully flex one thigh to the chest while standing on one leg.	The PSIS on the flexed side should move in an inferior direction. If it does not move or moves in a superior direction, this indicates a hypomobile joint or a "blocked" joint; this is a positive test.
	Sacroiliac compression (gapping) test (This is a pain provocation test.)	Client is in the supine position. Place your hands cross-armed on the ASIS, and repeatedly apply a downward and outward pressure to the ASIS as if you were trying to spread the two iliums apart.	Unilateral pain in the posterior leg, the PSIS, or the gluteals may indicate an anterior sprain to the SIJ. Pain elsewhere may indicate the involvement of other structures.

Orthopedic Tests for the Lumbar Spine and Sacrum *(Continued)*

Muscle	Trigger-Point Location	Referral Pattern	Chief Symptom
	Patrick's (Faber's) test (This is a pain provocation test.)	Client is in a supine position. Place the outside of the foot and ankle of the involved leg on the knee of the contralateral leg, and let it fall out to the side. Place one hand on the knee of the involved leg and the other hand on the ASIS of the uninvolved leg. Stabilize the ASIS, and apply pressure to the bent knee.	Pain in the SIJ of the involved side may indicate pathology and is considered a positive test.
	Gaenslen's test (This is a pain provocation test.)	Client is in a supine position close enough to the edge of the table that the hip extends beyond the edge. Have the client draw both legs up to the chest and slowly lower one into extension. *Note:* If the client cannot lie in the supine position, place him or her on the side and draw the bottom leg up to the chest; have the client hold the position. Bring the top leg into hyperextension while stabilizing the pelvis. Pain in the SIJ is considered a positive test.	Pain in the SIJ of the extended leg is considered a positive test and may indicate pathology.

chapter 7

Conditions of the Shoulder

chapter objectives

At the conclusion of this chapter, the reader will understand:

- the bony anatomy of the region
- how to locate the bony landmarks and soft tissue structures of the region
- where to find the muscles, as well as the origins, insertions, and actions of the region
- how to assess the movement and determine the range of motion for the region
- how to perform manual muscle testing to the region
- how to recognize dermatome patterns for the region
- trigger-point location and referral patterns for the region
- the following elements of each condition discussed:
  - background and characteristics
  - specific questions to ask
  - what orthopedic tests should be performed
  - how to treat the connective tissue, trigger points, and muscles
  - flexibility concerns

key terms

adhesive capsulitis
attrition tendonosis
capsular pattern
impingement tendonosis
painful arc
pseudothoracic syndrome
scapulohumeral rhythm
subacromial impingement syndrome

Introduction

The shoulder is one of two pairs of ball-and-socket joints in the body (the other set is located in the hip). Because of its complex anatomy, the shoulder has the greatest range of mobility compared to any other joint in the body (Beltran et al., 2003). Unfortunately, this greater mobility results in diminished stability. Two mechanisms contribute to the joint's stability:

Active mechanisms include the contractile tissues around the joint:
- The tendon of the long head of the biceps
- The rotator cuff muscles and tendons

Passive mechanisms include the support given by the inert tissues in the area:
- The size and shape of the glenoid fossa
- The labrum
- The joint capsule
- The glenohumeral ligaments (Beltran et al, 2003)

Because of this combination of high mobility and low stability, there is an increased risk of pathology, which explains why the shoulder is the most dislocated joint in the body.

Shoulder pain can originate from myriad causes, including not only intrinsic disease and dysfunction in the structures around the joint but also referrals from related areas such as the cervical spine, thorax, and soft tissue structures.

Shoulder dysfunction accounts for about 5% of visits to primary care physicians and is the third most common musculoskeletal complaint (Wilson, 2005). Assessment of shoulder dysfunction can be difficult in part because of the sophisticated interaction between the shoulder complex and other areas of the body. Shoulder injuries can arise from both traumatic and chronic overuse conditions, and they can be exacerbated by underlying postural concerns that lead to a predisposition to re-injury. While not comprehensive, this chapter addresses the complex components in order to provide an understanding of the overall functioning of the region. The chapter reviews basic anatomy and then moves into other areas, including:

> **Practical Tip**
>
> Remember that shoulder pain can originate from surrounding structures and not just from the shoulder.

- Specific bony landmarks that mark important areas for palpation
- Soft tissue structures, including muscles of the region
- Movements of the region
- Manual muscle tests for the shoulder
- Dermatome and trigger-point referral patterns for the involved muscles

ANATOMICAL REVIEW

Bony Anatomy of the Shoulder Girdle

"The humerus, scapula, clavicle, sternum and first eight thoracic ribs are the skeletal fundamentals of the shoulder" (Levy et al., 2002). The *humerus* is the long bone of the upper arm and has very differently shaped ends (Fig. 7-1). Its proximal end has a semiround head that articulates with the glenoid fossa of the scapula and a distal end that articulates with the ulna. At its proximal end are two prominences: the greater tuberosity, positioned laterally, and the lesser tuberosity, positioned anteriorly and medially. These are the attachment sites for the rotator cuff muscles and

Figure 7-1 Skeletal and surface anatomy structures of the shoulder girdle.

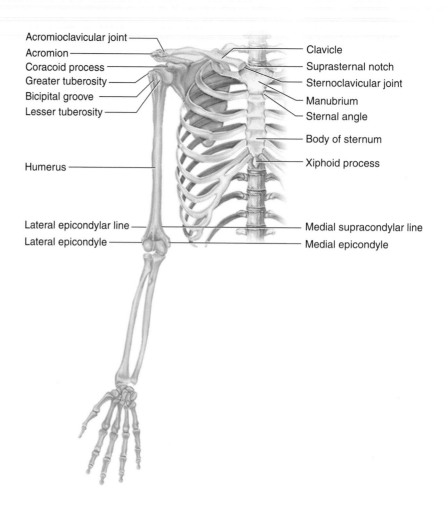

Acromioclavicular joint
Acromion
Coracoid process
Greater tuberosity
Bicipital groove
Lesser tuberosity
Humerus
Lateral epicondylar line
Lateral epicondyle

Clavicle
Suprasternal notch
Sternoclavicular joint
Manubrium
Sternal angle
Body of sternum
Xiphoid process
Medial supracondylar line
Medial epicondyle

create a groove between them to accommodate the tendon of the long head of the biceps brachii. The distal end has an hourglass-shaped notch that sits within the deep ulnar groove and forms the elbow joint.

The *scapula* is an important component within the shoulder girdle. It is a flat, triangular-shaped bone that lies over the 2nd through 7th ribs and has three distinct features (Fig. 7-2). The spine of the scapula lies on the posterior side of the bone and runs at a slightly upward angle from the medial aspect, about two-thirds up the medial border to the superior lateral aspect of the bone. It divides the scapula into unequal sections known as the *superior and inferior fossas,* both of which serve as sites for muscle attachments. As the spine moves to the superior lateral aspect, it ends in the next distinct feature, the *acromion process.* This flat end of the spine lies at the tip of the shoulder and articulates anteriorly with the clavicle to form the acromioclavicular joint.

The last feature is on the anterior aspect of the bone and projects through to the front of the shoulder. The *coracoid process* (see Fig. 7-1) serves as an attachment site for both trunk and arm muscles. The scapula is a unique bone because it does not articulate directly with the ribs and is held in place by numerous muscles.

The *clavicle* is the only bone that connects the axial and upper appendicular skeletons. It is an S-shaped bone that runs horizontally along the anterior part of the shoulder at the top of the thorax (see Fig. 7-1). Its medial edge is rounded and articulates with the manubrium of the sternum;

its lateral edge is flat and articulates with the acromion process of the scapula. The medial half of the bone bends in a convex direction, while the lateral portion of the muscle curves in a concave fashion. The part of the clavicle at which the curve changes from a convex curve to a concave curve creates a structural weak spot; therefore, the largest number of fractures occurs at this point.

The *sternum* is a bony plate that ties the rib cage together anteriorly and protects the heart. It is subdivided into three parts: the manubrium, the body, and the xiphoid process. The *manubrium* is the most superior part and articulates with the clavicle and 1st and 2nd ribs (see Fig. 7-1). Moving in an inferior direction, the *body* is the longest part of the sternum and articulates with the 3rd through 6th ribs directly and the 7th through 10th ribs indirectly via the costocartilage. The most inferior part, the *xiphoid process,* is the distal tip of the sternum and can damage the organs if it is broken off.

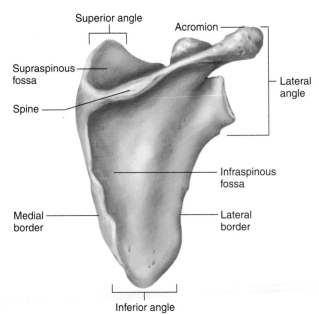

Figure 7-2 Posterior skeletal and surface anatomy structures of the scapula.

Bony Structures and Surface Anatomy of the Shoulder

Palpation of the shoulder area should take place in a systematic way and include the proximal humerus, clavicle, scapula, sternum, and ribs. Movement is often incorporated to make identification of the structures more accurate. We will start with the scapula, move to the clavicle, and palpate the humerus last (see Fig. 7-1).

Scapula

The *spine of the scapula* is on the posterior shoulder girdle on the upper half of the bone and runs in a transverse direction at a slight upward angle. The medial end lines up with T3, and the lateral end is the acromion process. To locate the spine, use the palm of your hand and place it on the upper half of the scapula. Palpate back and forth in a vertical fashion to find the distinct edge, and then use your fingertips to trace its borders to either end. Once you trace the spine to its medial edge, you can easily find the *medial border of the scapula.* It runs along the spinal column the entire length of the scapula and is palpated easier by placing the client's hand in the small of his or her back.

If you trace the medial border to its most superior part, you will encounter a sharp corner known as the *superior angle of the scapula.* This point is commonly tender and is the insertion for the levator scapula. Tracing inferiorly along the medial border until its inferior tip, you will feel another prominent corner, which is the *inferior angle of the scapula.*

The last structure on the posterior aspect of the bone is the *lateral border.* Using the inferior angle as a starting place, round the corner and move up the lateral edge of the bone to the axilla. This border may be more difficult to define since it is covered by thick muscles.

Practical Tip

Movement is very helpful in identifying structures in the shoulder.

As you move around to the anterior structures on the scapula, you encounter the *acromion process*. This is the flat, L-shaped lateral end of the spine of the scapula that forms the acromioclavicular joint with the clavicle. Place the palm of your hand on the lateral tip of the shoulder, and move it in a circular fashion, feeling for a flat, bony surface. Once you locate the general structure, use your fingertips to trace the borders. To ensure you are on the right structure, have the client move the shoulder. If you are on the acromion process, it should not move. If it does move, however, you are probably on the acromioclavicular joint or the head of the humerus.

The last structure on the scapula is the *coracoid process*, which lies on the anterior surface. It is located about 1 inch medial to the acromion and about a half-inch inferior to the clavicle. It feels like a small marble and will most likely be tender.

Clavicle

The *clavicle* is an S-shaped bone anterior to posterior. It has a convex curve medially and a concave curve laterally. The medial end is rounded and forms a joint with the sternum, while the lateral end is larger and flatter and forms a joint with the acromion process of the scapula. Starting at either end of the clavicle, trace the bone between its two ends. At the lateral end, the *acromioclavicular joint* can be a difficult structure to find on some clients. Start by tracing the clavicle to its lateral edge. Once you reach the end of the clavicle, you should feel a space where it meets the acromion process. This is the joint. You can also start by locating the acromion process and working your way medially until you feel a "step" up to the clavicle. The space before the step is the joint. You can ensure you are on the joint by having your client protract and retract the shoulders. You should feel it move.

At the other end of the clavicle, the *sternoclavicular joint* joins the axial to the upper appendicular skeleton. Trace the clavicle medially until you feel the joint space. It sits a little superior on the sternum and should be fairly prominent. You can also use the suprasternal notch as a starting point, and move just lateral until you feel the medial edge of the clavicle. In order to make the joint easier to feel, place a finger on the joint and have the client protract and retract the shoulders.

Sternum

Moving medially from the sternoclavicular joint onto the sternum, the *manubrium* is the most superior portion of the bone. The top of this structure is known as the *suprasternal* or *jugular notch* and is easily palpated. The first ribs also attach here on either side below the clavicle. Moving down the sternum, the *sternal angle*, also referred to as the *angle of Louis*, is the junction between the manubrium and the body of the sternum. To find it, start at the suprasternal notch and move in an inferior direction about 1 inch to 1½ inches. You will feel a ridge of bone, which is the angle and the landmark for the second rib. Continuing inferiorly, the *body of the sternum* is the largest portion of the sternum and runs inferiorly to the tip. It serves as the attachment for the last true rib via the costal cartilage. At the most inferior tip of the sternum lies the *xiphoid process*. It can differ in size and can point internally or externally or remain neutral.

Humerus

The last piece of the shoulder girdle is the humerus. The *humeral head* can be palpated in one of two ways. The first method is to stand behind the client and place one hand on the top of the shoulder while cupping the shoulder from the side with the other hand and placing your fingers around the front and your thumb around the back of the shoulder. With the client relaxed, slide the shoulder in an anterior and posterior direction; you will feel the head moving between your fingers and thumb. The second method of palpating the humeral head is to abduct the humerus to the end range and palpate in the axilla with your palm to find the round head of the humerus.

The next structure is the *greater tuberosity of the humerus*. It lies on the superior, lateral humerus and may be difficult to find. Using the acromion process, move off in an inferior direction and slightly medially until you find a large bony prominence. Once you have located it, use your fingers to palpate its borders. The *lesser tuberosity of the humerus* is smaller and deeper than the greater tuberosity. From the anterior portion of the acromion, move in an inferior direction onto the smaller tuberosity.

Between the two tuberosities is the *intertubercular* or *bicipital groove*. It runs in a vertical fashion and is home to the tendon of the long head of the biceps brachii. To locate it, have the client put his or her arm down by the side and bend the elbow to 90°. Locate the greater tuberosity, and laterally rotate the arm. Your finger should fall off the greater tuberosity into a groove. As you continue to rotate the arm, your finger will come up onto the lesser tuberosity. Rotate the arm medially and laterally to find the groove between the tuberosities.

Moving down from the head of the humerus, the *shaft* runs to the epicondyles. It can be directly palpated midway down the inside of the arm between the biceps brachii and the triceps brachii. At the distal end of the humerus on the medial side is the *medial epicondyle of the humerus*. Locate the bend in the elbow, and trace it in a medial direction until you find a round, bony structure. Just superior to the condyle is the *medial supracondylar line of the humerus*. Locate the medial epicondyle of the humerus, and palpate in a superior direction along the ridge. The *lateral epicondyle* is the distal lateral end of the humerus and may be more difficult to find than the medial epicondyle. Locate the bend in the elbow, and move laterally until you feel a round, bony prominence. From the lateral condyle, locate the *lateral epicondylar line* by palpating in a superior direction along the ridge.

> **✦ Practical Tip**
> You may have to move medially to find the greater tuberosity because the shoulder may be internally rotated.

> **✦ Practical Tip**
> Make sure you rotate the arm back and forth to a great enough degree to ensure that you don't miss the groove.

Soft Tissue Structures of the Shoulder

This section discusses the four separate joints that constitute the shoulder region (Fig. 7-3).

Glenohumeral Joint

The *glenohumeral joint* is the multiaxial ball-and-socket joint of the region and has the greatest degree of motion out of the four joints (see Fig. 7-3). It is formed by the humeral head and the glenoid fossa. As stated earlier, stability is sacrificed in exchange for motion. The humerus has three to

Figure 7-3 Soft tissue structures of the shoulder girdle.

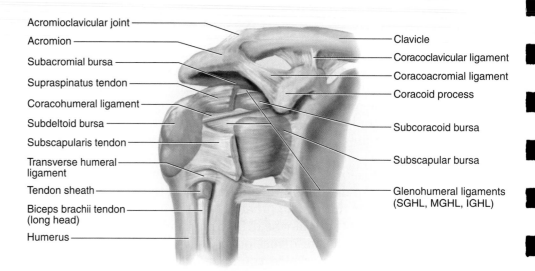

Acromioclavicular joint
Acromion
Subacromial bursa
Supraspinatus tendon
Coracohumeral ligament
Subdeltoid bursa
Subscapularis tendon
Transverse humeral ligament
Tendon sheath
Biceps brachii tendon (long head)
Humerus

Clavicle
Coracoclavicular ligament
Coracoacromial ligament
Coracoid process
Subcoracoid bursa
Subscapular bursa
Glenohumeral ligaments (SGHL, MGHL, IGHL)

four times the amount of surface area as the glenoid fossa. When combined with the shallowness of the joint, the humerus has been described as a basketball on a saucer or a golf ball on a tee. The relative shape of the humerus compared to that of the glenoid enables both rotation and linear motion, or translation.

A ring of fibrocartilage called the *glenoid labrum* attaches around the edge of the glenoid fossa and acts to deepen the socket (Fig. 7-4). Its most important function is to assist in anchoring the tendon of the long head of the biceps and the glenohumeral ligaments. The glenoid capsule encloses the joint and is attached around the periphery of the glenoid. It is quite loose and assists in enabling range of motion.

There are three anterior thickenings of the capsule that are classified as the glenohumeral ligaments (see Fig. 7-3). Each of the three ligaments contributes a different degree of stability to the joint depending on the position of the arm (Beltran et al., 2003):

1. *Superior glenohumeral ligament (SGHL):* Arises just anterior to the insertion of the long head of the biceps and inserts just superior to the lesser tuberosity on the humerus, lending stability to the superior part of the joint.

Figure 7-4 Soft tissue structures of the glenohumeral joint.

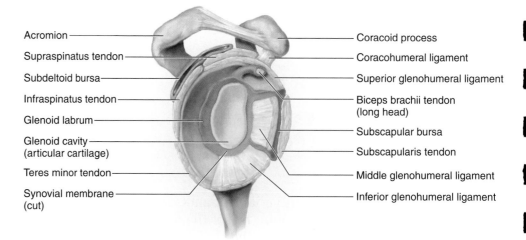

Acromion
Supraspinatus tendon
Subdeltoid bursa
Infraspinatus tendon
Glenoid labrum
Glenoid cavity (articular cartilage)
Teres minor tendon
Synovial membrane (cut)

Coracoid process
Coracohumeral ligament
Superior glenohumeral ligament
Biceps brachii tendon (long head)
Subscapular bursa
Subscapularis tendon
Middle glenohumeral ligament
Inferior glenohumeral ligament

2. *Middle glenohumeral ligament (MGHL):* Runs across the front of the joint to the anterior aspect of the humerus inferior to the SGHL, lending stability to the anterior portion of the joint.
3. *Inferior glenohumeral ligament (IGHL):* Has three portions that run between the inferior glenoid and the anatomical neck of the humerus. The IGHL is the most important stabilizing ligament of the shoulder; it is the main stabilizer against anterior/inferior dislocations, especially when the arm is in abduction and external rotation.

Acromioclavicular Joint

The lateral end of the clavicle and the acromion process of the scapula form the *acromioclavicular joint.* This joint enhances the motion of the glenohumeral joint and assists with freedom of movement in the area (see Fig. 7-3). It is considered a diarthrodial joint with limited movement and is surrounded by a thin capsule with a fibrocartilaginous disk between the two articulating surfaces. The superior and inferior acromioclavicular ligaments are strong ligaments that add stability to the joint. A third ligament supports the overall position of the joint and runs between the coracoid process and the acromion process. It is called the *coracoacromial ligament.*

Sternoclavicular Joint

The *sternoclavicular joint* is formed by the articulation of the medial end of the clavicle and the manubrium of the sternum (see Fig. 7-1). The clavicular component is larger than the sternum and tends to sit higher on the joint. The two surfaces are separated by an articular disk, which significantly strengthens the joint. It also absorbs shock and prevents the medial displacement of the clavicle. The joint is surrounded by a thin capsule that is reinforced by four strong ligaments:

- Anterior sternoclavicular
- Posterior sternoclavicular
- Costoclavicular
- Interclavicular

This proximal joint allows the distal clavicle to move in superior, inferior, anterior, and posterior directions, as well as allows some rotation.

Scapulothoracic Joint

While the *scapulothoracic joint* is not a true joint by definition, the articulation formed by the scapula on the wall of the thorax is critical to shoulder movement, so we include it as a joint.

This articulation is held in place entirely through soft tissue and has two important functions. First, the muscles attaching to the scapula stabilize the area during arm movements to provide a fixed base from which the shoulder can work. Second, the muscles move the scapula to assist in the proper positioning of the glenohumeral joint. Dysfunction will arise if the glenohumeral joint is not allowed to move properly.

There are several other relevant soft tissue structures in the shoulder region (see Fig. 7-4). The various bursae that surround the shoulder act to reduce friction between adjoining structures. The most important of these is the *subacromial bursa*, which is situated in the subacromial space and surrounded by the acromion process superiorly, the humeral head inferiorly, and the coracoacromial ligament anteriorly. It cushions the tendons of the rotator cuff muscles and can become a source of dysfunction if irritated.

The *coracoacromial ligament* is an important structure as well. It runs between the coracoid process and the acromion process of the scapula. It helps form the subacromial arch along with the undersurface of the acromion process and is a common site for impingement of the rotator cuff tendons (discussed later in the chapter).

The *brachial plexus* emerges from the cervical spine and consists of the nerve roots of C5 through T1. (Refer to Fig. 5-7, page 105.) As it leaves the neck and passes into the shoulder and arm, it starts as separate nerves and converges into three trunks. Just before the shoulder, the trunks split into anterior and posterior divisions. These divisions divide into cords as they enter the shoulder region and then branch to form the more familiar nerves that enter the arm. The posterior cord branches into the radial and axillary nerves; the lateral half of the medial cord converges with the medial half of the lateral cord to form the median nerve; and the rest of the medial cord becomes the ulnar nerve. The remaining part of the lateral cord becomes the musculocutaneous nerve.

There are a few additional soft tissue structures that are important to identify:

- *Brachial artery:* Lies along the medial humerus between the biceps and triceps brachii; it should be palpated carefully.
- *Cephalic vein:* Runs along the delto-pectoral interval, lateral to the biceps brachii and down the lateral humerus.
- *Basilic vein:* Runs superficially along the medial humerus between the biceps and triceps brachii.
- *Median cubital vein:* Runs along the cubital crease and connects the cephalic and basilic veins.
- *Epitrochlear lymph nodes:* Lie just above the medial epicondyle, along the medial supracondylar line. These lymph nodes are the last structures in the region. Use your fingers in a circular fashion to palpate these structures.

Muscles of the Shoulder Region

The muscles that are involved in the movement of the shoulder girdle are shown in Fig. 7-5. Refer to the Quick Reference Table "Muscles of the Shoulder Girdle" at the end of this chapter (page 269).

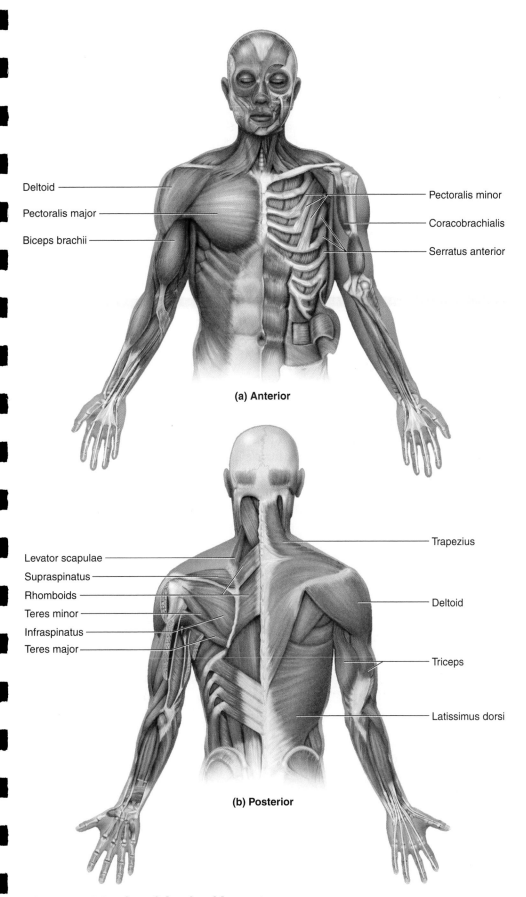

Deltoid

Pectoralis major

Biceps brachii

Pectoralis minor

Coracobrachialis

Serratus anterior

(a) Anterior

Levator scapulae

Supraspinatus

Rhomboids

Teres minor

Infraspinatus

Teres major

Trapezius

Deltoid

Triceps

Latissimus dorsi

(b) Posterior

Figure 7-5 Muscles of the shoulder region.

MOVEMENT AND MANUAL MUSCLE TESTING OF THE REGION

The shoulder is a complex joint with many simultaneous activities that are dependent on each other to prevent dysfunction. A thorough understanding of the baseline information of the region is important in performing an accurate assessment. This section discusses the information used to obtain that baseline.

Extensive range of motion is available at the shoulder. This is partially due to the laxity of the structures that create the glenohumeral joint, but it is also a result of the relationship among all the joints in the area. The coordination and combination of the various motions at the glenohumeral, acromioclavicular, sternoclavicular, and scapulothoracic articulations create the overall mobility of the region. This section explains the movements available at each of the joints in the shoulder, as well as the overall movement pattern of the shoulder complex.

Movements of the Region

Glenohumeral Joint

True glenohumeral movements occur before the contributions of the associated joints in the area. Actively distinguishing true glenohumeral motion can be difficult. Pin the scapula as best you can to the chest wall by placing your palm over the inferior angle and holding it in a secure position. The end of true glenohumeral movement comes when the inferior angle cannot be held anymore. The movements are assessed easier through passive methods, but their ranges are as follows:

- Flexion–90°
- Extension–45°
- Abduction–90° to 120°
- Adduction–45°
- Medial and lateral rotation–55°, and 40° to 45°, respectively

Sternoclavicular Joint

The sternoclavicular joint is important in shoulder motion and is often overlooked when discussing dysfunction in the area. It has a wide range of motion and can move in the following directions:

- Elevation–45° to 60°
- Depression–10°
- Protraction/retraction–20° to 30°
- Rotation–30° to 50°

Acromioclavicular Joint

The acromioclavicular is a gliding joint that has movement in three different planes. It has less motion than the other shoulder joints, but it still contributes to the overall mechanics of the shoulder complex:

- Protraction/retraction–20°

- Elevation–20°
- Rotation–45°

Scapulothoracic Joint

Because of the unique configuration of the scapulothoracic joint, we will not discuss the degrees of ranges of motion. Instead, we'll focus on the available movements at the articulation. The proper mobility at this joint contributes a large portion of the overall functioning of the shoulder. Its motions include:

- Elevation
- Depression
- Protraction
- Retraction
- Endorotation (downward rotation)
- Exorotation (upward rotation)
- Anterior tilt (inferior angle lifts off the rib cage)

Shoulder-Complex Movement

When assessing overall shoulder motion, place the client in a seated, standing, or supine position and perform the most painful movements last. While the client is performing the motions, watch for the combined participation of the various joints to accomplish the desired movement. Movements should be in a normal, coordinated sequence and should be smooth, with no apprehension. Movements should be observed from the front and back, and sometimes they should be performed in combination to determine the functional capacity of the client.

There are three combined movement patterns that can quickly screen for functionality (Fig. 7-6). They are known collectively as the *Apley*

> **Practical Tip**
>
> Watch the contributions of each joint to the overall movement of the shoulder.

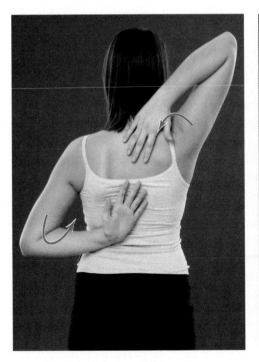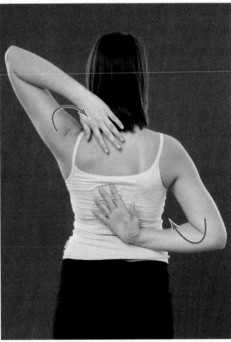

Figure 7-6 Apley scratch test.

scratch test and are also used to assess for adhesive capsulitis (addressed later in the chapter).

Apley Scratch Test

1. The first phase tests external rotation and abduction. Ask the client to reach behind the head and down the back as far as possible. Record how far the client can reach, repeat the movement for the opposite side, and compare the results.
2. The next phase assesses internal rotation and adduction. Have the client reach up behind the back as far as possible. Record the level, repeat the movement for the opposite side, and compare the results.
3. The third phase tests adduction and internal rotation. Have the client reach out in front of his or her body and touch the opposite shoulder. Repeat the movement for the opposite side, and compare the results.

The overall movements available at the shoulder complex are discussed below and are performed with the client standing.

Flexion—180° Starting with the arm at the side (0°), have the client raise the arm straight out in front of his or her body with the thumb up as far as possible.

Extension—45° to 60° Starting with the arm at the side (0°), have the client bring the arm back as far as possible. Make sure that the movement is coming from the shoulder and not the spine. Clients may lean forward to give the appearance of shoulder extension.

📖 **scapulohumeral rhythm** A ratio of movement between the scapulothoracic and glenohumeral joints.

Abduction—180° From the same starting position (arm at the side, 0°), have the client abduct the arm as far as possible. If the arm reaches 90°, have the client turn the palm up and continue farther. This motion utilizes a special relationship between the scapula and humerus. The **scapulohumeral rhythm** is a ratio of movement between the scapulothoracic and glenohumeral joints. Through the 180° of abduction, the ratio of movement of the humerus to the scapula is 2:1; that is, 120° occurs at the glenohumeral joint, and 60° is contributed by the scapulothoracic articulation. This rhythm occurs in three phases:

1. For the first 30° of abduction, there is little or no movement of the scapula and there is up to 15° of elevation of the clavicle. The scapula is said to be "setting" in this phase; thus, there is no ratio of movement.
2. During the next 60° of movement, the ratio becomes evident, with the scapula rotating 30°. The clavicle continues to elevate to 30° during this phase.
3. The last phase continues the 2:1 ratio with the humerus abducting to 120° and the scapula rotating to 60°. At this point, the clavicle rotates posteriorly 30° to 50° to allow the full range of motion. If the clavicle does not rotate and elevate, abduction is limited to 120°.

Lateral (External) Rotation—80° to 90° This is performed easiest with the client in the supine position and the arm abducted to 90° and the elbow flexed to 90°. As you look at the client from the side, the hand should be pointed toward the ceiling, which is considered 0° as a start point for this measurement. Let the client's hand fall backward toward the table, making sure the shoulder does not come off the table. This will provide a true measurement.

Medial (Internal) Rotation—70° to 90° Start with the client in the same position as that for lateral rotation and with the same start angle, but let the palm fall toward the table. Be careful that the client does not arch the back to add more movement.

Adduction—50° to 75° Starting with the client's arm at the side (0°), have the client bring the arm in front of the body. Be sure the client does not rotate the trunk to increase the movement.

Horizontal Adduction—135° With the arm abducted to 90°, which is the start position and a reference angle of 0° for this measurement, have the client bring the arm across the front of the body.

Horizontal Abduction—30° to 45° Starting with the arm abducted to 90°, which is the start position and a reference angle of 0° for this measurement, have the client bring the arm backward.

Passive Range of Motion

If the client has full range of motion actively, passive assessment is not necessary. If the active range is not full or the end-feels cannot be tested, each direction must be tested passively. If a client has full range of motion passively but not actively, muscle weakness or injury is likely the cause. If both active and passive ranges are limited, consider other causes, such as intra-articular blockages. The passive ranges are the same as those for the active movements, and they should be assessed with the client in either the supine or the seated position. It is important to ensure that the client is completely relaxed during this type of assessment.

Passive range-of-motion testing is better than active for assessing the range of motion at the true glenohumeral joint. With the client in the seated position, pin the scapula to the rib cage and take the humerus through flexion, extension, adduction, and abduction. The motion at the glenohumeral joint will occur before the scapula starts to move.

> **Practical Tip**
> Make sure the client is totally relaxed to facilitate passive testing.

Manual Muscle Testing

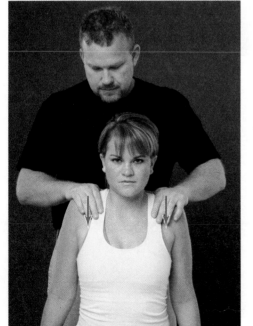

Motions at both the scapula and the humerus should be tested, as these bones work together to produce movement at the shoulder. With the client in the seated or standing position, create an isometric contraction by instructing the client not to allow you to move him or her. Strength should be tested at more than one range, and testing should be repeated several times to determine the presence of weakness or fatigue.

Scapular Tests

Elevation Have the client shrug the shoulders. Place your hands on top of the shoulders, and instruct the client to resist your pressing down. Repeat the process for varying degrees of elevation.

Depression Instruct the client to bend the arms to 90° and press the shoulders down. Place your hands under the client's elbows, and press up while the client resists. Repeat in several positions.

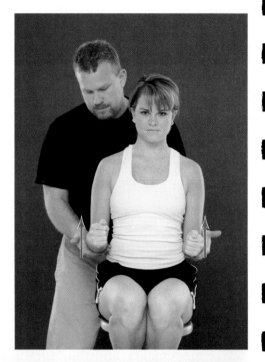

Protraction Stand in front of the client, and instruct him or her to round the shoulders. Place your hand on the front of the shoulders, and push backward while the client resists. Repeat in several positions.

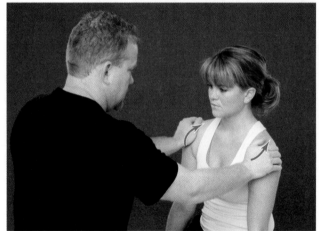

Retraction Stand behind the client, and instruct him or her to pinch the shoulder blades together. Place your hands on the back of the shoulders, and press them forward while the client resists. Repeat in several positions.

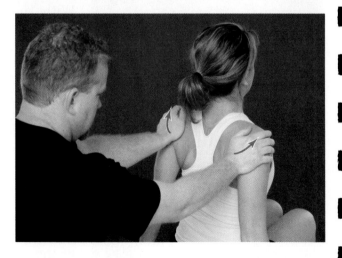

Flexion Have the client hang his or her arm down at the side, bend the elbow to 90°, and bring the shoulder into a slight amount of flexion. Stand behind the client, and place one hand on the shoulder and the other around the front of the biceps. Use your hand on the shoulder to stabilize the client; then pull on the upper arm while the client resists. Repeat using several different degrees of flexion as starting positions.

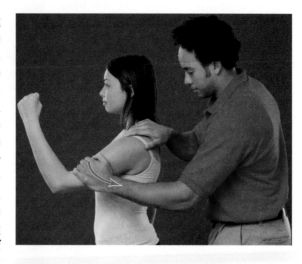

Extension Start with the client's arm bent to 90° and in slight extension. Place one hand on the client's shoulder and the other on the triceps. Push the client into flexion while he or she resists. Repeat using several different degrees of extension as starting positions.

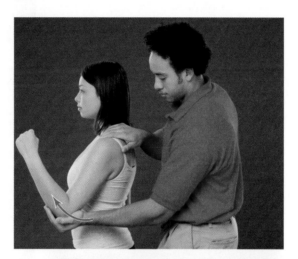

Abduction The client should have the elbow bent to 90° and the arm abducted slightly. Stand behind the client, and place one hand on the shoulder and the other on the distal humerus. Press the client's arm into his or her body while the client resists. Repeat using several different degrees of abduction as starting positions.

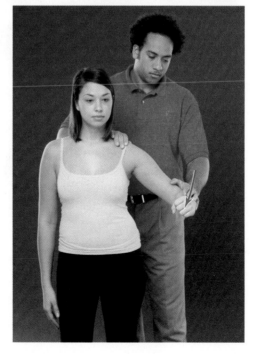

Adduction Stand behind the client, and begin with his or her arm slightly abducted, with the elbow flexed to 90°. Stabilize the client's shoulder with one hand; place the other hand on the medial side of his or her elbow, and move the arm into abduction as the client resists.

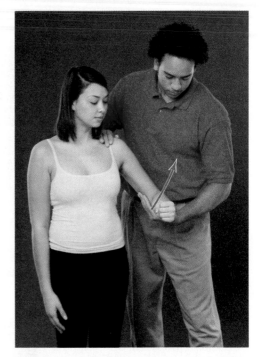

Lateral Rotation Stand behind the client, and place one hand on the shoulder to stabilize him or her. Keeping the client's arm against his or her side, have the client bend the elbow to 90°. Place your other hand on the lateral side of the distal forearm, and press medially while the client resists. Repeat using several different degrees of lateral rotation as starting positions.

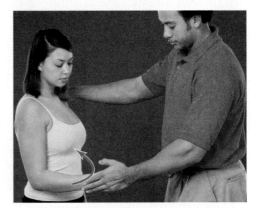

Medial Rotation Have the client bend the elbow to 90° and place his or her arm at the side. Stand in front of the client, and place one hand on the shoulder and one on the medial side of the distal forearm. Press the client into lateral rotation while he or she resists. Repeat using several different degrees of medial rotation as starting positions.

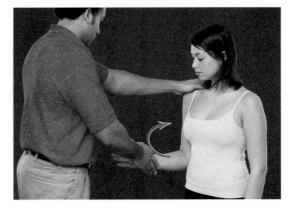

Elbow Flexion Stand next to the client, and have the client bend the elbow to 90° with the forearm supinated. Place one hand under the elbow to stabilize it and the other on the client's distal forearm. Press down on the forearm while the client resists. Repeat using different degrees of flexion as starting positions.

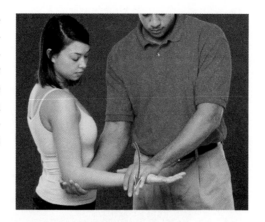

Elbow Extension Have the client bend the elbow to 120° and pronate the forearm. Stand on the side, and place one hand under the client's elbow and the other on the distal forearm. Press the client into flexion while he or she resists. Repeat using several different degrees of extension as starting positions.

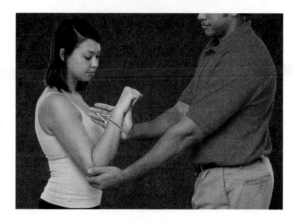

To ensure that there is no neurologic involvement, assess the myotomes for the shoulder as well. Perform the movements that were done for the manual muscle tests:

- *C4–scapular elevation:* Have the client shrug the shoulders and resist while you press down.
- *C5–shoulder abduction:* Have the client abduct the shoulders and resist while you move him or her into adduction.
- *C6–elbow flexion:* Flex the client's elbow to 90°, and have the client resist while you press the elbow into extension.
- *C7–elbow extension:* Flex the client's elbow to 90°, and have the client resist while you flex his or her arm.

DERMATOMES FOR THE SHOULDER GIRDLE

Dermatomes are the sensory areas innervated by the nerves and can be an indication of dysfunction in the area. Using a fingertip or blunt object, touch the area lightly bilaterally, and ask the client whether the sensations are equal. Include the neck, shoulder, anterior and posterior sides of the chest, and down both sides of the arms. Remember to stay in the middle of the dermatome to avoid overlap into adjacent dermatomes (Fig. 7-7). Any differences between sides can indicate pathology; moreover, dermatomes can vary from person to person. The dermatomes of the shoulder are summarized in Table 7-1.

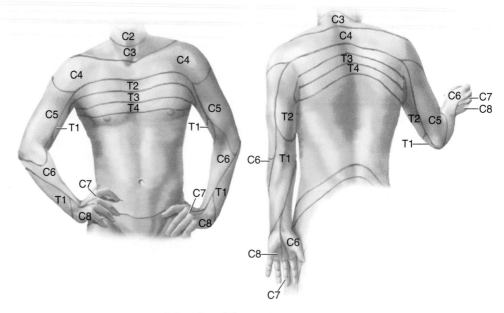

Figure 7-7 Dermatomes of the shoulder region.

Table 7-1 Dermatomes of the Shoulder Complex

C3	Base of the lateral neck
C4	Upper shoulder to base of neck; top of anterior and posterior chest
C5	Lateral upper arm
C6	Distal anterior biceps and lateral forearm
C7	Posterior shoulder down middle of posterior arm
T1	Half of the inside of the upper arm
T2	A 2-inch band running just below the clavicles
T3	A 2-inch band running just below the T2 dermatome
T4	A 2-inch band running across the nipple line

TRIGGER-POINT REFERRAL PATTERNS FOR MUSCLES OF THE REGION

Myofascial trigger points in the shoulder region are relatively common and can cause a variety of problems. The symptoms that these points create can mimic various conditions, resulting in misdiagnoses and often leading to more invasive treatments. These conditions include:

- **Pseudothoracic syndrome:** Occurs when three of four muscles (pectoralis major, latissimus dorsi, teres major, and subscapularis) have active trigger points. The points refer pain that is similar to the true thoracic outlet syndrome.

pseudothoracic syndrome The referral pattern created when three of four muscles (pectoralis major, latissimus dorsi, teres major, and subscapularis) have active trigger points.

- *Adhesive capsulitis (frozen shoulder):* Occurs when trigger points in the rotator cuff, particularly in the subscapularis, restrict motion just as if the shoulder were frozen.
- *Carpal tunnel syndrome:* Stems from the referral patterns of trigger points in the scalenes, the brachialis, and other muscles.

Because the symptoms created by myofascial trigger points in various shoulder muscles can be mistaken for other conditions, it is important for therapists to recognize their presentation. This ensures that the client will receive the appropriate treatment.

Trapezius

The *trapezius* (see Figs. 7-9 and 7-16) is the muscle most often affected by trigger points. There are three different divisions of the trapezius, each with its own trigger points. The two points in the upper fibers are approximately at the same level, one anterior and the other posterior. The anterior point is the most frequently identified point and refers behind, up, and over the ear in a ram's-horn pattern. The posterior point refers up the back of the neck to the area behind the ear. Both of these points contribute to tension headaches.

Moving inferiorly, the *middle trapezius* has two main points. One of these points may occur anywhere in the middle part of the muscle; the other is an attachment trigger point near the acromion. The point in the belly of the muscle refers superficial burning pain medially that will stay local to the point. The attachment point refers to the top of the shoulder or acromion.

The *lower trapezius* has one central point that is common but often overlooked. It is located about halfway along the lower border of the muscle and is key in inducing other trigger points in the upper back and neck. It refers sharply to the high cervical paraspinals, the mastoid process area, and the acromion. It also produces a deep ache in the suprascapular region.

Levator Scapula

The *levator scapula* is one of the most common muscles involved in shoulder and neck pain and is a unique muscle because of its spiral twist as

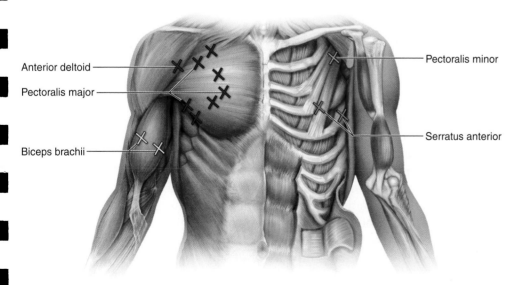

Figure 7-8 Trigger-point locations for the anterior deltoid, pectoralis major, biceps brachii, pectoralis minor, and serratus anterior.

Anterior deltoid

Pectoralis major

Biceps brachii

Pectoralis minor

Serratus anterior

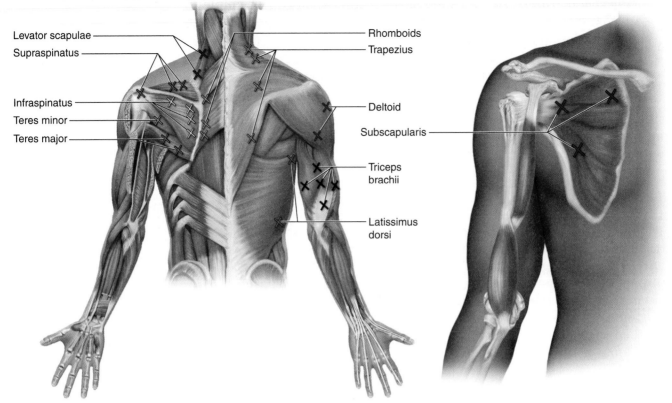

Figure 7-9 Trigger-point locations for the levator scapulae, supraspinatus, infraspinatus, teres minor, teres major, rhomboids, deltoids, trapezius, triceps brachii, and latissimus dorsi.

Figure 7-10 Trigger-point locations for the subscapularis.

it moves from the scapula to the neck. There are two main trigger points (see Figs. 7-9 and 7-11) associated with this muscle: one at the superior angle of the scapula and one about halfway up the muscle, where it emerges from underneath the upper trapezius. Typical symptoms include pain at the angle of the neck and stiffness with limited range of motion, which prohibits full movement of the head to either side. There may also be some referral into the posterior shoulder and medial scapular border.

Rhomboids

The *rhomboids* (see Figs. 7-9 and 7-11) often develop trigger points as a result of being in an overstretched position for long periods of time. The larger, stronger muscles on the anterior chest become shortened and pull the shoulders forward into a rounded position, which overloads the weaker posterior muscles. There are three main points that develop in this muscle. Pay attention to fiber direction when palpating the points to ensure that you are not finding the points in the trapezius.

All the points lie along the vertebral border, with one roughly at the level where the spine of the scapula meets the vertebral border. The other two are inferior to each other and lie about halfway down the vertebral border. Pain from these points concentrates around the vertebral border and does not radiate too far away. These points can also cause a snapping or crunching sound during movement of the scapula.

★ **Practical Tip**

Determining muscle fiber direction will ensure you are addressing the right structure.

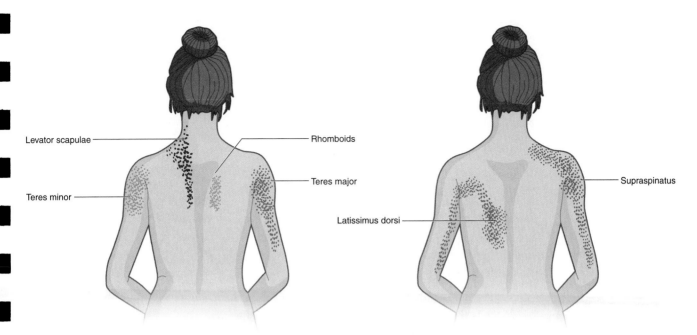

Figure 7-11 Trigger-point referrals for the levator scapulae, teres minor, teres major, and rhomboids.

Figure 7-12 Trigger-point referrals for the latissimus dorsi and the supraspinatus.

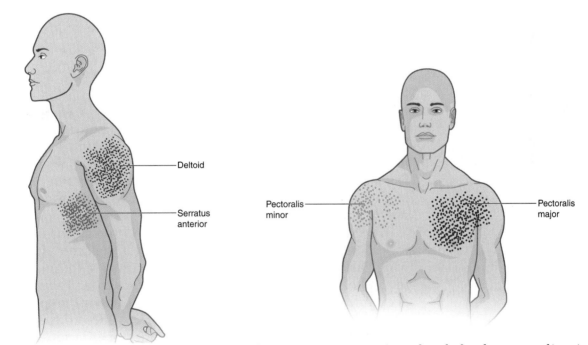

Figure 7-13 Trigger-point referrals for the deltoids and the serratus anterior.

Figure 7-14 Trigger-point referrals for the pectoralis minor and pectoralis major.

Rotator Cuff

The next group of muscles is collectively known as the *rotator cuff*. The first muscle of the group is the *supraspinatus* (see Figs. 7-9 and 7-12). Active trigger points in this muscle cause a deep ache of the shoulder and center around the middle deltoid. This ache can extend down the lateral side of the arm all the way to the lateral epicondyle of the elbow. There are three points along the same line of the muscle. The first two are in the

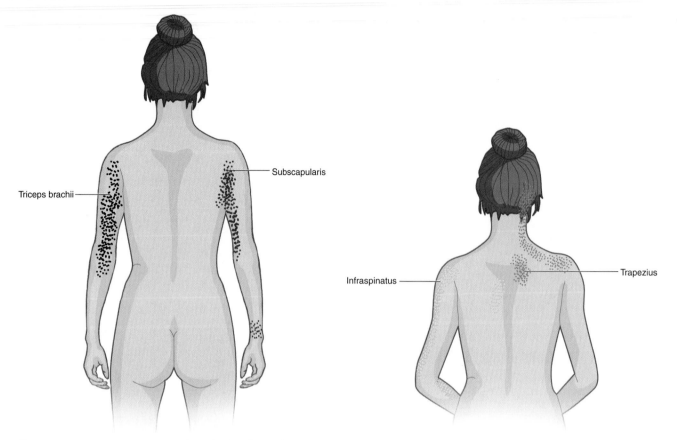

Figure 7-15 Trigger-point referrals for the subscapularis and the triceps brachii.

Figure 7-16 Trigger-point referrals for the trapezius and the infraspinatus.

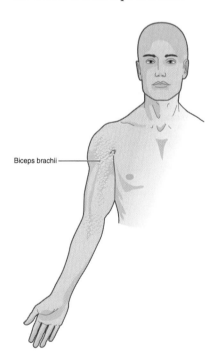

Figure 7-17 Trigger-point referrals for the biceps brachii.

belly of the muscle. One is close to the medial border, and the other is farther lateral, just before the muscle dives underneath the acromion. The third point is in the proximal tendon and may be difficult to locate. These points can be activated by carrying a heavy load at the side and will result in referred pain during abduction, as well as difficulty in performing overhead activities.

The next muscle of the rotator cuff is the *infraspinatus* (see Figs. 7-9 and 7-16). There are four points that can occur, all of which are in the belly. The first three points are located centrally in the belly, just under the spine of the scapula. They refer pain deep into the anterior shoulder and often down the anterior and lateral aspects of the arm, the lateral forearm, and the radial aspect of the hand. The fourth point is farther inferior and medial to the other three. It refers to the adjacent rhomboid area along the medial border of the scapula, and pain at this point may be difficult to distinguish from trapezius pain. All of these trigger points contribute to the client's inability to internally rotate and adduct the arm. Clients may also have trouble sleeping because lying on the painful side will compress the points and stimulate them.

The third muscle in the cuff is the *teres minor* (see Figs. 7-9 and 7-11). Clients with active trigger points in this muscle will complain of posterior shoulder pain that feels like an inflamed bursa around the posterior deltoid. The points refer just proximal to the deltoid tuberosity, which is why the client will compare it to bursitis. The points themselves lie about midbelly along the muscle and are relatively prominent and easy to find.

Completing the group of rotator cuff muscles, the *subscapularis* (see Figs. 7-10 and 7-15) contains trigger points that can be difficult to access manually. Trigger points in this muscle are often a significant contributor to "frozen shoulder." They can cause pain both at rest and during motion. Initially, clients are able to reach forward but not backward. As the trigger-point activity increases, abduction at the shoulder becomes severely restricted, sometimes to less than 45°, leading to the pseudodiagnosis of adhesive capsulitis. There are two lateral trigger points and one medial point in the muscle, and they may be difficult to access. The lateral points are located above one another. The superior point lies just inferior to the coracoid process; the inferior point is located about halfway up the lateral border of the scapula. The medial point is close to the superior medial edge of the muscle and may be better accessed from the prone position. The primary zone of referral for these points is the posterior shoulder. There can be some spillover into the posterior arm and elbow. One distinct characteristic of subscapularis trigger points is a straplike area of pain that encircles the wrist. The posterior side is often more painful than the anterior side.

Latissimus Dorsi

The next muscle extends from the lumbar spine to the shoulder. The *latissimus dorsi* (see Figs. 7-9 and 7-12) is frequently overlooked as a source of shoulder and thoracic pain. Active points in this muscle refer a constant aching to the inferior angle of the scapula and the surrounding thoracic region. Pain can also travel down the back of the shoulder, along the medial forearm to the ulnar side of the hand. There are two main points in the muscle. The more common point is located in the superior portion of the muscle at the posterior axial fold. A less common point is located along the midregion of the muscle and refers to the anterior shoulder and the lateral aspect of the trunk over the iliac crest.

Teres Major

Sometimes referred to as the "little lat" because it shares the same functions as the latissimus dorsi, the *teres major* (see Figs. 7-9 and 7-11) has three trigger points that can refer to the posterior shoulder and over the long head of the triceps. The first point is located medially along the muscle near its origin at the inferior angle of the scapula. The second point is located midmuscle in the posterior axillary fold, and the third point is located at the lateral musculocutaneous junction. The pain is primarily produced during movement and is usually mild at rest.

Deltoids

The *deltoids* (see Figs. 7-8, 7-9, and 7-13) consist of three heads and often develop trigger points in each of the divisions. Points in the anterior head lie along its medial border close to the cephalic vein. The middle head can develop multiple trigger points almost anywhere due to the fact that its motor end plates are widely distributed. The posterior deltoid trigger points are along the lateral border of the muscle, closer to the insertion.

Trigger points in the various heads of the muscle refer locally either in the same head or adjacent ones. Anterior points refer to the anterior deltoid and possibly spill over into the middle head. Points in the middle deltoid tend to refer central to the region, with some spillover to adjacent areas. Posterior points refer over the posterior shoulder and possibly into the arms. None of the trigger points in the deltoids refer any great distance.

Serratus Anterior

The *serratus anterior* (see Figs. 7-8 and 7-13) is commonly overlooked as a contributor to shoulder pain. It is a very large muscle that covers a lot of surface area. It can develop trigger points in the middle of any of its digitations but are most commonly located at about the 5th or 6th rib along the midaxillary line and refer to the anterolateral thorax. Pain can also be projected down the inside of the arm to the palm and ring finger. Another referral from trigger points in this muscle is interscapular pain over the distal half of the scapula. This particular referral pattern can be quite aggravating for the client and is often diagnosed as something else.

Biceps Brachii

Moving down the humerus, the *biceps brachii* (see Figs. 7-8 and 7-17) contains trigger points that primarily refer in a superior direction to the front of the shoulder but can also travel to the suprascapular region and the antecubital space. The trigger points in this muscle are usually found midbelly in either head. The pain that accompanies these points is typically superficial and does not present as deep shoulder pain; however, pain will occur during arm elevation above shoulder level. Other presentations include aching over the anterior arm and weakness.

Triceps Brachii

The antagonist to the biceps, the *triceps brachii* (see Figs. 7-9 and 7-15) can develop trigger points in all three of its heads in five locations, each with a unique referral pattern. The client may complain of diffuse pain posteriorly in the shoulder and upper arm. The points can affect movement but this is often overlooked by the client, especially if the client is able to make compensatory movements.

The first point is located in the central belly of the long head and refers upward over the posterior arm and shoulder, sometimes extending into the upper trapezius and down the posterior forearm. The second point is in the lateral portion of the medial head of the muscle. This point refers to the lateral epicondyle of the elbow and is often a component of tennis elbow. The third point is in the lateral head and refers centrally around the point over the posterior arm and sometimes down the posterior forearm into the 4th and 5th fingers. The fourth point is most likely an attachment point created from the other central points. It is located in the tendon and refers to the olecranon process. The last point is the least common and is most easily located from the anterior side. This point is in the medial portion of the medial head of the muscle and refers along the medial forearm and the palmar surface of the 4th and 5th fingers.

Pectoralis Major

The last two muscles in the shoulder region are the pectoralis major and minor. The *pectoralis major* (see Figs. 7-8 and 7-14) develops trigger points in five different areas, and each has a distinct referral pattern. The first area is in the clavicular head of the muscle, along the lateral edge; it refers pain over the anterior deltoid. The next area is the sternal section of the muscle. The points here lie in the belly of the sternal portion of the muscle, along the midclavicular line. The symptoms are often mistaken for a cardiac episode because they refer intense pain to the anterior chest and down the inner aspect of the arm, sometimes down to the hand. The third area for trigger points in the pectoralis major is along the lateral border of the muscle, about halfway between the origin and insertion. These points refer into the breast area and can cause tenderness and hypersensitivity of the nipple and intolerance to clothing. This occurs in both men and women but is more often found in women. The fourth area is along the medial sternum. Its points cause pain locally over the sternum, but the pain will not cross over to the opposite side.

Finally, the last area is only on the right side and does not cause significant pain. It is located just below the level of the 5th rib, midway on a line between the sternal margin and the nipple. It is known to contribute to certain cardiac arrhythmias, which are terminated on the trigger point's inactivation.

Pectoralis Minor

Lying underneath the pectoralis major, the *pectoralis minor* (see Figs. 7-8 and 7-14) can develop trigger points that may be difficult to discern from those of the major. There are two main points that occur along the belly of the muscle, one close to the insertion and one close to the origin. These points refer strongly over the anterior deltoid and down the medial arm, forearm, and hand. This pattern is similar to that of the clavicular trigger point in the pectoralis major. When the pectoralis minor becomes chronically shortened due to the trigger points, it can entrap the neurovascular bundle passing beneath it and mimic cervical radiculopathy. This is one of the distinct differences between trigger points in the major and minor. Refer to the Quick Reference Table "Trigger Points of the Shoulder Girdle" at the end of this chapter (page 272).

SPECIFIC CONDITIONS

Because of its many structures, movements, and potential pathologies, the shoulder complex can be extremely difficult to assess. Performing a thorough assessment will narrow down the focus of the treatment. Since many of the pathologies involve the same structures, there will be an overlap of treatment techniques. Remember that just because two people have the same condition does not mean they will require the same treatment. Each treatment should be customized to meet the specific needs of the individual.

Rotator Cuff Injuries

Background

Injuries to the rotator cuff are one of the most common types of shoulder problems. They can arise from a traumatic episode to the area but are more often caused by repetitive movements of the glenohumeral joint. This section discusses two of the more common rotator cuff injuries: impingement syndrome and tears to the supraspinatus tendon, two conditions that are intimately related to each other. Before discussing these specific injuries, it is necessary to review the functioning of the rotator cuff and other anatomy that is directly related to these conditions.

The tendons of four separate muscles form the rotator cuff:

1. Supraspinatus
2. Infraspinatus
3. Teres minor
4. Subscapularis

The cuff, which is a composite "sleeve" around the head of the humerus created from all the tendons, occupies the space between the humeral head and the coracoacromial arch. Its function is multifaceted. Individually, the muscles provide various movements of the glenohumeral joint. The supraspinatus abducts the humerus; the infraspinatus and teres minor extend and externally rotate the humerus; and the subscapularis internally rotates the humerus. While these roles are important, more critical is the muscles' combined function in regard to injury prevention: stabilizing the head of the humerus on the glenoid fossa of the scapula. When these muscles contract as a group, they compress the humeral head against the fossa, keeping it centered over the glenoid and creating a dynamic fulcrum for the deltoid muscles to produce movement. If there is any imbalance in the functioning of these muscles, an alteration in shoulder biomechanics will occur. This dysfunction of the cuff will cause the humeral head to shift or translate on the glenoid, eventually leading to problems in the shoulder.

In addition to muscle imbalances, other predisposing factors can contribute to shoulder problems. One factor is the anatomical shape of the acromion. The acromion can have three variations in shape:

- *Type I:* Relatively flat acromion; occurs in 17% to 32% of the population
- *Type II:* Curved acromion; occurs in 40% to 45% of the population
- *Type III:* Hooked acromion; occurs in 26% to 40% of the population

A higher incidence of rotator cuff injuries occurs in individuals with type II or type III acromions. These two morphologies reduce the already limited space within the coracoacromial arch.

Another anatomical factor is the so-called hypovascular zone in the supraspinatus tendon, about 8 mm proximal to its insertion. This zone corresponds to the most common site of rotator cuff injuries. Since vascularity decreases with age, there is an increase in the chance of injury to the rotator cuff in individuals over the age of 40.

These underlying conditions can lead to impingement syndrome. **Subacromial impingement syndrome** is defined as the "painful contact between the rotator cuff, subacromial bursa, and the undersurface of the anterior acromion" (Cohen et al., 1998). It is a mechanical phenomenon in which there is weakness

subacromial impingement syndrome A condition characterized by the painful contact between the rotator cuff, subacromial bursa, and undersurface of the anterior acromion.

or imbalance in the strength of the rotator cuff that allows superior translation of the humerus, resulting in the repetitive compression of the supraspinatus tendon into the coracoacromial arch. When the arm is abducted, the deltoids and supraspinatus pull the humeral head superiorly. The other rotator cuff muscles must produce force that cancels out this superior movement in order to prevent impingement. Other factors can also contribute to this syndrome, such as:

- Instability patterns in the glenohumeral joint
- The anatomical concerns listed earlier
- Glenohumeral capsular tightness
- Postural misalignments that change the position of the glenoid
- Dysfunctional scapular motion in which the acromion fails to rotate with the humerus

Initially, symptoms include deep pain in the shoulder that also occurs at night, crepitus, weakness, and pain over the subacromial space. Activity involving movements that are repetitive or are above 90° of flexion or abduction will exacerbate the symptoms. A characteristic sign of shoulder impingement is the presence of a "**painful arc**." As the client abducts the arm, no pain occurs between 0° and 45° to 60° because the structures are not being compressed (Fig. 7-18). Once the arm passes 60°, impingement of the structures begins, resulting in pain. This may prevent the client from abducting any further; however, if the client does abduct further, the pain will disappear after 120°. This is because the compressed structures have passed completely under the acromion and are no longer being impinged.

Repeated impingement of the rotator cuff structures will lead to tendon degeneration and the second rotator cuff injury: the eventual tearing of the supraspinatus tendon, or *rotator cuff tear.* The tears are almost always near the insertion and can be either partial or full thickness. Partial-thickness tears occur twice as often, with most full-thickness tears appearing in individuals who have a long history of shoulder problems and are typically over the age of 40. The signs and symptoms are the same for both impingement syndrome and rotator cuff tears, but more severe tears will present with significant weakness and some atrophy of the muscles. As previously stated, these two conditions are intimately related. A series of stages have been described that demonstrate how impingement syndrome progresses into a tear of the rotator cuff:

- *Stage I:* An initial injury to the supraspinatus tendon and surrounding structures causes inflammation with edema in the area. This results in pain during and after activity (especially abduction and flexion), point tenderness over the supraspinatus tendon, and a temporary thickening of the supraspinatus tendon and subacromial bursa. There is no palpable muscle defect, weakness, or loss of motion. While it can occur in any age group, it is most commonly seen in clients under the age of 25, and it is reversible.
- *Stage II:* This stage involves a permanent thickening of the supraspinatus tendon and subacromial bursa. Pain occurs more frequently during activity, throughout the painful arc (60° to 120° of abduction), and at night. The client has some range-of-motion loss and crepitus but

📖 painful arc The arc of the shoulder that is created during abduction and goes through a phase of no pain between 0° and 45° to 60°, pain between 60° and 120°, and then no pain again after 120°.

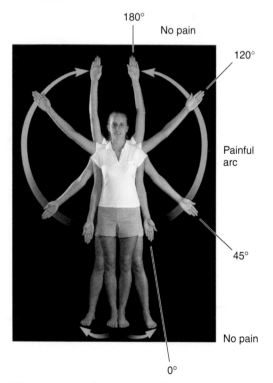

Figure 7-18 The phases of the painful arc.

still no palpable defect. This stage is common in individuals between 25 and 40 years of age.

- *Stage III:* Because of the repetitive impingement, this stage is characterized by a tear in the rotator cuff less than 1 centimeter (cm). When the client reaches this stage, he or she has had a long history of shoulder problems with significant weakness and a possibility of multidirectional instability. The client has significant pain on activity, which increases at night, with obvious atrophy of the rotator cuff. This stage typically occurs in individuals over the age of 40.
- *Stage IV:* This is a progression of the previous stage and is characterized by a tear in the rotator cuff that is greater than 1 cm. The client experiences significant motion reduction and weakness.

Assessment

Both shoulder impingement and tears to the rotator cuff are multifactorial and can have additional contributing pathologies in the surrounding joints and cervical region. Be sure to assess any related areas to ensure that proper treatment is administered.

Condition History Therapists should inquire about the following when taking the client's history:

Question	Significance
What is the client's age?	Many conditions in the shoulder can be age-related. Rotator cuff tears occur more in patients who are 40 years of age or older.
What was the mechanism of injury?	Most impingement and rotator cuff injuries occur as a result of repetitive micro-traumas; however, a fall on an outstretched hand or a blow to the tip of the shoulder can also cause a traumatic rotator cuff injury.
Are there any movements that cause pain?	Repetitive movements above 60° can be painful in a client who has impingement problems.
How is the pain qualified?	A deep, toothache-like pain that gets worse with activity and is bad at night can indicate what is known as *primary impingement*. Primary impingement is caused by chronic overuse and degeneration of the rotator cuff tendons. A "dead arm" feeling is an indicator of *secondary impingement,* which is a result of an underlying instability problem with the glenohumeral joint.
How does the injury affect the ability to function?	The more limited the functioning, the longer the client has had the condition.

| How long has the client had the problem? | Over a period of time, simple impingement syndrome can evolve into a more serious tear in the rotator cuff. |
| Is there any feeling of weakness or a change in sensation? | These symptoms can indicate neurologic involvement. |

Visual Assessment In order for the therapist to inspect the shoulder, the client must disrobe to the appropriate level (no shirt for males and a tank top or sports bra for females). This is a perfect opportunity to observe the functional capacity of the client: As the client disrobes, observe the quality of movement, compensation patterns, and symmetry of motions. From the front, observe the overall position of the head and neck in relation to the shoulders. Check for obvious swelling, bruising, or muscle atrophy. Look for a step deformity at the lateral end of the clavicle. This indicates an injury to the acromioclavicular joint and a sulcus sign, which may be an indication of instability. From the back, check the contour or the neck and note any atrophy in the musculature as well as any swelling or bruising. Check the position of the scapulae. Make sure that they are equal and that there is no winging. Assess the active and passive ranges of motion.

Palpation During shoulder palpation, be sure to include the neck and thoracic spine, since they can contribute to the dysfunction. Begin along the clavicle, palpating the sternoclavicular and acromioclavicular joints. Note any spasm or hypertonicity in the musculature of the area. Check the bicipital groove and subacromial space for tenderness, along with the coracoid process. Be sure the scapulae are positioned symmetrically on the thoracic spine. Complete the palpation of the area by locating the structures discussed earlier in the chapter.

Orthopedic Tests The information gathered from the history, visual assessment, palpation, and range-of-motion testing should give the therapist a good idea of which structures are involved. Orthopedic tests will add the missing data needed to provide a comprehensive assessment. Table 7-2 shows the tests and how to perform them.

Soft Tissue Treatment

As previously discussed, a wide range of motion in the shoulder results in diminished stability. Because the structures that make up the joint do little to offer stability, the muscles of the shoulder girdle not only are put into a locomotive role but are forced to create the stability in the area that the joint does not. This delicate balance between the various muscles of the area is frequently disrupted. Imbalance creates a domino effect and leads to the eventual breakdown of the system. The restoration of the balance between the muscles is vital in restoring proper biomechanical functioning. Once the correct biomechanics of the shoulder have been restored, any dysfunction in the area can be resolved. Other areas, including the back and neck, can contribute to problems in the shoulder; therefore, it is important to address these areas as needed.

| Table 7-2 | Orthopedic Tests for Rotator Cuff Injuries |

Orthopedic Test	How to Perform
Neer shoulder impingement test 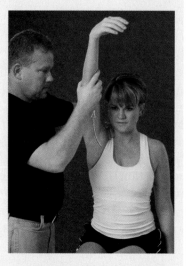 • This test is for shoulder impingement. *Note:* With this particular arm position, the greater tuberosity of the humerus will be "jammed" into the anterior inferior acromion.	Client is in the seated position. Standing at the client's side, use one hand to stabilize the posterior shoulder and use the other hand to grasp the client's arm at the elbow. Internally rotate the arm passively, and then flex it forcibly to its end range. Pain with motion, especially at the end of the range, indicates a positive test. It also indicates a possible impingement of the supraspinatus or long head of the biceps tendon.
Hawkins-Kennedy impingement test 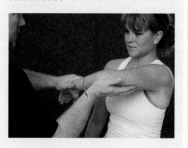 • This test is for shoulder impingement. *Note:* This test will cause the greater tuberosity of the humerus to contact the anteroinferior surface of the acromion and the coracoacromial arch.	Client is in the seated position. Forward flex the shoulder to 90°, and bend the elbow to 90°. Keeping the shoulder at 90° of flexion, place one hand under the bent elbow to support the arm and place the other at the wrist. Horizontally adduct the arm slightly across the chest, being careful not to lower the arm and internally rotate the shoulder. Pain that occurs with this test may indicate shoulder impingement.

Table 7-2 Orthopedic Tests for Rotator Cuff Injuries *(Continued)*

Empty-can test	Client is standing. Have the client abduct the arms to 90°.

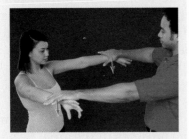

- This test is for rotator cuff tears, specifically in the supraspinatus.

Client is standing. Have the client abduct the arms to 90°.

Standing in front of the client, horizontally adduct the arms 30° and internally rotate the arms so that the client's thumbs point toward the floor (empty-can position).

Place your hands on the proximal forearms of the client, and apply downward force while the client resists.

Weakness or pain in the shoulder indicates a positive test and a possible tear of the supraspinatus tendon.

Drop-arm test

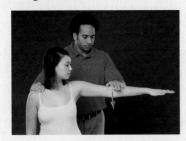

Client is in the standing position with his or her arms at 90° of abduction.

Instruct the client to slowly lower the arms down to the sides.

A positive test is indicated if the client cannot lower an arm smoothly or has increased pain during the motion.

An alternative test is to place the arms in 90° of abduction and apply downward force at the distal humerus while the client resists.

A test is positive if the client cannot hold an arm up and drops it to the side.

If either variation of test elicits a positive result, this may be an indication of a more severe tear of the supraspinatus tendon.

Connective Tissue One common imbalance in the region occurs from the chronic posture of protracted shoulders. Over time, the connective tissue restricts the motion of the shoulder girdle; thus, addressing the area becomes vital.

Prone Position Begin by assessing the superficial fascia of the back from superior to inferior, from medial to lateral, and at various angles, paying special attention to the posterior shoulder girdle. A common pattern of restriction of the posterior shoulder is from the superior angle of the scapula down at a 45° angle toward the lateral border. Move into any restriction in the various directions until it releases. The incorporation of active and passive movements is very effective in this area. Passively apply pressure in the direction of the restriction, and then passively move the limb in the opposite direction, effectively pulling the tissue under the hand that is applying the pressure. Active motion can be applied in the same manner, with the client actively moving the limb in the direction opposite the restriction.

Once the superficial fascia has been addressed, move into the deeper layers and begin to strip out the borders of the muscles in the area. Be sure to address any muscle that attaches to either the scapula or the humerus. The lateral border of the lower trapezius is best identified by placing the fingertips on the lateral portion of the rib cage and pressing toward the opposite shoulder. Once the border is located, it can be stripped out by separating your hands along the border while keeping the fingertips on the border. Pay special attention to the muscles of the posterior rotator cuff and the deltoids. The posterior deltoid becomes tight because of the protracted posture of the shoulder.

One muscle that often gets left out when treating the shoulder is the latissimus dorsi. Because of its insertion on the humerus, it can affect the overall motion of the shoulder and should not be ignored. Another muscle that often gets left out is the triceps brachii. The long head attaches on the scapula and can play a role in restricting motion.

Supine Position Addressing the connective tissue in this position contributes a great deal to correcting the underlying postural concerns that create some of the muscle imbalance issues. Essentially, almost everything we do requires reaching in front of us. This constant movement pattern leads to the tightening of the connective tissue, which exacerbates the postural concerns.

Begin by assessing the superficial fascia of the chest, anterior shoulder, and upper arm in various directions, including any associated area as necessary. Move into any restrictions that are found in the various directions. One effective method of treating the chest is to place the arm over the head, which aligns the muscle fibers of the pectoralis major. Focus on strokes that will mimic shoulder retraction and encourage the reversal of the rounded shoulder posture by moving up and out from the sternum toward the shoulder.

Incorporating movement is also beneficial in this position. While standing at the client's side and facing his or her head, hold the wrist with the outside hand and lift the arm so that the hand is straight up toward the ceiling. Start at the edge of the drape, and apply pressure with the inside hand toward the shoulder. During the stroke, move the client's arm up and out at various angles to address restriction in different parts of the muscle. Another good technique involves abducting the client's arm to 90° or as far as possible and flexing the elbow by grasping the wrist. Perform a stroke from the medial portion of the chest toward the shoulder while you internally and externally rotate the arm, paying special attention to the anterior deltoid. Address the lateral border of the chest and axilla from either a superior or an inferior direction, depending on the restrictions. Once the superficial restrictions have been addressed, strip out the individual muscles that are involved in the shoulder. It is important to create space between the pectoralis major and and the pectoralis minor. With the arm abducted, find the lateral edge of the pectoralis major, and run your fingertips along the border from superior to inferior. This area is generally tender, so make sure to address the client's comfort.

Another area that is necessary to define is the inferior border of the clavicle and sternoclavicular joint. Defining this area will remove any restrictions around the joint and address the clavicular attachment of the pectoralis major. The biceps brachii should also be defined, especially where it crosses under the anterior deltoid. This area is also very tender, so use caution. Finally, make sure the border between the lateral scapula and the rib cage is stripped out. This will address the portion of the rotator cuff and teres major that may not have been worked on in the prone position.

Side-Lying Position The best way to reach the subscapularis on the anterior surface of the scapula and the serratus anterior is to have the client in a side-lying position. These two muscles contribute a great deal to shoulder girdle motion and often get stuck together; therefore, removing their restrictions is extremely beneficial. Once the restrictions have been assessed, move into them until they release.

Both active and passive movements are effective in this position as well. After the superficial concerns have been cleared up, work into the individual muscles in the area. The posterior deltoid is treated effectively in this position. Support the humerus with one hand, and use the thumb to trace its borders.

Since they lie under the scapula, the subscapularis and serratus anterior are not completely accessible. Support the humerus with one hand, and find the lateral border of the scapula with the other, using your fingertips or thumb and making sure you are lateral to the teres major. Because this area can be tender, a more comfortable approach for the client may be to leave your hand stationary and protract the client's shoulder by pulling it onto your thumb or fingertips. Move up and down the border of the scapula, and use passive movement, pulling the arm at different angles. The emphasis should be on creating space between the scapula and the rib cage. If the pressure is directed up into the anterior scapula, the focus will be on the subscapularis; if the pressure is down onto the rib cage, the focus will be the serratus anterior.

Tissue Inconsistencies Trigger points in the muscles of this area can be major contributors to the improper biomechanics that are causing dysfunction. Special attention should be given to the muscles that cause protraction of the shoulder, such as the pectoralis minor and serratus anterior. These muscles contribute to the underlying postural concerns, and releasing them will benefit the client. Be sure to expand the treatment area into the neck if necessary, and do not forget about the biceps and triceps brachii. They are traditionally thought of as arm muscles, but they can affect the shoulder as well. The use of movement during the releasing of the points will help with the neuromuscular reeducation of the muscles and will help relieve the client's associated discomfort.

Muscle Concerns

The focus of the muscular work should be on restoring normal biomechanics to the area and further removing any imbalances between the muscles. Utilize strokes that incorporate movement at every opportunity.

Prone Position The posterior rotator cuff and any involved back muscles are best addressed in this position. Working between the shoulder blades with the forearm or elbow is very effective for the rhomboids and trapezius. Start at the head of the table, and run your forearm down the back; or start at the side of the table, and run your forearm up the back between the scapulae.

One effective technique for the posterior cuff is to hang the arm off the front of the table and perform a stroke using a loose fist from the inferior angle of the scapula up toward the shoulder. This technique addresses the muscles in a parallel direction. To treat the muscles perpendicularly, keep the client's arm in the same position and stand facing his or her shoulder. Drag your loose fist down from the medial border of the scapula toward the table, taking care not to slip and pinch the tissue into the table. Strip out each muscle using active movement to increase the stroke's effectiveness.

Another technique that helps increase shoulder mobility is to place the client's hand in the small of his or her back. If the client lacks the range to place the hand on the back, have the client slide the hand up his or her side. As the client relaxes the arm, the medial border of the scapula will become prominent. Cup the front of the shoulder with your front hand, and grasp the medial border of the scapula with your fingertips. Passively retract the scapula with the hand that is cupping the shoulder, and distract the scapula with the hand on the medial border. Compress and distract the scapula in various directions to increase the mobility.

When addressing the triceps in the prone position, an effective technique is to hang the arm off the side of the table. This allows the muscle to be compressed into the table for the most effective stroke possible. Perpendicular compressive effleurage works well in this application. Both active and passive movements can easily be added in this position by using the techniques described in Chapter 3.

Supine Position The muscles that control the protraction of the shoulder can be treated effectively in the supine position. An effective method of treating the pectoralis major is to stand at the side of the client and hold the wrist in the manner described for the connective tissue work. Passively abduct the arm at various angles while performing strokes from the medial aspect of the muscle to the lateral. This addresses the different orientations of the fibers.

The biceps brachii can be treated in the supine position by holding the wrist with one hand and working the muscle with the other. Movement can easily be incorporated into this part of the treatment by flexing and extending the client's arm or having the client do so. From the biceps, move into the anterior deltoids, which can be very tight.

To treat the pectoralis minor, abduct the arm to find the lateral edge of the pectoralis major. Place your fingertips underneath the pectoralis major, and adduct the arm; this will place slack in the muscle. Place your other hand on top of the client's shoulder, and passively depress it onto your fingertips. As the muscle begins to loosen, change the direction of your fingers to address different portions of the muscle. Be sure that pressure is directed onto the rib cage. You can incorporate active movement by having the client raise his or her arm to 90°. Protract the shoulder toward the ceiling, or, conversely, have the client reach down toward the feet and depress the shoulder.

Side-Lying Position With the client in this position, have the client make a fist and place his or her arm over the head, resting the fist on the table. Stand at the client's hips, and face the head of the table. Perform a stroke between the lateral border of the scapula and the chest, up the axillary line, to treat the serratus anterior.

To treat the subscapularis, hold the client's wrist and place your thumb or fingers along the lateral edge of the scapula, making sure you are lateral to the teres major. Passively protract the client's shoulder by pulling it onto your thumb or fingers. Change the direction of both your fingers and the pull of the arm to address the entire muscle. Direct pressure up into the anterior scapula for the subscapularis and down onto the ribs for the serratus anterior. Incorporate active motion by having the client reach with the arm while you protract the shoulder in different directions.

Access the medial edge of the anterior scapula by having the client move so that his or her back is at the edge of the table. Place the client's top hand in the small of his or her back. This will cause the medial edge to stick out, and you can access the anterior medial edge by grasping it and curling your fingers around the medial border.

Stretching

Because of the chronic posture patterns of the shoulder, the anterior structures will typically be tighter. The posterior muscles may feel tight because they are being chronically lengthened. This is why it is important to stretch the anterior structures first and then move to the posterior ones. All of these stretches are performed with the client in the seated position; however, they can be modified if the client has any limitations.

Chest To stretch the chest, have the client sit up straight and place his or her arms straight out in front of the body with the palms together (Fig. 7-19). As the client exhales, have him or her open the arms as far as possible. Assist at the end by reaching over the top of the client's arms and gently pulling at the elbows. Have the client return to the starting position and repeat for one to two sets of 10 repetitions. As the tissue loosens, have the client raise the arms 10° to 15° for three different angles.

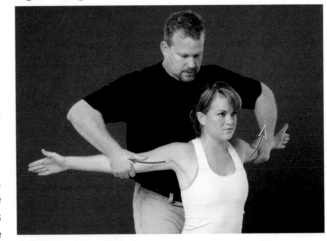

Figure 7-19 Pectoralis stretch.

Pectoralis Minor To stretch the pectoralis minor, have the client interlock the fingers behind the head and bring the elbows together in front of his or her body (Fig. 7-20). As the client exhales, have him or her move the elbows back as far as possible.

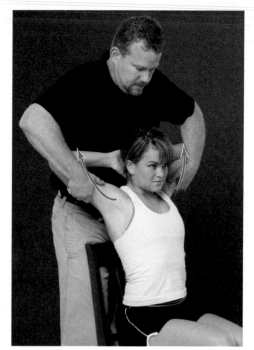

Figure 7-20 Pectoralis minor stretch.

At the end of the range, gently assist in an upward and backward direction at a 45° angle by either reaching under or over the top and holding at the elbows. Repeat for one to two sets of 8 to 10 repetitions.

Anterior Arm and Shoulder Moving to the anterior arm and shoulder, have the client sit up straight and place the arms at the sides (Fig. 7-21). Without bending at the waist, the client should exhale and extend the arms as far back as possible, keeping them close to the sides with the elbows locked. At the end of the range, assist gently in the same direction by holding the forearms, and then return to the starting position. Repeat for 10 repetitions.

Anterior Shoulder A similar stretch for the anterior shoulder is to have the client interlace the fingers behind the back with palms facing away from the body (Fig. 7-22). While exhaling, the client should lift the arms upward as far as possible. At the end of the range, gently assist the client in the same direction by holding under the forearms, and then return to the starting position. Make sure the client does not lean over to compensate. If necessary, the client may flex his or her neck 15° for comfort. Repeat for one to two sets of 10 repetitions.

Rotators While the rotators of the shoulders can be stretched in various positions, the safest is the prone position.

Internal Rotators For the internal rotators, have the client lie prone and hang the arm off the table at 90° with the elbow bent (Fig. 7-23). Place a folded towel under the front of the shoulder to prevent the humerus from translating anteriorly. Place the hand or forearm of the side closest to the table on the scapula of the client to stabilize the posterior shoulder. While exhaling, the client should rotate the arm and bring the hand up as far as possible. At the end of the range, gently assist the client by grasping the wrist and pulling. Release to the starting position, and then repeat for one to two sets of 10 repetitions.

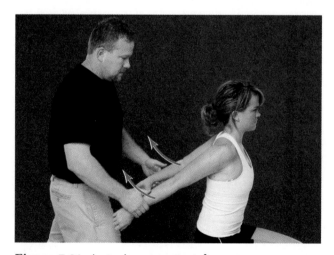

Figure 7-21 Anterior arm stretch.

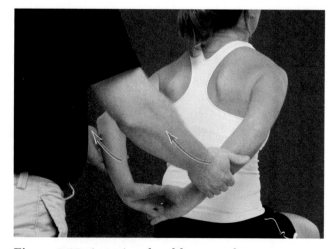

Figure 7-22 Anterior shoulder stretch.

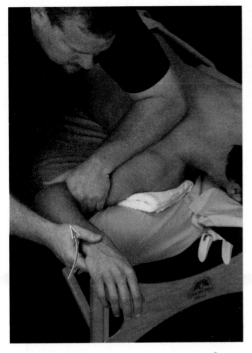

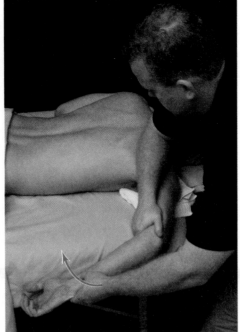

Figure 7-23 Internal rotator stretch.　　**Figure 7-24** External rotator stretch.

External Rotators To stretch the external rotators, begin in the same position as that for the internal rotators, except stand at the head of the table and face the feet. Use the folded towel under the front of the shoulder for this stretch. While exhaling, the client should rotate the shoulder inward, bringing the palm up as far as possible (Fig. 7-24). To make sure the client's arm does not adduct, apply firm pressure to the scapula. At the end of the range, gently assist in the same direction by grasping the wrist and pulling up, and then return to the starting position. Repeat for one to two sets of 10 repetitions.

Posterior Shoulder Once the anterior muscles are loosened, you can move to the posterior muscles. To stretch the posterior shoulder, have the client reach the arm in front of his or her body with the thumb up (Fig. 7-25). While exhaling, the client should reach across the front of the chest toward the top of the shoulder, keeping the arm parallel to the ground. At the end of the motion, gently assist by grasping the elbow and compressing the arm into the chest. To make sure the client does not rotate the trunk to compensate, stabilize the opposite shoulder. Return to the starting position, and then repeat for one to two sets of 10 repetitions.

Another stretch for the posterior shoulder begins by having the client place the arm to be stretched on the opposite shoulder. Stabilize the shoulder being stretched to prevent it from shrugging or moving out of the neutral position (Fig. 7-26). As the client exhales, he or she should walk the fingers down his or her back as far as possible. At the end of the range, gently assist the client by placing your hand on the elbow. Return the arm to the starting position, and then repeat for 8 to 10 repetitions.

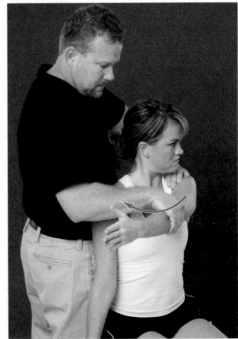

Figure 7-25 Posterior shoulder stretch with arm straight.

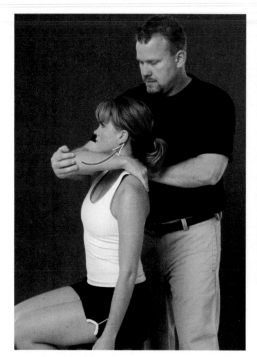 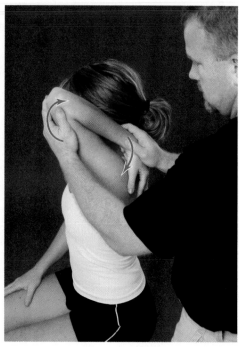

Figure 7-26 Posterior shoulder stretch with arm bent.   **Figure 7-27** Triceps stretch.

Triceps Brachii The last stretch is for the triceps brachii. Have the client reach straight out in front of his or her body with the palm facing up (Fig. 7-27). Have the client bend the elbow. While exhaling, the client should reach over the shoulder as far as he or she can. At the end of the movement, assist the client by standing at his or her side. Placing one hand on the wrist to keep the arm bent and the other hand under the elbow, continue the motion, keeping the arm bent and the shoulder moving straight back. Return to the starting position, and then repeat for 5 to 10 repetitions. Once the triceps has been stretched directly backward, repeat the process with the elbow swung out to 45° so that the client is reaching down his or her back at an oblique angle. Assist the client for 5 to 10 repetitions, returning to the starting position each time.

Biceps Brachii Tendonopathy

Background

Injuries to different parts of the tendon of the long head of the biceps brachii can occur for a variety of reasons. Although injury can occur to both the short and long heads of the muscle, this section addresses pathology involving the tendon of the long head of the biceps. In order to understand the pathology of this tendon, we must first understand its role in the overall functioning of the shoulder.

The tendon of the long head of the biceps plays an important role in the properly functioning shoulder. It arises from inside the glenohumeral joint at the supraglenoid tubercle and superior labrum, where the glenohumeral ligaments converge (see Fig. 7-4) (Beall et al., 2003). The tendon travels at an oblique angle over the humeral head. It exits the joint capsule at the level of the humeral neck and moves inferiorly through the bicipital groove, continuing down the groove until it merges with the tendon from the short head coming off the coracoid process. The tendon is surrounded by a synovial sheath and is held in the groove by the coracohumeral ligament.

Since the biceps brachii is one of several muscles that cross two joints, it makes sense that the muscle performs functions at both locations. At the elbow, its primary function is supination; it contributes to flexion as a secondary function. Its function at the shoulder joint, however, is less clear (Levy et al., 2001). While studies agree that the long head of the biceps is important in shoulder function, it generally functions as a stabilizing structure and not a movement generator. Electromyographic studies performed on the shoulder showed minimal or no activity of the biceps during various shoulder motions. Based on these studies, as well as cadaveric research, the role of the long head of the biceps seems to be that it stabilizes the anterior and superior portions of the glenohumeral joint and assists in maintaining a normal relationship between the humeral head and glenoid fossa (Beall et al., 2003). This role increases as the stability of the glenohumeral joint decreases (Morag et al., 2005).

Because of this, injuries to the long head of the biceps are usually associated with other pathological processes in the shoulder. Isolated injuries to the tendons occur primarily from blunt traumas causing a primary injury to the tendon or from congenital factors affecting the groove through which the tendon runs. As the tendon passively slides within the groove, the friction it creates causes the tendon to become irritated and inflamed. This leads to tendonitis.

Injury to the biceps tendon often occurs as a result of a related shoulder pathology, the most common of which is impingement of the rotator cuff. The primary mechanism of injury is repetitive motion that includes overhead movement or activity. The biceps tendon and the rotator cuff structures make contact with the coracoacromial arch. This type of tendonopathy is classified as **impingement tendonosis,** wherein the intracapsular portion of the tendon is compressed against various structures.

Another classification of tendonopathy is known as **attrition tendonosis,** which is the result of a narrow bicipital groove and affects the extracapsular portion of the tendon.

Despite the cause, clients will generally present with vague anterior shoulder pain with a possible radiation to the proximal upper arm or deltoid insertion (Pfahler et al., 1999). There may be focused discomfort over the bicipital groove during internal and external rotation. This often makes it difficult to distinguish the difference between a biceps tendon injury and impingement.

Additional damage to the tendon can occur as the associated condition worsens. Continued damage to the rotator cuff will increase compression of the biceps tendon and further the pathologic process, which can result in partial tearing of the tendon. If the process is not resolved, a complete rupture of the tendon of the long head may occur. This will result in a "Popeye" deformity due to the distal displacement of the belly of the biceps.

Another condition that can arise from untreated associated pathologies is the subluxation or dislocation of the tendon from the groove. The

Practical Tip

The stabilizing role of the shoulder muscles increases as the joint stability decreases.

impingement tendonosis Pathology of the biceps tendon in which the intracapsular portion of the tendon is compressed against various structures.

attrition tendonosis Pathology of the biceps tendon caused by a narrow bicipital groove and resulting in irritation of the extracapsular portion of the tendon.

primary structures holding the tendon in the groove are the coracohumeral ligament and the insertion tendon of the subscapularis. The tendon may become displaced if these structures are damaged. Repeated subluxations can fray the tendon and will also lead to its eventual rupture.

As the shoulder loses stability from underlying pathology, a superior labrum anterior to posterior (SLAP) lesion can occur. This affects the labrum and typically begins where the biceps tendon inserts into the labrum at the supraglenoid tubercle. With increasing instability comes an increase in the severity of the lesion, which eventually makes its way down the superior part of the biceps tendon. Clients with this disorder typically present with shoulder pain but have a distinct clicking within the joint on movement. This injury is beyond the scope of this text; if it is suspected, the client should be referred to another health care provider.

Assessment

Tendonopathy of the long head of the biceps brachii can be difficult to discern. Since it can present with the same symptoms as rotator cuff injuries, and is often caused by associated shoulder pathology, practitioners should perform a thorough assessment of the area, including the neck if warranted.

Condition History Inquire about the following when taking the client's history:

Question	Significance
What is the client's age?	Biceps tendonopathy in a young client may be the result of trauma or improper mechanics during overhead activities or an anatomical anomaly.
What was the mechanism of injury?	Since isolated injuries to the biceps tendon don't often occur, the nature of the injury can lend useful information.
Are there any movements that cause pain?	Overhead movements will typically cause pain.
Is there any sound or sensation?	A popping sound or sensation can indicate a rupture of the tendon.
Where is the pain?	Biceps injury may present more anterior pain.
How long has the client had the problem?	Long-standing pain can indicate a more severe problem.

Visual Assessment Make sure the client is disrobed to the appropriate level. Observe the client's functional capacity during movement. Note dysfunctional movement patterns and the quality of the client's movement. Check for obvious swelling, bruising, or muscle atrophy along with passive and active ranges of motion. From the front, observe the overall position of the head and neck in relation to the shoulders. Notice any excessive rotation of the shoulders, which could indicate a possible underlying pathology. Check the biceps brachii for any obvious deformity that would suggest a rupture.

Palpation Begin by checking the overall shoulder for hypertonicity of the musculature. Check the sternoclavicular and acromioclavicular joints, and make sure the scapulae sit evenly on the thoracic spine. Focus your attention over the bicipital groove and the greater and lesser tuberosities, being careful not to exacerbate any discomfort in the area. Palpate the coracoid process and the short head of the biceps tendon. Concentrate on the structures listed earlier in the chapter, expanding the area as necessary.

Orthopedic Tests Biceps tendonopathy typically arises as a result of additional shoulder pathology; therefore, it is necessary to perform the orthopedic tests for impingement and rotator cuff tears. Table 7-3 shows the orthopedic tests and how to perform them.

Table 7-3   Orthopedic Tests for Biceps Brachii Tendonopathy

Orthopedic Test	How to Perform
Speed's test 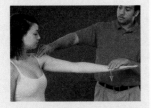 *Note:* This test was first described by J. Spencer Speed when he experienced pain in the proximal shoulder while he was performing a straight-leg-raise test on a patient. He was subsequently diagnosed with bicipital tendonitis and the test has been used ever since (Bennett, 1998).	Have client flex the shoulder to 90° and fully extend the elbow. Place one hand on the bicipital groove and the other hand on the client's distal forearm. Force the client's arm into shoulder extension while he or she resists. *Note:* Placing the client's arm in this position and applying an eccentric load forces the biceps tendon to act as a suspensor cable from its insertion. The presence of inflammation will cause pain, which is considered a positive sign. An alternate method is to flex the client's arm to 60°. Resist forward flexion. *Note:* This position will create upward force and may cause the biceps tendon to impinge into the acromion or other structures, subsequently causing pain. The presence of pain is considered a positive test.

Table 7-3   Orthopedic Tests for Biceps Brachii Tendonopathy (Continued)

Orthopedic Test	How to Perform
Yergason's test 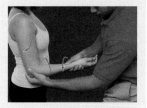 *Note:* Although both tests are helpful, Speed's test has shown to be more reliable at detecting pathology.	Have the client flex his or her elbow to 90° while keeping it stabilized against the torso and pronating the forearm. Place one hand on the client's forearm, and instruct him or her to simultaneously supinate the forearm, externally rotate the shoulder, and flex the elbow while you resist. Pain is an indicator of a positive test, as is the tendon snapping out of its groove.
Ludington's test 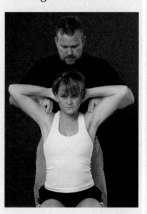 *Note:* This test is used for detecting a rupture in the tendon of the long head of the biceps.	Have the client clasp his or her hands on top of or behind the head, using the fingers to support the weight of the head. Place your fingers on the biceps tendon in the groove. Have the client alternately contract the biceps while you feel for the contraction. There is likely a rupture if you do not feel a contraction, which is a positive sign.

Soft Tissue Treatment

Since bicipital tendonopathy may have arisen as a result of other pathologies, it is necessary to address those conditions before the pathology with the biceps tendon can be resolved. Treatment will be based first on the underlying pathology. For example, if the underlying pathology is a rotator cuff tear, use the soft tissue treatments for that particular condition, followed by the techniques for biceps tendon pathology. Be aware of the phase of the injury to the tendon. It may be necessary to use more conservative treatments until the injury has moved out of the acute phase. Make sure to thoroughly treat any areas that are contributing to the dysfunction.

Connective Tissue Dysfunctional posture patterns can be an underlying factor in this condition. Since connective tissue plays a major role in postural patterns, treating it can offer significant benefit.

Prone Position In addition to the general treatment of the shoulder and associated areas, treatment of the triceps can also be performed effectively in the prone position. Moreover, the triceps is an important muscle to treat since it is the antagonist to the biceps brachii.

Hang the arm off the side of the table, and assess the superficial connective tissue of the posterior arm and shoulder in various directions. Move into any restrictions until they are cleared. As you move deeper, strip out the border between the long head of the triceps and the posterior deltoid.

Supine Position Assess the superficial tissue of the anterior arm and shoulder in various directions. Grasp the wrist with one hand to control the arm, and incorporate movement while moving into any restrictions. Separate the biceps brachii from the underlying muscles, and strip out each head of the muscle. Create separation between the anterior deltoid and the biceps. Use caution, as it is likely this area will be tender. Perform direct connective tissue treatment to the biceps tendon if the tissue can tolerate it. Strip out any restrictions around the tendon, and remove any adhesions. Strip out underneath the insertion of the pectoralis major to remove any restrictions between the two tendons.

Side-Lying Position Use this position to treat the deltoids directly. Stand at the head of the table facing inferiorly. Place the client's arm at his or her side, and strip out each head of the deltoids.

Tissue Inconsistencies Trigger points should be addressed in all the associated muscles, depending on the underlying pathology involved. Specific points that should be addressed are in the biceps brachii, anterior deltoid, pectoralis minor, and pectoralis major.

Muscle Concerns

The elimination of the underlying pathology that is contributing to the formation of bicipital tendonitis should be addressed. The emphasis should be on restoring normal shoulder kinematics. Remove any excess tension through the tendon as it passes through the groove to lessen the pressure on the structures involved.

Prone Position Focus on the triceps in this position by hanging the arm off the table to optimize the work to the muscle. Both active and passive movements can easily be incorporated while the arm is in this position. Apply perpendicular compressive effleurage while the client extends his or her arm. Use parallel thumb stripping starting at the olecranon process to strip out the borders of the three heads of the triceps while the client actively flexes and extends his or her arm. Be sure to address the posterior shoulder girdle using the techniques described for treating impingement syndrome.

Supine Position The biceps tendon can be directly treated in this position. Take the client's wrist with one hand to control the arm, and work deep into the biceps brachii from distal to proximal, easing the pressure as you pass over the anterior shoulder. Perpendicular compressive effleurage is a good stroke to use in this position. Make sure the biceps is facing up, and work proximally and distally.

Movement can also be easily incorporated into the work for the biceps. Parallel thumb stripping while the client is extending the arm will separate the heads of the biceps and remove any restrictions. Working under the anterior deltoid at its border with the biceps will remove adhesions between the two muscles. This border may be painful, so it is important to warm it up properly. Address the associated muscles of the trunk such as the pectoralis major and minor to remove restrictions.

Side-Lying Position This position is effective for treating the deltoids directly. Place the client's arm along his or her side, and work down onto the lateral shoulder. The pectoralis minor may be accessed from this position. Stand in front of the client, and support his or her arm while abducting it in front. Work along the lateral border of the pectoralis major, sliding behind it onto the pectoralis minor. You can have the client move while you are applying pressure to increase the effectiveness of the stroke.

Stretching

As with the other treatments of this condition, it is beneficial to stretch the entire shoulder girdle to address any underlying conditions that may be contributing to problems with the biceps tendon. Use the stretches for impingement syndrome to address the shoulder, placing special emphasis on the anterior shoulder and biceps, as seen in Figs. 7-19 to 7-27.

Anterior Shoulder To stretch the anterior shoulder, have the client sit up straight and place the arms at the sides (see Fig. 7-21). Without bending at the waist, the client should extend the arms as far back as possible, keeping them close to the sides with the elbows locked, while exhaling. At the end of the range, assist gently in the same direction by grasping the forearms, and then return to the starting position. Repeat for 10 repetitions.

For a similar stretch, have the client interlace the fingers behind the back with palms facing away from the body (see Fig. 7-22). While exhaling, the client should lift the arms upward as far as possible. At the end of the range, gently assist in the same direction by grasping under the forearms and returning the client to the starting position. Make sure the client does not lean over to compensate. The client may also flex his or her neck 15° for comfort. Repeat for one to two sets of 10 repetitions.

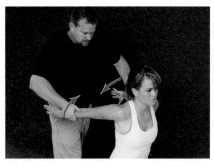

Figure 7-28 Anterior shoulder stretch.

Biceps Brachii To stretch the biceps brachii, have the client sit up straight, abduct his or her arms 90° to the side, and turn the thumbs down (Fig. 7-28). With the palms facing each other, horizontally abduct the arms and adduct the scapula. At the end of the range, gently assist in the same direction as the client exhales. Hold for 2 seconds and release. If the client cannot raise the arms to 90°, have him or her raise them as far as possible, gradually raising them higher as they loosen. Repeat for 5 repetitions per level. Make sure the anterior shoulder is sufficiently loose before performing this stretch.

Adhesive Capsulitis (Frozen Shoulder)

Background

The term *frozen shoulder* has been used as a catchall term for a variety of clinical conditions, including subacromial bursitis, calcifying tendonitis, and rotator cuff tears (Pearsall et al., 1998). Shoulder problems are the third-largest segment of musculoskeletal disorders seen in primary health care, trailing lower-back and neck disorders (Wiffen, 2002). Adhesive capsulitis constitutes almost 50% of stiff shoulders in a shoulder clinic and affects between 2% and 5% of the general population. Although various terms are employed to describe frozen shoulder, they all describe the same condition: the painful restriction of both active and passive motions of the glenohumeral and scapulothoracic joints (Pearsall et al., 1998). There are many conditions that will result in a stiff and painful shoulder, but movement is limited only by pain and not by capsular contraction as it is with adhesive capsulitis.

Frozen shoulder was first described by Codman in 1934 as a "class of cases which I find difficult to define, difficult to treat, and difficult to explain from the point of view of pathology. Yet these cases form a fairly distinct clinical entity" (Bunker, 1998). Even though he could not explain the entire pathological process, Codman recognized that clients with this condition had numerous things in common. These points are summarized in Table 7-4.

Table 7-4 Codman's Characteristics of Frozen Shoulder

Slow onset

Pain near the deltoid insertion

Inability to sleep on the affected side

Painful and incomplete elevation and external rotation

Both spasmodic and adherent restrictions

Atrophy of the rotator cuff

Little local tenderness

It was not until 1945 that Neviaser coined the term "**adhesive capsulitis**" and tried to explain the pathologic anatomy. He described adhesive capsulitis as an "insidious condition that begins with pain, then gradual restriction of all planes of movement in the shoulder" (Mitsch et al., 2004). Neviaser believed that an inflammatory process in the capsule and synovium of the joint led to the formation of adhesions within the shoulder joint, and he identified four stages of adhesive capsulitis, described in Table 7-5.

In 1969, Lundberg created two classifications for adhesive capsulitis based on pain and motion requirements. Primary frozen shoulder is idiopathic in nature, and clients have no significant findings in the history, clinical examination, or radiographic information to explain the loss of motion or pain. If a client has a predisposing condition such as a

adhesive capsulitis An insidious condition that begins with pain and progresses to a loss of motion in all planes.

Table 7-5 Four Stages of Adhesive Capsulitits

Stage	Characteristics
1	Clients present with pain described as achy at rest and sharp at end ranges of motion, similar to the presentation of impingement syndrome.
	Symptoms are present for fewer than 3 months, and a loss of motion begins in flexion, internal rotation, and abduction.
	This loss of range is due to pain levels rather than capsular restrictions.
2	Clients present with symptoms that they have experienced for 3 to 9 months.
	Their pain is a result of the inflammation of the synovium and a reduction in capsular volume.
	These patients show a continued reduction in the range of motion in the same directions as stage 1.
3	Client's symptoms have been present for 9 to 14 months.
	The painful phase is over, but the shoulder is still stiff due to capsular adhesions.
4	This final stage is also known as the *thawing phase.*
	Symptoms have usually been present for 15 to 24 months.
	This stage is characterized by slow progressive improvement of the client's range of motion in response to the use of the shoulder and arm.
	Full range may never be regained, but normal everyday activities are possible.

trauma or surgery to explain his or her symptoms, the client is classified as having secondary frozen shoulder.

The etiology of adhesive capsulitis remains elusive; however, several predisposing factors can increase the occurrence of the condition:

- The incidence of adhesive capsulitis in the diabetic population increases to 10% to 20% and up to 36% in insulin-dependent diabetics.
- Other conditions that have shown a higher rate of frozen shoulder include thyroid disease, stroke or myocardial infarction, autoimmune diseases, cervical disk disease, chest or breast surgery, hormonal changes, and any condition that requires long periods of immobilization.
- There is an association between frozen shoulder and another fibrosing condition, Dupuytren's disease, wherein there is a contracture of the palmar fascia. This relationship was first recognized in 1936 by Schaer when he discovered that 25% of patients with frozen shoulder also had Dupuytren's. One study reported a 58% rate of correlation (Smith et al., 2001).

- The prevalence of frozen shoulder is greater in women than men, and the nondominant side is more typically involved. The most common age range affected is 40 to 70, and there is a 20% to 30% chance that patients will develop symptoms in the opposite shoulder.

Disagreement exists as to whether the underlying pathologic process of adhesive capsulitis is inflammatory or fibrosing in nature. Recently, there has been significant evidence indicating that the pathologic processes are an initial synovial inflammatory condition with the subsequent occurrence of capsular fibrosis, making adhesive capsulitis both an inflammatory and a fibrosing condition. To understand this pathology, we must look at the healing process. In Chapter 3, we described the three stages of healing: inflammatory, repair and regeneration, and remodeling and scar formation. The initial inflammatory trigger is not known for frozen shoulder. This inflammation causes a hypertrophy and increased vascularity of the synovial membrane, resulting in pain and loss of motion. It is the last two stages of healing that hold the key to the dysfunction of the biology of frozen shoulder.

Contractures can occur as a result of physiologic or pathologic processes. An example of a physiologic process occurs when the edges of a healing wound pull together. A pathologic process includes an imbalance between scar formation and remodeling, resulting in the abnormal formation of a contracture (Bunker, 1998). Recall that the main cell of scar tissue formation is the fibroblast. Fibroblast activity is controlled by a certain type of cell messenger called *cytokines.* Cytokines are involved in the initiation and termination of scar tissue formation and remodeling (Hannafin et al., 2000). There seem to be elevated levels of cytokines and fibrogenic growth factors in frozen-shoulder tissue. An increase in scar tissue formation is only one side of the coin. The other side is the failure of tissue remodeling. The task of remodeling is left to a family of enzymes that act as collagenases and are now referred to as *matrix metaloproteinases (MMPs)* (Bunker, 1998). It seems that in adhesive capsulitis these enzymes are inhibited and a failure of the remodeling of the scar tissue takes place, leaving contractures that restrict shoulder motion.

Assessment

Depending on whether adhesive capsulitis is primary or secondary, there may be other underlying conditions that have caused the pathology. Two aspects need to be assessed in all clients: pain and contracture (Bunker, 1998). Performing a thorough assessment, using the various pieces, and integrating the results into an overall picture of the condition will ensure that the proper treatment is given. Remember, your assessment may differ depending on what stage the frozen shoulder is in. You may need to expand the assessment to associated areas if it is determined that they are involved.

Condition History Prior to the physical assessment, inquire about the following when taking the client's history:

Question	Significance
What is the client's age?	Frozen shoulder tends to favor a certain age group (40 to 70).

Question	Significance
When did the symptoms start, and how long have they been there?	This will help identify what stage the pathology is in.
Was there any trauma to the shoulder?	This can lend information about whether the condition is primary or secondary.
Does the client have any other health problems?	This will determine any associated conditions.
Where is the pain located?	This will help identify involved structures.
Are there any positions or motions that increase or decrease the pain?	This will help identify involved structures.
Is there any radiculopathy?	This will help determine neurologic involvement.
What is the loss of function?	This can help identify reductions in common movement patterns.

Visual Assessment Ensure that the client is disrobed to the appropriate level. You can observe the client in a seated or standing position. Notice the positions of the arm and the head and neck. Depending on the stage, the shoulder may be elevated to guard against the pain. In later stages, a common appearance is the loss of the normal axillary fold due to the contracture. Check for muscle atrophy or obvious deformity, along with any swelling and discoloration. Assess active and passive ranges of motion, and note abnormalities.

Palpation Areas may or may not be tender, depending on the stage of the condition. Later stages will show more hypertonicity in the musculature. Generally, there is not a lot of point tenderness in the shoulder area, although the biceps brachii tendon may be tender to direct palpation (Beam, 2000). Begin with the neck, and work your way down onto the shoulder girdle, palpating the anterior side first. Include the structures discussed earlier in the chapter, and be sure to use a systematic approach, noting any tenderness, tightness, swelling, or bruising.

Orthopedic Tests To ensure a complete assessment, include tests for associated shoulder conditions, such as the Hawkins-Kennedy and empty-can tests (see Table 7-2 on pages 244 and 245). To fully understand frozen shoulder, it is important to realize that shoulder function involves both the scapulothoracic articulation and the glenohumeral joint (Pearsall et al., 1998). The primary symptom of frozen shoulder is the progressive loss of range of motion. It stands to reason that special orthopedic tests for the condition assess range of motion.

There is a consistent pattern of motion loss referred to as a **capsular pattern**. "A capsular pattern is a proportional motion restriction that is unique to every joint that indicates irritation of the entire joint" (Mitsch et al., 2004).

Adhesive capsulitis causes the most restriction in external rotation, followed by abduction and then internal rotation. The therapist should assess each movement individually; however, Apley's scratch test will provide a quick scan of the entire shoulder girdle movement at once. Table 7-6 explains how to perform this test.

📖 **capsular pattern**
A proportional motion restriction that is unique to every joint that indicates irritation of the entire joint.

Table 7-6 Orthopedic Test for Adhesive Capsulitis

Orthopedic Test	How to Perform
Apley's scratch test (see Fig. 7-6 on page 225) • The test combines internal rotation with adduction and external rotation with abduction. *Note:* This test will provide valuable information about the functional capacity of the client and whether he or she can perform certain tasks.	Have the client reach behind his or her head and down the back as far as possible with one hand, while you assess external rotation and abduction. Have the client reach up behind the back as far as possible while you assess internal rotation and adduction. Record the level for each hand, and repeat for the opposite side. Reduced range of motion that affects functioning is considered a positive test.

Soft Tissue Treatment

The primary objectives for treatment should be to relieve pain and restore motion (Pearsall et al., 1998). The techniques used may vary depending on the stage of the condition. The goal for stage 1 is to interrupt and control the inflammatory process and limit pain. Methods such as rest and ice should be implemented to reduce discomfort and facilitate healing. Stage 2 goals include reversing and preventing motion restrictions. Once the client has reached stage 3, emphasize treating the significant loss of motion and abnormal scapulohumeral rhythm.

Connective Tissue As the pathology progresses, connective tissue can play a larger role in the dysfunction; therefore, it is important to address it.

Prone Position Assess the superficial fascia of the back from superior to inferior, from medial to lateral, and at various angles as described earlier. The incorporation of active and passive movements is effective in this area.

Once you have addressed the superficial fascia, move into the deeper layers and begin to strip out the borders of the muscles in the area. Pay special attention to the posterior rotator cuff.

Supine Position Addressing the connective tissue in this position helps treat underlying pathologies that are contributing to the loss of range of motion. Begin by assessing the superficial fascia of the chest, anterior shoulder, and upper arm, including any associated areas as necessary. The use of movement is also beneficial in this position. Make sure you stay within the client's comfort level, depending on his or her restrictions. Use the techniques described for the earlier conditions.

Once you have addressed the superficial restrictions, strip out the individual muscles that are involved in the shoulder. A good area to define is the inferior border of the clavicle and sternoclavicular joint. Defining this area will remove any restrictions around the joint and address the clavicular attachment of the pectoralis major. Finally, make sure the border between the lateral scapula and the rib cage is stripped out. This will address the portion of the rotator cuff and teres major that may not have been worked on in the prone position.

Side-Lying Position The subscapularis and the serratus anterior are best accessed in this position. These two muscles contribute a great deal to shoulder girdle motion and often get stuck together; therefore, removing their restrictions is very beneficial. Once the superficial restrictions have been assessed, move into them until they release. Both active and passive movements are effective in this position as well. Since they lie under the scapula, the subscapularis and serratus anterior are not completely accessible. Support the humerus with one hand, and find the lateral border of the scapula with the other using your fingertips or thumb. Because this area can be tender, a more comfortable approach for the client may be to leave your hand stationary and protract the shoulder onto your thumb or fingertips. Move up and down the border of the scapula, and use passive movement pulling the arm at different angles.

Tissue Inconsistencies Because of the long duration of this condition, excessive guarding of the musculature is typical. This will, however, lead to the presence of trigger points in just about every muscle of the shoulder girdle. Use figures 7-8 to 7-17 to identify the muscles that should be treated. Incorporating motion can increase the effectiveness of your pressure. It will also help reeducate the muscles' firing patterns.

Muscle Concerns

The synergistic relationship of the muscles in the shoulder girdle can be easily upset, and this imbalance is a major contributor to adhesive capsulitis. Addressing the involved muscles and restoring the normal biomechanics to the area should be a major part of the overall treatment procedure.

Prone Position The focus of this work should be to remove any restrictions in the posterior rotator cuff and the lateral border of the scapula. Abduct the arm as far as it will go. Use a loose fist, starting at the spine of the scapula and working perpendicularly across the scapula toward the lateral border. Try to incorporate as many strokes with movement as possible. The area has typically been immobile for a long period of time, and the client's active participation will help with the neurologic input to the muscle.

Another technique that works well in this position is to place the hand in the small of the back and let the elbow fall to the table. If the client is not able to place the hand on the lumbar spine, slide the hand up the side of the body as far as it will go. Cup the anterior shoulder with one hand, and lift up. The medial edge of the scapula should swing, and you can grasp it with your other hand. Distract the scapula as much as possible, and perform various movements with it to help break up any adhesions between the scapula and the thorax. This will also improve its mobility.

Supine Position Focus on the muscles that control the position of the shoulder, such as the pectoralis major and minor and the anterior deltoid. Once they have been addressed, work the lateral border of the scapula thoroughly, again incorporating as much movement as possible.

Side-Lying Position This position allows the best access to the serratus anterior and subscapularis. Have the client abduct the arm as far as possible or flex it forward and rest it on the table. Work between the axillary border of the scapula and the lateral border of the pectoralis major; this will directly address the serratus anterior. Side lying is also the position for stripping out the muscles that run along the lateral scapula. To access the deeper parts of the subscapularis and serratus anterior, support the client's arm with your hand and place your thumb along the lateral border of the scapula, just anterior to the teres major and latissimus dorsi. Passively protract the client's arm onto your thumb, staying within the client's comfort level. You can change the angle of pull to address different portions of the muscle. If tolerable, the client can perform active motions while you hold pressure on the muscle. If you focus your pressure upward into the scapula, you will affect the subscapularis muscle; if you direct the pressure down onto the rib cage, you will affect the serratus anterior.

Stretching

Adhesive capsulitis results in the global loss of mobility in the shoulder. Perform all the stretches discussed for the previous conditions in order to restore balance to the musculature. For maximum results, be sure the client always contracts the muscle opposite the one being stretched.

Shoulder Extensors There are some additional stretches that can be beneficial for this condition. While the client is in the seated position, have the client lock the elbows with the palm facing the body (Fig. 7-29). Stabilize the same-side shoulder with your hand so that it does not shrug, and have the client forward flex the arm while exhaling. At the end of the range of motion, gently assist in the same direction for 2 seconds, and then return to the starting position. Repeat this for one to two sets of 10 repetitions.

Shoulder Adductors For a similar stretch, place the client in the seated position. Have the client lock the elbow with the palm facing forward while you place your hand on the same-side shoulder to stabilize it (Fig. 7-30). Instruct the client to abduct the arm as far as possible while exhaling. At the end of the range of motion, gently assist at the elbow in the same direction. Return to the starting position, and then repeat for 10 repetitions.

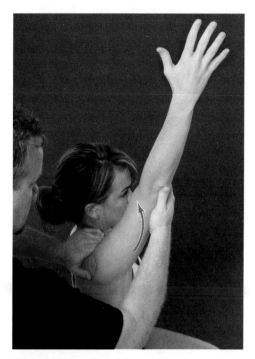

Figure 7-29 Shoulder extensor stretch.

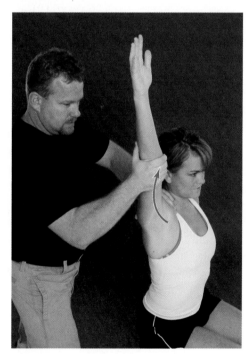

Figure 7-30 Shoulder adductor stretch.

SUMMARY

The shoulder is a very complex region of the body, with several different structures that must act in a symbiotic relationship to provide us with the freedom of motion that we enjoy. The anatomical review at the beginning of the chapter listed all the various structures involved in the region and explained how to palpate them. The next section discussed the movements of the areas, pointing out that the motion actually comes from four separate joints working in unison. The chapter presented several conditions that can affect the shoulder, as well as the assessment and treatment techniques for each. It showed how the various structures are interrelated, and it emphasized that dysfunction in one structure leads to dysfunction in all.

REVIEW QUESTIONS

1. What bones make up the shoulder girdle?
2. What is the size of the humeral head compared to that of the glenoid fossa?
3. What function does the glenoid labrum perform?
4. What are the three ligaments of the glenohumeral joint, and which one provides the most stability?
5. What is the most vulnerable position of the shoulder?
6. What is the scapulohumeral rhythm?
7. What muscles make up the rotator cuff?
8. What are the three variations of acromion shapes, and how does the shape affect the shoulder?
9. What is the painful arc?
10. What is the function of the long head of the biceps brachii at the shoulder?
11. What is a SLAP lesion?
12. What are Codman's characteristics of frozen shoulder?
13. What is the condition that involves the palmar fascia and is associated with frozen shoulder?
14. What is the capsular pattern of a joint?

CRITICAL-THINKING QUESTIONS

1. Discuss how the increased range of motion available in the shoulder results in a decrease in stability.
2. Discuss the importance of the scapulohumeral rhythm.
3. Discuss the importance of the proper functioning of the rotator cuff.
4. Describe the process of the progression from shoulder impingement to a rotator cuff tear.
5. What is the importance of correcting postural concerns when treating shoulder conditions?
6. Why is an isolated chronic injury to the biceps tendon rare?
7. Discuss the process involved in the progressive loss of range of motion in adhesive capsulitis.

Bony Structures of the Shoulder Girdle

Spine of the scapula	This part of the scapula is on the posterior shoulder girdle. It is in the upper half of the bone and runs in a transverse direction at a slight upward angle. The medial end is in line with T3, and the lateral end is the acromion process. Place the palm of your hand on the upper half of the scapula, and palpate in a vertical fashion to find the edge. Use your fingertips to trace its borders.
Medial border of the scapula	This border runs along the spinal column. Trace the spine of the scapula to its medial edge, and move up and down along the border. To make it easier to find, place your client's hand in the small of his or her back.
Superior angle of the scapula	Trace the spine of the scapula to its medial edge. Trace superior and slightly lateral to the superior angle.
Inferior angle of the scapula	This is the inferior tip of the bone. It is found by tracing the spine to the medial edge and running in an inferior direction until the inferior corner is felt.
Greater tuberosity of the humerus	This structure lies on the superior lateral humerus and may be difficult to find. Using the acromion process, move inferior and a little lateral until you find a large, bony prominence. Use your fingers to palpate its borders.
Intertubercular (bicipital) groove	This groove runs in a vertical fashion between the greater and lesser tuberosities of the humerus. Have your client put the arm at the side and bend the elbow to 90°. Locate the greater tuberosity, and laterally rotate the arm. Your finger should fall off the greater tuberosity into a groove and, as you continue to rotate the arm, will come up onto the lesser tuberosity. Rotate the arm medially and laterally to find the groove between the tuberosities.
Lesser tuberosity of the humerus	This structure is smaller and deeper than the greater. From the bicipital groove, move medially onto the bump, which is the lesser tuberosity. You may need to laterally rotate the arm to help locate this structure.
Coracoid process	This bone part lies on the scapula and is located about 1 inch medial to the acromion and about ½ inch inferior to the clavicle. It feels like a small marble or a pea and will most likely be tender.
Humeral head	Abduct the humerus to the end range. Palpate in the axilla with your palm to find the round head of the humerus.
Humeral shaft	The shaft runs from the head of the humerus to the epicondyles. It can be palpated midway down the inside of the arm, in between the biceps brachii and the triceps brachii.
Suprasternal notch	This is the notch or indentation at the top of the sternum. It is also known as the *jugular notch.*
Sternoclavicular joint	Using the suprasternal notch, move just lateral and you will feel the medial edge of the clavicle. You can also trace the clavicle medially until the joint space is found. It sits a little superior on the sternum. In order to make the joint easier to feel, place a finger on the joint and have your client protract and retract the shoulders.
Manubrium	This is the most superior portion of the sternum. The top of this structure is the suprasternal or jugular notch. The first ribs attach on either side below the clavicle.

Bony Structures of the Shoulder Girdle *(Continued)*

Clavicle	This is an S-shaped bone anterior to posterior and runs between the sternum and the scapula. It has a convex curve medially and a concave curve laterally. The lateral end is larger and flatter and forms a joint with the acromion process of the scapula. Trace the bone from the sternum to the scapula.
Acromioclavicular joint	Trace the clavicle to its lateral edge. You should feel a space where it meets the acromion process. You can also locate the acromion process and work your way medially until you feel a "step" up to the clavicle. The space before the step is the joint. You can have your client protract and retract the shoulders to feel the joint move.
Acromion process	Place the palm of your hand on the lateral tip of the shoulder, and move it in a circular fashion. You will feel a flat, bony surface. Use your fingertips to trace the borders. If you are unsure, have your client move the shoulder. If you are on the process, it should not move. If it moves, you are probably on the AC joint or head of the humerus.
Sternal angle (angle of Louis)	Start at the suprasternal notch and move in an inferior direction. You will feel a ridge of bone about 1 inch to 1½ inches down. This is the junction between the manubrium and the body of the sternum. It is a landmark for the second rib.
Body of the sternum	This is the largest portion of the sternum and runs inferiorly to the tip. The last true rib attaches here via the costal cartilage.
Xiphoid process	This process is the end tip of the sternum. It differs in size and can point internally or externally or remain neutral. Trace the sternum in an inferior direction to its end, and press in.

Soft Tissue Structures of the Shoulder Girdle

Brachial artery	This artery lies along the medial humerus, in between the biceps and triceps brachii.
Cephalic vein	This vein runs along the delto-pectoral interval, lateral to the biceps brachii and down the lateral humerus.
Basilic vein	This vein runs along the medial humerus, in between the biceps and triceps brachii.
Median cubital vein	This vein runs along the cubital crease and connects the cephalic and basilic veins.
Medial epicondyle of the humerus	Locate the cubital crease, and trace in a medial direction until you find a round, bony structure.
Medial supracondylar line of the humerus	Locate the medial epicondyle of the humerus, and palpate in a superior direction along a ridge.
Epitrochlear lymph nodes	These nodes lie above the medial epicondyle, along the medial supracondylar line. Use your fingers in a circular fashion to palpate this structure.

Muscles of the Shoulder Girdle

Muscle	Origin	Insertion	Action	How to Palpate
Posterior Muscles				
Trapezius	External occipital protuberance; ligamentum nuchae; spinous processes C7-T12	Lateral third of the clavicle, spine, and acromion process of the scapula	Upper fibers: elevation of the scapula; lateral flexion of the head to same side; rotation of the head to opposite side; exorotation of the scapula; bilateral extension of the head Middle fibers: retraction of the scapula Lower fibers: depression and exorotation of the scapula	Client in prone or standing position; resist shoulder elevation for the upper trapezius, shoulder retraction for the middle trapezius, and shoulder depression for the lower trapezius
Rhomboids	Spinous processes C6-T5	Vertebral border of the scapula from the spine to the inferior angle	Elevation, retraction, and endorotation of the scapula	Client in prone position; retract the shoulders and palpate between the medial border of the scapula and the spine
Levator scapulae	Transverse processes C1-C4	Superior angle and superior part of vertebral border of the scapula	Unilateral: elevation of the scapula; lateral flexion of the head and neck; rotation of the head and neck to same side; endorotation of the scapula Bilateral: extension of the head and neck	Client in prone position; find the superior angle of the scapula, have client shrug shoulder, trace the muscle toward the first four cervical vertebrae
Supraspinatus	Supraspinous fossa of the scapula	Greater tuberosity of the humerus	Abduction of the arm at the shoulder (first 15°); stabilization of the humerus in the glenohumeral joint	Client in seated position; palpate deep to the upper trapezius during slight shoulder abduction
Infraspinatus	Infraspinous fossa of the scapula	Greater tuberosity of the humerus	Adduction, lateral rotation, extension, and horizontal abduction of the arm at the shoulder	Client in prone position; abduct shoulder and elbow to 90°, resist external rotation, and palpate just inferior to the spine of the scapula

Muscle	Origin	Insertion	Action	How to Palpate
Posterior Muscles (Continued)				
Teres minor	Axillary border of the scapula	Greater tuberosity of the humerus	Adduction, lateral rotation, extension, and horizontal abduction of the arm at the shoulder	Client in prone position; abduct shoulder and elbow to 90°, resist external rotation, and palpate between the teres major and the infraspinatus
Subscapularis	Subscapular fossa	Lesser tuberosity of the humerus	Internal rotation of the humerus	Client in side-lying position; palpate underneath scapula
Teres major	Inferior angle of the scapula	Lesser tubercle of the humerus	Adduction, medial rotation, and extension of the arm at the shoulder	Client in prone position with the hand in the small of the back; have client lift hand off the back, and palpate at the inferior angle of the scapula
Serratus anterior	Ribs, upper 8 or 9 pair	Vertebral border of the scapula and costal surface of the subscapular fossa	Protraction of the shoulder girdle; abduction of the arm by exorotation of the scapula	Client in side-lying position; resist protraction of shoulder girdle
Latissimus dorsi	Spinous processes of lower 6 thoracic vertebra, thoracolumbar aponeurosis, posterior iliac crest, lower 3 to 4 ribs, and inferior angle of the scapula	Medial lip of the bicipital groove of the humerus	Adduction, extension, and medial rotation of the arm at the shoulder	Client in prone position; abduct arm to 90°, and hang it off the table; resist adduction and internal rotation of the arm
Anterior Muscles				
Pectoralis major	Medial half of the clavicle; sternum; and cartilage of the first 6 ribs	Lateral lip of the bicipital groove of the humerus	Adduction, flexion, medial rotation, and horizontal adduction of the arm at shoulder Lower fibers: extension of the arm at shoulder	Client in supine position; abduct the arm to 90°, and flex the elbow to 90°; resist horizontal adduction of arm at shoulder

Muscle	Origin	Insertion	Action	How to Palpate
Anterior Muscles (Continued)				
Pectoralis minor	Anterior surface of the 3rd through 5th ribs	Coracoid process of the scapula	Protraction, depression, and endorotation of the scapula	Client in supine position; palpate through pectoralis major while client protracts and depresses the shoulder
Arm Muscles				
Deltoids	Anterior: lateral third of the clavicle Middle: acromion process Posterior: spine of the scapula	Deltoid tuberosity of the humerus	Anterior: flexion, medial rotation, and horizontal adduction of the shoulder Middle: abduction of the shoulder Posterior: extension, lateral rotation, and horizontal abduction of the shoulder	Client in seated or side-lying position Anterior deltoid: resist flexion of the shoulder Middle deltoid: resist abduction of shoulder Posterior deltoid: resist extension of the shoulder
Biceps brachii	Supraglenoid tubercle through bicipital groove (long head); coracoid process of the scapula (short head)	Radial tuberosity and bicipital aponeurosis	Flexion of the supinated elbow; supination of the forearm and flexion of the arm at the shoulder	Client in supine position; resist flexion of a supinated forearm at the elbow
Triceps brachii	Infraglenoid tubercle of the humerus (long head) and proximal end (lateral head) and distal end (medial head) of the shaft of the humerus	Olecranon process of the ulna	Extension of the forearm at the elbow; extension of the arm at the shoulder	Client in prone position; hang the arm off of the table; resist extension of the arm at the elbow
Coracobrachialis	Middle of the humeral shaft on the medial surface	Coracoid process of the humerus	Flexion and adduction of the arm at the shoulder	Client in supine position; abduct the arm to 90°, and externally rotate it; flex the elbow to 90°, and resist horizontal adduction

Trigger Points of the Shoulder Girdle

Muscle	Trigger-Point Location	Referral Pattern	Chief Symptom
Trapezius	1. Upper fibers: one anterior and the other posterior 2. Middle trapezius: one occurs anywhere in the middle part of the muscle; the other is an attachment trigger point near the acromion 3. Lower: one central point halfway along the lower border of the muscle	1. Anterior: behind, up, and over the ear in a ram's-horn pattern Posterior: up back of neck to behind the ear 2. Belly: superficial burning pain; stay local to the point Attachment: top of the shoulder or acromion 3. Sharply to the high cervical paraspinals, mastoid process area, and acromion; deep ache in the suprascapular region	1. Major contributors to tension head-aches 2. Induces other trig-ger points in the up-per back and neck
Rhomboids	1. Level where the spine of the scapula meets the vertebral border 2. Inferior to each other, about halfway down the vertebral border	Pain concentrates around the vertebral border; does not radiate too far away	Superficial aching pain at rest, not influ-enced by movement; snapping or crunching noises
Levator scapulae	1. Superior angle of the scapula 2. Halfway up the muscle	Posterior shoulder and medial scapular border	Pain at the angle of the neck; stiffness pre-venting turning head fully to either side
Supraspinatus	Two in belly of muscle: one close to the medial border; the other farther lateral Third point in proximal tendon	Deep ache centering on the mid-dle deltoid; can extend down the lateral side of the arm to lateral epicondyle of the elbow	Referred pain that is usually felt strongly during abduction of the arm and dully at rest
Infraspinatus	Three located cen-trally in belly, under the spine of the scapula Fourth farther infe-rior and medial to the other three	Refer pain deep into anterior shoulder and possibly down the anterior and lateral aspect of the arm, lateral forearm, and radial aspect of the hand Refer to adjacent rhomboid area along the medial border of the scapula; may be difficult to dis-tinguish from trapezius pain	All contribute to in-ability to internally rotate and adduct arm; can result in trouble sleeping

Trigger Points of the Shoulder Girdle *(Continued)*

Muscle	Trigger-Point Location	Referral Pattern	Chief Symptom
Teres minor	Midbelly along muscle and relatively prominent	Refers just proximal to deltoid tuberosity	Posterior shoulder pain that feels like inflamed bursa
Subscapularis	Two lateral points located above one another, with superior point lying inferior to the coracoid process and inferior point halfway up lateral border of scapula Medial point close to superior medial edge of the muscle	Posterior shoulder; spillover into posterior arm and elbow; strap-like area of pain that encircles the wrist, with the posterior side more painful than the anterior	Significant contributor to "frozen shoulder"; pain both at rest and in motion; initially, clients are able to reach forward but not backward; abduction becomes severely restricted
Latissimus dorsi	1. Superior portion of muscle at posterior axial fold 2. Midregion of the muscle	Pain down back of shoulder, along medial forearm to the ulnar side of hand Anterior shoulder and lateral aspect of the trunk over iliac crest	Constant aching to the inferior angle of the scapula and the surrounding thoracic region
Teres major	1. Medially along muscle near origin 2. Midmuscle in posterior axillary fold 3. Lateral musculocutaneous junction	Posterior shoulder and over the long head of the triceps	Pain primarily produced during movement and usually mild at rest
Deltoids	1. Anterior: along medial border, close to the cephalic vein 2. Middle: almost anywhere 3. Posterior: along lateral border of the muscle, closer to the insertion	Anterior: refer to the anterior deltoid; spillover into middle head Middle: refer central to the region with some spillover to adjacent areas Posterior: refer over posterior shoulder and possibly into the arms	Pain on shoulder motion; weakness on abduction

Trigger Points of the Shoulder Girdle *(Continued)*

Muscle	Trigger-Point Location	Referral Pattern	Chief Symptom
Serratus anterior	Middle of any of its digitations but usually at about the 5th or 6th rib along the midaxillary line	Anterolateral thorax; pain projected down inside of the arm to palm and ring finger; interscapular pain over the distal half of the scapula	Chest pain; shortness of breath
Biceps brachii	Midbelly in either head	Primarily in superior direction to front of shoulder; can also travel to suprascapular region and antecubital space	Pain during arm elevation above shoulder level; other presentations include aching over the anterior arm and possible weakness
Triceps brachii	1. Central belly of the long head of the muscle 2. Lateral portion of the medial head of the muscle 3. Lateral head 4. Attachment point created from other points 5. Medial portion of the medial head of the muscle	1. Upward over the posterior arm and shoulder, sometimes extending into the upper trapezius and down the posterior forearm 2. Lateral epicondyle of the elbow 3. Centrally around the point over the posterior arm; sometimes down the posterior forearm into the 4th and 5th fingers 4. Olecranon process 5. Medial forearm and palmar surface of the 4th and 5th fingers	Diffuse pain posteriorly in the shoulder and upper arm; can affect movement but is often overlooked by the client because of compensatory movements
Pectoralis major	1. Clavicular head of the muscle along lateral edge 2. Sternal portion of the muscle along midclavicular line 3. Lateral border of the muscle about halfway between origin and insertion 4. Medial sternum	1. Pain over anterior deltoid 2. Intense pain to anterior chest and down inner aspect of arm 3. Breast area; can cause tenderness and hypersensitivity of nipple and intolerance to clothing 4. Pain locally over sternum but will not cross over to the opposite side	Can be mistaken for a cardiac episode; associated with contributing to certain cardiac arrhythmias; interscapular back pain; pain in the anterior shoulder

Trigger Points of the Shoulder Girdle *(Continued)*

Muscle	Trigger-Point Location	Referral Pattern	Chief Symptom
	5. Only on the right side, just below 5th rib midway on line between sternal margin and nipple		
Pectoralis minor	1. In belly, close to insertion 2. In belly, close to the origin	Strongly over anterior deltoid and down the medial arm, forearm, and hand	Pain with no distinction between that of pectoralis major

Orthopedic Tests for the Shoulder Region

Condition	Orthopedic Test	How to Perform	Positive Sign
Shoulder impingement	Neer shoulder impingement test *Note:* With this particular arm position, the greater tuberosity of the humerus will be "jammed" into the anterior inferior acromion.	Client is in the seated position. Standing at the client's side, use one hand to stabilize the posterior shoulder and grasp the client's arm at the elbow with the other. Internally rotate the arm passively, and then flex it forcibly to its end range.	Pain with motion, especially at the end of the range, indicates a positive test. This also indicates a possible impingement of the supraspinatus or long head of the biceps tendon.
	Hawkins-Kennedy impingement test *Note:* This test will cause the greater tuberosity of the humerus to contact the anteroinferior surface of the acromion and the coracoacromial arch.	Client is in the seated position. Forward flex the shoulder to 90°, and bend the elbow to 90°. Keeping the shoulder at 90° of flexion, place one hand under the bent elbow to support the arm and place the other at the wrist. Horizontally adduct the arm slightly across the chest, being careful not to lower the arm, and internally rotate the shoulder.	Pain that occurs with this test may indicate shoulder impingement.
Rotator cuff tear	Empty-can test *Note:* This test is specifically for the supraspinatus.	Client is standing. Have the client abduct the arms to 90°. Standing in front of the client, horizontally adduct the arms 30° and internally rotate the arms so that the client's thumbs point toward the floor (empty-can position). Place your hands on the proximal forearms of the client, and apply downward force while the client resists.	Weakness or pain in the shoulder indicates a positive test and a possible tear of the supraspinatus tendon.
	Drop-arm test	Client is in the standing position with his or her arms at 90° of abduction. Instruct the client to slowly lower the arms down to the sides. An alternative test is to place the arms in 90° of abduction and apply downward force at the distal humerus while the client resists.	A positive test is indicated if the client cannot lower the arms smoothly or has increased pain during the motion.

Condition	Orthopedic Test	How to Perform	Positive Sign
			Alternative version: A test is positive if the client cannot hold an arm up and drops it to the side. If either variation of test elicits a positive result, this may be an indication of a more severe tear of the supraspinatus tendon.
Biceps tendonitis/tendonosis	Speed's test Note: This test was first described by J. Spencer Speed when he experienced pain in the proximal shoulder while he was performing a straight-leg-raise test on a patient. He was subsequently diagnosed with bicipital tendonitis, and the test has been used ever since (Bennett, 1998).	Have client flex the shoulder to 90° and fully extend the elbow. Place one hand on the bicipital groove and the other hand on the client's distal forearm. Force the client's arm into shoulder extension while he or she resists. *Note:* Placing the client's arm in this position and applying an eccentric load forces the biceps tendon to act as a suspensor cable from its insertion. Alternate method is to flex the client's arm to 60°. Resist forward flexion. *Note:* This position will create upward force and may cause the biceps tendon to impinge into the acromion or other structures, subsequently causing pain.	The presence of inflammation will cause pain, which is considered a positive sign. Alternate version: The presence of pain is considered a positive test.
	Yergason's test *Note:* Although both tests are helpful, Speed's test has shown to be more reliable at detecting pathology.	Have the client flex his or her elbow to 90° while keeping it stabilized against the chest and pronating the forearm. Place one hand on the client's forearm and instruct him or her to simultaneously supinate the forearm, externally rotate the shoulder, and flex the elbow while you resist.	Pain is an indicator of a positive test, as is the tendon snapping out of its groove.

Orthopedic Tests for the Shoulder Region *(Continued)*

Condition	Orthopedic Test	How to Perform	Positive Sign
Biceps tendon rupture	Ludington's test *Note:* This test is used for detecting a rupture in the tendon of the long head of the biceps.	Have the client clasp his or her hands on top of or behind the head, using the fingers to support the weight of the head. Place your fingers on the biceps tendon in the groove. Have the client alternately contract the biceps while you feel for the contraction.	There is likely a rupture if you do not feel a contraction, which is a positive sign.
Adhesive capsulitis	Apley's scratch test The test combines internal rotation with adduction and external rotation with abduction. *Note:* This test will provide valuable information about the functional capacity of the client and whether he or she can perform certain tasks.	Have the client reach behind his or her head and down the back as far as possible with one hand while you assess external rotation and abduction. Have the client reach up behind the back as far as possible while you assess internal rotation and adduction. Record the level for each hand and repeat for the opposite side.	Reduced range of motion that affects functioning is considered a positive test.

chapter 8

Conditions of the Elbow, Forearm, Wrist, and Hand

chapter outline

chapter objectives

At the conclusion of this chapter, the reader will understand:

- the bony anatomy of the region
- how to locate the bony landmarks and soft tissue structures of the region
- where to find the muscles, and the origins, insertions, and actions of the region
- how to assess the movement and determine the range of motion for the region
- how to perform manual muscle testing to the region
- how to recognize dermatome patterns for the region
- trigger-point location and referral patterns for the region
- the following elements of each condition discussed:
  - background and characteristics
  - specific questions to ask
  - what orthopedic tests should be performed
  - how to treat the connective tissue, trigger points, and muscles
- flexibility concerns

key terms

carpal tunnel syndrome

carrying angle

de Quervain's tenosynovitis

double-crush syndrome

gunstock deformity

lateral epicondylitis

medial epicondylitis

resting position

triangular fibrocartilage complex (TFCC)

Introduction   It is hard to imagine performing daily activities without the use of our arms and hands, which together complete the kinetic chain of the upper extremity. The upper extremity assists with tasks such as lifting and carrying; however, it also functions to protect the body during collisions, falls, and injuries.

The elbow functions as the link between the powerful movement of the shoulder and the fine motor control of the hand. The shoulder positions the hand in space, while the elbow adjusts the height and length of the arm and rotates the hand into position.

Because the wrist and the hand are the most active and intricate parts of the upper extremity, they are also vulnerable to injury and do not respond well to trauma. And, in addition to performing numerous functional tasks, the hand is an important sensory organ that provides information about our surroundings such as temperature, texture, shape, and motion. Under certain circumstances, the hands and the upper extremities also assist in communication when used for things such as sign language.

Assessing and treating the elbow, forearm, wrist, and hand can be challenging because of the complexity of the joints; moreover, the sources of dysfunction in these areas can arise from myriad causes. Each component of the upper extremity must work in harmony with related components for the entire structure to function properly.

Any disruption of balance, regardless of cause, can lead to dysfunction and disability. In addition, this region is susceptible to both chronic and traumatic injuries. The elbow is second only to the shoulder as the most dislocated joint in the body, and it is second to the knee in overuse injuries. The wrist can sustain acute injuries through falls or blunt force on a hyperextended joint, and it is also subject to injuries from chronic overuse conditions.

> **✳ Practical Tip**
>
> Remember that the components of the upper extremity rely heavily on one another's proper functioning to complete the movement.

As with the other regions of the body, it is essential for massage practitioners to have a thorough knowledge and understanding of the anatomy and physiology of the region. By taking an extensive history and conducting a thorough assessment, the therapist will be able to properly identify and treat most conditions. While this chapter is not a comprehensive study of the elbow, forearm, wrist, and hand, it does provide a general understanding of the region, its functions, and how to recognize, assess, and treat some common pathologies. In addition to reviewing the structures, this chapter discusses:

- Specific bony landmarks for palpation
- Soft tissue structures, including the muscles of the region
- The movements of the region, and basic biomechanics of the elbow, forearm, and wrist
- Manual muscle tests for the region
- Dermatome and trigger-point referral patterns for the involved muscles
- Some common causes of dysfunction and how to assess and treat them using soft tissue therapy

ANATOMICAL REVIEW

Bony Anatomy of the Elbow and Forearm

The elbow is often viewed as a simple hinge joint, but it actually comprises three bones: the humerus, the radius, and the ulna (Fig. 8-1). Since the previous chapter addressed the proximal humerus, this section focuses on the distal portion of the bone.

Humerus

Lateral epicondylar line

Lateral epicondyle

Medial supracondylar line

Radial head

Radial tuberosity

Medial epicondyle

Ulna

Radius

Olecranon fossa

Olecranon process

Ulnar groove

Ulnar border

As you move distally along the humerus toward its articulation with the elbow, it flares on both its lateral and medial borders to create two angular surfaces, the lateral and medial supracondylar ridges, and then continues to form the lateral and medial epicondyles (see Fig. 8-1). Just below the epicondyles are two smooth condyles at the distal end of the humerus that form articulations with the other bones in the area. The lateral condyle is known as the *capitulum*. Its shape is rounded, and it articulates with the head of the radius. Its medial counterpart, the *trochlea*, is shaped like a pulley; it articulates with the ulna.

The distal humerus also has three distinct depressions, one posterior and two anterior. The largest is on the posterior side and is called the *olecranon fossa*. This accommodates the olecranon process of the ulna when the elbow is extended. The two fossae on the anterior surface are the *coronoid fossa* on the medial side, which accommodates the coronoid process of the ulna in elbow flexion, and the *radial fossa* on the lateral side, which accommodates the head of the radius.

The forearm comprises two bones: the radius on the lateral side and the ulna on the medial side (see Fig. 8-1). The proximal radius, known as the *head,* is a distinctive round disk that rotates on the humerus at the capitulum and at the radial notch on the ulna. Continuing distally is a small neck between the head and the next distinguishing feature, the radial tuberosity. This large bump serves as the attachment for the biceps brachii. As it continues distally, the shaft of the radius curves slightly at its wider end.

The second forearm bone is the medially placed ulna. Its proximal end is also unique and allows articulations with both the humerus and the radius. A distinct C-shaped notch called the *trochlear,* or semilunar, *notch,* articulates with the trochlea of the humerus. Directly opposite the notch on the posterior side of the ulna is the olecranon process, which fits into the olecranon fossa during extension. The distal border of the trochlear notch is the coronoid process, which fits into the coronoid fossa during flexion. Just medial and distal to the coronoid process is the radial notch, which accommodates the radial head. The ulna continues along the radius and is narrower at its distal end.

Bony Structures and Surface Anatomy of the Elbow and Forearm

Palpation of this area should include the distal humerus through the proximal radius and ulna. As with the shoulder, it is important to incorporate movement frequently to help distinguish the structures in the area.

Distal Humerus

Using a systematic approach, start from the distal humerus and work toward the forearm (see Fig. 8-1). The *medial epicondyle of the humerus* is located at the distal end of the humerus on the medial side. Find the bend in the elbow, and trace it medially until you feel a round, bony structure. The *medial supracondylar line of the humerus* is located just superior to the condyle. To find this, palpate in a superior direction from the epicondyle to locate the ridge. The *lateral epicondyle* may be more difficult to find than the medial epicondyle. It is located at the distal lateral end of the humerus. Locate the bend in the elbow and move laterally until you feel a round, bony prominence. From the lateral condyle, locate the *lateral epicondylar line* by palpating in a superior direction along the ridge.

Proximal Forearm

The *olecranon process of the ulna* is located on the posterior side of the elbow. This is the very prominent process on the proximal tip of the ulna and can be seen best when the elbow is flexed. It serves as the insertion for the triceps brachii. The *olecranon fossa*, which is hidden when the elbow is extended, is located on the distal posterior humerus; it joins with the ulna to form the elbow joint. Bend the client's arm to 90°, and palpate in the divot just above the olecranon process. Using the olecranon process and medial epicondyle, palpate at the midpoint of a line between those two points to locate the *ulnar groove* or *sulcus*. This structure is home to the ulnar nerve, which runs very superficially at this point.

Moving back around to the front of the elbow, the *radial tuberosity* can be difficult to find and is not directly palpable. Locate the cubital crease, and have the client bend the arm to 90°. Perform an isometric contraction of the biceps brachii, and locate the tendon, tracing it onto the forearm. Have the client relax. Palpate lateral and deep to the tendon, staying medial to the brachioradialis.

The *radial head* may also be difficult to locate. Have the client flex the elbow to 90°. Locate the lateral epicondyle of the humerus, and move distally along the radius about one finger's width; palpate for the round head. To make sure you are in the right place, passively supinate and pronate the client's forearm; the radial head will rotate beneath your thumb.

To find the *ulnar border*, start at the olecranon process and trace distally along the ulna.

Part II Regional Approach to Treatment

Soft Tissue Structures of the Elbow and Forearm

Three articulations make up the elbow joints: the humeroulnar, humeroradial, and proximal radioulnar joints; however, their close relationships classify them as one compound synovial joint (Fig. 8-2). Additionally, these joints are surrounded by one synovial capsule.

- *Humeroulnar joint:* A joint formed by the trochlea of the humerus and the semilunar notch of the ulna (see Fig. 8-2). Its primary motion capabilities are flexion and extension, although some individuals are capable of a small amount of hyperextension.

- *Humeroradial joint:* A modified hinge joint, but sometimes classified as a gliding joint (see Fig. 8-2), that is composed of the radial head, which articulates on the capitulum of the humerus. In addition to flexion and extension, internal and external rotation occurs during supination and pronation.

- *Proximal radioulnar joint:* A pivot joint that is formed by the head of the radius. It articulates with the radial notch of the ulna; the head rotates in the notch during supination and pronation.

Several strong ligaments add stability to the area, including the medial and lateral collateral ligaments, which support the humeroulnar and humeroradial joints, respectively.

The *medial collateral ligament* (see Fig. 8-2) is the most important ligament for stability in the elbow. It runs from the medial epicondyle of the humerus to the ulna in a fan shape and is divided into three distinct bands. To feel the ligament, palpate transversely from the medial epicondyle onto the proximal ulna. The anterior oblique band is the primary restraint against valgus forces and is taut throughout the entire range of motion. The transverse band does not provide a great deal of support to the medial elbow, and the posterior oblique is a capsular thickening that is taut beyond 60° of flexion.

The complex *lateral collateral ligament* supports the lateral side of the elbow (see Fig. 8-2). To locate this ligament, palpate between the lateral epicondyle and the radial head. This ligament complex consists of four components:

- *Radial collateral ligament:* Resists varus forces on the elbow and terminates on the annular ligament. It is the most important of the four ligaments.

- *Ulnar collateral ligament:* Resists valgus forces on the elbow and is the posterior portion of the radial collateral ligament. It is separate from the other three ligaments.

- *Annular ligament:* Encircles the radial head and allows for rotation of the radial head in the radial notch.

- *Accessory ligament:* Assists the annular ligament during a varus stress.

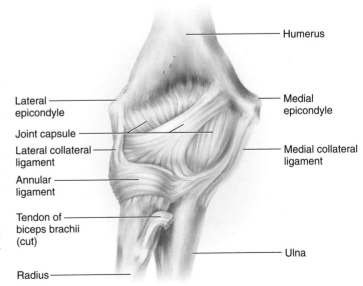

Figure 8-2 Soft tissue structures of the elbow and forearm.

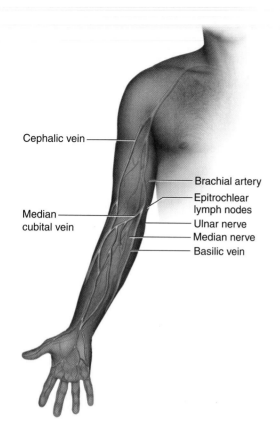

Cephalic vein

Median
cubital vein

Brachial artery
Epitrochlear
lymph nodes
Ulnar nerve
Median nerve
Basilic vein

Figure 8-3 Soft tissue structures and surface anatomy of the elbow and forearm.

There are several other soft tissue structures in the region, as well (Fig. 8-3). The *brachial artery* lies along the medial humerus, between the biceps and triceps brachii, and marks the point of the brachial pulse. The *cephalic* and *basilic* are two of the major veins in the area. The cephalic vein runs along the delto-pectoral interval, lateral to the biceps brachii and down the lateral humerus. The basilic vein runs along the medial humerus, between the biceps and triceps brachii next to the brachial artery. A third vein, the *median cubital vein*, runs along the cubital crease and connects the cephalic and basilic veins. Just proximal to the medial epicondyle are the *epitrochlear lymph nodes*, which lie along the medial supracondylar line and are palpated using the fingers in a circular fashion. The *ulnar nerve* travels on the posterior humerus and runs through the ulnar groove before it enters the forearm. It is superficial at this location and is often referred to as the "funny bone."

The *median nerve* is also palpable in the elbow. Locate the biceps tendon, and press medial and deep to it watching for radicular symptoms. Lastly, the *olecranon bursa* lies directly on top of the olecranon process, just under the skin. It is not palpable unless it is enlarged from a hematoma, chronic irritation, or rheumatoid synovitis.

Bony Anatomy of the Forearm, Wrist, and Hand

The wrist is one of the most intricate areas of the body. It comprises a series of individual small bones that have articulations with each other, as well as with the distal radius and ulna, and the metacarpals in the hand (Fig. 8-4).

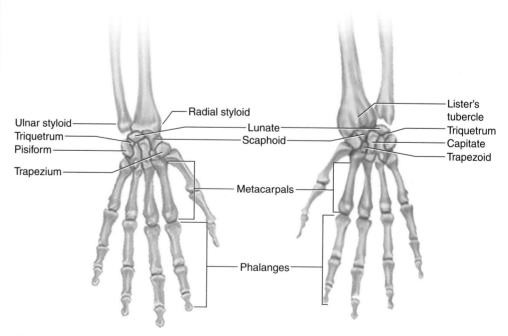

Ulnar styloid
Triquetrum
Pisiform
Trapezium

Radial styloid
Lunate
Scaphoid

Metacarpals

Phalanges

Lister's tubercle
Triquetrum
Capitate
Trapezoid

Figure 8-4 Skeletal and surface anatomy structures of the distal forearm, wrist, and hand.

At the distal forearm, the end of the radius is quite wide and the ulna is quite small (see Fig. 8-4). The distal radius is flared and has a bony point known as the *styloid process* on its lateral side. On the medial side of the bone, a notch articulates with the medial surface of the distal ulna to form the distal radioulnar joint. There are two shallow depressions that articulate with the scaphoid and lunate bones of the wrist. The distal ulna is shaped differently. The shaft narrows considerably and terminates in a knoblike head that has a medial styloid process. The ulna does not articulate directly with any of the carpal bones. Rather, it articulates through a cartilaginous disk (discussed later).

The carpal bones that form the wrist are arranged in two rows of four bones each (see Fig. 8-4). The proximal row of carpals articulates with the radius. From lateral to medial, they are the scaphoid, the lunate, the triquetrum, and the pisiform. The pisiform is actually a sesmoid bone and "floats" on the triquetrum, acting as a pulley for the flexor carpi ulnaris muscle. The scaphoid is the bone most often fractured in the wrist, while the lunate is the bone most often dislocated. This proximal row of carpals also articulates with the distal row of bones. From lateral to medial, they are the trapezium, the trapezoid, the capitate, and the hamate.

Lastly are the hand and finger bones (see Fig. 8-4). The metacarpals of the hand are numbered I to V from thumb to pinky. The phalanges are the finger bones. There are two phalanges in the thumb and three phalanges in each finger (II–V).

Bony Structures and Surface Anatomy of the Forearm, Wrist, and Hand

Palpation of this area can be difficult because of its small size and the close proximity of the structures. Movement assists with accurate identification.

Distal Forearm

Start with the distal forearm, and work down into the wrist and hand (see Fig. 8-4). The *ulnar styloid* is the projection on the medial side of the distal ulna just before the wrist. On the radius, the *radial styloid* is the most distal end of the radius and is a palpable bony prominence just proximal to the wrist.

Lister's tubercle is an important point of reference used to locate several other structures. It sits between the radial and ulnar styloid processes on the dorsal radius and is in line with the 3rd metacarpal. To ensure you are on the process, have the client flex and extend the wrist. Lister's tubercle will not move; if it does move, you are on the proximal row of carpals.

Carpals

The carpal bones are very small and can be difficult to palpate. If possible, use larger landmarks as starting points to give better frames of reference. Beginning with the proximal row of carpals, the *scaphoid* makes up the floor of the anatomical snuffbox. Start at the radial styloid, and move distally into a divot. The scaphoid can be tender in some people and will become more prominent with ulnar deviation and less prominent with radial deviation. From the scaphoid, the next bone medially is the *lunate*.

> **Practical Tip**
>
> Because of the close proximity of structures in this area, work your way to the structure you are locating from both an inferior and a superior direction to ensure accurate palpation.

This bone lies in line with Lister's tubercle and the 3rd metacarpal. Start at Lister's tubercle, and move in a distal direction to the lunate, which will become more prominent with wrist flexion. The *triquetrum* is located just distal to the ulnar styloid in the proximal row of carpals. Find the indentation on the side of the wrist just distal to the ulnar styloid, and palpate while radially deviating the wrist to make the bone more prominent. The last bone in the proximal row of carpals is located on the palmar side of the wrist. The *pisiform* feels like a small pea at the base of the hypothenar eminence. It is distinct and relatively easy to palpate.

The distal row of carpals has its own challenges in palpation. The *trapezium* lies in the distal row of carpals and is somewhat difficult to find. One method is to locate the scaphoid and move just distal to it. A more accurate method is to trace the metacarpal of the thumb in a proximal direction to its base. Once you move off the metacarpal, you will be on the trapezium; move the thumb to ensure you are on the proper structure. The *trapezoid* lies next to the trapezium and is at the base of the 2nd metacarpal. Trace the 2nd metacarpal to its base, and move off into the row of carpals onto the trapezoid. The *capitate* lies between the lunate and the 3rd metacarpal. Trace the 3rd metacarpal to its base, and passively extend the wrist. Place your finger in the divot that is created; you will then be on the bone. The *hamate* is easy to find on the dorsal side of the hand at the base of the 4th and 5th metacarpals. On the palmar side, locate the "hook" by placing the interphalangeal joint of the thumb on the pisiform, pointing the tip of the thumb toward the web space between the thumb and the first finger. Flex the interphalangeal joint, and the tip of the thumb will fall onto the hook and can be felt using a fair amount of pressure.

Metacarpals and Phalanges

Find the *metacarpals* by squeezing in the middle of the hand to locate each bone. Trace proximally and distally to define each bone's edges. Lastly, identify the *phalanges* by palpating each of the finger bones.

Soft Tissue Structures of the Forearm, Wrist, and Hand

Since the distal forearm, wrist, and hand have numerous individual bones that make up the structures in the area, the soft tissue links many of the structures and has an important function. The distal radioulnar joint is a pivot joint that allows for the rotation of the radius over the ulna and enables supination and pronation. At the distal end of the ulna is a fibrocartilage disk called the **triangular fibrocartilage complex (TFCC)**. It extends from the ulnar side of the radius to the styloid process of the ulna. The disk adds stability to the wrist and helps bind the distal radius and ulna together. Together, this disk and the radius form the radiocarpal joint with the proximal row of carpals.

Several ligaments are formed by thickenings of the joint capsule surrounding the wrist (Fig. 8-5). There are two collateral ligaments:

- *Radial collateral ligament:* Runs from the radial styloid process to the scaphoid and trapezium; it limits ulnar deviation.
- *Ulnar collateral ligament:* Runs from the ulnar styloid to the triquetrum and pisiform; it limits radial deviation.

📖 triangular fibrocartilage complex (TFCC) A small meniscus resting on the ulnar side of the wrist opposite the thumb. The complex serves as a site of connection of ligaments as well as a spacer or cushion between the carpal bones and the end of the forearm.

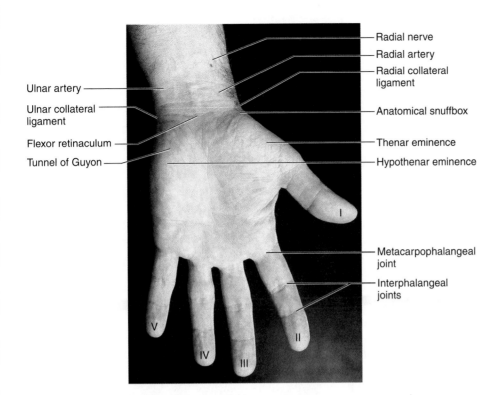

Figure 8-5 Ligaments and soft tissue structures of the wrist and hand.

Radial nerve
Radial artery
Radial collateral ligament
Anatomical snuffbox
Thenar eminence
Hypothenar eminence
Metacarpophalangeal joint
Interphalangeal joints

Ulnar artery
Ulnar collateral ligament
Flexor retinaculum
Tunnel of Guyon

The dorsal radiocarpal and palmar radiocarpal ligaments limit wrist flexion and extension, respectively.

Similar to ligaments, bands of connective tissue lie over extrinsic tendons and their sheaths. These retinacula hold the tendons down and prevent the tendons from popping up or "bow-stringing" when they turn corners at the wrist. In addition, there are both a flexor retinaculum and an extensor retinaculum; however, the joints of the hand and fingers are beyond the scope of this text.

Several other important soft tissue structures are in the region, as well (see Fig. 8-5). The *radial artery* is the pulse just proximal to the ventral wrist on the radius. From this pulse, find the *radial nerve* by palpating just proximal to the radial styloid process in a transverse direction. On the ventral side of the forearm, the *ulnar artery* is just proximal to the wrist on the ulna. This pulse is not as strong as the radial pulse, so it is not necessary to use a lot of pressure to palpate it.

As it moves into the hand, the ulnar nerve travels through a structure called the *tunnel of Guyon*, which is formed by a ligament connecting the hook of the hamate and the pisiform bone. At the base of the thumb is an area called the *anatomical snuffbox*, which is so-named because snuff, or powdered tobacco, would be placed in this area to be sniffed into the nostrils. This structure is formed by the scaphoid at its base, the extensor pollicis longus along the index finger, and the abductor pollicis longus and extensor pollicis brevis along the thumb. To make these tendons more prominent, extend the thumb and look for the depression at the wrist.

There are two muscular areas on the palm, one on the medial and one on the lateral side. The *thenar eminence* lies over the base of the thumb and forms the lateral palm and heel of the hand. It comprises the abductor pollicis brevis, flexor pollicis brevis, opponens pollicis, and adductor pollicis muscles. The medial side of the palm and heel of the hand is known as the *hypothenar* eminence and lies over the base of the 5th metacarpal.

It comprises the abductor digiti minimi, flexor digiti minimi brevis, and opponens digiti minimi muscles.

Muscles of the Elbow, Forearm, Wrist, and Hand

The muscles that have an involvement in the elbow, forearm, wrist, and hand are shown in Fig. 8-6. Refer to the Quick Reference Table "Muscles of the Elbow, Forearm, Wrist, and Hand" at the end of this chapter (page 330).

Figure 8-6 Muscles of the elbow, forearm, wrist, and hand.
(a) Anterior.
(b) Posterior.

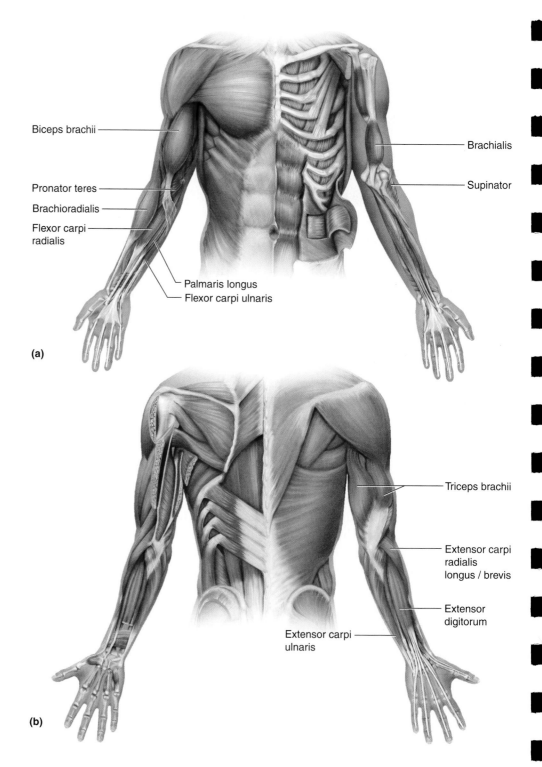

Biceps brachii

Pronator teres

Brachioradialis

Flexor carpi radialis

Palmaris longus
Flexor carpi ulnaris

Brachialis

Supinator

(a)

Triceps brachii

Extensor carpi radialis longus / brevis

Extensor digitorum

Extensor carpi ulnaris

(b)

Part II Regional Approach to Treatment

MOVEMENT AND MANUAL MUSCLE TESTING OF THE REGION

There are some general assessment tools that can help therapists establish a baseline for more specific assessments regardless of the dysfunction.

Movements of the Region

Elbow and Proximal Forearm

Since they are enclosed within the same joint capsule, the articulations between the humerus, ulna, and radial head are commonly viewed as one joint. The motions at the humeroulnar joint are limited to flexion and extension, and the radiohumeral and radioulnar joints allow rotation for supination and pronation. To gather baseline information, determine which active and passive movements are allowable at the joints.

To test the active range at the elbow, place the client in the seated position for all activities. Stabilize the client's upper arm against the body to prevent compensation.

- *Flexion:* Have the client bend the arm with the palm face up. The client should be able to obtain the normal range, which is 140° to 150°. The movement will usually stop due to soft tissue approximation.
- *Extension:* Have the client straighten the arm. It should stop at 0°; however, some individuals will have as much as 10° of hyperextension. This is considered normal if it is equal on both sides and there is no history of trauma. Loss of extension is indicative of intra-articular pathology.
- *Supination:* Start this test with the client's arm in the neutral position, which is the elbow bent to 90° and the thumb pointing up. From this position, the client should be able to supinate, or turn the palm up, 90°.
- *Pronation:* Starting from the same position as above, the client should be able to pronate, or turn the palm down, 80° to 90°.

Keep in mind that for both supination and pronation, only 75° of the range comes from the radioulnar joints; the remaining 15° occurs at the wrist. Assess any repetitive, sustained, or combined movements that cause the client pain.

Passive Range of Motion Apply a small amount of overpressure at the end of the range of motion to test the end-feel in the same directions as those used with active motion. Place the client in the positions that were used for active testing, and stabilize the shoulder to prevent compensation. Distinct end-feels will occur at various joints.

- *Flexion:* Soft tissue approximation from the biceps brachii contacting the forearm.
- *Extension:* Bone-to-bone end-feel from the olecranon process and olecranon fossa.
- *Supination/pronation:* Tissue stretch from the radioulnar ligaments and interosseous membrane.

Manual Muscle Testing Muscle strength in the elbow is greatest between 90° and 110° of flexion, with the forearm supinated. That strength is reduced to 75% of maximum at 45° and 135°. Perform the tests below with the client seated and with the arm bent to 90°. Perform an isometric contraction by instructing the client not to allow you to move him or her.

- *Flexion:* Place the shoulder in a neutral position with the elbow bent to 90°. Stabilize the upper arm, and move the client into extension by applying force just proximal to the wrist while the client resists. Repeat the test with the forearm supinated, pronated, and in neutral to emphasize the different muscles of flexion.
- *Extension:* Begin in the same starting position as that for flexion. Apply an upward force just proximal to the wrist while the client resists.
- *Pronation/supination:* Place the client's arm in the neutral position as described earlier, and place your hand under his or her elbow for support. Apply resistance using a handshake grip, or apply it on the palmar surface of the forearm during pronation and the dorsal surface during supination.

The myotomes of the area include movements at the wrist, which are discussed at the end of the section.

Distal Forearm and Wrist

Because of the various joints in the region, a variety of movements are available at the wrist. Be conscious of the numerous structures in the region, and take the appropriate amount of time to thoroughly assess the area. During wrist extension, most of the movement (40°) occurs at the radiocarpal joint, with the midcarpal joint contributing 20°. This is reversed for wrist flexion, where the midcarpal joint contributes 50° and the radiocarpal joint contributes 35°. For radial deviation, movement occurs between the proximal and distal rows of carpals, whereas ulnar deviation takes place at the radiocarpal joint. Remember to gather information using active and passive range-of-motion tests. Perform the painful movements last.

For the active ranges of motion at the wrist, the client may be in either the seated or the standing position. Place the client's forearm on a table for support, and stabilize the forearm of the wrist being tested.

- *Flexion:* With the forearm pronated, have the client bend the wrist toward the floor. The normal range should be 80° to 90°.
- *Extension:* Starting from the same position as that used for flexion, have the client bend the wrist up toward the ceiling. Normal range is 70° to 90°.
- *Ulnar deviation:* With the wrist in a neutral position, have the client bend the wrist toward his or her pinky finger. Make sure no accessory movement such as flexion or pronation occurs, as accessory movement will alter the results. Normal range for ulnar deviation is 30° to 45°.
- *Radial deviation:* Starting in the neutral position, have the client move the wrist toward the thumb. Make sure no accessory movement occurs. Normal range is 15°.

Test any combined or repetitive movements that the client complains are causing discomfort.

Passive Range of Motion If the active range of motion is normal, passive range can be tested by applying a small amount of overpressure at the end of the range. If the amount of motion is limited, use overpressure to assess the end-feel of the joint.

- *Flexion/extension:* For flexion, place the forearm on a table with the wrist hanging off the end, palm down. Stabilize the forearm to prevent any unwanted movement. Flex the wrist, pressing on the dorsal surface of the hand. The end-feel should be firm from the tissue stretch. Start in the same position for extension. Extend the hand while pushing on the palm. The end-feel will be firm from the tissue stretch in this direction as well.

- *Radial/ulnar deviation:* Place the hand and forearm on the table, palm down. Stabilize the forearm to prevent unwanted movement. Radially deviate the wrist while applying pressure to the pinky side of the hand. There should be a hard end-feel from the bone-to-bone contact of the scaphoid and radial styloid. When the wrist is ulnarly deviated with pressure on the thumb side of the hand, the end-feel is firm from the radial collateral ligament's being stretched.

Manual Muscle Testing To perform manual muscle tests to the wrist, place the forearm on the table for support or place a hand under the forearm if a table is not available.

- *Flexion:* With the hand supinated, press the hand into extension by pressing on the palm while the client resists.

- *Extension:* With the hand pronated, press the hand into flexion with pressure on the dorsal surface of the hand while the client resists.

- *Ulnar deviation:* With the hand in neutral, move the hand into radial deviation while the client resists.

- *Radial deviation:* With the hand in neutral, move the hand into ulnar deviation while the client resists.

There are additional manual muscle tests that will assess the myotomes of the area. They will help identify neurologic involvement.

- *C5—shoulder abduction:* Have the client abduct the shoulders and resist while you move them into adduction.

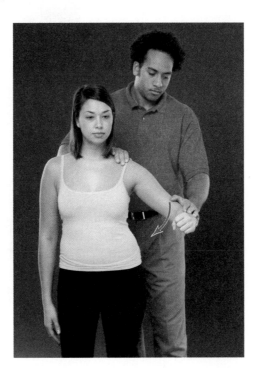

> **Practical Tip**
> Be sure not to use too much pressure when testing extension, as the tendons can be injured at the wrist.

- *C6—elbow flexion/wrist extension:* Flex the client's elbow to 90°, and have him or her resist while you press it into extension. To test wrist extension, extend the wrist and have the client resist while you move it into flexion.

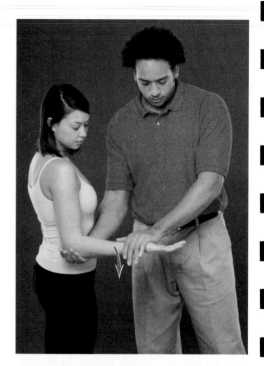

- *C7—elbow extension/wrist flexion:* Flex the client's elbow to 90°, and have him or her resist while you flex the arm. To test wrist flexion, flex the wrist and have the client resist while you move it into extension.

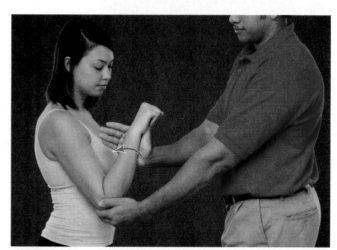

- *C8—ulnar deviation:* With the hand in neutral, move the hand into radial deviation while the client resists.

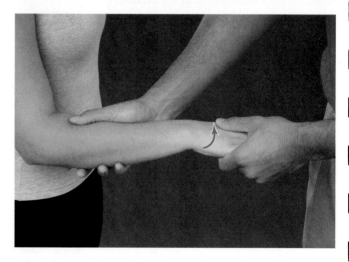

- *T1—abduction/adduction of the fingers:* To test abduction, have the client spread the fingers and resist while you squeeze them together. To test adduction, have the client hold the fingers together while you try to spread them apart.

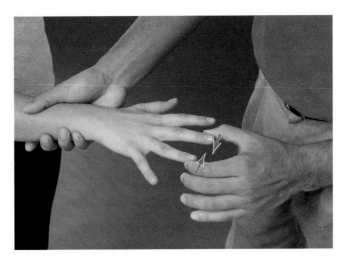

DERMATOMES FOR THE ELBOW, FOREARM, WRIST, AND HAND

Assessing the dermatomes will provide information on sensory changes in an area that can indicate dysfunction in the sensory nerve root. When addressing this region, keep in mind that there is a great deal of variability in the distribution patterns and that these are peripheral nerves; therefore, it is important to assess the entire upper limb as well (Fig. 8-7). Remember to stay in the middle of the dermatome to avoid overlap of the areas. Use a blunt object, and touch the dermatome lightly. Ask the client whether there are any discrepancies between the sides of the body. Discrepancies can indicate pathology. The dermatomes for the elbow, forearm, and wrist are summarized in Table 8-1.

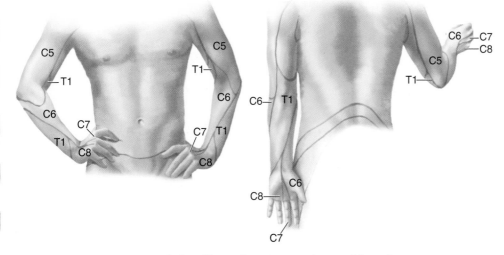

Figure 8-7 Dermatomes of the elbow, forearm, wrist, and hand.

Table 8-1 Dermatomes of the Elbow, Forearm, and Wrist

C5	Lateral shoulder and arm to the thenar eminence, stopping at the thumb; overlaps the dorsal distal wrist
C6	Lateral forearm starting at the elbow; down the wrist, including the thumb and palmar side of the first finger
C7	Middle of the triceps brachii; down the dorsal forearm and the first two fingers; palmar surface of the first two fingers
C8	Medial distal forearm just below the elbow, including both sides of the lateral hand, and 4th and 5th fingers
T1	Medial side of the arm from the midhumerus to the midforearm

TRIGGER-POINT REFERRAL PATTERNS FOR MUSCLES OF THE REGION

As we have seen in previous chapters, myofascial trigger points can cause dysfunction and create referral patterns of pain that are often mistaken for other conditions. Remember, however, that trigger points can coexist with other conditions that may be the source of the primary problem; therefore, a thorough assessment of the area is warranted to ensure that proper treatment is given.

Some of the more common pathologies that can be associated with trigger points in this region include carpal tunnel syndrome, lateral epicondylitis, osteoarthritis, de Quervain's tenosynovitis, and various nerve compression conditions. This section discusses the symptoms and char-

Figure 8-8 Trigger-point locations for the biceps brachii, pronator teres, brachioradialis, flexor carpi radialis, palmaris longus, flexor carpi ulnaris, brachialis, and supinator.

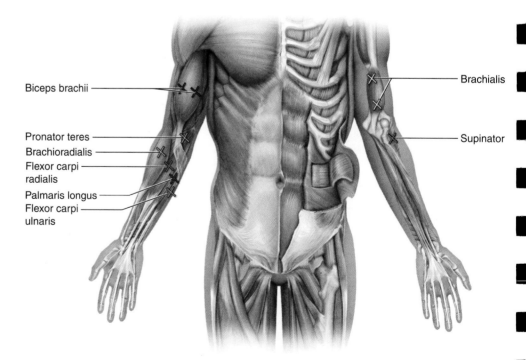

Biceps brachii

Pronator teres

Brachioradialis

Flexor carpi radialis

Palmaris longus

Flexor carpi ulnaris

Brachialis

Supinator

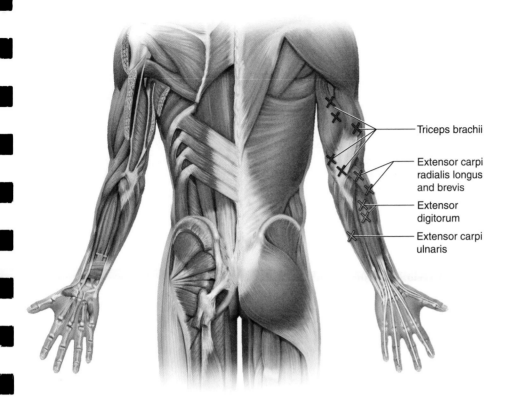

Triceps brachii

Extensor carpi radialis longus and brevis

Extensor digitorum

Extensor carpi ulnaris

acteristics of some myofascial trigger points contained in the major muscles of the region.

Biceps Brachii

The *biceps brachii* (see Figs. 8-8 and 8-14) contains trigger points that primarily refer in a superior direction to the front of the shoulder, but these trigger points can also travel to the suprascapular region and the antecubital space. The distal referral to the antecubital space is of interest in this section. In addition to pain, some other symptoms that occur distally in the dorsal surface of the forearm and hand include deep tenderness, numbness, pallor, and weakness. The trigger points in this muscle are usually found midbelly in either head. The pain that accompanies these points typically is superficial and does not present as deep pain.

Brachialis

The *brachialis* (see Figs. 8-8 and 8-15) is deep to the biceps and contains numerous trigger points that are covered by the biceps. The proximal point lies about halfway up the humerus on the lateral edge of the biceps brachii. This point is accessible without displacing the biceps. The distal points are located just proximal to the elbow and must be located by moving the biceps out

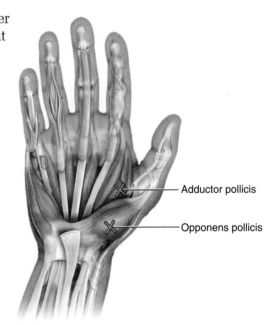

Adductor pollicis

Opponens pollicis

Figure 8-10 Trigger-point locations for the opponens pollicis and adductor pollicis.

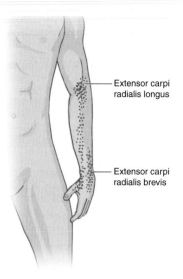

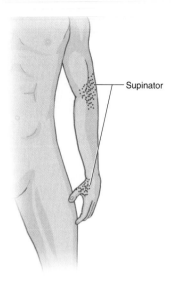

Figure 8-11 Trigger-point referrals for the extensor carpi radialis longus and extensor carpi radialis brevis.

Figure 8-12 Trigger-point referrals for the supinator.

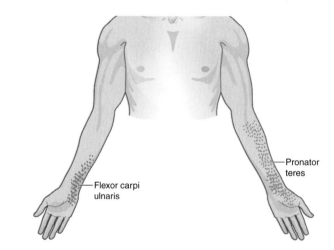

Figure 8-13 Trigger-point referrals for the flexor carpi ulnaris and pronator teres.

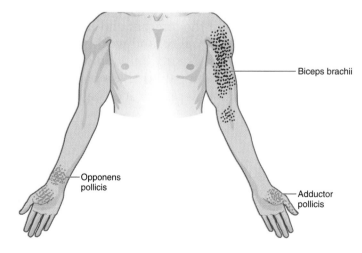

Figure 8-14 Trigger-point referrals for the biceps brachii, opponens pollicis, and adductor pollicis.

Part II Regional Approach to Treatment

of the way. These distal points are generally attachment points from tension in the midfiber points. The trigger points in this muscle refer primarily to the base of the thumb, the dorsal carpometacarpal joint, and the dorsal web space of the thumb. Additional areas of referral may occur in the antecubital space and the front of the shoulder. Clients with brachialis trigger points will complain of a diffuse soreness at the base of the thumb and pain in the front of the shoulder; however, these symptoms will not affect motion. Passive motion will increase elbow pain; active motion will not.

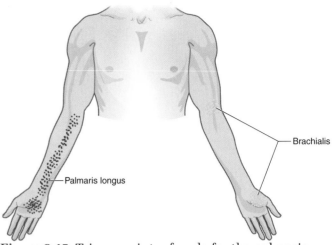

Figure 8-15 Trigger-point referrals for the palmaris longus and brachialis.

Triceps Brachii

The *triceps brachii* (see Figs. 8-9 and 8-17) can develop trigger points in all three of its heads and can affect movement; however, clients often overlook this, particularly when they are able to make compensatory movements. The first point, in the central belly of the long head, refers upward over the posterior arm and shoulder and down the posterior forearm. The second point is located in the lateral portion of the medial head of the muscle. It refers to the lateral epicondyle of the elbow and down the radial aspect of the forearm; it is often a component of tennis elbow. The third point is located in the lateral head and refers centrally around the point over the posterior arm, occasionally moving down the posterior forearm into fingers IV and V. The fourth point is located in the tendon and refers to the olecranon process. The last point is the least common and is most easily located from the anterior side. It is in the medial portion of the medial head of the muscle; it refers along the medial forearm and the palmar surface of fingers IV and V. Clients with triceps trigger points will complain of vague posterior pain in the shoulder and upper arm.

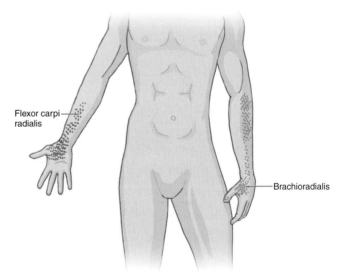

Figure 8-16 Trigger-point referrals for the flexor carpi radialis and brachioradialis.

Wrist Extensors

This section addresses only the major muscles of the forearm. The first are the *wrist extensors*. The *extensor carpi radialis longus* (see Figs. 8-9 and 8-11) refers pain into the lateral epicondyle and the dorsal anatomical snuffbox. This point can be activated by a repetitive forceful handgrip. It is located in the muscle just distal to the elbow on the radial side of the dorsal forearm. The next wrist extensor is the *extensor carpi radialis brevis* (see Figs. 8-9 and 8-11). Its trigger point lies about 2 inches

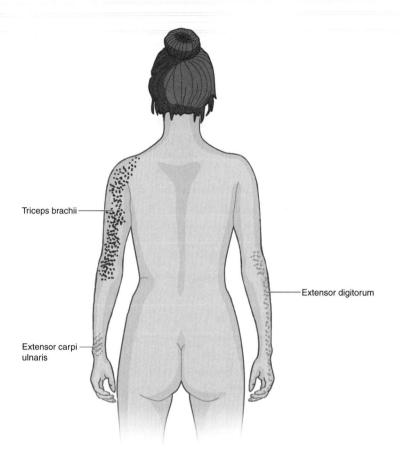

Figure 8-17 Trigger-point referrals for the triceps brachii, extensor carpi ulnaris, and extensor digitorum.

distal to the cubital crease on the ulnar side of the brachioradialis in the muscle mass of the brevis, but distal to the point of the longus. This point refers pain to the dorsal surface of the hand and wrist and is one of the most common sources of posterior wrist pain. The *extensor carpi ulnaris* (see Figs. 8-9 and 8-17) produces a trigger point less often than the previous two muscles. If present, however, it refers to the ulnar side of the posterior wrist. The point lies about 3 inches distal to the lateral epicondyle along the ulnar side of the forearm.

The *brachioradialis* (see Figs. 8-8 and 8-16) does not have any action at the wrist, but it refers pain to the wrist. It projects its pain pattern to the wrist and the web space between the thumb and the first finger. The muscle can also refer pain up over the lateral epicondyle. The points are usually located in the deeper layers of the muscle and lie directly along the proximal radius, just distal to the elbow when the forearm is in a neutral position. When more than one muscle is involved, it is hard to delineate which symptoms are caused by the wrist extensors and which are a result of trigger points in the brachioradialis.

The *extensor digitorum* (see Figs. 8-9 and 8-17) originates alongside the previous forearm muscles, the extensor carpi radialis longus and brevis as well as the extensor carpi ulnaris, but it acts on the fingers instead of the wrist. It projects pain down the dorsal forearm and into the finger that is moved by the involved fibers; however, the pain will stop short of the distal phalanx. Trigger points in the fibers of the middle finger are extremely common because this finger is used in almost all of the hand's activities. The point is located about 1½ inches distal to the head of the radius. Clients may complain of pain in the hand, as well as pain and stiffness in the involved fingers. The points in the ring finger present in a similar fashion, with pain radiating down the dorsal forearm to the ring finger; however, this pain will also refer proximally to the lateral epicondyle. These points are located deep in the proximal muscle and can be hard to palpate.

Supinator

The *supinator* (see Figs. 8-8 and 8-12) contributes most frequently to the symptoms of lateral epicondylitis. Its trigger points lie on the ventral aspect of the radius between the biceps brachii tendon and the brachioradialis. Clients with this trigger point will complain of aching in the lateral epicondyle and the dorsal web space between the thumb and the first finger.

Palmaris Longus

On the flexor side of the forearm, the *palmaris longus* (see Figs. 8-8 and 8-15) contains trigger points that refer a superficial prickling pain that is centered in the palm of the hand and stops short of the fingers and thumb. Clients with these points may complain of difficulty handling things in the palm, such as tools. The point lies in the midbelly of the muscle, and its palpation can cause a twitch response of wrist flexion.

Wrist Flexors

The *wrist flexors* can be a common source of referred pain, especially near their common attachment at the medial epicondyle. Clients will typically complain of difficulty in activities such as cutting heavy material with scissors or using shears. The *flexor carpi radialis* (see Figs. 8-8 and 8-16) has a point that lies in the midfiber portion of the belly and refers pain that centers on the radial side of the ventral crease in the wrist. The *flexor carpi ulnaris* (see Figs. 8-8 and 8-13) has a similar referral pattern, but it centralizes over the ulnar side of the ventral crease. Its point is also in the midfiber portion of the belly and is superficial enough to be palpable.

Pronator Teres

The last muscle on the flexor side of the forearm is the *pronator teres* (see Figs. 8-8 and 8-13). Clients with trigger points in this muscle will complain of the inability to supinate the cupped hand and will usually compensate by rotating the arm at the shoulder. Its point lies just medial to the medial epicondyle, distal to the cubital crease. It refers pain deep in the ventral wrist and forearm.

Adductor Pollicis and Opponens Pollicis

Clients with trigger points in the *adductor pollicis* and *opponens pollicis* (see Figs. 8-10 and 8-14) muscles may be unable to perform fine finger manipulations, such as holding a pen or buttoning a shirt. The adductor pollicis contains a trigger point that may cause aching along the outside of the thumb and hand, distal to the wrist. This pain may also affect the web space and thenar eminence. Its point is located in the web space and found by palpating from the dorsal side of the web space just inside the metacarpal of the thumb. Use caution, as there is often extreme spot tenderness and referred pain in this area. The opponens pollicis contains a trigger point that lies in the thenar eminence, about halfway down. It is found by palpating across the direction of the fiber and will elicit pain to the palmar surface of most of the thumb and a spot on the ventral side of the wrist at the radius. Trigger points located in both of these muscles are often mistaken for other conditions or are present in conjunction with other conditions. The most common pathologies associated with these points are carpal tunnel syndrome and de Quervain's tenosynovitis, both of which are discussed later in the chapter.

Refer to the Quick Reference Table "Trigger Points of the Elbow, Forearm, Wrist, and Hand" at the end of this chapter (page 333).

SPECIFIC CONDITIONS

Elbow and wrist pathologies can arise from a variety of causes. While a comprehensive study of the etiologies is beyond the scope of this text, we focus here on some common sources of dysfunction and address the various components of assessment and treatment. Since dysfunction can arise from other areas of the body, it is important for practitioners to thoroughly assess each client to ensure that the proper treatment or referral is provided. As with other conditions, several of the same structures are involved in causing various dysfunctions, so treatments will overlap; however, it is important to individualize treatment for each client.

Elbow: Lateral Epicondylitis (Tennis Elbow)

Background

lateral epicondylitis A condition considered to be a cumulative trauma injury that occurs over time from repeated use of the muscles of the arm and forearm that leads to small tears of the tendons.

While "the pathophysiology of **lateral epicondylitis** is poorly understood" (Gabel, 1999), tennis elbow is one of the most common conditions of the arm. It occurs in about 1% to 3% of the population and is most prevalent in the 30- to 55-year-old age range. Generally, work- or sports-related injuries cause tennis elbow, and micro-traumas occur primarily in the extensor carpi radialis brevis, originating from excessive, monotonous, repetitive eccentric contractions and gripping activities (Stasinopoulos, 2004). The condition tends to be chronic, with only 20% of cases arising from acute injuries. The average duration is between 6 months and 2 years, and most clients seek medical attention a few weeks or months after symptoms begin, when it becomes evident that the problem may not resolve on its own.

The complaint associated with lateral epicondylitis is well defined and consists of pain over the lateral condyle and a decrease in grip strength, both of which may limit everyday activities. Lateral epicondylitis pain can be re-created in one of three ways:

- Digital palpation of the lateral epicondyle
- Resisted wrist extension and/or resisted middle-finger extension with the elbow extended
- Gripping an object

Since 80% of cases are chronic, there exists a consistent cycle of inflammation and scar tissue formation. Because of this cycle, one would expect to see evidence of inflammatory tissue in studies; however, studies of chronically affected tissue have found no evidence of inflammatory cells present or of an increase in fibroblasts, vascular hyperplasia, and immature collagen. This evidence has led some to reclassify this condition as a tendonopathy, instead of a tendonitis, due to a failed tendon healing response or degenerative process occurring, especially as the condition moves into the long-term chronic phase.

Assessment

The pathology of lateral epicondylitis has numerous sources. Examine all the possible etiologies by expanding the assessment to include other regions as necessary.

Condition History Therapists should inquire about the following while taking the client's history:

Question	Significance
What is the client's age?	Tennis elbow is more common between the ages of 30 and 50.
How did the pain arise?	The cause of the pain can help determine the structures involved and whether there is any associated trauma.
What was the mechanism of injury?	This will help determine whether the condition is chronic or acute and which structures may be involved.
How long has the client had the problem?	This will help determine whether the condition is chronic.
How is the pain qualified?	Nerve symptoms present differently than muscular conditions.
When does the pain occur?	This will help identify the involved structures.
Are there any movements that cause pain?	This will help identify the involved structures.
How does the injury affect the ability to function?	This will help determine the severity of the condition.

resting position The position of elbow flexion of 70°. This position allows the most amount of space possible within the joint.

carrying angle The angle that is formed by the long axis of the humerus and the long axis of the ulna.

gunstock deformity An exaggerated cubital varus that occurs as a result of trauma to the distal humerus.

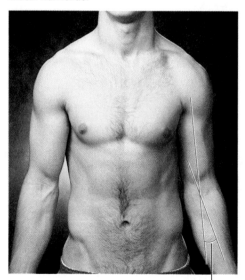

Carrying angle

Figure 8-18 The carrying angle.

Is there a feeling of weakness or a change in sensation?

This will determine whether there is nerve involvement.

Is there numbness or tingling?

This will determine whether there is nerve involvement.

Visual Assessment Both arms should be clearly visible to compare the involved side with the uninvolved side. Include the neck and shoulder in the visual comparison in case there are pain referral issues.

First, observe the position of the arm and how the client is holding it. Check for obvious deformity, swelling, and bruising. If a client holds the arm in the **resting position** at slight elbow flexion of 70°, this may indicate the presence of swelling, as this position allows for maximum joint volume to accommodate fluid. Notice the alignment of the olecranon relative to the epicondyles of the humerus. In a normal flexed elbow, the three structures form an isosceles triangle. When the elbow is extended, the structures should form a straight line.

Next, observe the client's **carrying angle**, which is created when the arm is in the anatomical position. It is the angle that is formed by the long axis of the humerus and the long axis of the ulna. In an adult, normal carrying angle is 5° to 10° in males and 10° to 15° in females (Fig. 8-18). If the angle is greater than 15°, this is called *cubital valgus;* if the angle is less than 5°, this is called *cubital varus.* If there has been trauma to the distal humerus, an exaggerated cubital varus occurs. This is referred to as a **gunstock deformity** because the angle the arm makes resembles the stock of a rifle.

To complete the visual assessment, inspect the cubital fossa for swelling and compare the entire region for symmetry. The dominant side may be slightly larger due to muscle hypertrophy.

Palpation Begin by focusing on the elbow and the structures listed earlier in the chapter. Determine the presence of swelling, temperature differences, deformity, point tenderness, and muscle spasm. Start at the distal humerus, and work distally on the proximal forearm. Expand palpation to related areas as necessary.

Orthopedic Tests The lateral epicondylitis test has three variations. Perform them after assessing both sides for ranges of motion, dermatomes, and myotomes. Table 8-2 shows the tests and how to perform them.

Soft Tissue Treatment

Tennis elbow arises primarily from chronic overuse of the forearm extensors. A cycle of inflammation and scar tissue formation creates a huge muscle imbalance in the area, which causes severe dysfunction.

Focus treatment on reducing inflammation in the area, removing muscle restrictions, restoring muscular balance, and increasing muscle length. This will remove stress in the area and restore optimal function to the elbow. Address associated areas as necessary, taking into account the phase of the injury and appropriate treatment.

Table 8-2 Orthopedic Tests for Lateral Epicondylitis

Orthopedic Test	How to Perform
Cozen's test 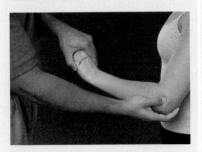 *Note:* This is the most common of these tests.	Have the client pronate the forearm and then extend and radially deviate the wrist. Support the client's forearm, and place your thumb over the lateral epicondyle. Try to move the wrist into flexion while the client resists. Sudden severe pain in the area of the epicondyle indicates a positive test.
Mill's test 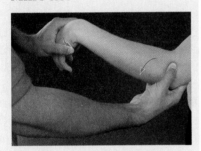	Support the client's forearm, and place your thumb over the lateral epicondyle while you simultaneously passively pronate the forearm, fully flex the wrist, and slowly extend the elbow. Pain over the lateral epicondyle indicates a positive test.
Tennis elbow test 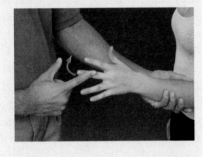	Support the client's forearm, and place his or her third finger into slight extension. Apply force on the finger to move it into flexion while the client resists. This will place an eccentric load on the extensor digitorum muscle. Pain over the lateral epicondyle indicates a positive test.

Connective Tissue Part of the cycle of lateral epicondylitis is scar tissue formation. Scar tissue will greatly restrict the muscle in which it forms; therefore, removing excessive adhesions and creating a more functional scar is beneficial to the treatment process.

Prone Position The triceps brachii and the ventral side of the forearm are treated effectively in this position:

1. If the client has no restrictions, begin by hanging the arm off the side of the table so that just the upper arm remains on the table, orienting the triceps face up.
2. Assess the superficial connective tissue vertically, horizontally, and at various angles to determine the restrictions.

3. Once located, move into the restrictions until they release. Internally and externally rotate the arm to address the entire muscle.

Passive and active movements are effective and easy to apply in this position. Stroke from the elbow toward the shoulder, while passively extending and flexing the client's elbow. This will effectively "pull" the tissue under the pressure of the hand and help release the restriction. The client can also actively flex and extend the elbow while you perform the strokes in various directions. This will help release restrictions by generating heat and softening the connective tissue.

Perpendicular compressive effleurage is effective for this muscle in this position. Once the superficial tissues have been released, move into defining the three heads of the triceps brachii. When defining the long head of the triceps, remove any restrictions between the triceps and the posterior deltoid.

Place the forearm back on the table, and assess the superficial tissue in various directions. Move into the restrictions until they release. Be sure to secure the hand when working from the wrist to the forearm so that the arm does not bend.

Because of the size of the forearm, perpendicular compressive effleurage works well. Pay special attention to the flexor retinaculum at the wrist. Excessive connective tissue buildup can exacerbate wrist dysfunction. Use thumb strokes in both parallel and perpendicular directions to isolate the structure.

When moving into the deeper layers, strip out each wrist flexor using your thumbs or fingers. Spread the palm with your hands to open up the fascia. Work along either side of the thumb, deep in the thenar eminence and into the web space.

Supine Position Begin by assessing the superficial tissue of the anterior upper arm in parallel, perpendicular, and oblique directions. Once the restrictions have been identified, hold the wrist in one hand and bend the elbow to help control the position of the humerus and to put slack in the muscles. Move into the restrictions until they release. Control the wrist and incorporate passive movement by flexing, extending, and rotating the humerus to maximize the effectiveness of the strokes.

After the superficial layers have been released, strip out the two heads of the biceps by finding the split in the muscle and moving proximally and distally. Separate the bicep from the underlying brachialis. Bending the elbow softens the biceps brachii so that it can be pushed aside and the brachialis can be identified, allowing the therapist to strip along the border between the two muscles to create space.

Once the anterior humerus has been sufficiently treated, pronate the forearm and place it on the table. Assess the superficial tissue of the forearm in various directions to determine the restrictions. Be sure to hold the hand when doing the strokes to ensure that the elbow does not bend. Address the extensor retinaculum, as it can be a common site of restrictions. Strip out each extensor when moving into deeper tissues, and pay special attention to identifying the brachioradialis.

Side-Lying Position There is no clinical advantage to placing the client in this position, unless the client specifically requests it or it is warranted by other factors.

Tissue Inconsistencies Trigger points can mimic or exacerbate tennis elbow and often exist in conjunction with dysfunction in the region. Using movement to treat trigger points in this area is effective. Be sure to treat the muscles of the upper arm in addition to those of the forearm, since they cross the elbow. Examine the wrist extensors for trigger points, as well as the extensor carpi radialis brevis, which is usually involved in tennis elbow.

Muscle Concerns

Focus treatment on relieving tension in the elbow and the wrist extensors in order to relieve pressure on the lateral epicondyle. Movement can be incorporated easily because the size of this area is more manageable.

Prone Position With the arm hanging off the table, focus on the triceps brachii. Some effective strokes include the advanced techniques that incorporate active movement, as discussed in Chapter 3. Applying perpendicular compressive effleurage as the client extends the elbow will exaggerate the broadening phase of the muscle contraction and help break up adhesions between muscle fibers. To focus on the lengthening phase of the muscle contraction, administer deep parallel stripping while the client flexes the elbow; slowly inch up the muscle. This intense stroke will effectively separate restrictions as well as define the borders of adjacent tissues.

With the forearm on the table, deep effleurage to the wrist flexors will help loosen the overall forearm. Using the forearm to administer a stroke from the elbow toward the wrist is effective in this position. Be sure to stay within the client's comfort level, especially when moving closer to the wrist. Once you have loosened up the overall forearm, secure the hand while you strip out each flexor from distal to proximal.

Supine Position The involved structures are effectively treated in this position.

1. Begin by working the biceps brachii and brachialis, using various strokes that do and do not incorporate movement.
2. Once the upper arm has been sufficiently addressed, place the pronated forearm on the table and work from distal to proximal.
3. Move the hand off the side of the table to incorporate movement into the techniques. The tissues are typically shortened in this condition; therefore, deep parallel stripping to the extensors during wrist flexion is effective.
4. Be sure to strip out the brachioradialis by bending the elbow and supporting the forearm with your hands while stripping out the borders with the thumbs.

Another technique that incorporates movement includes standing or sitting at the client's side and flexing the elbow to 90°. Hold the wrist, and run your thumb down the posterior forearm, between the radius and the ulna, from the wrist toward the elbow. Passively pronate the forearm while performing the stroke, stopping to focus on restrictions in the muscle. Be aware of the client's comfort level; this technique can cause discomfort.

Side-Lying Position There is no clinical advantage to placing the client in this position, unless the client specifically requests it or it is warranted by other factors.

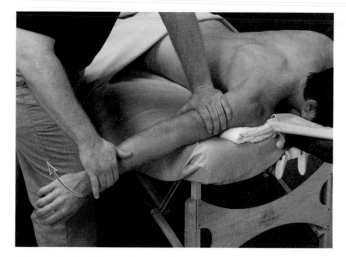

Figure 8-19 Biceps brachii stretch.

Stretching

The chronic nature of tennis elbow and the repetitive scarring that occurs reduce flexibility in the area. Stretching the involved muscles helps remove tissue restrictions in the region.

Biceps Brachii To stretch the distal end of the biceps brachii (Fig. 8-19), start with the client in the prone position with the arm abducted to 90°. Hang the client's forearm off the table, but allow the table to support the humerus. Stand at the side of the client, facing his or her head, and use your inside hand to stabilize the humerus. Have the client extend the elbow as far as possible while exhaling. Assist at the end by grasping the wrist and continuing the movement. Repeat for one to three sets of 10 repetitions, depending on the severity of the condition.

Triceps Brachii To stretch the triceps brachii (Fig. 8-20), start with the client in the seated position. Have the client reach straight out in front of his or her body with the palm facing up. While exhaling, the client should bend his or her elbow and reach over the shoulder as far as possible. At the end of the movement, assist in the same direction by standing at the client's side and placing one hand on the wrist to keep the arm bent and the other hand under the elbow.

Continue the motion, keeping the arm bent and the shoulder moving straight back. Return to the starting position, and repeat for 5 to 10 repetitions. Once the triceps has been stretched directly backward, repeat the process with the elbow swung out to 45° so that the client is reaching down his or her back at an oblique angle. Assist the client for 5 to 10 repetitions, returning to the starting position each time.

> ★ Practical Tip
>
> Make sure the arm travels straight back over the shoulder and does not swing out to the side.

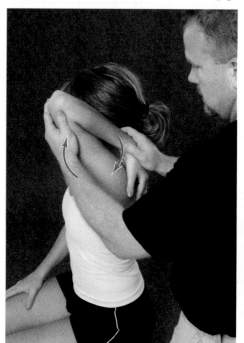

Figure 8-20 Triceps brachii stretch.

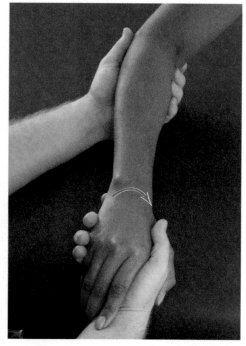

Figure 8-21 Forearm supinator stretch.

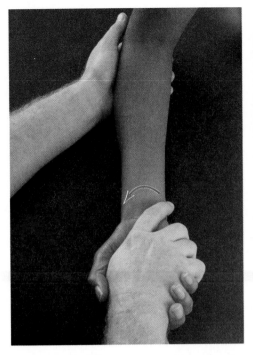
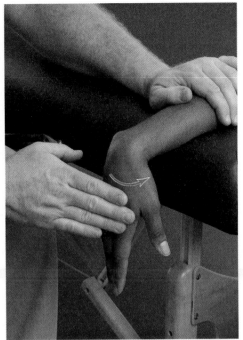

Figure 8-22 Forearm pronator stretch.   **Figure 8-23** Wrist extensor stretch.

Supinators To stretch the muscles that supinate the forearm, place the client in the seated position. The table should support the forearm, and the hand should hang off the side of the table. Bend the arm to 90°, and grasp the client's hand as if giving a handshake (Fig. 8-21). While resisting slightly, have the client keep the elbow at his or her side and then exhale and pronate the hand. At the end of the range, grasp the client's other hand and assist with pronation in a gentle stretch. Return to the starting position, and repeat for one to three sets of 10 repetitions.

Pronators To stretch the pronators (Fig. 8-22), start with the client in the seated position with the elbow bent to 90°, and grasp the client's hand as if giving a handshake. Apply slight resistance while the client exhales and supinates the forearm. At the end of the range, grasp the forearm and assist in the same direction for a gentle stretch. Repeat for one to three sets of 10 repetitions.

Wrist Extensors To stretch the wrist extensors, place the client in the seated position and place the forearm on the table for support. Stabilize the forearm just proximal to the wrist (Fig. 8-23). Have the client slowly flex the wrist while exhaling. At the end of the motion, assist in the same direction for a gentle stretch. To avoid any injury to the extensor tendons, pay attention to the amount of pressure applied.

Ulnar Deviators To stretch the ulnar deviators, place the client in the seated position and place the forearm on the table for support. Stabilize the forearm just proximal to the wrist (Fig. 8-24). Keep the palm facing down, and grasp the hand. Have the client move the wrist into radial deviation while exhaling. Assist the motion at the end of the range to administer a gentle stretch. Repeat for two sets of 10 repetitions.

> **Practical Tip**
> To avoid any injury to the tendons, be aware of the amount of pressure used while stretching the wrist extensors.

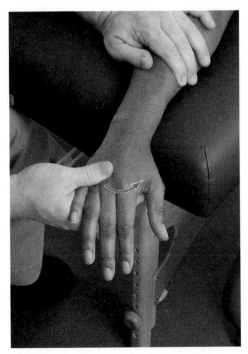

Figure 8-24 Ulnar deviator stretch.

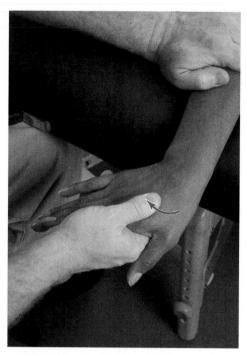

Figure 8-25 Radial deviator stretch.

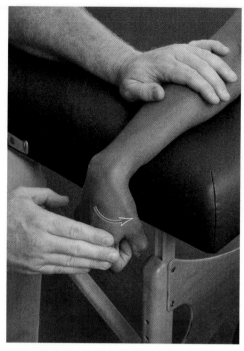

Figure 8-26 Wrist and finger extensor stretch.

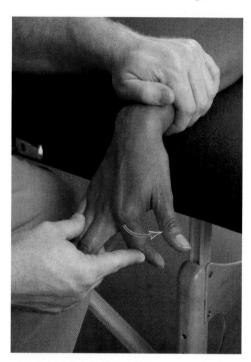

Figure 8-27 Finger extensor stretch.

Radial Deviators To stretch the radial deviators, place the client in the seated position and place the forearm on the table for support. Stabilize the forearm just proximal to the wrist (Fig. 8-25). Grasp the hand, and have the client move into ulnar deviation while exhaling. Assist the motion at the end of the range, and repeat for two sets of 10 repetitions.

Finger Extensors The last stretch for tennis elbow involves another technique for the wrist extensors, but it emphasizes the finger extensors (Fig. 8-26). With the client in the seated position, place the forearm on the table for support, with the wrist hanging off the side. Stabilize the forearm just proximal to the wrist. Have the client make a tight fist and slowly flex the wrist. At the end of the range, gently assist in the same direction to provide a stretch. Pay attention to the amount of pressure, and apply pressure slowly to avoid causing injury. To emphasize the finger extensors, start with the wrist flexed. While holding the wrist in flexion, have the client flex each finger; assist at the end of the range (Fig. 8-27). Repeat both phases for two sets of 10 repetitions.

medial epicondylitis An overuse injury affecting the flexor-pronator muscle origin at the anterior medial epicondyle of the humerus.

Elbow: Medial Epicondylitis (Golfer's Elbow)

Background

Far less common than lateral epicondylitis, **medial epicondylitis** is also an overuse injury of the wrist and forearm, involving primarily the pronator teres and the flexor carpi radialis (Gabel, 1999). Its symptoms are similar to those of its lateral counterpart and include:

- Pain and tenderness over the medial epicondyle
- Pain and tenderness just distal along the tendinous origin of the flexor-pronator origins
- Swelling
- Discoloration
- Point tenderness over the humeroulnar joint
- Increased pain with resisted wrist flexion, pronation, and valgus stress at 30° of flexion

In addition to the flexor carpi radialis and pronator teres, other affected tissues can include the flexor carpi ulnaris and palmaris longus origin tendons. Medial epicondylitis arises from repeated flexion and pronation combined with a repeated valgus force on the elbow. There are several pathologies that are associated and often coexist with medial epicondylitis, including ulnar collateral ligament sprains, ulnar neuropathy, and medial elbow intra-articular damage. To ensure that proper treatment is administered, it is necessary to rule out the presence of other conditions via a thorough history and assessment.

Assessment

Since medial epicondylitis can arise from and coexist with a variety of other elbow pathologies, assessment should include additional regions as necessary.

Condition History Therapists should inquire about the following while taking the client's history:

Question	Significance
What was the mechanism of injury?	Helps determine whether the condition is chronic or acute.
Is there any noise, weakness, or change in sensation that accompanies the condition?	Helps identify structures that may be involved.
Are there any repetitive movements involved?	Helps determine the etiology of the condition.
How long has the client had the problem?	Helps determine whether the condition is chronic.
What is the pain like? What are its boundaries? If it radiates, is it worse at night?	Helps identify structures that may be involved.
Are there any specific motions that increase or decrease the pain?	Helps identify structures that may be involved.
Are there any limitations in motion?	Helps determine where the dysfunction is.

| What are the client's normal activities? | New activities can lead to pathologies. |
| Is there any numbness or tingling? | This will determine whether there is nerve involvement. |

Visual Assessment The visual assessment for medial epicondylitis is essentially the same as that for lateral epicondylitis. Compare both arms for symmetry. Include associated areas such as the neck and shoulder in case there are pain referral issues. Place the arms in the anatomical position to observe the carrying angle, which is created by the long axis of the humerus and the long axis of the ulna. The normal carrying angle is 5° to 10° in adult males and 10° to 15° in adult females (see Fig. 8-18). Cubital valgus is present if the angle is greater than 15°; cubital varus is present if the angle is less than 5°. An exaggerated cubital varus that has resulted from trauma to the distal humerus is referred to as a gunstock deformity; therefore, check for obvious deformity, swelling, and bruising.

Observe both flexed elbows to see the alignment of the olecranon relative to the epicondyles of the humerus. Normally, the three structures form an isosceles triangle when flexed and form a straight line when extended. Finally, bilaterally compare the cubital fossa for swelling and the entire region for symmetry, as the dominant side may be slightly larger due to muscle hypertrophy.

Palpation Start at the distal humerus and work distally onto the proximal forearm, palpating the structures listed earlier in the chapter. Expand the palpation to related areas to determine the presence of swelling, temperature differences, deformity, point tenderness, and muscle spasm.

Orthopedic Tests The orthopedic test for medial epicondylitis is the medial epicondylitis test, or golfer's elbow test, and it has two methods: a passive technique and an active technique. Table 8-3 lists both methods and explains how to perform them.

Soft Tissue Treatment

The primary mechanism of this injury is an overuse condition. Because of the nature of overuse injuries, soft tissue work is very beneficial. Focus on removing restrictions in the tissue to relieve stress on the area. Consider the state of the injury, and treat any related dysfunctions.

Connective Tissue The nature of repetitive motion injuries includes a cyclical pattern of inflammation and the formation of scar tissue. Connective tissue work is beneficial for removing restrictions that have formed as a result of the scarring. The wrist flexors tend to be larger in comparison to the extensors—a result of being used more frequently. Since they are larger and stronger, they may develop adhesive restrictions in addition to scarring. Even if there is no current injury, connective tissue work to this area can be beneficial as a maintenance technique.

Prone Position Medial epicondylitis is best treated with the client in the prone position. If the client has no restrictions, begin by hanging the forearm off the side of the table, with the upper arm remaining on the table. Treating the muscles of the upper arm also positively affects the forearm muscles:

Table 8-3 Orthopedic Tests for Medial Epicondylitis

Orthopedic Test	How to Perform
Medial epicondylitis test (passive) 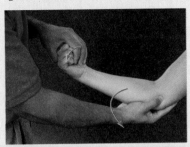	Bend the client's elbow to 90°, and stabilize it against the client's body. With the client's forearm supinated, palpate the medial epicondyle and slowly extend the client's elbow and wrist. Pain over the medial epicondyle is considered a positive test.
Medial epicondylitis test (active) uses the same procedure as passive testing	Bend the client's elbow to 90° and stabilize it against the client's body. Extend the elbow and wrist while the client resists. Pain over the medial epicondyle is considered a positive test.

1. Assess the superficial connective tissue vertically, horizontally, and at various angles to determine the restrictions. Once located, move into the restrictions by directing the stroke along the restrictions until they release.
2. Internally and externally rotate the arm to address the entire muscle. Passive and active movements are effective and easy to apply in this position using the techniques described in the previous section. The most effective stroke that incorporates active movement is perpendicular compressive effleurage during elbow extension.
3. Once the superficial tissues have been released, move into defining the three heads of the triceps brachii, taking care to remove any restrictions between the triceps and the posterior deltoid.
4. Place the forearm back on the table, and assess the superficial connective tissue in various directions as described previously. When moving into the deeper layers, focus on separating out the individual wrist flexors using parallel thumb stripping with active movement. Move the hand off the table to enable full range of motion at the wrist. While the client extends the wrist, strip out the wrist flexors.

Pay special attention to the flexor retinaculum to release any restrictions, using the treatments described for lateral epicondylitis.

Supine Position Although the wrist extensors are not directly related to this condition, it is important to address them so that any imbalances between the groups are removed.

1. Begin by assessing the superficial tissue of the humerus. Release any restrictions in the biceps brachii, and identify each head as you move into the deeper layers.

2. Remove any restrictions between the biceps and the brachialis by flexing the elbow to create slack in the biceps and moving it aside in order to identify the border between the two muscles.

3. Move into the forearm by pronating it and placing it on the table. Assess the superficial tissue, and address it as necessary. Identify the brachioradialis, as it is a common source of dysfunction. Strip out each wrist extensor to remove any restrictions. Be sure to address the extensor retinaculum.

Side-Lying Position There is no clinical advantage to placing the client in this position, unless the client specifically requests it or it is warranted by other factors.

Tissue Inconsistencies Trigger points in this area can be debilitating and can mimic other conditions; therefore, addressing them is vital. Investigate the muscles of the upper arm for trigger points, as well, since they function at the elbow. Additionally, focus on the wrist flexors, using the information discussed earlier in the chapter to help identify the location of the points. Expand the treatment areas to include the entire forearm as necessary.

Muscle Concerns

Treatment should focus on removing pressure on the medial epicondyle and restoring balance to the forearm. Utilize the same strokes as those described for treating lateral epicondylitis. Movement can also be easily incorporated when treating this region.

Prone Position Treatment for medial epicondylitis is similar to treatment for lateral epicondylitis. To address the triceps, hang the arm off the table and place it face up. Petrissage, perpendicular compressive effleurage, and parallel thumb stripping work well at treating the triceps and will help remove any overall tension in the area.

To treat the forearm in this position, place it on the table so that the ventral surface is face up. Once the superficial tissue has been released, using the forearm to administer a stroke from the elbow toward the wrist is effective. Be sure to stay within the client's comfort level, especially as you move closer to the wrist. Apply a finishing stroke from the wrist to the elbow to ensure the return of circulation to the heart. Securing the hand and performing deep thumb-stripping strokes to the flexors is also effective in this position.

Supine Position The techniques described to treat lateral epicondylitis can also be applied here. One effective technique is to "milk" the forearm. Bend the client's elbow, and hold the hand to control the arm. Perform alternating effleurage strokes from the wrist to the elbow, grasping the entire forearm. Apply more pressure with the thumb over the desired muscle to affect specific muscles. From here, separate out the brachioradialis by running one thumb down each side of the muscle.

Side-Lying Position There is no clinical advantage to placing the client in this position, unless the client specifically requests it or it is warranted by other factors.

Stretching

The forearm is usually a chronically tight region of the body because of excessive use during daily activities, and stretching the entire region is beneficial regardless of the condition. To begin, perform the stretches that were discussed for lateral epicondylitis (see Figs. 8-19 to 8-27).

Wrist Flexors Three stretches specific to the wrist flexors have a direct effect on medial epicondylitis. Perform them with the client in the seated position. Place the client's arm on the table, and stabilize the forearm.

1. For the first stretch, have the client exhale and extend the wrist as far as possible, keeping the forearm pronated (Fig. 8-28). Once the client reaches the end of the range, assist in the same direction by placing the therapist's hand on the palmar surface of the client's hand and the entire length of the fingers, keeping them straight. Return to the starting position, and repeat for one to two sets of 10 repetitions.

2. The next stretch addresses the same muscles but at the proximal attachments (Fig. 8-29). Position the client as described above but with the forearm supinated. While exhaling, the client should extend the wrist toward the floor until he or she reaches the end of the range. At the end of the movement, assist in the same direction by placing the therapist's hand on the palmar surface of the client's hand and the entire length of the fingers. Release the stretch, and repeat for one to two sets of 10 repetitions.

3. For the final stretch, position the client as described above but with the forearm pronated (Fig. 8-30). Secure the client's hand, and allow movement of only one finger at a time. While exhaling, the client should extend one finger until the end range. Assist at the end of the range in the same direction. If the client can move to 90°, place the wrist in slight extension to achieve a greater stretch, and repeat. Perform one to three sets of 10 repetitions per finger.

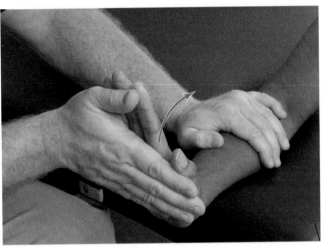

Figure 8-28 Wrist flexor stretch—distal attachments.

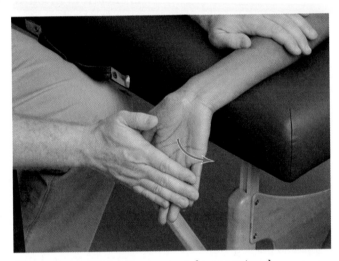

Figure 8-29 Wrist flexor stretch—proximal attachments.

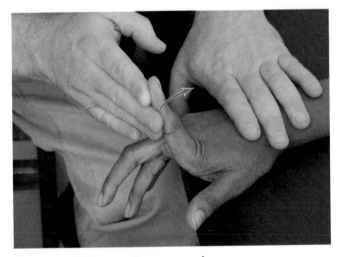

Figure 8-30 Finger flexor stretch.

Wrist: de Quervain's Tenosynovitis

Background

While other conditions we have discussed are complicated in their presentation and pathology, **de Quervain's tenosynovitis** is a relatively common, uncomplicated, and noncontroversial musculoskeletal disorder (Moore, 1997) that essentially involves a tenosynovitis of the first dorsal compartment.

To review, a ligamentous structure helps hold the extrinsic tendons down as they move from the forearm to the wrist. The dorsal or extensor retinaculum forms six fibro-osseous compartments with the underlying bones, with de Quervain's affecting the first compartment. Not all tendons have sheaths. Depending on their location, as the tendon approaches an area of potential irritation, its outer covering forms a synovial sheath. This sheath is filled with synovial fluid and wraps around the tendon to reduce friction as it slides back and forth. The tendons involved in this condition are the abductor pollicis longus and the extensor pollicis brevis, which form a portion of the anatomical snuffbox. As these tendons move through the sheath, they create friction between the bony compartment and the sheath. This irritation causes a localized inflammation that, over time, results in the thickening of the retinaculum and the sheaths, causing a stenosing of the compartment. Even though tenosynovitis is typically classified as an inflammatory condition, the main pathology in de Quervain's is the stenosis of the first dorsal compartment. This stenosis will impair the gliding of the tendons and may result in physical deformity or granulation tissue formation on the tendon.

This pathology, which was first described by Swiss surgeon Fritz de Quervain in 1895, manifests itself as pain over the radial styloid and radial side of the thumb that increases with hand or thumb motion. The pain may also radiate up the forearm or down the thumb and may intensify during forceful grasping or twisting. It is usually constant and often intense. There may be localized swelling over the base of the thumb and even occasional snapping or catching of the thumb during motion. Other symptoms may include stiffness, neuralgia, decreased function, and sleep disturbances.

The etiology of this condition is multifaceted. Several theories propose a range of causes, from a defect in the tendons, either from trauma or congenital origins, to increasing friction in the compartment to repetitive motion injuries. Generally, de Quervain's tenosynovitis is thought to arise from overexertion of the thumb usually due to a new, unaccustomed activity. Historically, the most frequently reported activity responsible for the condition was household chores. Other activities ranged from flyfishing to playing the piano. This condition often affects women between the ages of 35 and 55 in a gender ratio of 10:1. It is also more common in the dominant hand.

Assessment

Since there is no definitive method for identifying de Quervain's tenosynovitis, it is important to perform a thorough assessment of the entire region to ensure that the proper treatment is administered.

Condition History Therapists should inquire about the following when taking the client's history:

Question	Significance
What is the client's age?	This condition is more prevalent between the ages of 35 and 55.
What are the client's occupation and normal activities?	New and/or repetitive motions can cause or exacerbate symptoms.
What was the mechanism of injury?	This condition tends to be chronic, so an acute mechanism may indicate another pathology.
How long has the client experienced the pain?	This condition generally has a slow onset.
Where is the pain?	Pain over the radial styloid or at the base of the thumb is indicative of de Quervain's.
How does the injury affect the ability to function?	This will help determine the extent of the injury.
Which is the client's dominant hand?	This condition affects the dominant hand more often.

Visual Assessment To begin, observe the client's willingness to use the affected hand as he or she moves around the treatment facility. Note the contours of the forearms and hands, and record any deviations. A natural hand position shows a small amount of flexion with a slight arch in the palm, while the normal functioning position of the wrist is 20° to 35° of extension, with 10° to 15° of ulnar deviation. Check for wounds or scars on both sides of the hands and wrists, and notice the palmar creases. The absence of these creases is an indication of swelling.

Inspect the continuity of the carpals, metacarpals, and phalanges, and note any discrepancies. Abnormal presentation of the hands and fingers can indicate a more serious condition and should be investigated for potential referral.

Palpation Palpate from proximal to distal in an organized pattern, addressing the most painful areas last. Note any swelling, bruising, temperature changes, or obvious deformity. Investigate crepitus for a possible fracture, especially if it is directly over a bone. Include all the structures covered at the beginning of the chapter, and expand to related areas as necessary.

Orthopedic Tests Perform specific orthopedic tests once baseline information has been established from the history, visual assessment, palpation, motion assessments, and dermatomes.

The only specific test for de Quervain's tenosynovitis is Finkelstein's test. Table 8-4 lists the test and explains how to perform it.

Soft Tissue Treatment

As with medial epicondylitis and lateral epicondylitis, de Quervain's tenosynovitis arises from repetitive motion and therefore benefits greatly

> ⋆**Practical Tip**
>
> Pay attention to the palm of the hand, as the absence of creases is an indication of swelling.

Table 8-4 Orthopedic Test for de Quervain's Tenosynovitis

Orthopedic Test	How to Perform
Finkelstein's test 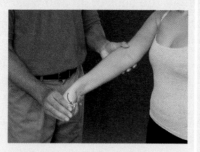 *Note:* This test often produces positive results in otherwise normal wrists; therefore, results should be correlated with the other evaluative findings.	Place the client in the seated or standing position. Instruct the client to make a fist and then tuck his or her thumb inside. With the wrist in neutral, administer the active version of the test by instructing the client to perform ulnar deviation; administer the passive version of the test by stabilizing the forearm and ulnarly deviating the wrist. Pain over the tendons of the abductor pollicis longus and extensor pollicis brevis at the wrist indicates a positive result.

from soft tissue work. Focus on removing restrictions within the synovial sheath around the involved tendons. In addition, address the entire muscle to remove tension in the muscle itself. Address associated areas as necessary, taking into account the phase of the injury and incorporating the appropriate treatment.

Connective Tissue The chronic nature of de Quervain's tenosynovitis increases connective tissue restrictions. Begin treatment with the involved structures, and radiate out to the surrounding areas as necessary.

Prone Position Place the client's arm on the table with the forearm facing up. Assess the superficial tissue in various directions, and then move into the restrictions. Continue to treat the ventral forearm in this position using the techniques discussed for the two previous conditions. Be sure to address the flexor retinaculum and the palmar surface of the hand in this position.

Supine Position The involved structures are most effectively treated in this position. Assess and treat the superficial fascia as described for the two previous conditions. One useful technique involves emphasizing the separation of the brachioradialis. Place the client's hand in neutral, and support the forearm with one hand. Perform a superficial stroke to the muscle from the radial styloid to the elbow. Once the superficial tissue has been released, strip out on both sides of the muscle to identify it.

For another useful technique, extend the client's elbow, and place it on the table with the wrist in neutral and hanging off the table. Instruct the client to ulnarly deviate the wrist while you administer a stroke from the thumb to the wrist.

For a more specific technique, instruct the client to tuck his or her thumb into a fist and ulnarly deviate it, similar to Finkelstein's test. On a stretch, administer specific strokes to the tissue of the involved tendons. This will break up the adhesions between the tendon sheaths and the tendons. Be sure to strip out around the thumb on both sides to remove any restrictions.

Side-Lying Position There is no clinical advantage to placing the client in this position, unless the client specifically requests it or it is warranted by other factors.

Tissue Inconsistencies Trigger points in this area can mimic other conditions; therefore, addressing them is vital. Focus on the muscles in the forearm and thumb, using the information discussed earlier in the chapter to help identify the location of the points. Expand the treatment areas to include the entire forearm as necessary.

Muscle Concerns

While de Quervain's is primarily a tendon problem, address the entire muscle to alleviate any tension on the tendons. Additionally, treat the hand and forearm to restore normal mechanics to the area.

Prone Position With the forearm on the table and sufficiently warmed up, administer a forearm stroke from the elbow to the wrist to address the deeper wrist and finger flexors. Strip out the individual wrist and finger flexors from the wrist to the elbow, while incorporating movement to enhance the effectiveness. Work into the thenar and hypothenar eminences to release tension in the hand. Perform a parallel thumb stroke to the thenar eminence while the client adducts and abducts the thumb. Trace out the web space along the thumb and first finger to address some of the additional muscles.

Supine Position Use the techniques discussed for lateral epicondylitis and medial epicondylitis to warm up the forearm. Alternating effleurage to "milk" the forearm is effective for this condition. Specific thumb strokes to the brachioradialis are beneficial as well. Focus on stripping out the tendons of the abductor pollicis brevis and extensor pollicis longus using movement.

Side-Lying Position There is no clinical advantage to placing the client in this position, unless the client specifically requests it or it is warranted by other factors.

Stretching

Overuse injuries typically produce scar tissue and adhesions, which will reduce the functional range of motion and limit the movement patterns of the involved structures. Stretching will help remove those restrictions and restore normal motion. Begin by stretching the entire forearm and fingers, using the methods described for the two previous conditions (see Figs. 8-19 to 8-30). Several stretches that are especially beneficial to de Quervain's are discussed below; administer them with the client in the seated position, with the forearm resting on the table.

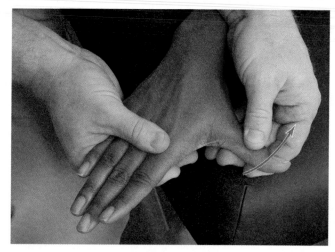

Figure 8-31 Thumb web space stretch.

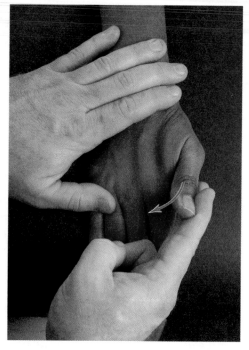

Figure 8-32 Thumb abductor stretch.

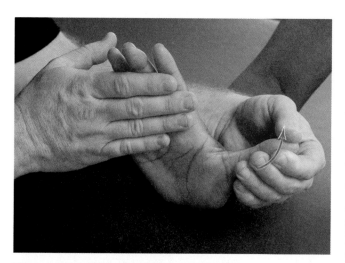

Figure 8-33 Thumb adductor stretch.

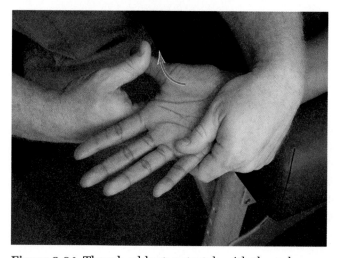

Figure 8-34 Thumb adductor stretch with the palm up.

Thumb Stretches

Stretch 1: The first stretch is for the web space of the thumb (Fig. 8-31). Stabilize the client's hand and fingers with one hand, and grasp the client's thumb with the other. Instruct the client to abduct the thumb away from the first finger while exhaling. At the end of the movement, assist in the same direction, repeating for one to two sets of 10 repetitions.

Stretch 2: Starting from the position used for stretch 1, support the client's hand and fingers. Instruct the client to move the thumb toward the index finger, across the top of the hand, while exhaling (Fig. 8-32). At the end of the movement, grasp the thumb and assist in the same direction for 2 seconds. Return to the starting position, and complete one to two sets of 5 to 8 repetitions.

Stretch 3: There are two methods for this stretch. For the first method, begin by having the client extend the wrist and abduct the thumb so that it is at a 90° angle in relation to the index finger (Fig. 8-33). Support the client's hand in this position, and instruct the client to horizontally abduct the thumb away from the palm while exhaling. Assist in the same direction at the end of the range. "Stretch 4," below, explains the second method for this stretch.

Stretch 4: Have the client supinate the forearm so that the palm is facing up (Fig. 8-34). Support the client's palm and fingers with one hand, and support the thumb with the other. Instruct the client to horizontally abduct the thumb toward the floor while exhaling. Assist in the same direction at the end of the range. Increase the distance between the thumb and the index finger, and repeat the stretch in various positions. Repeat both methods (stretches 3 and 4) for one to two sets of 10 repetitions.

Stretch 5: For the last stretch, instruct the client to tuck his or her thumb into a fist (Fig. 8-35) and to ulnarly deviate the wrist while you assist at the end of the range. Pay attention to the amount of pressure, as this is the most intense and direct stretch for this condition. Modify the stretch by adding slight flexion or extension along with the deviation. Repeat for one to two sets of 5 to 8 repetitions.

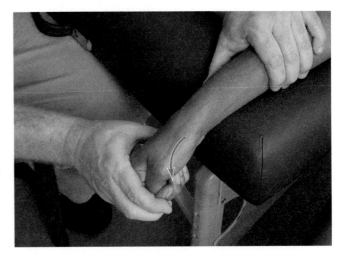

Figure 8-35 Thumb extensor stretch.

Wrist: Carpal Tunnel Syndrome

Background

Carpal tunnel syndrome is part of a larger group of pathologies known as *nerve entrapment injuries.* It is the most common of the entrapment injuries and affects about 3% of adults in the United States, resulting in 400,000 to 500,000 surgeries at a cost in excess of $2 billion annually. Sir James Paget was the first to coin the term *carpal tunnel syndrome* in 1865. Today, the condition contributes to unpleasant symptoms, loss of employee productivity, and increased workers' compensation costs (Field, 2004). Before moving on to the specifics of this condition, let's review the anatomy and physiology of the carpal tunnel.

The osteoligamentous tunnel is formed by the eight carpal bones discussed earlier in the chapter and the fibrous band of tissue called the *flexor retinaculum.* The alignment of the carpal bones forms an arch and has four securing points for the retinaculum at the four outer carpal bones: the scaphoid and trapezium radially and the pisiform and hamate ulnarly. This structure is taut when the wrist is flat and relaxed when the thumb is moved into opposition. This tunnel houses nine tendons (four of the flexor digitorum superficialis, four of the flexor digitorum profundus, and one of the flexor pollicis longus), the synovial sheath, and the median nerve.

Carpal tunnel syndrome is brought on by increased pressure in the tunnel, which can arise from two causes: a decrease in available space or an increase in the size of the tendons and other structures that pass through the tunnel. Sometimes, the condition is caused by a combination of the two. An increase in pressure causes compression of the perineural and intraneural vasculature, resulting in an ischemic condition. The resulting metabolic dysfunction damages the median nerve, which causes an inflammatory response in the area and the depositing of connective tissue. This thickens the retinaculum and the synovial sheaths in the tunnel and causes the vasculature to increase in size. Thus begins a vicious cycle. If the pressure is not relieved, the tissue will die.

Carpal tunnel syndrome presents as pain, numbness, and tingling along the median nerve distribution (the palmar surface of the thumb,

carpal tunnel syndrome A type of nerve entrapment injury that is brought on by increased pressure in the carpal tunnel. This can arise from two causes: a decrease in available space or an increase in the size of the tendons and other structures that pass through the tunnel. Symptoms include pain, numbness, and tingling along the median nerve distribution.

index, and middle fingers and sometimes the radial aspect of the ring finger). These symptoms usually start gradually and are more severe at night. The symptoms may also radiate up the arm, elbow, and shoulder as they worsen. As the condition progresses, symptoms may also occur during the day, and a weakness in grip strength may surface, making it difficult to perform certain tasks. The client may "flick" the wrists to relieve symptoms.

Carpal tunnel syndrome has a variety of causes, but the crux of the problem lies with increased intracarpal canal pressure, which produces carpal tunnel symptoms. Nonspecific flexor tendonopathies are the most common cause of the pathology. With finger flexion, shearing forces can cause hyperplasia and fibrosis to the tenosynovium around the flexor tendons and the median nerve. Symptoms are typically exacerbated with repetitive wrist movements.

Metabolic conditions, pathologic changes, and other congenital predispositions all contribute to carpal tunnel syndrome, as well. Some of these include:

- Diabetes
- Acromegaly
- Thyroid conditions
- Rheumatoid arthritis
- Gout
- Vitamin deficiencies
- Tumors
- Trauma
- Body fluid changes from pregnancy
- Edema
- Congestive heart failure
- Obesity
- Bone spurs

Other congenital predispositions include small carpal canals, ganglion cysts, and a condition called *cervical spondylitis,* which can entrap the median nerve at the proximal end and result in what is known as **"double-crush syndrome"**: the same nerve entrapped at two different locations.

Carpal tunnel afflicts more women, between the ages of 40 and 60, than men. It primarily affects the dominant hand and, in cases of bilateral syndromes, affects the dominant side more.

Assessment

Carpal tunnel syndrome can arise from myriad etiologies. It is important to remember that the problem may not lie specifically in the tunnel itself. A thorough assessment will help rule out other causes and ensure that proper treatment is given.

Condition History Therapists should inquire about the following when taking the client's history:

Question	Significance
What is the client's age?	This condition is more prevalent between the ages of 40 and 60.
What is the client's occupation?	Repetitive motions exacerbate symptoms.
How long has the client had the problem?	This condition progresses gradually.

double-crush syndrome A diagnosis of a compressed or trapped nerve in one area and a second entrapment in another location, with both entrapments contributing to symptoms.

Where is the pain?	Pain typically occurs over the median nerve distribution and can radiate proximally.
Is there a loss of function?	Long-standing symptoms can result in atrophy of the thenar muscles, causing a decrease in grip strength.
Which is the client's dominant hand?	This condition affects the dominant hand more often, and in bilateral cases it will affect the dominant hand to a greater degree.
Is there any previous injury to the area?	Trauma such as a Colles' fracture or carpal fracture can lead to carpal tunnel syndrome.
Does the client have any other medical conditions?	Several metabolic, congenital, and pathologic conditions can cause or exacerbate carpal tunnel syndrome.
When does the pain occur?	Carpal tunnel pain is typically worse at night.

Visual Assessment To begin, observe the client's behavior in using the affected side. Notice if the client is flicking the hand or has trouble gripping things. Note the position of the hand and the skin creases. A natural hand position shows a small amount of flexion with a slight arch in the palm, while the normal functioning position of the wrist is 20° to 35° of extension, with 10° to 15° of ulnar deviation. Check for muscle atrophy along the thenar eminence, as well as swelling in the wrist and hand. Observe the carpals, metacarpals, and phalanges and note any discrepancies. Abnormal presentation of the hands and fingers can indicate a more serious condition and should be investigated for potential referral.

Palpation Note any swelling, bruising, temperature changes, or obvious deformity. Palpate the distal forearm through the carpals to the metacarpals, and record any discrepancies. Pay particular attention to the ventral side of the forearm and the palmar side of the hand. Since the condition can arise as a result of a double-crush injury, be sure to palpate the structures of the neck if necessary. Include all the structures covered at the beginning of the chapter, and expand to related areas as necessary.

Orthopedic Tests Perform specific orthopedic tests once baseline information has been established from the history, visual assessment, palpation, motion assessments, manual muscle tests, dermatomes, and myotomes. There are various tests for carpal tunnel syndrome, all of which aim to increase intracarpal canal pressure in order to reproduce symptoms. Table 8-5 shows these tests and how to perform them.

Soft Tissue Treatment

Depending on the cause of the pathology, massage can be very beneficial. Focus on reversing the condition that is causing a decrease in the space in the carpal tunnel. Be sure to work the forearm, as the structures in the forearm pass through the tunnel.

Table 8-5 Orthopedic Tests for Carpal Tunnel Syndrome

Orthopedic Test	How to Perform
Tinel-sign test 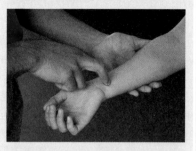 *Note:* Developed by French neurologist Jules Tinel in 1915, this test is one of the best-known and most widely used health care clinical assessment tools.	Client is in seated or standing position. Supinate his or her forearm so that the palm is facing up. Tap your fingertip over the carpal tunnel at the wrist. Tingling and/or numbness along the median nerve distribution indicates a positive result.
Phalen's test 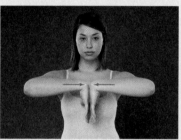	Client is in seated or standing position. Instruct the client to flex the wrists as far as possible. Push the backs of the hands together, and hold the position for 1 minute. Be sure the client does not shrug the shoulders, as this may compress the median nerve at the thoracic outlet. Tingling and/or numbness along the median nerve distribution indicates a positive result.
Carpal tunnel compression test 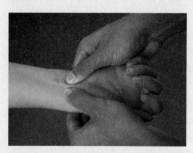	Client is in seated or standing position. Using both thumbs, place even pressure over the carpal tunnel and hold for at least 30 seconds. Tingling and/or numbness along the median nerve distribution indicates a positive result.

Connective Tissue Since repetitive motion can be a factor in this condition, there will be a buildup of connective tissue that may decrease the intracarpal canal space; therefore, addressing the connective structures in the area is beneficial.

Prone Position Place the client's arm on the table, and assess the superficial tissue of the forearm in various directions. Move into any restrictions to release the tissue. Treat the deeper structures using the techniques discussed previously. Using stripping strokes to separate the muscles that have tendons that run through the tunnel is also very beneficial. To treat the flexor retinaculum directly, place your thumbs in opposite directions parallel to the tissue, and spread the tissue to help lengthen it. You can also work perpendicular to the fibers to remove adhesions within the retinaculum. Move into the palmar fascia, and treat it by spreading the palm open, incorporating movement to remove restrictions.

Supine Position This position is not the most efficient for treating the carpal tunnel directly. Assess the superficial tissue in various directions, and use the techniques discussed previously to release the connective tissue; this will help remove any overall restrictions in the forearm and wrist.

Side-Lying Position There is no clinical advantage to placing the client in this position, unless the client specifically requests it or it is warranted by other factors.

Tissue Inconsistencies Trigger points in the muscles in this region can mimic carpal tunnel syndrome; therefore, it is important to remove any adhesions and trigger points to ensure that appropriate treatment is administered. Address all the muscles listed earlier in the chapter, paying special attention to the:

- Brachioradialis
- Radial wrist extensors
- Palmaris longus
- Flexor carpi radialis
- Opponens pollicis
- Adductor pollicis

Muscle Concerns

Treat the entire length of the muscle to ensure the most effective release of tension in the area. While the tendons are the structures that pass through the tunnel, tension can be present proximally in the muscle belly.

Prone Position Warm up the area using various strokes such as petrissage and effleurage, as well as some advanced strokes such as perpendicular compressive effleurage. Once the area is sufficiently warmed up, move into the deeper structures using the techniques discussed previously, such as the elbow-to-wrist forearm stroke. Once the forearm is loose, move distally into the hand, working the thenar and hypothenar eminences and the web space.

Supine Position The purpose of working the arm in this position is primarily to loosen the forearm. Use the techniques discussed previously to address the various superficial and deeper tissues.

Side-Lying Position There is no clinical advantage to placing the client in this position, unless the client specifically requests it or it is warranted by other factors.

Stretching

Stretching for carpal tunnel syndrome will remove restrictions between the structures that pass through the tunnel. Perform all the stretches discussed previously in order to restore balance to the musculature (see Figs. 8-19 to 8-35). For maximum results, be sure that the client always contracts the opposite muscle from the one being stretched. Focus on the stretches for the wrist flexors and finger flexors, and include stretches for the shoulder and neck if necessary.

SUMMARY

This chapter has brought to light the importance of the elbow-to-hand region of the body and the region's level of integration into the overall functioning of the upper extremity. The chapter began with an anatomical review of the region and descriptions of how to locate various bony landmarks and soft tissue structures. Various components such as range-of-motion testing and dermatome assessment were discussed in order to help the therapist obtain a thorough baseline for the region. The section on specific conditions noted the interrelation between the areas and explained how the presentations of the pathologies were similar. For each condition, the background, assessment techniques, and treatment recommendations were given to help the therapist effectively work on the condition.

REVIEW QUESTIONS

1. What three bones constitute the elbow?
2. List the three joints of the elbow and the components of each articulation.
3. What is the name of the superficial nerve that is nicknamed the "funny bone"?
4. What are the movements of the elbow, wrist, and hand region?
5. List the eight bones of the wrist.
6. What is the function of the triangular fibrocartilage complex?
7. What is the function of the retinaculum at the wrist?
8. What is the common mechanism of injury for lateral epicondylitis?
9. What are the three ways to re-create the pain of tennis elbow?
10. Define the carrying angle at the elbow, and list the three variations.
11. What are the two primary muscles involved in medial epicondylitis?
12. What is the difference between tenosynovitis and tendonitis?
13. List the structures that pass through the carpal tunnel.

CRITICAL-THINKING QUESTIONS

1. Explain the thinking in reclassifying tennis elbow as a degenerative condition rather than an inflammatory one.
2. Why would someone hold his or her elbow in the resting position?
3. Explain the double-crush phenomenon.
4. For carpal tunnel syndrome, explain why it is important to treat the entire upper extremity instead of just the wrist and hand.
5. What are some possible disadvantages to having carpal tunnel surgery?
6. Why is it important to release the forearm when treating carpal tunnel syndrome?

QUICK REFERENCE TABLES

Bony Structures of the Elbow

Medial epicondyle of the humerus	This is the medial distal humerus and is in line with the cubital crease. Locate the cubital crease, and trace in a medial direction until you find a round, bony structure.
Medial supracondylar line of the humerus	Locate the medial epicondyle of the humerus, and palpate in a superior direction along a ridge.
Lateral epicondyle	This is the distal lateral end of the humerus. Locate the cubital crease, and move laterally until you feel a round, bony prominence. This may be more difficult to find than the medial epicondyle.
Lateral epicondylar line	Using the lateral epicondyle, palpate in a superior direction along the ridge.
Olecranon process of the ulna	This is the very prominent process on the proximal tip of the ulna. It is best seen when the elbow is flexed, and it is the insertion of the triceps brachii.
Olecranon fossa	This fossa is located just proximal to the olecranon process on the humerus and forms the elbow joint with the ulna. Bend your client's arm to 90°, and palpate just above the process. You will be in a divot that will disappear when the arm is extended.
Ulnar groove/sulcus	This structure is home to the ulnar nerve. Locate the medial epicondyle of the humerus and the olecranon process of the ulna, and palpate the midpoint and the groove.
Ulnar border	Using the olecranon process, trace distally along the ulna.
Radial tuberosity	This structure can be difficult to find and is not directly palpable. Locate the cubital crease, and have your client bend the arm to 90°. Perform an isometric contraction of the biceps brachii, and locate the tendon. Have your client relax, and move lateral and deep to the tendon, staying medial to the brachioradialis.
Radial head/radiohumeral joint line	This structure can be difficult to find. Have your client flex the elbow to 90°. Locate the lateral epicondyle of the humerus. Move distally along the radius about one finger's breadth. To make sure you are on the structure, passively supinate and pronate the forearm; the radial head will rotate beneath your thumb.

Soft Tissue Structures of the Elbow

Medial collateral ligament of the elbow	This ligament is difficult to find and runs from the medial epicondyle of the humerus to the ulna in a fan shape.
Lateral collateral ligament of the elbow	This ligament runs from the lateral epicondyle of the humerus to the head of the radius. It becomes continuous with the annular ligament.
Brachial artery	This artery lies along the medial humerus, in between the biceps and triceps brachii.
Cephalic vein	This vein runs along the delto-pectoral interval, lateral to the biceps brachii and down the lateral humerus.
Basilic vein	This vein runs along the medial humerus, in between the biceps and triceps brachii.
Median cubital vein	This vein runs along the cubital crease and connects the cephalic and basilic veins.
Epitrochlear lymph nodes	These nodes lie above the medial epicondyle along the medial supra-condylar line. Use your fingers in a circular fashion to palpate this structure.
Median nerve	This nerve is found by locating the biceps tendon and pressing medial and deep.

Bony Structures of the Wrist and Hand

Ulnar styloid	This is on the medial side of the distal ulna, just above the wrist.
Radial styloid	This is the most distal end of the radius and is a palpable bony prominence just proximal to the wrist.
Lister's tubercle of the radius	This bony process sits between the radial and ulnar styloid processes on the dorsal radius. It is in line with the 3rd metacarpal. To make sure you are on the process, have your client flex and extend the wrist. If you are on Lister's tubercle, it will not move.
Scaphoid	This bone makes up the floor of the anatomical snuffbox and lies in the proximal row of carpals. Move distal to the radial styloid and into a divot. The scaphoid will become more prominent with ulnar deviation and less prominent with radial deviation.
Trapezium	This bone lies in the distal row of carpals and is somewhat difficult to find. Trace the metacarpal of the thumb in a proximal direction to its base. Once you move off the metacarpal, you will be on the bone. To make sure, move the thumb.
Lunate	This bone lies in the proximal row of carpals in line with Lister's tubercle and the 3rd metacarpal. Move off Lister's tubercle in a distal direction, and you will be on the lunate. The bone will become more prominent with wrist flexion.
Capitate	This bone lies in the distal row of carpals in between the lunate and the 3rd metacarpal. You can find this bone by extending the wrist and placing your finger in the divot created at the base of the 3rd metacarpal.
Triquetrum	This bone is located just distal to the ulnar styloid in the proximal row of carpals. Find the indentation on the side of the wrist just distal to the ulnar styloid. While palpating, radially deviate the wrist to make the bone more prominent.
Pisiform	This bone is on the palmar side of the hand at the base of the hypothenar eminence. It is very distinct and relatively easy to palpate.
Hamate	This bone is easy to find on the dorsal side of the hand at the base of the 4th and 5th metacarpals. On the palmar side, locate the "hook" by placing the interphalangeal joint of the thumb on the pisiform, pointing the tip toward the web space. The tip will fall onto the hook and can be felt by using a fair amount of pressure.
Trapezoid	This bone lies in the distal row of carpals and is located at the base of the 2nd metacarpal.
Metacarpals 1–5	These are the bones of the hands.
Phalanges 1–5	These are the bones of the fingers. There is a proximal and distal phalange of the thumb and a proximal, middle, and distal phalange of digits 2–5.

Soft Tissue Structures of the Wrist and Hand

Radial artery	This pulse is found just proximal to the ventral wrist on the radius.
Radial nerve	This nerve can be palpated just proximal to the radial styloid process. Move ½ inch proximally, and palpate in a transverse direction.
Ulnar artery	This pulse is found just proximal to the ventral wrist on the ulna.
Tunnel of Guyon	This tunnel is formed by a ligament connecting the hook of the hamate and the pisiform bone. The tunnel houses the ulnar nerve as it moves into the hand.
Anatomical snuffbox	This structure is formed by the scaphoid at its base, the extensor pollicis longus along the index finger, and the abductor pollicis longus and extensor pollicis brevis along the thumb. To make these tendons more prominent, extend the thumb and look for the depression at the wrist.
Metacarpal phalangeal (MCP) joints	These are the joints between the metacarpals and the proximal phalanges. They are very flexible.
Interphalangeal joints	These are the joints between the phalanges.
Thenar eminence	This structure lies over the base of the thumb and forms the lateral palm and heel of the hand. It comprises the abductor pollicis brevis, flexor pollicis brevis, opponens pollicis, and adductor pollicis muscles.
Hypothenar eminence	This structure lies over the base of the 5th metacarpal and forms the medial palm and heel of the hand. It comprises the abductor digiti minimi, flexor digiti minimi brevis, and opponens digiti minimi muscles.

Muscles of the Elbow, Forearm, Wrist, and Hand

Muscle	Origin	Insertion	Action	How to Palpate
Arm Muscles				
Triceps brachii	Long head: infra-glenoid tubercle of the humerus Lateral head: proximal end of the shaft of the humerus Medial head: distal end of the shaft of the humerus	Olecranon process of the ulna	Extension of the forearm at the elbow and of the arm at the shoulder	Client in the prone position; hang arm off the table, and resist extension of the arm at the elbow
Biceps brachii	Long head: supraglenoid tubercle through bicipital groove Short head: coracoid process of the scapula	Radial tuberosity and bicipital aponeurosis	Flexion of the supinated elbow; supination of the forearm and flexion of the arm at the shoulder	Client in the supine position; resist flexion of a supinated forearm at the elbow
Brachialis	Distal half of the anterior surface of the humerus	Coronoid process and tuberosity of the ulna	Flexion of the forearm at the elbow	Client in the supine position; resist flexion of a pronated forearm at the elbow; palpate lateral and medial to the biceps brachii
Forearm Muscles				
Pronator teres	Medial epicondyle of the humerus and coronoid process of the ulna	Middle of the lateral shaft of the radius	Pronation of the forearm and flexion of the elbow	Have client pronate forearm against resistance; palpate just medial to the biceps brachii insertion
Supinator	Lateral epicondyle; annular ligament; proximal ulna	Lateral surface of the proximal radius	Supination of the forearm	Forearm in neutral; palpate between brachioradialis and wrist extensors

Muscle	Origin	Insertion	Action	How to Palpate
Forearm Muscles (Continued)				
Brachioradialis	Lateral supracondylar ridge of the humerus	Styloid process of the radius	Flexion of the forearm at the elbow in a neutral position	Client in the seated position; resist flexion of the neutral forearm
Extensor carpi radialis longus and brevis	Lateral supracondylar ridge of the humerus	Longus: Base of the 2nd metacarpal Brevis: Base of the 3rd metacarpal	Extension and radial deviation of the wrist	Client in the seated position; have client extend wrist, and palpate just lateral to the brachioradialis
Extensor digitorum	Lateral epicondyle of the humerus	Base of the middle phalanges of fingers II–V	Extension of the proximal phalanges of fingers II–V	Client in the seated position; have client extend wrist, and palpate just lateral to the extensor carpi radialis longus
Extensor carpi ulnaris	Lateral epicondyle of the humerus	Base of the 5th metacarpal	Extension and ulnar deviation of the wrist	Client in the seated position; have client extend wrist, and palpate lateral to the extensor digitorum along the ulnar border
Flexor carpi radialis	Medial epicondyle of the humerus	Base of the 2nd and 3rd metacarpals	Flexion and radial deviation of the wrist	Client in the seated position; have client flex wrist; the tendon will be prominent in line with the 2nd metacarpal; trace the muscle up toward the medial epicondyle of the humerus
Palmaris longus	Medial epicondyle of the humerus	Palmar aponeurosis and the flexor retinaculum	Flexion of the wrist	Have client flex the wrist and abduct the thumb; the tendon will be palpable on the midline of the anterior surface of the wrist

Muscle	Origin	Insertion	Action	How to Palpate
Forearm Muscles (Continued)				
Flexor carpi ulnaris	Medial epicondyle of the humerus	Pisiform and the hamate bones	Flexion and ulnar deviation of the wrist	Have client flex wrist; the tendon will be palpable on the lateral ulna in line with the pisiform bone
Hand Muscles				
Adductor pollicis	2nd and 3rd metacarpals; capitate	Base of the thumb	Adduction of the thumb; assists flexion of thumb	Deep in palmar web space
Opponens pollicis	Trapezium and flexor retinaculum	Shaft of the 1st metacarpal	Opposition of the thumb	Base of thenar eminence
Abductor pollicis longus	Posterior radius and ulna deep to the extensors	Base of the 1st metacarpal	Abduction and extension of the thumb	Forms radial tendon of the anatomical snuffbox
Extensor pollicis brevis	Interosseous membrane; posterior radius and ulna	Base of the proximal phalanx of the thumb	Extension of the thumb	Forms radial tendon of the anatomical snuffbox

Trigger Points of the Elbow, Forearm, Wrist, and Hand

Muscle	Trigger-Point Location	Referral Pattern	Chief Symptom
Biceps brachii	Midbelly in either head	Primarily in the superior direction to the front of the shoulder; can also travel to the suprascapular region and antecubital space	Pain during arm elevation above shoulder level; other presentations include aching over the anterior arm and possible weakness
Brachialis	1. Proximal point: halfway up the humerus on the lateral edge of the biceps brachii; accessible without displacing the biceps 2. Distal points: just proximal to the elbow; located by moving the biceps out of the way (Distal points are generally attachment points.)	Primarily to the base of the thumb, dorsal carpometacarpal joint, and dorsal web space of the thumb; additional areas may occur in the antecubital space and the front of the shoulder	Diffuse soreness at the base of the thumb and pain in front of the shoulder; passive motion will increase elbow pain, but active motion will not
Triceps brachii	1. Central belly of the long head of the muscle 2. Lateral portion of the medial head of the muscle 3. Lateral head 4. Attachment point created from other points 5. Medial portion of the medial head of the muscle	1. Upward over the posterior arm and shoulder, sometimes extending into the upper trapezius and down the posterior forearm 2. Lateral epicondyle of the elbow 3. Centrally around the point over the posterior arm; sometimes down the posterior forearm into the 4th and 5th fingers 4. Olecranon process 5. Medial forearm and palmar surface of the 4th and 5th fingers	Diffuse pain posteriorly in the shoulder and upper arm; can affect movement but is often overlooked by the client because of compensatory movements

Trigger Points of the Elbow, Forearm, Wrist, and Hand *(Continued)*

Muscle	Trigger-Point Location	Referral Pattern	Chief Symptom
Extensor carpi radialis longus	Just distal to the elbow on the radial side of the dorsal forearm	Pain into the lateral epicondyle and the dorsal anatomical snuffbox	Pain in the lateral epicondyle; can be activated by a repetitive forceful handgrip
Extensor carpi radialis brevis	Two inches distal to the cubital crease on the ulnar side of the brachioradialis in the muscle mass of the brevis, but distal to the point in the longus	Pain to the dorsal surface of the hand and wrist	One of the most common sources of posterior wrist pain
Extensor carpi ulnaris	Three inches distal to the lateral epicondyle along the ulnar side of the forearm	Ulnar side of the posterior wrist	Posterior wrist pain
Brachioradialis	In deeper layers of muscle; lie directly along the proximal radius, just distal to the elbow when the forearm is in a neutral position	Pain to the wrist and the web space between thumb and first finger; can also refer pain up over the lateral epicondyle	Pain in the wrist
Extensor digitorum	About 1½ inches distal to the head of the radius	Pain down the dorsal forearm and into the finger that is moved by the involved fibers; pain will stop short of the distal phalanx; points in the ring finger present with pain radiating down the dorsal forearm to the ring finger and proximally to the lateral epicondyle	Pain in the hand, as well as pain and stiffness in the involved fingers
Supinator	On the ventral aspect of the radius between the biceps brachii tendon and the brachioradialis	Symptoms of lateral epicondylitis	Aching in the lateral epicondyle and the dorsal web space between thumb and first finger
Palmaris longus	In midbelly of muscle (Palpation can cause a twitch response of wrist flexion.)	Superficial prickling pain centered in palm of hand; stops short of fingers and thumb	Difficulty handling things in the palm, such as tools

Trigger Points of the Elbow, Forearm, Wrist, and Hand *(Continued)*

Muscle	Trigger-Point Location	Referral Pattern	Chief Symptom
Flexor carpi radialis	Midfiber portion of the belly	Pain centers on the radial side of the ventral crease in the wrist	Difficulty in activities such as cutting heavy material with scissors or using shears
Flexor carpi ulnaris	Midfiber portion of the belly; superficial enough to be palpable	Similar to flexor carpi radialis but centralizes over the ulnar side of the ventral crease	Difficulty in activities such as cutting heavy material with scissors or using shears
Pronator teres	Just medial to the medial epicondyle, distal to the cubital crease	Pain deep in the ventral wrist and forearm	Inability to supinate the cupped hand; client will usually compensate by rotating arm at shoulder
Adductor pollicis	Web space; found by palpating from the dorsal side of the web space just inside the metacarpal of the thumb	Aching along the outside of the thumb and hand, distal to the wrist; may also affect web space and thenar eminence	Unable to perform fine finger manipulations, such as holding a pen or buttoning a shirt
Opponens pollicis	Thenar eminence about halfway down	Pain to the palmar surface of most of the thumb and to a spot on the ventral side of the wrist at the radius	Unable to perform fine finger manipulations, such as holding a pen or buttoning a shirt

Orthopedic Tests for the Elbow, Forearm, Wrist, and Hand

Condition	Orthopedic Test	How to Perform	Positive Sign
Lateral epicondylitis	Cozen's test *Note:* This is the most common of these tests.	Have the client pronate the forearm; then extend and radially deviate the wrist. Support the client's forearm, and place your thumb over the lateral epicondyle. Try to move the wrist into flexion while the client resists.	Sudden severe pain in the area of the epicondyle indicates a positive test.
	Mill's test	Support the client's forearm, and place your thumb over the lateral epicondyle while you passively pronate the forearm, fully flex the wrist, and slowly extend the elbow.	Pain over the lateral epicondyle indicates a positive test.
	Tennis elbow test	Support the client's forearm, and place his or her 3rd finger into slight extension. Apply force on the finger moving it into flexion while the client resists. This will place an eccentric load on the extensor digitorum muscle.	Pain over the lateral epicondyle indicates a positive test.
Medial epicondylitis	Medial epicondylitis test (passive)	Bend the client's elbow to 90°, and stabilize it against the client's body. With the client's forearm supinated, palpate the medial epicondyle and slowly extend the client's elbow and wrist.	Pain over the medial epicondyle is considered a positive test.
	Medial epicondylitis test (active)	Bend the client's elbow to 90°, and stabilize it against the client's body. Extend the elbow and wrist while the client resists.	Pain over the medial epicondyle is considered a positive test.
de Quervain's tenosynovitis	Finkelstein's test *Note:* This test will often produce positive results in otherwise normal wrists; therefore, results should be correlated with the other evaluative findings.	Place the client in the seated or standing position. Instruct the client to make a fist and then tuck his or her thumb inside. With the wrist in neutral, administer the active version of the test by instructing the client to perform ulnar deviation; administer the passive version of the test by stabilizing the forearm and ulnarly deviating the wrist.	Pain over the tendons of the abductor pollicis longus and extensor pollicis brevis at the wrist indicates a positive result.

Orthopedic Tests for the Elbow, Forearm, Wrist, and Hand *(Continued)*

Condition	Orthopedic Test	How to Perform	Positive Sign
Carpal tunnel syndrome	Tinel-sign test *Note:* Developed by French neurologist Jules Tinel in 1915, this is one of the best-known and most widely used health care clinical assessment tools.	Client is in the seated or standing position. Supinate his or her forearm so that the palm is facing up. Tap your fingertip over the carpal tunnel at the wrist.	Tingling and/or numbness along the median nerve distribution indicates a positive result.
	Phalen's test	Instruct the client to flex the wrists as far as possible. Push the backs of the hands together, and hold the position for 1 minute. Be sure the client does not shrug the shoulders, as this may compress the median nerve at the thoracic outlet.	Tingling and/or numbness along the median nerve distribution indicates a positive result.
	Carpal tunnel compression test	Client is in the seated or standing position. Using both thumbs, place even pressure over the carpal tunnel and hold for at least 30 seconds.	Tingling and/or numbness along the median nerve distribution indicates a positive result.

QUICK REFERENCE TABLE

chapter *9*

Conditions of the Hip and Knee

chapter objectives

At the conclusion of this chapter, the reader will understand:

- bony anatomy of the region
- how to locate the bony landmarks and soft tissue structures of the region
- where to find the muscles, and the origins, insertions, and actions of the region
- how to assess the movement and determine the range of motion for the region
- how to perform manual muscle testing to the region
- how to recognize dermatome patterns for the region
- trigger-point location and referral patterns for the region
- the following elements of each condition discussed:
  - background and characteristics
  - specific questions to ask
  - what orthopedic tests should be performed
  - how to treat the connective tissue, trigger points, and muscles
  - flexibility concerns

KEY TERMS

acetabulum
angle of inclination
anteversion
chondromalacia patella
iliotibial band friction syndrome (ITBFS)
ligamentum teres

meralgia paresthetica
patellar tendonosis
patellofemoral pain syndrome (PFPS)
piriformis syndrome
quadriceps angle (Q angle)
screw-home mechanism

Introduction

The hip and the knee compose an important part of the lower extremity. While constructed differently, they are interrelated and dysfunction in one can affect the other. The hip and the knee provide a stable foundation that allows the upper body and the trunk to perform activity. Since humans interact with their surroundings through bipedal locomotion, limitations in either of these regions can be devastating.

The hip's strong, bony stability helps protect it from injury. It is one of the body's two ball-and-socket joints, and it is one of the largest and most stable joints in the body. During locomotion, however, the hip can be subjected to forces that are four to seven times the body's weight, thus making the joint vulnerable to stress-related injuries (Anderson et al., 2000). While injuries to the hip are not as common as injuries to the lower extremities, the overall prevalence of hip pain in adults has increased over time (Paluska, 2005). Yet 30% of hip-related pain still remains without a clear etiology.

There are three reasons why it is difficult to determine the origin of hip pain:

1. The joint is not superficial. Pain may be felt across a broader region, making it more difficult to determine which structures are involved.
2. Hip pain is often referred from the surrounding structures, and dysfunction in the sacrum, the lumbar spine, and the groin can all refer pain into the hip.
3. There is debate as to the specific topographic area that can be defined as the "hip" (Birrell et al., 2005).

Not surprisingly, the prevalence of hip pain depends largely on the assessment methods used, and, unfortunately, no gold standard of assessment exists.

Quite different from the hip, the knee is prone to traumatic injury because of its anatomy. It is located at the ends of the two longest bones in the body, the femur and tibia, which act as two long lever arms, exposing the joint to large torques. Because these two long bones are stacked on one another, the knee has to rely on soft tissue structures, such as ligaments and muscles, to provide stability. This intricate balance between static and dynamic structures makes the knee a complicated area to assess. All the relevant structures must be considered, including related areas that may refer pain into the knee, such as the lumbar spine, hip, and ankle.

Entire texts are written on the pathology of the hip and knee. While this chapter is not a comprehensive review of these regions, it does provide a thorough assessment of the dysfunctions and some of the more common pathologies in the regions. In addition, this chapter covers:

- Specific bony landmarks for palpation
- Soft tissue structures, including the muscles of the region
- The movements of the region, and basic biomechanics of the hip and knee
- Manual muscle tests for the hip and knee
- Dermatome and trigger-point referral patterns for the involved muscles
- Some common causes of dysfunction, and how to assess and treat them using soft tissue therapy

ANATOMICAL REVIEW

Bony Anatomy of the Hip

When discussing the bony anatomy of the hip, it is necessary to include part of the pelvis because it articulates with the femur to form part of the hip (Fig. 9-1). The portion of the pelvis that is commonly referred to as the "hip bone" is the innominate bone. It is sometimes called the *os coxae* and is created by the fusion of three separate bones: the ilium, the ischium, and the pubis. These bones fuse by the age of 15. The articulations with the other os coxae at the pubic symphysis and with the sacrum at the sacroiliac joint form the pelvic girdle. The three bones fuse at a point known as the **acetabulum**, a unique name derived from its resemblance to the vinegar cups used in ancient Rome. This is an important structure because it forms the pelvic portion of the hip joint and articulates with the head of the femur.

The largest of the three coxal bones is the *ilium;* it extends from the iliac crest to the superior portion of the acetabulum (see Fig. 9-1). The medial surface of the ilium has a depression known as the *iliac fossa,* and the lateral surface has three ridges: the anterior, posterior and inferior gluteal lines, which serve as attachment points for the gluteals. At the most superior point of the ilium is the iliac crest. It terminates at the anterior superior iliac spine (ASIS) in the front and the posterior superior iliac spine (PSIS) in the back. Below the superior spines are the anterior and posterior inferior iliac spines, as well as the greater sciatic notch, which lies below the posterior inferior iliac spine.

The next portion of the innominate bone is the *ischium;* it accounts for the inferoposterior portion of the bone and the posterior two-fifths of the acetabulum (see Fig. 9-1). It has a stout body that is marked with a prominent spine with a small indentation below: the lesser sciatic notch. At

acetabulum The point at which the three bones of the pelvis (ilium, ischium, and pubis) fuse. It forms the pelvic portion of the hip joint and articulates with the head of the femur.

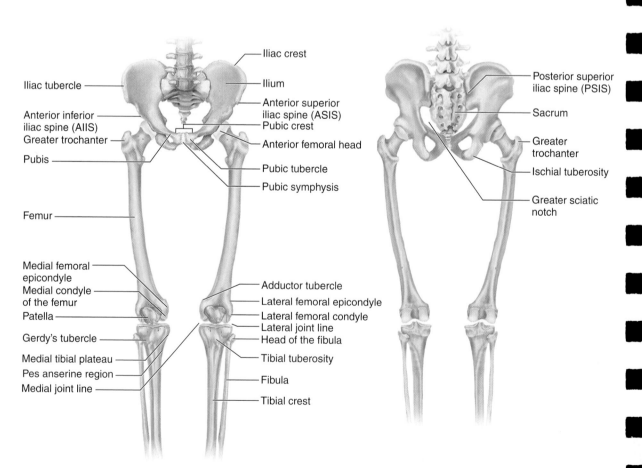

Figure 9-1 Skeletal and surface anatomy structures of the pelvis, femur, and knee.

the bottom of the bone is a large, rough projection, the ischial tuberosity. This is the common origin for the hamstrings, and it supports the body's weight in the seated position, giving it the nickname the "sits bone." The ischium extends anteriorly via the ramus of the ischium and joins the inferior ramus of the next bone, the pubis.

The *pubis* is the most anterior portion of the innominate bone and forms the anterior portion of the acetabulum, where it joins the ilium and the ischium (see Fig. 9-1). A superior ramus extends from the acetabulum and joins with the inferior ramus to form the body of the pubis. The superior and inferior rami of the pubis and ischium, along with the body of the ischium, form an important space known as the *obturator foramen.*

The next bone that forms the hip is the *femur,* which is the longest, heaviest, and strongest bone in the body (see Fig. 9-1). The head of the femur is nearly spherical and forms an ideal ball-and-socket joint with the acetabulum. The head of the femur is angled in the socket at approximately 125° in the frontal plane. This **angle of inclination** allows the femur to angle downward medially, thereby bringing the knees closer together to provide a better base of support.

Inferior to the head is an elongated neck that is smaller in diameter than the rest of the bone, followed by two large processes known as the *greater* and *lesser trochanters.* These massive, roughened structures serve as muscle attachments for the hip and are connected by the intertrochanteric crest anteriorly and the intertrochanteric line posteriorly. Inferior to the trochanters is a long shaft that extends distally. The major feature of this shaft is a posterior ridge known as the *linea aspera.* It serves as the attachment site for various thigh muscles and branches into smaller lateral and medial ridges at its distal end.

📖 **angle of inclination** The angle of the head of the femur in the socket. It is approximately 125° in the frontal plane, allowing the femur to angle downward medially, which brings the knees closer together to provide a better base of support.

Bony Structures and Surface Anatomy of the Hip

When palpating this region, include other relevant areas such as the lumbar spine to rule out any involvement of the structures in those areas. The client must be properly draped to ensure that the correct structures are being palpated.

Beginning on the innominate bone (see Fig. 9-1), find the *iliac crest* by placing the palms of the hands in the flank area just below the ribs. Press down and in to feel the top of the crests, using the fingertips to trace the edges. From the crest, move in an anterior direction and locate two prominent structures, the *iliac tubercles,* which are the widest points on the pelvis. Continuing in an anterior direction, find the *anterior superior iliac spines (ASIS)*, which are very prominent. These are the most anterior structures on the pelvis. To locate, place the client in the supine position. Place the palms of your hands on the front of the client's hips and feel for two bony prominences.

The *anterior inferior iliac spine (AIIS)* is not generally palpable. Move about a half-inch inferior to the ASIS, and press in. The AIIS is located at the origin of the rectus femoris, where the thigh blends into the trunk. At the other end of the iliac crest are the *posterior superior iliac spines (PSIS).* These are the most posterior aspects of the iliac crest and are found by tracing the crest in a posterior direction until reaching the most posterior part. They are commonly referred to as the "dimples" in the low back and help to form the sacroiliac joint with the sacrum.

Medial to the PSIS is the *sacrum*. This bone consists of four to five fused vertebrae and sits inferior to the lumbar spine. Once on the bone, use the fingertips to trace its lateral edge in an inferior direction.

Around the front of the body, find the *pubic crest* by placing the fingertips in the umbilicus and resting the hand in an inferior direction on the abdomen. Slowly press down and in; the heel of the hand will hit a bony ledge. Use the fingertips to trace its edges. Between the two pubic bones is the *pubic symphysis*, which is the joint formed by the two pubic bones. On either edge of the pubic crest are small bumps known as the *pubic tubercles*. From the crest, move to either edge to find the tubercles.

Moving to the femur, the *anterior femoral head* lies at the midpoint of the inguinal ligament. Using the palm of the hand, press just inferior to the midpoint of the ligament until you feel a hard, round object. Externally rotate the client's thigh to make the structure a little more palpable. An important landmark in this area is the *greater trochanter of the femur*, which lies on the proximal lateral thigh. To locate, have the client lie in the prone position and place the palm of the hand over the client's lateral hip. Bend the knee to 90°, and press in on the hip while rotating the client's leg medially and laterally. You should feel a large, bony structure rotating under your hand; use the fingertips to trace its borders.

From the greater trochanter, move medially to find the *ischial tuberosity*. This structure is on the inferior ischium and is the common origin for the hamstrings. Using the gluteal fold, place the web space of the hand with the thumb pointing medially along the fold, and press in. The thumb should be on the tuberosity.

The *greater sciatic notch* lies approximately in the middle of the hip. To locate, draw an imaginary line and find the midpoint between the posterior superior iliac spine on the opposite side of the notch and the greater trochanter on the side of the notch you are trying to locate. Press in to feel a depression; this is the greater sciatic notch.

Soft Tissue Structures of the Hip

As stated earlier, the hip joint is one of two ball-and-socket joints of the body; the other is located in the shoulder. The acetabulum and the head of the femur form the hip joint (Fig. 9-2). The acetabulum forms half of a sphere and opens outward, forward, and downward; the head of the

Figure 9-2 Soft tissue structures of the hip.

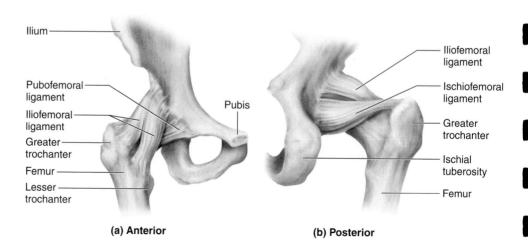

Ilium

Pubofemoral ligament

Iliofemoral ligament

Greater trochanter

Femur

Lesser trochanter

Pubis

Iliofemoral ligament

Ischiofemoral ligament

Greater trochanter

Ischial tuberosity

Femur

(a) Anterior

(b) Posterior

Part II Regional Approach to Treatment

femur forms two-thirds of a sphere. While the hip is inherently stable, it is less mobile than the shoulder. The surfaces of both bones are covered with articular cartilage to reduce friction, and a U-shaped fibrocartilaginous labrum lies around the edge of the acetabulum, which contributes additional stability to the joint.

The capsule surrounding the joint is extremely dense and strong. It runs from the acetabulum to the trochanters of the femur and attaches along the intertrochanteric crest and line. The capsule is reinforced with three major ligaments (see Fig. 9-2):

- *Iliofemoral ligament:* Runs from the AIIS to the intertrochanteric line, supporting the anterior region of the joint. Also known as the *Y ligament of Bigelow,* the iliofemoral is the strongest ligament in the body.

- *Ischiofemoral ligament:* Helps support the posterior aspect of the hip joint and limits extension by using its spiral shape to wind tight during extension.

- *Pubofemoral ligament:* Arises from a thickening of the capsule's inferior region. It prevents excessive abduction of the femur and also assists in limiting extension.

Lastly, the ligament of the head of the femur, also known as the **ligamentum teres**, runs from the acetabulum to the center of the head of the femur. It does not add stability to the joint. Rather, it contains a small artery that supplies the head of the femur.

ligamentum teres A small ligament that runs from the femoral head to the acetabulum. It does not add stability to the joint but contains a small artery that supplies the head of the femur.

Additional Soft Tissue Structures (See Fig. 9-3)

On the anterior side of the hip, the *inguinal ligament* is located on a line between the ASIS of the ilium and the pubic tubercles; it serves as the inferior edge of the oblique abdominal muscles. Inferior to the ligament is a region known as the *femoral triangle*; it is bound by three structures. Have the client bend his or her hip and knee; then place the foot across the opposite knee, and let it fall out. The triangle is bound superiorly by the inguinal

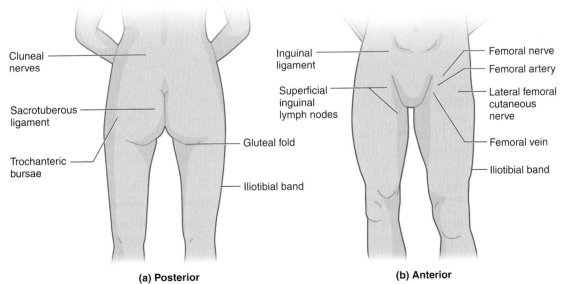

(a) Posterior

Cluneal nerves

Sacrotuberous ligament

Trochanteric bursae

Gluteal fold

Iliotibial band

(b) Anterior

Inguinal ligament

Superficial inguinal lymph nodes

Femoral nerve

Femoral artery

Lateral femoral cutaneous nerve

Femoral vein

Iliotibial band

Figure 9-3 Additional soft tissue structures of the hip.

ligament, laterally by the sartorius muscle, and medially by the adductor longus muscle. Within the triangle are three important structures:

- *Femoral artery:* In the middle of the triangle; found by pressing in with the fingers and feeling for a strong pulse
- *Femoral nerve:* Just lateral to the femoral artery
- *Femoral vein:* Just medial to the femoral artery

Using the femoral triangle as a reference, locate the *superficial inguinal lymph nodes,* which consist of two chains. The horizontal chain runs just inferior to the inguinal ligament from lateral to medial. The vertical chain starts at the medial edge of the horizontal chain and runs inferior along the lateral border of the adductor longus. Both chains can be palpated in a circular fashion with the fingertips and will feel like clusters of grapes.

The *lateral femoral cutaneous nerve* lies inferior to the ASIS and medial to the tensor fascia latae. It is located approximately around the origin tendon for the rectus femoris muscle and may be tender. Continuing around to the posterior side of the hip, the *iliotibial band* is made of dense fascia and lies directly over the vastus lateralis. A portion of the band runs deep and inserts along the femur, separating the hamstrings from the quadriceps. It serves as the tendon of insertion for the gluteus maximus and the tensor fascia latae; it is palpated easiest at the knee. Have the client lie on his or her side, and then locate the edges of the band on the lateral thigh, tracing it from the knee to the hip. Directly on the lateral side of the hip is the *trochanteric bursa.* It is generally not palpable and is found by palpating just posterior and behind the greater trochanter.

At the base of the hip on the posterior side of the thigh is the *gluteal fold*, which is formed by the thigh as it meets the hip. Have the client lie in the prone position, and locate the fold at the base of the gluteus maximus muscle and the top of the hamstrings. From the ischial tuberosity, the *sacrotuberous ligament* runs to the inferior lateral angle of the sacrum. Using the ischial tuberosity, move in a superior and medial direction and press in. To ensure it is indeed the correct ligament, have the client cough; the ligament will tighten.

The last structures are the *cluneal nerves*, which are located along the iliac crest between the PSIS and the iliac tubercles. Find the midpoint along the iliac crest, and palpate these vertically oriented nerves in a transverse direction.

Bony Anatomy of the Knee

The knee comprises the distal femur, the proximal tibia, and the patella (see Fig. 9-1).

Distal Femur

The distal end of the femur flares out to create two attachment surfaces for muscles and ligaments known as the *medial* and *lateral epicondyles.* At their most superior edge is the termination of the linea aspera, which forms the medial and lateral supracondylar lines. Continuing distally, the medial and lateral condyles are the articular surfaces that articulate with

---

⭑ Practical Tip

Make sure you let the client know what you are doing, and be sure that it is within the client's comfort level.

the tibia. The condyles are separated by the intercondylar notch and have a smooth depression on the anterior side of the distal femur called the *patellar surface,* wherein the patella glides during motion.

Proximal Tibia

The proximal end of the tibia creates the distal portion of the knee (see Fig. 9-1). Two broad, flat condyles, one medial and one lateral, accommodate the condyles of the femur. The tibial condyles are separated by a ridge called the *intercondylar eminence,* which matches the femur's intercondylar notch. A rough anterior projection called the *tibial tuberosity* serves as the insertion for the quadriceps muscle group. Just inferior to the lateral tibial plateau is a depression called the *fibular articular surface,* which accepts the head of the fibula. Extending distally is a prominent ridge called the *tibial crest,* also known as the "shin."

Patella

The patella (see Fig. 9-1) completes the knee joint and is actually a large, triangular-shaped sesmoid bone that lies within the quadriceps tendon. It has a broad superior base and a narrow, pointed inferior apex. The anterior surface of the bone is relatively smooth, while the posterior aspect has several facets covered in hyaline cartilage that form the articular surface, which articulates with the femur.

While the fibula is not technically part of the knee, it deserves mentioning. The long, thin fibula runs along the lateral side of the leg; it serves primarily as a site for muscle attachment and has no real weight-bearing function. The proximal end, which is thicker and broader, is the head. It articulates with the fibular notch of the tibia to form the proximal tibiofibular joint. The shaft of the fibula is narrow and runs distally to the ankle.

Bony Structures and Surface Anatomy of the Knee

The landmarks of the knee provide a tremendous amount of information during the assessment process (see Fig. 9-1). This area is bonier than the hip, and the structures are generally easier to palpate. The most recognizable bone is the *patella,* or the kneecap; it is located dead center on the anterior knee. Use the palm of the hand on the anterior knee to locate the patella, and then trace its borders with the fingers. From the patella, move distally onto the tibia to a large bony prominence called the *tibial tuberosity.* This large, bony prominence is located about 1 to 1½ inches distal to the inferior pole of the patella on the tibia. Just lateral to the tibial tuberosity, a smaller tubercle known as the *lateral tibial tubercle (Gerdy's tubercle)* is the insertion for the iliotibial band. Continuing inferiorly, locate the *tibial crest* by tracing from the tibial tuberosity down the midline of the tibia. This is a relatively sharp edge of bone and can be tender.

Starting back up at the patella, have the client sit with his or her knee flexed to 90°. Move off the patella onto the soft tendon, and locate the midpoint. Slide off the tendon in a medial direction into a depression. This depression is the *medial joint line*; trace the line around the entire medial side of the knee (see Fig. 9-1).

From the anteromedial joint line, move distally about a half-inch, staying above the concavity of the tibia to locate the *medial tibial plateau*. Roll the fingers in an inferior direction into the concavity of the tibia; this is the *pes anserine region* of the knee. This area on the tibia is the insertion for the sartorius, gracilis, and semitendinosus; it has a bursa that lies between the tendons and the tibia.

Using the medial joint line as a beginning point, palpate the *medial condyle of the femur* by pressing up and just medial to the patella. The hard surface is the condyle. Walk the fingers up past the condyle and around the medial side of the knee to locate the *medial epicondyle*. The femur will start to dip in toward the midline. This is the epicondyle. Continue upward from the epicondyle as the femur dips inward. There is a bony prominence deep on the femur known as the *adductor tubercle*; it is one of the attachments of the adductor magnus.

As with the medial side, locate the *lateral joint line* with the client's knee flexed to 90° (see Fig. 9-1). Locate the midpoint of the patellar tendon, and move off laterally until you feel a depression. Once in the joint line, press up and in just lateral to the patella to locate the *lateral femoral condyle,* which is typically more prominent on the lateral side than on the medial side. To locate the *lateral femoral epicondyle,* move up from the lateral joint line along the lateral side of the knee. The femur will start to dip in toward the midline; this is the epicondyle. Trace the lateral joint line to its most lateral point, and palpate inferior to the lateral tibial crest to find the *head of the fibula*. The last landmark of the knee is the *shaft of the fibula*. Trace from the fibular head down the lateral side of the leg to the lateral malleolus. It may or may not be possible to palpate the bone directly.

Soft Tissue Structures of the Knee

Structurally, the knee comprises two separate articulations (Fig. 9-4). The tibiofemoral joint is the largest and most complex joint in the body. It is considered a modified hinge joint that is capable of rotation as well as lateral gliding. The medial and lateral condyles of the femur are different sizes, which causes the tibia to rotate laterally during the last few degrees of extension and produces a phenomenon known as the "**screw-home mechanism.**" This locking brings the knee into its most stable position of extension.

The other articulation is the patellofemoral joint, which is formed by the patella riding in the trochlear groove of the anterior distal femur. The posterior surface of the patella has three distinct facets, the medial, lateral, and odd, which contact the groove at different times during movement.

The capsule that surrounds the joint is thin and weak. It surrounds the medial, lateral, and posterior sides of the joint. The anterior portion of the joint is covered by the quadriceps tendon and contains the patella. To find the *quadriceps tendon,* move superior just off the superior edge and palpate the tendon. Inferior to the patella is the *patellar ligament*. This is the tendon of insertion for the quadriceps muscles and lies between the inferior pole of the patella and the tibial tuberosity. Have the client flex his or her knee to 90°, and then palpate between these two points.

There are several additional structures that add stability to the joint. On each side of the joint are two collateral ligaments, the *lateral collateral ligament (LCL)* and the *medial collateral ligament (MCL)*:

- *LCL:* Runs from the lateral epicondyle of the femur to the head of the fibula; it is separate from the lateral meniscus. It resists varus forces and reinforces the lateral side of the joint. The LCL lies directly on the lateral side of the knee. To locate, have the client bend the hip and knee; then place the foot across the opposite knee and let it fall out. Locate the lateral joint line, and palpate laterally until feeling a distinct cordlike structure.

- *MCL:* Formed by two layers, with the deep layer merging with the joint capsule and medial meniscus, thereby connecting the femur to the tibia. The superficial layer originates just above the adductor tubercle and is separate from the deep layer. Both layers attach inferiorly at the pes anserine region and resist valgus forces. To locate, use the joint line and move in a medial direction until reaching the middle of the joint. Because the ligament runs in a vertical fashion, it is best palpated in a transverse direction; however, it is not always easily palpated because of its structure.

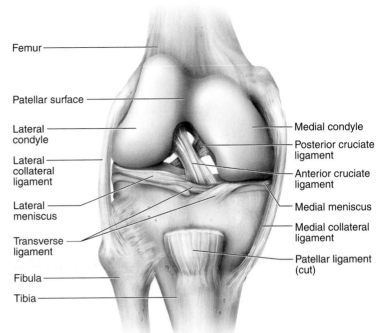

Figure 9-4 Soft tissue structures of the knee.

Two other important ligaments are considered intracapsular because they lie within the articular capsule but are extrasynovial because they lie outside the synovial cavity. The *anterior cruciate ligament (ACL)* and the *posterior cruciate ligament (PCL)* are the major ligaments of the knee and are so-named because they cross each other in the joint:

- *ACL:* Runs from the posterior femur to the anterior tibia. It serves to prevent the anterior translation of the tibia on the femur, hyperextension of the knee, and the excessive internal or external rotation of the tibia on the femur.

- *PCL:* Runs from the front of the femur to the back of the tibia. Smaller and stronger than the ACL, it is the primary stabilizer of the knee. It serves to resist posterior translation of the tibia on the femur and hyperflexion of the knee joint.

Within the joint, the space between the femur and the tibia is partially filled by two disks of fibrocartilage called the *menisci*. They are firmly attached to the tibial condyles and are thicker on the periphery, thus deepening the tibial plateaus. They have several functions, which are listed in Table 9-1.

The *medial meniscus* is C-shaped and is attached to the MCL and the semimembranosus muscle. It is injured more frequently than the lateral meniscus. To find the medial meniscus, locate the medial joint line and press in deep while the client internally rotates the tibia. The meniscus will move into the thumb during internal rotation and will move away during external tibial rotation. The *lateral meniscus* is almost a complete

Table 9-1 Functions of the Menisci

Deepen the articulation, and shift to fill in the gaps during motion

Assist in lubrication and nourishment of the joint

Reduce friction during motion

Increase the surface area of contact between the femur and the tibia

Provide shock absorption

Help prevent hyperextension of the joint

Prevent the joint capsule from entering the joint and locking the knee

circle and is smaller than the medial meniscus. It is much more mobile than the medial meniscus, making it less prone to injury. It is found by locating the lateral joint line and pressing in deep as the client externally rotates the tibia. The meniscus will move into the thumb during external rotation and will move away during internal tibial rotation.

The last structure is not located within the knee joint but can be injured along with the knee. The *peroneal nerve* sits just behind the head of the fibula and is found by palpating behind the head of the fibula as the client internally rotates the tibia.

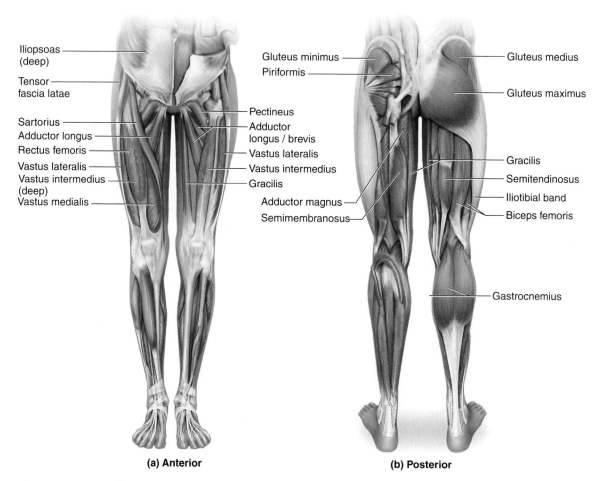

(a) Anterior   (b) Posterior

Figure 9-5 Muscles of the pelvis, hip, and knee.

Muscles of the Hip and Knee

The muscles that either are directly attached to the hip or knee or have an affect on the area are shown in Fig. 9-5. Refer to the Quick Reference Table "Muscles of the Hip, Thigh, and Knee" at the end of this chapter (page 393).

MOVEMENT AND MANUAL MUSCLE TESTING OF THE REGION

This section discusses gathering baseline information for the purpose of assessing specific conditions of the region.

Movements of the Region

Hip

The position of the knee can affect the hip's range of motion, so it is important to place the knee in a flexed position when appropriate. The range of motion of the hip is limited by bony and soft tissue restraints, and although the hip is a ball-and-socket joint, it is very stable. The proper assessment of various movements requires that the client assume different positions. Consider the client's limitations when deciding on positioning, and always perform painful movements last.

The hip is capable of six movements, which are assessed in the following manner:

- *Flexion (110° to 130°):* Have the client lie in the supine position and bring the knee to the chest, keeping the knee flexed.
- *Extension (10° to 15°):* Have the client lie in the prone position and lift the thigh off the table. Make sure that the motion arises only from the hip and that the lumbar spine does not extend as well.
- *Abduction (30° to 40°):* This can be assessed in two different positions. For the supine position, make sure the pelvis is neutral by checking the ASISs to see that they are aligned; have the client abduct the thigh as far as possible. The measurement is stopped when the pelvis begins to move. For the side-lying position, be sure the pelvis is "stacked" and not tilted in either direction; have the client abduct the hip until the pelvis begins to tilt.
- *Adduction (30°):* This can also be measured in two different ways. For the side-lying position, have the client bend the top leg and place the foot on the table in front of the straightened bottom leg, at the knee. Ensure that the pelvis is not tilted, and instruct the client to adduct the bottom leg off the table. End the measurement when the pelvis starts to move. For the supine position, level the pelvis by checking the ASISs; have the client lift the leg and bring it in front of the other leg, stopping the measurement when the pelvis begins to move.
- *Internal (medial) rotation (30° to 40°):* This can be assessed from either the seated or the prone position. For the seated position, have the client hang the leg off the table; place a towel under the thigh if necessary

> **Practical Tip**
> Keeping the hips stacked will produce a more accurate assessment of the range of motion.

to ensure that the thigh is level with the table. Have the client move the lower leg outward; this will internally rotate the hip. Be sure to prevent compensatory movements of the pelvis or lumbar spine. For the prone position, have the client bend the knee and let the lower leg fall out to the side. The measurement is stopped when the pelvis begins to move.

- *External (lateral) rotation (40° to 60°):* This can be assessed using the same positions as those for internal rotation. For the seated position, ensure that the thigh is parallel to the table, and have the client move the lower leg inward. Ensure that there are no compensatory movements, and stop the measurement when the pelvis moves. For the prone position, have the client bend the knee and rotate the lower leg inward across the other leg; stop the measurement when the pelvis begins to move.

Passive Range of Motion Perform passive assessment if the client's active range of motion is not full and you are unable to assess the end-feel of the joint. Take the joint to the end of its range, and apply a small amount of overpressure to assess the end-feel.

- *Flexion:* With the client in the supine position, have the client place the hand in the small of the back to prevent the pelvis from compensating. Flex the thigh, and allow the knee to bend. The normal end-feel is soft due to the tissue approximation of the thigh with the abdomen.
- *Extension:* Place the client in the prone position, and stabilize the pelvis. Extend the hip, and feel for the normal end-feel, which is firm due to the stretching of the anterior joint capsule and associated ligaments.
- *Adduction and abduction:* Place the client in the supine position for both of these tests. The pelvis should be level. For adduction, lift the thigh and bring it across the opposite leg. The end-feel is firm due to the restriction of the soft tissue structures. For abduction, move the thigh outward. The end-feel is also firm due to the tightness in the joint capsule and ligaments.
- *Internal and external rotation:* Place the client in the supine position for these tests. Flex the client's hip and knee to 90°; rotate the leg out to assess internal hip rotation and in to assess external hip rotation. The end-feel in both directions is firm due to the restrictions of the soft tissues.

Manual Muscle Testing When testing the strength of the hip muscles, stabilize the pelvis to prevent any muscle substitution. The hip muscles are extremely strong; therefore, remember to place the joint in the proper position, and instruct the client to resist movement. As with active movement, perform the most painful movements last.

- *Flexion:* Since several muscles cross the hip, it is important to perform the test in more than one position. With the client in the supine position, keep the knee straight, and raise the entire leg about halfway. Instruct the client to hold the leg in that position while you push the client into extension. The pressure should be applied at the lower leg unless there is knee pathology, in which case the pressure should be

⁕Practical Tip

Be sure to test the hip in various positions to assess the individual muscles of the area.

Part II Regional Approach to Treatment

applied proximal to the knee. With the client seated and the knee hanging off the table, have the client pick up the thigh and hold it off the table. Place the client's hand just proximal to the knee, and push on the top of the thigh back toward the table.

- *Extension:* This direction is also tested in more than one position to isolate various muscles. Place the client in the prone position, and instruct him or her to bend the knee to 90° and lift the thigh off the table and hold it. Press on the client's distal thigh, and try to push it down while the client resists. For the second test, have the client hold the leg straight and lift it off the table. Press down on the lower leg while the client resists.

- *Adduction:* Have the client lie on the side that is being tested and support the top leg by holding it at the knee. Instruct the client to raise the bottom leg off the table to meet the top leg and hold it there. Apply downward pressure on the medial epicondyle of the femur of the bottom leg while the client resists. An alternate test is to place the client in the supine position and start with both legs abducted. Apply pressure to the inside of the knee being tested, and instruct the client to resist the movement.

- *Abduction:* This test is performed with the client lying on the side, with the side being tested facing up. Have the client bend the bottom leg slightly for stability and abduct the top leg. Stabilize the client's pelvis and torso while applying pressure to the lateral knee. Instruct the client to resist the movement.

- *Internal and external rotation:* For these tests, place the client in a seated position with the legs hanging straight down off the table and a towel under the thigh to ensure that it is parallel to the table. For external rotation, stabilize the outside of the thigh of the leg being tested with one hand, and apply force at the distal lower leg to move it outward while the client resists. For internal rotation, stabilize the inside of the thigh of the leg being tested with one hand, and apply force to the outside of the lower leg to move it inward while the client resists.

- *Knee flexion and extension:* It is important to test these movements since the muscles that perform them cross the hip as well. Refer to the section below to see how to perform the tests.

Knee

The knee's range of motion is easier to assess because the knee performs fewer movements. Flexion and extension are easily measured; however, tibial rotation is more difficult to measure and must be approximated.

- *Flexion (135°):* Have the client lie in either the supine or the prone position and flex the knee as far as possible.

- *Extension (0° to -10°):* This is best tested with the client in the sitting position, but it can also be assessed with the client in the supine position. Have the client lie supine or sit on the edge of a table with the leg hanging down. Straighten the leg as far as possible. The presence of a condition known as *genu recurvatum,* or hyperextension of the knee, may result in extension past 0°. This is particularly prevalent in women.

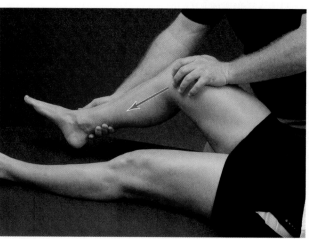

Practical Tip

Hyperextension of the knee will make it more susceptible to injury.

- *Tibial internal (medial) rotation (20° to 30°):* From the sitting position, the client should hang the leg off the table. Instruct the client to turn the foot in and internally rotate the tibia.
- *Tibial external (lateral) rotation (30° to 40°):* From the sitting position, the client should externally rotate the tibia by turning the foot outward.

Passive Range of Motion If the range of motion at the knee is not full, assess the passive range of motion by applying a slight overpressure at the functional end of the range.

- *Flexion and extension:* Place the client in the supine position for these assessments. For extension, place the hand closest to the client's feet under the ankle and the other hand just proximal to the knee. Apply gentle force to straighten the knee. The end-feel should be firm due to tissue stretch. Test flexion by grasping the client's ankle and bending the heel toward the gluteals. The end-feel should be soft due to tissue approximation of the calf and thigh.
- *Tibial medial and lateral rotation:* This is performed with the client in a seated position with the leg hanging off the table. Rotate the tibia in either direction to determine the end-feel, which should be firm as a result of the tissue stretch.

Manual Muscle Testing When testing the strength of the knee muscles, use several different joint angles to assess different portions of the muscles. Make sure that there is no contribution of the surrounding muscles other than those being tested.

- *Extension:* Place the client in the seated position with the leg hanging off the table. Extend the leg to the desired starting position, and instruct the client to resist while you apply force just proximal to the anterior ankle pushing the leg into flexion. Repeat at several starting angles.
- *Flexion:* Place the client in the prone position, and bend the knee to the desired starting position. Have the client resist while you pull him or her into extension, placing your hand just above the heel. Repeat at various starting positions.
- *Ankle plantar flexion:* This must be tested since the gastrocnemius has a function at the knee. With the client in the supine position and the leg straight, stabilize the anterior lower leg with one hand and press into the bottom of the foot with the other while instructing the client to resist.

Along with these manual muscle tests, there are specific tests to determine whether there is a neurologic component to any strength deficits. The tests to these myotomes are performed the same way as the other manual muscle tests:

- *L1-L2—hip flexion:* Have the client lie in the supine position. Flex the thigh to 40° while supporting the lower leg off the table. Place the other hand just proximal to the client's knee. While the client resists, try to move him or her into hip extension. Make sure the client does not increase his or her lumbar lordosis during this test.

- *L3—knee extension:* This can be performed with the client's leg hanging off the table. If the client is in the supine position, place one hand under the knee of the leg being tested and rest the other hand on the thigh of the opposite leg. Flex the client's knee to 30°, and apply force at the midshaft of the tibia while he or she resists.

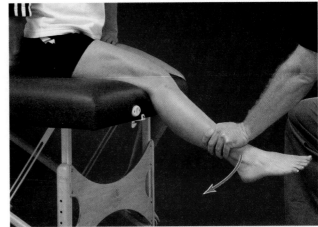

- *L4—ankle dorsiflexion:* Have the client lie in the supine position. Place his or her feet at 90° relative to the leg. Hold the tops of the feet, and push the client into plantar flexion while he or she resists.

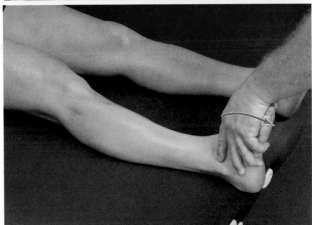

- *L5—great-toe extension:* Place the client in the supine position, and have him or her hold the great toes in a neutral position. Apply force to the tops of the toes while the client resists.

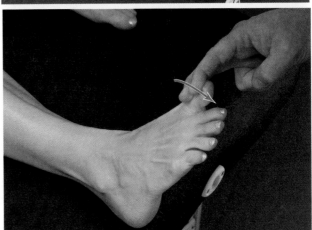

- *S1—ankle plantar flexion, ankle eversion, hip extension tests:*
  - *Ankle plantar flexion:* Have the client lie in the supine position and hold his or her feet in a neutral position. Have the client resist as you apply force on the bottom of the feet to push him or her into dorsiflexion.

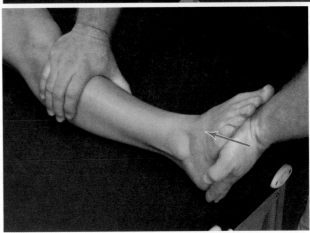

- *Ankle eversion:* Have the client resist as you apply force to the outside of the foot to move it into inversion.

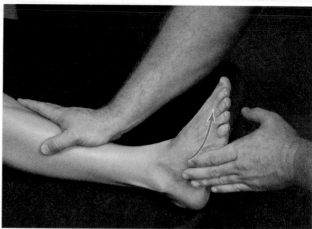

- *Hip extension:* This test is administered only if the client is unable to perform the other two. Have the client lie in the prone position and flex his or her knee to 90°. Lift the client's thigh off the table, and instruct the client to hold it there. Apply downward force to the thigh.

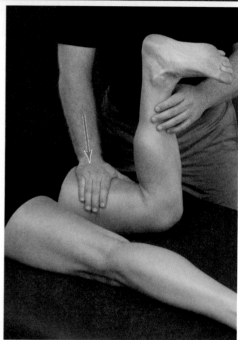

- *S1-S2—knee flexion:* Keep the client in the prone position, and flex the knee to 90°. Place the hand just proximal to the ankle, and apply force into extension while the client resists.

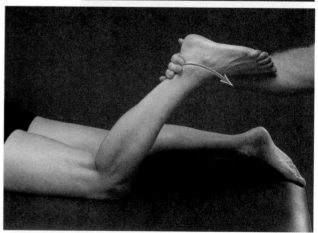

DERMATOMES FOR THE HIP AND KNEE

To assess any dysfunction in cutaneous sensations, check the dermatomes for any diminished functioning (Fig. 9-6). Use a blunt object, such as a fingertip, and a sharp instrument, such as the tip of a pen, to touch the various dermatomes. Ask the client to distinguish between the two

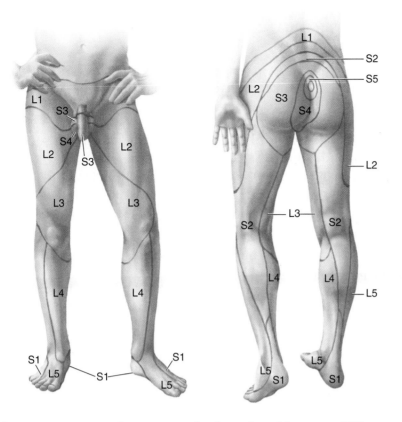

Figure 9-6 Dermatomes of the hip and knee.

types of instruments and to note whether the sides are different. Any discrepancies can be an indication of pathology, which will vary among individuals. Remember to stay in the middle of the dermatome to avoid any overlap between segments. The dermatomes for the hip and knee are summarized in Table 9-2.

Table 9-2 Dermatomes of the Hip and Knee

L1	Side of the hip over the trochanter; front of the hip into the groin
L2	Back, just over the PSIS running toward the trochanter; front of the thigh to the knee
L3	Back, upper gluteal along the iliac crest; front of the thigh, knee, and medial lower leg
L4	Inner gluteal; lateral thigh, running to the medial lower leg below the knee; top of the foot on the great-toe side, including the toes
L5	Gluteal; back and side of the thigh; lateral aspect of the lower leg; top of the foot on the lateral side, including the toes; distal medial sole of the foot including the first three toes
S1	Gluteal; back of the thigh and lateral lower leg; distal lateral sole of the foot, including the last two toes
S2	Same as S1
S3	Groin; inner thigh to the knee

TRIGGER-POINT REFERRAL PATTERNS FOR MUSCLES OF THE REGION

As with other regions, trigger points in the muscles of the hip and thigh can cause referral pain that mimics other conditions. It is important to consider all the possible etiologies of a condition to ensure that proper treatment is administered.

Earlier, the text noted that the hip muscles can develop trigger points that may affect the lumbar spine and sacrum. In addition, trigger points in the hip can affect the surrounding structures of the pelvis and the thigh.

Gluteus Maximus

There are three points in the *gluteus maximus* (see Figs. 9-7 and 9-9) that can refer pain. All the points refer to the general gluteal region; they do not travel any considerable distance and will cause pain and restlessness after long periods of sitting, as well as pain while walking uphill.

1. The first point is along the lateral edge of the sacrum about halfway down. Its referral pattern is a semicircular pattern up along the sacrum and natal cleft to the sacroiliac joint and down along the gluteal fold.

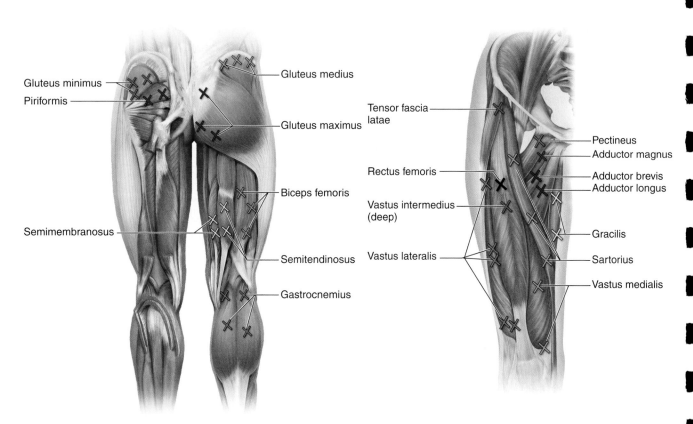

Figure 9-7 Trigger-point locations for the gluteus maximus, gluteus medius, gluteus minimus, piriformis, semitendinosus, semimembranosus, biceps femoris, and gastrocnemius.

Figure 9-8 Trigger-point locations for the tensor fascia latae, rectus femoris, vastus lateralis, vastus intermedius (deep), pectineus, vastus medialis, adductor magnus, adductor brevis, adductor longus, gracilis, and sartorius.

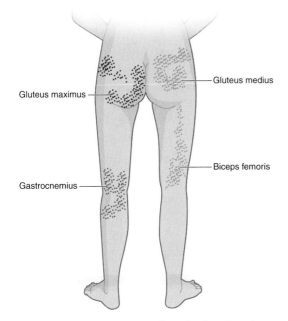

Figure 9-9 Trigger-point referrals for the gluteus medius, gluteus maximus, biceps femoris, and gastrocnemius.

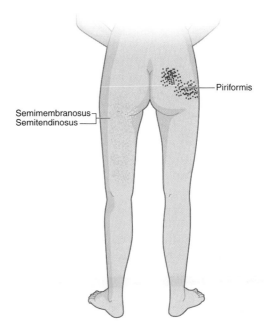

Figure 9-10 Trigger-point referrals for the semimembranosus, semitendinosus, and piriformis.

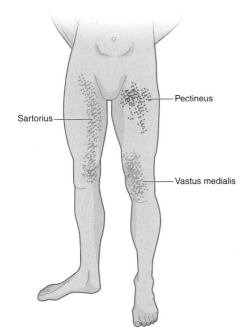

Figure 9-11 Trigger-point referrals for the pectineus, sartorius, and vastus medialis.

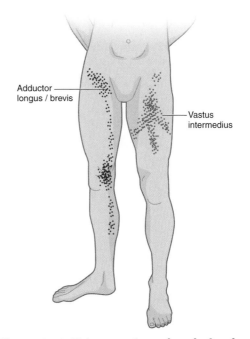

Figure 9-12 Trigger-point referrals for the adductor longus/brevis and the vastus intermedius.

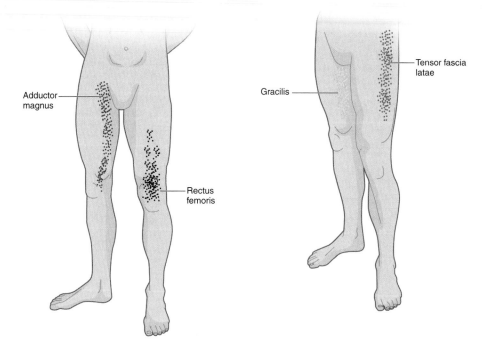

Figure 9-13 Trigger-point referrals for the adductor magnus and the rectus femoris.

Figure 9-14 Trigger-point referrals for the gracilis and the tensor fascia latae.

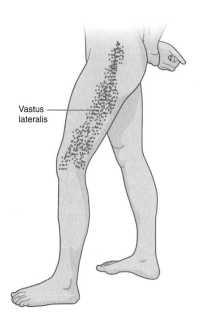

Figure 9-15 Trigger-point referrals for the vastus lateralis.

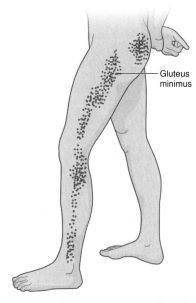

Figure 9-16 Trigger-point referrals for the gluteus minimus.

2. The second point is the most common and is located just superior to the ischial tuberosity. It refers to the entire buttock both superficially and deep, encompassing the entire sacrum and moving laterally just under the iliac crest.
3. The last point is located medial to the ischial tuberosity and refers to the coccyx; it is also often mistaken for problems with the coccyx.

Gluteus Medius

The *gluteus medius* (see Figs. 9-7 and 9-9) also has three points that can cause problems. Active trigger points in this muscle will cause the client to complain of pain on walking and sitting in a slumped position, as well as difficulty sleeping on the affected side.

1. The first point is located just inferior to the posterior iliac crest, near the sacroiliac joint. It refers along the crest and up into the sacroiliac joint and lumbar spine, over the sacrum, and can extend over much of the buttock.
2. The second point is located midway along the length of the muscle, just inferior to the iliac crest. Its referral is more lateral and to the midgluteal region, extending into the upper lateral thigh.
3. The last point is located just inferior to the crest, near the anterior superior iliac spine. Pain from this point travels along the crest and encompasses the lower lumbar and sacral region.

Gluteus Minimus

The last gluteal muscle, the *gluteus minimus* (see Figs. 9-7 and 9-16), has multiple trigger points located in both the anterior and posterior portions of the muscle. Common symptoms include hip pain that can affect gait, difficulty lying on the affected side, and difficulty standing after prolonged sitting. The two points are located in the anterior portion of the muscle, inferior to the anterior iliac crest. They refer pain to the lower lateral buttock and down the lateral thigh, along the peroneals sometimes as far as the ankle. The posterior points lie along the superior edge of the muscle and refer to most of the buttock and down the back of the thigh and into the calf.

Piriformis

Deep to the gluteals is the *piriformis* (see Figs. 9-7 and 9-10). It is another muscle that can lead to the misdiagnosis of sciatica because of its relationship with the nerve. Symptoms from trigger points in this muscle include pain and numbness in the low back, groin, buttock, hip, and posterior thigh and leg. These areas can be aggravated by prolonged sitting or through activity. There are two points located along the length of the muscle, one just lateral to the sacrum and the other just before the greater trochanter. The referral is over the sacroiliac region for the medial point and the posterior hip joint for the lateral point.

Tensor Fascia Latae

Covering the most anterior aspect of the gluteus medius, the *tensor fascia latae* (see Figs. 9-8 and 9-14) is often forgotten but can contribute to significant problems nonetheless. It is often termed "pseudotrochanteric bursitis" because of its referral pattern over the greater trochanter and down the anterolateral aspect of the thigh.

Clients will complain of deep hip pain that is exacerbated during movement of the hip. They are aware primarily of the pain around the greater trochanter and do not tolerate long periods of sitting with the hips flexed to 90° or more. The pain prohibits walking at a rapid pace and lying on the affected side. The point can become active through a sudden trauma such as landing on the feet from a high jump or through a chronic overload such as jogging on a foot that overpronates. It is located in the proximal third of the muscle and is found through the flat palpation method.

Practical Tip

Always keep in mind the possibility of a trigger point mimicking a pathology.

Sartorius

The trigger points in the sartorius muscle do not present in the same manner as those in other muscles. Instead, the pain from trigger points in the *sartorius* (see Figs. 9-8 and 9-11) refers up and down the thigh and in the knee region. It is described as a burst of superficial sharp or tingling pain and not the usual deep aching pain that is associated with other muscles. Clients will rarely present with pain that is caused solely by the sartorius. Rather, such pain usually occurs in conjunction with surrounding related muscles. The points are located superficially throughout the length of the muscle and do not limit range of motion or cause mechanical dysfunction. They are usually discovered with flat palpation after trigger points in related muscles are inactivated. Trigger points in this muscle can contribute to **meralgia paresthetica**. This condition arises as a result of the entrapment of the lateral femoral cutaneous nerve as it exits the pelvis. Symptoms include burning pain and paresthesias in the distribution of the nerve. Trigger points in the proximal portions of the sartorius can exacerbate these symptoms, while their inactivation can alleviate the symptoms.

meralgia paresthetica A condition that arises as a result of the entrapment of the lateral femoral cutaneous nerve as it exits the pelvis. Symptoms include burning pain and paresthesias in the distribution of the nerve.

Pectineus

Moving medially along the thigh, the *pectineus* (see Figs. 9-8 and 9-11) forms the floor of the femoral triangle and has a corduroy-like texture when palpated. The trigger points in this muscle are located just distal to the superior pubic ramus in the proximal portion of the muscle. Symptoms from this point include deep-seated groin pain just distal to the inguinal ligament that may continue to distribute to the anteromedial thigh. In addition to feeling pain, the client may also notice a limitation in abduction, especially in a seated "butterfly" position. As with the sartorius, this muscle is rarely the isolated source of pain and will be discovered only when trigger points in functionally related muscles are inactivated.

Adductor Longus and Brevis

Continuing medially along the thigh, the next two muscles have no real distinction in their pain patterns. The *adductor longus* and *adductor bre-*

vis (see Figs. 9-8 and 9-12) both refer proximally and distally. Symptoms of these points are typically noticed with vigorous activity or overload and not at rest. Trigger points in the proximal portion of the muscle refer deep into the groin and upper thigh, while the distal points refer to the upper medial knee and spill over onto the tibia.

Adductor Magnus

Sitting deep to all the adductors, the *adductor magnus* (see Figs. 9-8 and 9-13) is the largest of all the adductors. It has two main point locations that have very different referral patterns. The first point is more common and is located in the midportion of the muscle. It refers proximally into the groin and distally over the anteromedial aspect of the thigh almost to the knee. Clients will complain of deep groin pain, which may be misconstrued as pelvic pain, although no specific pelvic structure is identifiable. The second point is located in the proximal portion of the muscle, just below the ischial tuberosity. This pain refers proximally to the pelvis and is described as generalized internal pelvic pain; however, pain may also affect the pubic bone, the vagina, and the rectum. Regardless of the point's location, clients will have difficulty finding a comfortable position for the leg while sleeping.

Gracilis

Trigger points in the *gracilis* (see Figs. 9-8 and 9-14), the most medial adductor, are also not a common instigator of pain but are found when treating related muscles. The points are located in the midbelly of the muscles and refer locally around the points in a proximal and distal direction. The client will primarily complain of superficial, hot, stinging pain in the medial thigh. No change in position will reduce the symptoms; however, walking tends to relieve the pain.

Quadriceps Femoris Group

The quadriceps femoris muscles lie on the anterior thigh and form the quadriceps femoris group. As a group, trigger points in these muscles refer pain to the thigh and knee region. The trigger points may be activated through acute overloads, as in eccentric contractions, and may be perpetuated through exercise programs that encourage concentric strengthening of the muscles around the knee.

The first muscle of the group is the only one that crosses two joints. The *rectus femoris* (see Figs. 9-8 and 9-13) contains a trigger point that is located in the proximal end of the muscle, just under the anterior inferior iliac spine; it refers to the distal end of the muscle at the knee around the patella and sometimes deep into the joint. Clients will complain of pain in the front of the knee that awakens them at night, as well as the inability to find a comfortable position. Since this muscle is rarely lengthened at both attachments during normal daily activities, clients have trouble finding a movement that relieves the symptoms until they have been taught how to stretch the muscle fully.

The next muscle in this group is the *vastus medialis* (see Figs. 9-8 and 9-11), and it has two common trigger-point locations. The first point, which is more common, is located in the distal aspect of the muscle and refers to the front of the knee. The second point is located toward the proximal end of the muscle and refers along the anteromedial aspect of the thigh in a linear distribution. Clients with these points will complain of an initial deep ache in the knee that often interrupts sleep. Over a period of several weeks or months, pain will be replaced by an inhibition in the muscle. These unexpected episodes of weakness will cause the knee to buckle and will result in the client's falling.

The next muscle of the group is deep to the rectus femoris. The *vastus intermedius* (see Figs. 9-8 and 9-12) is sometimes called the "frustrator" because its points cannot be directly palpated. Its points are located in the proximal end of the muscle, near its origin, and refer distally over the thigh almost to the knee, with the most intense pain at the midthigh. Clients will complain of pain as well as difficulty extending the knee, especially after they have been immobile for extended periods of time. Pain occurs primarily during movement and rarely at rest.

The last muscle of the group is the largest. The *vastus lateralis* (see Figs. 9-8 and 9-15) has five main trigger-point locations located along the lateral thigh. These points can refer pain throughout the full length of the thigh and to the outside of the knee. The first point is located on the anterior aspect of the distal end of the muscle. It refers pain down the lateral aspect and into the knee. This point can also cause the patella to become immobilized, subsequently affecting gait. The second point is located in the posterior aspect of the distal end of the muscle. It also refers to the lateral knee, but primarily up the lateral thigh and down the lateral aspect of the lower leg. The third point is at the midthigh level on the posterolateral aspect of the muscle and generates pain in the lateral half of the popliteal space.

The next group of trigger points can cause severe pain over the entire length of the lateral thigh, sometimes as high as the iliac crest. They are located directly on the lateral aspect of the thigh. The last point is located at the proximal attachment at the greater trochanter and refers locally around the point. The client will complain of pain during walking and difficulty lying on the involved side, which disturbs sleep.

Hamstring Group

The hamstring group of muscles is located on the posterior thigh. The hamstrings consist of three muscles. Trigger points in the hamstrings cause pain while walking to the point that a client may limp. Another common complaint is pain over the posterior proximal thigh, buttock, and back of the knee while sitting. This thigh pain can mimic sciatica and result in a misdiagnosis. The two hamstrings on the medial side, the *semimembranosus* and *semitendinosus* (see Figs. 9-7 and 9-10) contain trigger points in the distal portion of the muscle. They refer primarily up to the gluteal fold and may spill over down the medial thigh to the medial calf. The lateral muscle of the hamstring, the *biceps femoris* (see Figs. 9-7 and 9-9), contains trigger points in the distal portion of both heads of the muscle and refers primarily to the back of the knee, with spillover distally below the lateral calf and proximally to the lateral thigh.

Gastrocnemius

The last muscle is in the *gastrocnemius* (see Figs. 9-7 and 9-9) in the lower leg; it crosses the knee joint and can cause pain in the area. It has trigger points in both heads of the muscle that tend to cluster in four locations. The first two points are located just proximal to the middle of the medial and lateral heads of the muscle. The point in the medial head is the most common. It refers primarily to the instep of the ipsilateral foot and will spill over down the medial aspect of the calf. The lateral point is the next most common and refers in a general pattern around the point. Both of these points are associated with calf cramping at night. The other two points lie behind the knee, near the medial and lateral attachment points of the femoral condyles. These points also refer to the general location around the point and cause posterior knee pain. Refer to the Quick Reference Table "Trigger Points of the Hip and Knee" at the end of this chapter (page 397).

SPECIFIC CONDITIONS

The hip and the knee are two very different regions of the body, and both can incur injuries from a variety of sources. Inherently, the stability of the hip is more susceptible to pathologies arising from chronic conditions than from acute trauma, although acute conditions can occur. While it is less stable than the hip, the knee is also susceptible to numerous pathologies from chronic conditions. The assessment of this region may be isolated to either the hip or the knee, or it may include the entire lower limb. Depending on the condition, the same structures can be involved in both regions, so similar treatments for both may be warranted. As with other regions, each client's treatment should be individualized to the situation.

Hip: Piriformis Syndrome

Background

Piriformis syndrome is part of a larger group of pathologies known as *nerve entrapment syndromes.*

Since its first mention in 1928 by Yeoman, there has been skepticism on whether piriformis syndrome actually exists, particularly because the condition is rare, it has a nonspecific clinical presentation, and there is no specific diagnostic technique to determine its presence. It is estimated that piriformis syndrome is the cause of up to 6% of all low-back pain and sciatica. Based on its location and its relationship with the sciatic nerve, Yeoman theorized that fibrosis of the piriformis along with sacro-iliac periarthritis could cause sciatica. In order to understand this theory, it is first necessary to look at the specific anatomy in the area.

The sciatic nerve arises from the lumbosacral plexus created by the ventral rami of L4 to S3. As the nerve leaves the sacrum, it travels through the sciatic notch of the pelvis, passing in proximity to the piriformis muscle before continuing between the ischial tuberosity and greater trochanter of the femur. It passes distally deep in the posterior thigh, branching

piriformis syndrome A nerve entrapment condition that involves the compression of the sciatic nerve and its branches by the piriformis. It can arise from trauma and chronic conditions and is characterized by pain in the hip and along the distribution of the sciatic nerve.

at the popliteal fossa into the tibial and peroneal nerves. The piriformis muscle is triangular-shaped and arises from the anterior sacrum. It inserts at the greater trochanter of the femur. Its relationship with the sciatic nerve is unique.

There are six different orientations that the two structures can take in relation to one another, as listed in Table 9-3. This anatomical relationship, combined with a causative factor, can lead to the syndrome.

Table 9-3 Anatomical Relationship of the Sciatic Nerve to the Piriformis

1. An undivided nerve passing under the muscle (This is the most common.)
2. A divided nerve passing through and below the muscle
3. A divided nerve passing through and above the muscle
4. A divided nerve passing above and below the muscle
5. An undivided nerve passing through the muscle
6. An undivided nerve passing above the muscle

Piriformis syndrome arises from a variety of causes and can involve both trauma and chronic overuse. Traumatic causes make up about 50% of the cases; however, the severity of the incident is not dramatic and may have occurred several months prior to the appearance of the first symptoms.

The initial trauma will lead to a spasm of the muscle and the release of inflammatory substances that can irritate the nerve, such as prostaglandins, histamines, and serotonin. When it comes to overuse causes, the muscle is involved throughout the entire gait cycle and is thus prone to hypertrophy, which can also put pressure on the nerve. Other etiologies include leg-length discrepancies, piriformis myositis, or abnormalities in either the muscle or the nerve. Its symptoms include posterior hip and gluteal pain along with radicular symptoms. There may be an increase in symptoms at night, difficulty walking up stairs, and pain with any activity that requires external hip rotation. This condition is six times as likely to affect women as men. There are six cardinal features of the condition overall:

- A history of trauma to the sacroiliac and gluteal region
- Pain in the sacroiliac joint, greater sciatic notch, and piriformis muscle that extends down the leg and causes difficulty walking
- Acute pain caused by stooping or lifting that is relieved by traction of the limb
- A tender, palpable mass over the piriformis
- A positive result from Lasegue's test
- Gluteal atrophy

Assessment

Because the etiology of piriformis syndrome is suspect and because it has a nonspecific clinical presentation, a thorough assessment is warranted to

Practical Tip

Remember that the initial trauma to the piriformis muscle could have occurred long before the symptoms arise.

ensure that proper treatment is administered. Since this syndrome falls under the broader classification of entrapment syndromes, be sure to expand the assessment area to related structures as needed.

Condition History Therapists should inquire about the following while taking the client's history:

Question	Significance
What is the client's gender?	Piriformis syndrome affects six times more women than men.
What is the history of injury in associated areas?	A history of low-back or pelvis pain can help identify the structures involved.
Is there a history of trauma? If so, what was the mechanism of injury, and how long ago did the incident occur?	Knowing the mechanism of injury can help identify the structures involved. Remember that symptoms may not present themselves for some time.
What is the presentation of the pain and other symptoms? Does the pain follow the sciatic nerve distribution, or are there any other symptoms, such as snapping, that occur?	This helps determine the involved structures.
What is the progression of the condition? Are the pain and the other symptoms getting better, worse, or staying the same?	This helps determine the severity of the condition.
What makes the condition better or worse?	This helps determine the severity of the condition.
What is the client's normal activity level?	Certain movement patterns or repetitive movements, such as those that require external rotation at the hip, can lead to the development of this condition.
Are there any movements that feel abnormal?	Compression of the sciatic nerve can lead to hip weakness.

Visual Assessment Ideally, the client should be observed entering the facility to notice any faulty gait patterns and obvious abnormalities. For someone with hip pain, the length of the step is typically shortened to minimize the amount of time weight is distributed on the involved leg. Additionally, the body weight is lowered carefully while the knee is bent to absorb any shock. Try to observe any swinging of the limb, which is an indicator of stiffness in the joint. Once the client is in the treatment room, he or she should be suitably disrobed in preparation for a proper visual assessment.

> **Practical Tip**
> The type of deviation in a gait pattern can be an indicator of where the pathology is located.

1. Begin by assessing posture from the front, side, and posterior views. Observe for any differences in the bony or soft tissue contours, and check for swelling. This may be difficult due to muscle bulk or excess soft tissue.

2. Look for unequal leg length, muscle contractures, or any type of scoliosis that will affect the position of the hips. Notice whether the client is willing to evenly distribute his or her weight, whether the limbs are symmetric, and whether there is any rotation.

3. Check the color and texture of the skin, and notice any scars, bruising, or other deformities.

Palpation For completeness, palpate the structures in the lumbar spine and the pelvis that were discussed in Chapter 6 (pages 159–165) because of their possible involvement at the hip. Begin with the lumbar spine and pelvis, and then move into the hip, paying special attention to the tension of the musculature in the area. Check for differences in tissue temperature, tone, deformity, point tenderness, and swelling between the sides. Check the iliopsoas for hypertonicity, as it has a significant effect on the movement of the sacroiliac joint, which can affect piriformis tightness. Palpate the structures discussed earlier in the chapter, and expand the area as necessary.

Orthopedic Tests Since this is a controversial condition, a variety of related tests for other pathologies—such as Lasegue's test, Gillet's test, and the slump test (see Chapter 6, pages 179–180 and 199)—may be used to rule out other conditions. Ruling out other possible pathologies, in combination with the information gathered from the history, visual assessment, range of motion, dermatomes, and myotomes, will ensure that the proper treatment is administered.

There is only one test for piriformis syndrome, and its goal is to re-create the symptoms of the condition by increasing the pressure on the sciatic nerve. Table 9-4 lists the test and explains how to perform it.

Table 9-4   Orthopedic Test for Piriformis Syndrome

Orthopedic Test	How to Perform
Piriformis test 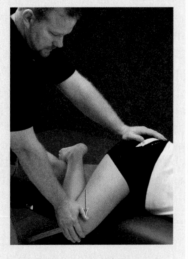	Client is in the side-lying position. Flex the top hip to 60°, and flex the knee so that the foot of the top leg rests on the knee of the bottom leg. Stand at the knee of the client, and stabilize the hip with one hand; then press the bent knee down toward the floor. If the piriformis is tight or is entrapping the sciatic nerve, this test will either increase the pain or re-create the symptoms, both of which indicate a positive test.

Soft Tissue Treatment

Whether this syndrome develops as a result of a trauma or chronic overuse, the primary structures involved are the muscles in the area; therefore, soft tissue work will be beneficial. The focus of the work should be on balancing the pelvis and removing muscle restrictions and tension in the hip rotators, as this will remove the pressure on the sciatic nerve.

Connective Tissue The symptoms of piriformis syndrome may not present for a long time. This will allow connective tissue restrictions to develop, which may exacerbate the condition. Spending some time releasing any connective tissue restrictions in the area will be beneficial to the client.

Prone Position Since the hip and low back are interdependent on each other, it is a good idea to include the lumbar spine in the treatment. Assess the superficial connective tissue of the lumbar spine from superior, inferior, medial, and lateral directions to determine the areas of restriction. Once the direction of the restrictions is determined, move into them until they release. Change the direction to include oblique angles to identify restrictions in those patterns, and move into them until they release as well. Drape the hip with the back, as described in Chapter 2, and assess superficial restrictions in the gluteals. To release them, stand at the side of the table opposite the side being worked, and work across from the PSIS to the greater trochanter.

Once the superficial restrictions are released in the low back and superior gluteals, move into the deeper layers and define the borders of the various muscles in the area. One important area to release is the border between the gluteus maximus and the gluteus minimus. Start at the PSIS and move on a line to the greater trochanter, separating the two muscles.

Two other important areas to focus on are the PSIS and the insertion of the hip rotators at the greater trochanter. Dysfunction in the sacroiliac joint can affect the piriformis, so ensuring its mobility by defining the PSIS and removing any restrictions can be beneficial for piriformis syndrome as well. Release the hip rotator insertions by tracing around the greater trochanter with the fingertips.

After releasing the connective tissue in the hip, move to the hamstring and inferior gluteals. Drape the bottom half of the hip with the leg, and assess the superficial tissue in all directions. Move into any restrictions until they release. Keep in mind that the hamstrings are a large muscle group and may take some time to release. Incorporating active engagement of the muscles can hasten the release. Once the superficial tissue has been released, strip out and define each hamstring to ensure that the hamstrings are not hindering any motion at the pelvis.

Supine Position Treating the connective tissue in this position is important because doing so will address any restrictions that may be indirectly related to the piriformis. As discussed previously, dysfunction in the pelvis can exacerbate this condition, so treating the muscles that affect the pelvis will ensure that the client receives the proper treatment.

Begin by assessing the superficial tissue of the quadriceps and adductors in all directions, moving into any restrictions until they release.

Work into the deeper layers by defining the quadriceps and adductors. For the adductors, flex the client's hip and knee, and externally rotate the hip for direct access to the adductors. Support the knee with a cushion so that the client is able to relax the leg. Pay special attention to the border between the rectus femoris and the vastus lateralis, as this area is usually tight. Be aware of the client's tolerance level because the adductors are typically a sensitive area. Move to the abdomen and release the connective tissue around the anterior iliac crest and along the inguinal ligament. Restrictions in these areas can have a dramatic effect on the pelvis.

Side-Lying Position This is the most effective position for directly addressing the hip. The superficial connective tissue should be sufficiently released from the other positions, but it should be checked to be sure. This is an ideal position for defining the borders of the gluteal muscles and the piriformis. Be sure to reorient yourself to the muscle in this position. This is also an ideal position for defining the borders of the tensor fascia latae.

Tissue Inconsistencies Several muscles are involved in this area; therefore, treating the trigger points can be a large task. Using the trigger-point section earlier in the chapter as a guide, begin with the muscles that are directly related to piriformis syndrome, such as the gluteals and rotators of the hip. Move into the surrounding areas of the hamstrings, quadriceps, adductors, and lumbar spine. Finally, expand to any compensatory musculature. Be sure to keep the intensity at 7 out of 10 on a pain scale, and use active and passive release techniques when appropriate.

Muscle Concerns

This region of the body functions as an integral part of our everyday lives, and any dysfunction can bring about drastic changes. The primary focus of treatment should be to remove pressure placed on the sciatic nerve by the piriformis muscle. Such pressure can be caused by the piriformis or through indirect compensation of the muscle due to problems in related areas; therefore, including associated areas is essential to providing effective treatment.

Prone Position With the client in this position, treat the muscles that attach to the iliac crest, sacrum, pelvis, and greater trochanter. Focus on the gluteals by using a loose fist and performing a stroke from the sacrum toward the table. Secure the sacrum, and do not pinch the tissue into the table. An effective stroke for the hip rotators is to bend the knee to 90° and place a loose fist in the tissue between the greater trochanter and the sacrum. Rotate the leg internally and externally while either holding static compression or performing a stroke in an inferior direction, down from the iliac crest. Perform fingertip friction along the lateral edge of the sacrum to release the gluteus maximus and just inferior to the iliac crest to release the gluteus medius and minimus. Use a forearm from either a superior or an inferior direction to effectively treat the lumbar spine.

Move into the hamstrings, and use a combination of the strokes discussed in earlier chapters to thoroughly treat the area. Use a forearm to treat the entire thigh, using deep effleurage, and stay aware of the client's tolerance level. Perpendicular compressive effleurage and deep parallel stripping work well on the hamstrings. To perform perpendicular compressive effleurage, place the heels of the hands on the middle of the muscle. Lean laterally so that you won't get kicked as the client moves his or her leg.

As the client slowly flexes the knee, slide the hands apart, finishing the stroke when the client finishes the contraction. Start at the distal end and work toward the proximal end. For deep parallel stripping, use either a broad surface such as a loose fist or a specific surface such as the thumbs or fingertips. Have the client flex the knee to 90°. Place your fist on the client's hamstrings at the knee, applying pressure in a proximal direction. As the client slowly extends the leg, your hand will move up the muscle a short distance. Repeat this process until the entire muscle is covered.

Supine Position Use this position to treat the quadriceps, adductors, and iliopsoas. Begin by treating the quadriceps with various strokes to loosen the tissue. Move deeper by using a loose fist or forearm, staying aware of the client's tolerance level. To incorporate movement, hang the client's leg off the side of the table at the knee, being sure to adjust the drape accordingly. Perform perpendicular compressive effleurage by placing the heels of the hands on the middle of the muscle and spreading them apart as the client slowly extends the leg. Position yourself so that you will not get kicked by the client. Begin at the distal end of the thigh, and move proximally until the entire muscle group has been addressed. For deep parallel stripping, begin in the same position, but have the client extend the knee to start. Place a fist or thumbs at the distal end of the muscle, directing the stroke proximally. As the client's knee flexes, your hand will move up the muscle a small distance. Repeat this process until the entire distance up the thigh has been covered. Repeat this process for each muscle in the group.

To treat the adductors, flex the client's knee and hip, and externally rotate the hip, supporting it with a bolster or pillow. Be specific to each muscle, using the various strokes discussed in the chapter. For the iliopsoas, have the client bend the knees to about 45° and place the feet on the table. Instruct the client to take a deep breath. Slide the fingertips in along the inside of the bowl of the pelvis, beginning at the ASIS as the client exhales and staying lateral to the edge of the rectus abdominus muscle. Once a restriction in the muscle has been identified, direct the pressure down toward the table. Have the client slowly extend the leg, keeping the heel on the table as he or she slides it as far as possible and brings it back up. Repeat this process several times.

Side-Lying Position Treat the muscle of the hip by performing radiating strokes out from the greater trochanter to the sacrum and iliac crest using a loose fist. If necessary, climb on the table behind the client, positioning the front leg at the client's midback and the knee at the client's thigh (Fig. 9-17). This will enhance biomechanics and provide more leverage if needed.

Another effective technique is to perform a forearm stroke to the hip and lateral thigh. Stand behind the client, and place a forearm at the anterior hip between the greater trochanter and the ASIS. Drag the forearm posteriorly, staying between

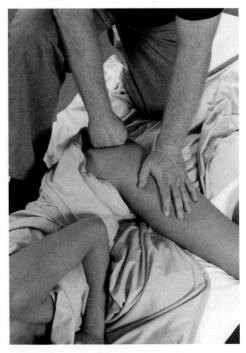

Figure 9-17 Side-lying work to the hip.

the greater trochanter and the sacrum, to the ischial tuberosity. Once at the tuberosity, move the forearm up and over the trochanter so that the elbow is not dragged directly over the bone. Continue the stroke down the lateral thigh as far as possible while maintaining proper body mechanics.

An effective technique for the hip rotators is to anchor the fingertips at the greater trochanter and perform cross-fiber effleurage to the hip rotators from the anterior to posterior hip. Repeat the stroke at increasing radii from the trochanter. This is also an effective way to address the tensor fascia latae. In this position, the muscle is on a line between the ASIS and the greater trochanter, and both parallel and cross-fiber strokes can be easily administered.

Stretching

Piriformis syndrome stems from the entrapment of the sciatic nerve by the piriformis muscle, so removing tension in the muscle is beneficial. The stretches in this section will benefit the piriformis as well as any other muscles that are contributing to the pathology. While this condition primarily affects the hip, the stretches for the lumbar spine in Chapter 6 are also beneficial for the overall flexibility of the region.

Gluteus Maximus Have the client lie in a supine position (Fig. 9-18). Move the leg not being stretched across the midline, and internally rotate it. Instruct the client to take a deep breath and exhale as he or she flexes the hip of the side being stretched toward the opposite shoulder. If the client experiences a pinching sensation in the groin, have him or her circumduct the leg out and up toward the same shoulder before bringing it across. Stabilize the other leg while assisting the stretch once the client has reached the end of the range of motion. Return to the starting position with the thigh pointing straight up. Hold the stretch for 2 seconds, and perform one to two sets of 10 repetitions.

Hip Rotators There are three different stretches for the hip rotators:

1. To stretch the hip external rotators, place the client in the prone position and secure the client by using a seat belt across the sacrum to prevent compensation (Fig. 9-19). Sit on the table, and bend the client's

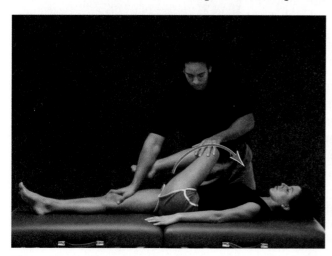

Figure 9-18 Gluteus maximus stretch.

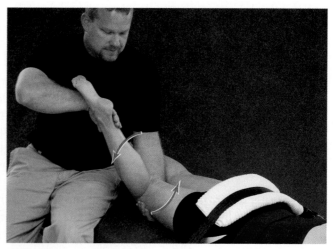

Figure 9-19 External hip rotator stretch.

knee to 90°. Cup the front of the thigh at the knee with one hand, and hold the foot with the other. Instruct the client to take a deep breath and exhale as he or she internally rotates the thigh. At the end of the range, assist the motion by applying pressure to rotate the thigh. To address the various external rotators, perform the stretch in three different positions: First have the legs together, and then abduct the client's thigh two times, 10° each time. It is important not to apply too much pressure to the ankle, as it will put too much stress on the knee. Return to the starting position, and perform one to two sets of 10 repetitions at each angle.

✦ Practical Tip

Be sure not to put too much pressure on the ankle.

2. To stretch the internal rotators of the hip (Fig. 9-20), begin with the client in the same position as that for the external hip rotators. Bring the leg that is not being stretched about 15° across the midline, and internally rotate it. Place the top hand under the front of the client's thigh just above the knee and the other hand on the outside of the foot. Instruct the client to take a deep breath and exhale as he or she externally rotates the thigh. At the end of the range, assist the client in the same direction by rotating the thigh with the hand that is supporting it while applying gentle pressure to the outside of the lower leg. This stretch should be performed in three positions, extending and adducting the thigh 5° two additional times. Have the client contract the abdominals and rotate the thigh slowly so as to not irritate the back. Perform one to two sets of 10 repetitions at each position.

3. The last rotator stretch targets the piriformis directly. Begin with the client in the supine position (Fig. 9-21). Have the client bring the leg that is not being stretched across the midline and internally rotate it. Instruct the client to bend the knee, bring it toward the bottom rib of the opposite side, and hold it with his or her hand. Keep a 90° bend in the knee. Instruct the client to internally rotate the thigh and move the foot toward the table while exhaling. Keep the knee at 90°, and prevent the thigh from performing any movement other than rotation. Assist in the same direction at the end of the range by applying force to the outside of the lower leg. Return to the starting position, and repeat for one to two sets of 10 repetitions.

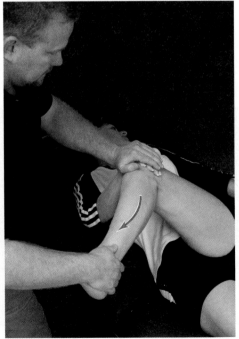

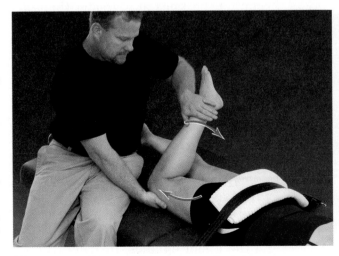

Figure 9-20 Internal hip rotator stretch.

Figure 9-21 Piriformis stretch.

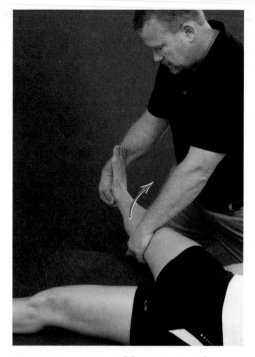

Figure 9-22 Hip adductor stretch.

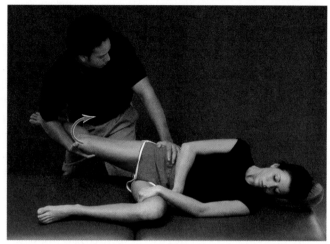

Figure 9-23 Iliopsoas stretch.

Adductors Moving into the thigh, stretch the adductors with the client in a supine position, and externally rotate and abduct the leg not being stretched for stability (Fig. 9-22). Stand at the side of the client, and instruct him or her to internally rotate the leg being stretched as far as possible. While exhaling, the client should abduct the leg as far as possible. Meet the leg as it comes off the table, supporting it at the inside of the knee and the heel. Assist in the same direction after the client has reached the end of the range. Hold the stretch for 2 seconds, and return to the starting position. Repeat for one to two sets of 10 repetitions.

Iliopsoas To stretch the iliopsoas, have the client lie on his or her side and pull the bottom leg up to the chest and hold it (Fig. 9-23). Place the hand that is closest to the client's head on the client's hip to keep it from rolling backward. The client's bottom hand will support the thigh at the knee, keeping the knee at a greater-than-90° angle. Instruct the client to extend the top thigh back as far as possible, and assist him or her in the same direction at the end range. Repeat for two sets of 10 repetitions. This stretch will also affect the proximal rectus femoris. The other muscles of the quadriceps group are discussed later in the chapter.

Hamstrings Stretch the hamstrings with the client in the supine position. Have the client slightly bend the leg that is not being stretched (Fig. 9-24). As the client exhales, instruct him or

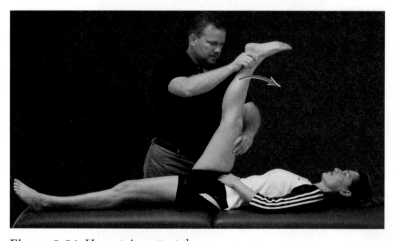

Figure 9-24 Hamstring stretch.

her to lock the knee and lift the entire lower limb off the table as high as possible. At the end of the motion, assist in the same direction with one hand just above the client's anterior knee to help it stay straight and one hand under the distal lower leg. It is very important to make sure that the client keeps the knee as straight as possible to get the most effective stretch. Return to the starting position, and repeat for two to three sets of 10 repetitions. Isolate the individual hamstrings by internally and externally rotating the thigh and performing the stretch the same way.

Hip: Iliotibial Band Friction Syndrome

Background

Iliotibial band friction syndrome (ITBFS) is a common overuse injury that usually presents as lateral knee pain. It is caused by excessive friction between the distal iliotibial band and the lateral condyle of the femur, and it results in inflammation and pain. ITBFS is the most common cause of lateral knee pain in runners, contributing to as many as 12% of all running-related overuse injuries (Fredericson et al., 2005). The iliotibial band is a continuation of the tendons of the tensor fascia latae and gluteus maximus muscles. It travels down the lateral side of the thigh and is connected to the linea aspera through the deep lateral intermuscular septum, and then it fans out at its distal end to insert primarily at Gerdy's tubercle. It also has insertions on the lateral border of the patella and the lateral retinaculum.

Iliotibial band friction syndrome has a very clear pathophysiology and occurs when the distal iliotibial band, which lies anterior to the femoral condyle in knee extension, slides posteriorly over the condyle when the knee flexes between 0° and 30°. The area where the condyle and iliotibial band (ITB) come into contact is called the *impingement zone,* and the greatest point of friction occurs when the knee is in 30° of flexion. This repetitive sliding over the condyle can cause the band to thicken and the space deep to the band, known as the *lateral synovial recess,* to become inflamed and filled with fluid. Pain presents 2 to 3 centimeters above the lateral joint line over the lateral condyle of the femur and tends to be worse between foot strike and midstance of the gait cycle. Pain may increase after running or walking downhill.

Few studies show a direct relationship between biomechanical factors and the development of this syndrome; however, individuals with genu varum at the knee, excessive pronation at the foot, leg-length discrepancies, patellar tracking problems, and weak hip abductors seem to be more prone to the condition.

Assessment

Fortunately, ITBFS has a very clear pathology, so it is relatively easy to assess clinically; however, it can be a challenge to treat. Assessment of this condition includes components from both the hip and the knee, but since the ITB functions as the tendon of insertion for the gluteus maximus and tensor fascia latae, it should be included in the hip assessment section. Performing a thorough assessment will ensure that no related areas are contributing to the condition.

iliotibial band friction syndrome (ITBFS) A common overuse injury caused by excessive friction between the distal iliotibial band and the lateral condyle of the femur, resulting in inflammation and pain.

Practical Tip
A classic sign of ITBFS is that the pain over the lateral knee gets worse as the activity continues.

Condition History Therapists should inquire about the following when taking the client's history:

Question	Significance
Was there trauma involved?	ITBFS is traditionally a chronic overuse condition and not usually associated with direct trauma.
Where is the pain?	Pain will present over the lateral epicondyle of the femur.
Is there any clicking or popping?	A tight ITB can cause a snapping noise as it moves over the greater trochanter. This is referred to as *external snapping.*
When does the pain occur?	Typically, the pain will become worse as the duration of the activity increases.
What are the client's normal activities and habits?	This condition will normally affect clients who perform some type of repetitive behavior such as running or cycling.

Visual Assessment Depending on how long the client has been experiencing symptoms, there may be no obvious outward visual signs. Observe the client's gait to see whether there is any compensation for pain, especially from foot-strike through midstance, as this is when the pressure on the ITB is the greatest. The client may limp or walk with the leg straighter than normal to minimize discomfort. Observe posture from the anterior and posterior to determine whether there is any genu varus of the knees or excessive pronation of the foot, both of which are predisposing factors. Check for any obvious deformity, swelling, or bruising over the leg, especially directly over the lateral femoral epicondyle.

Palpation Check the overall tension in the muscles of the area. The quadriceps, hamstrings, and iliotibial band will generally be hypertonic if there is pathology in the area. Feel for swelling and deformities, noting any inconsistencies. Include all the structures covered earlier in the chapter, and expand the area for compensation as needed.

Orthopedic Tests After completing the visual assessment, the history, and the assessment of active and passive ranges of motion, dermatomes, and myotomes, use orthopedic tests to complete the picture of the pathology and ensure that the proper treatment is given. Two orthopedic tests are used to determine the presence of ITBFS, as shown in Table 9-5.

> **Practical Tip**
>
> Be sure to keep the hips stacked for an accurate test.

Soft Tissue Treatment

This condition involves muscle tendon tension; therefore, treatment using soft tissue techniques is extremely beneficial. Even though the pain presents at the knee, the entire leg must be treated due to the ITB's relationship to the muscles of the area, particularly the gluteus maximus and tensor fascia latae. The focus should be to remove any tension in the ITB in order to reduce friction at the femoral epicondyle.

Table 9-5 Orthopedic Tests for ITBFS

Orthopedic Test	How to Perform
Ober test 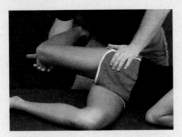 *Note:* First described in 1936, this test is widely accepted for this condition (Gajdosik et al., 2003). It is used to determine the length of the iliotibial band, which can predispose a client to developing pathology in the area or can exacerbate an existing condition.	Place the client on his or her side with the bottom hip and knee bent to 90° for stability. Stand behind the client. With the hand closest to the client's head, stabilize the client's hip so that he or she does not roll anteriorly or posteriorly and the iliums are on top of or "stacked" on each other. Instruct the client to bend the top knee to 90°. Support the client's leg at the knee with the other hand. Keep the leg parallel to the table, and passively extend the client's hip slightly. While keeping the client's hips stacked, slowly lower the top leg. The client's leg should drop below horizontal. If it doesn't, this is an indication of tightness in the iliotibial band and constitutes a positive test.
Noble compression test 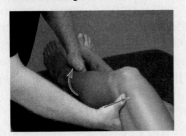 *Note:* This is a pain provocation test and is used to determine involvement at the knee.	Place the client in a supine position with the hip flexed to 45° and the knee flexed to 90°. Apply pressure with the thumb either to the lateral epicondyle of the client's femur or about ½ inch above the epicondyle. Passively extend the client's leg while maintaining pressure. When the leg approaches about 30° of flexion, the client will report feeling pain similar to that which occurs during activity. This indicates a positive test.

Connective Tissue The iliotibial band is a large strap of connective tissue that runs the length of the lateral thigh. Since this is a long tendon, connective tissue work is ideal for this condition. Remember that some tension is normal for the band, so it will only release to a certain extent.

Prone Position Begin working on the gluteals by draping the top of the hip with the back and assessing the superficial restrictions. Move into any restrictions until they release by standing at the side of the table opposite the side on which you are working, and work across from the PSIS to the greater trochanter.

Once the superficial restrictions have been addressed, release the deeper restrictions between the muscles of the hip, particularly the border between the gluteus maximus and the gluteus minimus, by moving on a line from the PSIS to the greater trochanter, separating the two muscles. Address the restrictions around the PSIS and the insertions of the hip rotators at the greater trochanter.

Move to the hamstrings and assess the superficial tissue in all directions. Move into any restrictions until they release. Be patient—this may take longer than expected because this is a large muscle group; however, actively engaging the muscles can speed up the process. Once the superficial tissue has been released, strip out and define each hamstring to ensure that the hamstrings are not hindering motion at the pelvis.

In this position, the distal ITB can be accessed quite easily. Redrape the leg slightly; then flex and externally rotate the hip and flex the knee so that the lateral side of the knee is facing up toward the ceiling. Strip out on either side of the band, paying attention to the client's tolerance level.

Supine Position Assess the superficial tissue of the quadriceps and adductors in all directions, moving into any restrictions until they release. Define the individual muscles in the quadriceps and adductors, paying special attention to the border between the vastus lateralis and rectus femoris. The lateral quadrant around the patella and lateral joint line should be addressed both generally and specifically to remove any connective tissue restrictions, as the iliotibial band attaches to the patella and Gerty's tubercle. The anterior border of the ITB can be easily accessed in this position and separated from the vastus lateralis as much as possible.

Side-Lying Position In this position, the ITB is facing directly up and can therefore be treated effectively. Assess the superficial tissue of the hip as well as the lateral thigh, and move into any restrictions. Identify the border between the tensor fascia latae and the gluteus medius to separate the two. The insertion tendons around the greater trochanter can be treated effectively in this position by using the fingertips to define the trochanter. Try to lift off the ITB from the lateral thigh by stripping along its borders from insertion to origin. This may be difficult since the deep intermuscular septum attaches the ITB to the femur.

Another useful technique is to mobilize the ITB. Begin by hooking into the posterior border and applying anterior force as the client externally rotates the hip; then hook into the anterior border to the band and apply posterior force as the client internally rotates the hip. Move up and down the thigh to mobilize the entire length of the band.

Tissue Inconsistencies The entire thigh can be affected by this pathology, even though only two muscles are attached to the ITB. Many of the trigger points can mimic the pain of this syndrome, so they must be released. Address the trigger points of all the muscles listed earlier in the chapter, beginning with the gluteus maximus and tensor fascia latae. Move into the quadriceps and hamstrings, keeping the intensity at 7 out of 10 on a pain scale and using movement to increase the treatment's effectiveness.

Muscle Concerns

Removing tension imbalances between the muscles of the hip and leg should be a primary focus when treating this pathology. It may be necessary to include compensatory regions in the treatment, depending on how long the client has had the condition and its severity. Incorporating movement can enhance the treatment, as well.

Prone Position Focus on the gluteals and hip rotators in this position. Bend the knee to 90°, and place a loose fist in the tissue between the greater trochanter and the sacrum. Hold static compression, or perform a stroke from the sacrum down to the table while rotating the leg internally and externally. Friction along the lateral edge of the sacrum is effective at helping to release the gluteus maximus.

Once the area is warmed up, use a forearm effleurage stroke to treat the entire thigh, staying aware of the client's tolerance level. Two useful strokes on the hamstrings are perpendicular compressive effleurage and deep parallel stripping while incorporating active movement. To perform perpendicular compressive effleurage, place the heels of the hands on the middle of the muscle. Slide the hands apart as the client slowly flexes the knee, finishing the stroke when the client finishes the contraction. Start at the distal end, and work toward the proximal end. For deep parallel stripping, have the client flex the knee to 90°, and place either the fist or the thumbs on the hamstrings at the knee, applying pressure in a proximal direction. As the client slowly extends the leg, move up the muscle a short distance. Repeat this process until the entire muscle is covered.

Supine Position Focus on the quadriceps in this position, and make sure they are thoroughly warmed up using various strokes. Use a forearm or loose fist to work into the deeper layers of the muscle. Incorporate movement by hanging the client's leg off the side of the table at the knee, adjusting the drape accordingly. Use both perpendicular compressive effleurage and deep parallel stripping, as described for piriformis syndrome. Position yourself at the lateral side of the leg so that you do not get kicked as the client extends the leg. Friction around the iliotibial band, patella, and lateral joint line is helpful at removing tension in the area.

Side-Lying Position This position is ideal for treating the hip and lateral thigh. Perform radiating strokes out from the greater trochanter to focus on the gluteals and hip rotators. Climb on the table if necessary, as described earlier, to enhance body mechanics (see Fig. 9-18). Thumb-stripping strokes can be applied to the tensor fascia latae very effectively in this position to address restrictions in the muscle. Perform a forearm stroke to the hip and lateral thigh by standing behind the client and placing a forearm at the anterior hip between the greater trochanter and the ASIS. Run the forearm posteriorly, staying between the greater trochanter and the sacrum, to the ischial tuberosity. Once at the tuberosity, move the forearm up and over the trochanter, continuing down the lateral thigh as far as possible while maintaining proper body mechanics. Another direct way to address the ITB is to stand at the client's knee and perform strokes from the knee toward the hip. Compression broadening is very effective in this position. Defining strokes to the distal ITB while the client flexes and extends the knee will release restrictions in the area.

Stretching

Increasing flexibility in the ITB is beneficial for treating this condition; however, finding a stretch that effectively accomplishes this goal can be

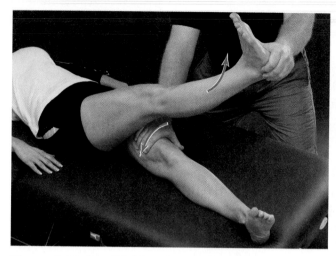

Figure 9-25 Iliotibial band stretch—phase 1.

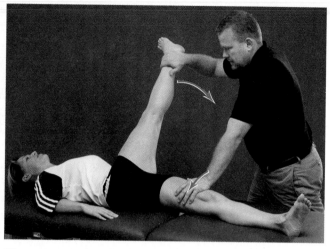

Figure 9-26 Iliotibial band stretch—phase 2.

challenging. There are many stretches that can be effective for the ITB, including those discussed below. In addition to using these specific stretches, use the stretches for the gluteals, hip rotators, quadriceps, and hamstrings (see Figs. 9-18 to 9-24) to ensure the overall flexibility of the region.

Stretch 1: The first stretch has two phases and is performed with the client in the supine position. For the first phase, instruct the client to move the leg that is not being stretched across the midline and internally rotate the thigh (Fig. 9-25). Have the client take a deep breath and, while exhaling, externally rotate the leg being stretched and lift it up and across the other leg while keeping the knee locked. It is important to make sure that the client keeps the knee locked and only lifts the leg high enough to clear the leg on the table. Using your top hand, assist as the client internally rotates the leg, and assist the leg moving across in the same direction by grasping the heel when it reaches the end of the range. Return to the starting position, and repeat for two sets of 10 repetitions.

For the second phase, begin in the position used for the first phase (Fig. 9-26). Have the client externally rotate the leg being stretched, lift it straight up, and bring it straight across the other hip. Maintain the internal rotation of the client's leg that is not being stretched while assisting the stretch in the same direction at the client's end range. Instruct the client to hold the table or use a seat belt across the hips to ensure that the hip does not come off the table too much. Repeat for two sets of 10 repetitions.

Stretch 2: The next stretch is a modified yoga pose known as the *one-legged king pigeon pose* (Fig. 9-27). Have the client get on his or her hands and knees so that the back is flat. Have the client bring the knee of the leg that is being stretched to the center of the body at the level of the chest. Cross the entire opposite leg over the leg that is being stretched, and slide backward. The client will feel this more in the hip and can shift his or her body weight and the angle of the back leg to adjust the stretch. Even though the pain is at the knee in ITBFS, it is important to stretch the entire hip complex. To focus the stretch down the outside of the thigh, before sliding back, straighten

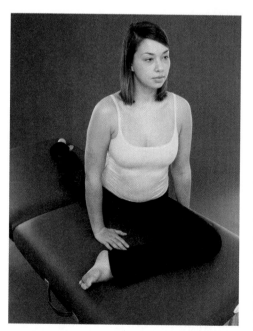

Figure 9-27 The pigeon yoga pose.

the leg that is bent as far as possible; then slide back. The straighter the leg gets, the more the iliotibial band stretches. Hold this pose for 30 seconds, and repeat several times for each leg.

Knee: Patellofemoral Dysfunction

Dysfunction in the patellofemoral articulation can lead to a pain syndrome known as **patellofemoral pain syndrome (PFPS)**. This is anterior knee pain caused by abnormal motion of the patella in the trochlear groove, which results from biochemical and/or physical changes within the patellofemoral joint (Green, 2005). The patellofemoral joint is one of the highest-loaded musculoskeletal components in the body and is therefore one of the most difficult areas in which to restore normal functionality after injury (Dye, 2005). Symptoms of patellofemoral problems can include:

- Anterior knee pain exacerbated by squatting
- Sitting for prolonged periods of time (movie theater sign)
- Ascending or descending stairs
- Point tenderness over the lateral facet of the patella
- Crepitus
- Possible catching or locking at the knee
- A sensation of stiffness or swelling

The dysfunction in the joint is a conglomeration of several factors that can result in a variety of conditions. These pathologies are often looked at as individual conditions but actually fall under this broader umbrella.

The patellofemoral articulation consists of the patella, the quadriceps and patellar tendons, and the four muscles of the quadriceps group. There are other soft tissue structures that help hold the patella in check, such as the medial and lateral retinacula and fibers from the iliotibial band. The articular side of the patella has various facets that contact the trochlear groove of the femur at different points during movement.

The patella's job is to protect the anterior portion of the knee and absorb joint forces, as well as enhance the mechanical advantage of the extensor mechanism of the quadriceps. As the knee moves, the surface of contact between the patella and the trochlear groove of the femur constantly changes to optimize the efficiency of the lever by magnifying either force or displacement. As the knee flexes, the patella moves downward until, at 90°, only the top portion is in contact with the femur. This reverses during extension until, at 0°, there is no contact between the patella and the femur. On the surface, movement of the patella during flexion and extension seems simple; however, the stability of the patellofemoral joint occurs as a result of a complex interaction between a range of factors, both static and dynamic (Farahmand et al., 2004). Any disruption of these factors can result in a variety of pathologies that have plagued the medical community.

The misalignment of the patellofemoral joint may arise from anatomical factors that are outside the body's control. The shape of the patella itself can affect its function: If the articular facets are misshapen or the patella is smaller or larger than normal, its mobility in the trochlear notch can be affected. The depth of the trochlear groove can affect how the patella tracks: The more shallow the groove, the less stable the patella, due to the lateral facet of the patella being poorly buttressed by the lateral face

patellofemoral pain syndrome Anterior knee pain caused by abnormal motion of the patella in the trochlear groove, which results from biochemical and/or physical changes within the patellofemoral joint.

of the sulcus of the trochlear notch; hence, the greater the chance to have a tracking problem.

Soft tissue structures can affect the functioning of the joint, as well. Normally, the length of the patellar tendon should be as long as the long axis of the patella, resulting in the inferior pole of the patella lining up with the upper margins of the femoral trochlea. If the patellar tendon is longer than normal, the patella rides higher in the trochlea. This condition is known as *patella alta.* Because the patella rides higher on the femur, it has a greater chance of mistracking. A quick way to check for patella alta is to have the client seated with the hip and knee at 90°. The patella should normally be perpendicular to the floor. In patella alta, however, it will be angled 45° to the floor. If there is an abnormally short tendon, the patella rides lower in the groove, resulting in a condition known as *patella baja,* which can also lead to instability of the patella in the groove. A tight lateral retinaculum, ITB, or vastus lateralis tendon will result in the lateral pull of the patella or the tilting up of the medial edge of the patella, thereby causing an uneven load distribution and excessive pressure on the lateral facet.

Imbalance in the musculature around the knee can cause the patella to track one way or the other. The vastus medialis has fibers in its distal end that attach to the superomedial aspect of the patella about one-third of the way down the patella at a 55° angle. This region of the muscle is known as the *vastus medialis obliquus (VMO)* and is arguably the most important muscle around the knee in regard to patellar mechanics (Grelsamer et al., 1998). It is the only muscle that dynamically moves the patella medially and restrains the patella's tendency to track laterally. In normal knees, the VMO should fire at the same time or just before the vastus lateralis to maintain proper tracking; however, in abnormal knees, the VMO fires late, a phenomenon that can be caused by pain or swelling. An accumulation of only 20 to 30 milliliters of excess fluid within the capsule can neurologically inhibit the VMO, compared to 50 to 60 milliliters of fluid for the rest of the extensor mechanism. The late firing of the vastus medialis allows the larger, stronger vastus lateralis to have a greater effect on the patella, pulling it laterally.

Another cause of patellofemoral dysfunction is the posture of various structures around the knee and at the hip. At the hip, **anteversion** will lead to an internal rotation of the femur, resulting in a misalignment known as *squinting patella,* which means that the patellas are oriented as if they were looking at each other even though the feet are pointed straight ahead. This misalignment can also come from an internally rotated femur or tibia and causes an increased valgus force at the knee, leading to lateral tracking tendencies.

"Frog-eyed" patella is so-named because the patellas are aligned as if they were looking away from each other. This originates from the hip as a result of retroversion or from an externally rotated femur or tibia. The orientation of the knee can also be a factor in misalignments. The presence of genu valgum, or "knock-knees," can place excessive strain on the medial facet of the patella due to the increase in lateral forces created by the posture. Genu varus, or "bowlegged," posture can increase the compressive forces on the lateral facet of the patella. Also, a difference in the length of the legs can cause an abnormal posture at the knee.

There are two types of leg-length discrepancies: true leg-length discrepancy and functional leg-length discrepancy: True shortening comes from an anatomical or structural change in the lower leg, which is either a congenital

anteversion An excessive internal rotation of the shaft of the femur in relation to the neck.

condition or the result of trauma. Functional shortening is typically a result of compensation for a posture, such as scoliosis or unilateral foot pronation. These differences in leg length cause abnormal rotations and postures in the hip and knee and can contribute to a variety of pathologies.

A measurement taken at the knee can help identify a tracking problem. The **quadriceps angle (Q angle)** is a measurement of the patellofemoral mechanics that is a reasonable estimate of the force between the quadriceps group and the patellar tendon (Herrington et al., 2004). The concept was first described in 1964 by Brattstrom and is one of the few measurements of the patellofemoral joint mechanics that does not require sophisticated equipment (Wilson et al., 2002). The angle is formed by the intersection of two lines (Fig. 9-28). One line is drawn from the anterior superior iliac spine (ASIS) through the midpoint of the patella. The other line is drawn from the midpoint of the patella through the tibial tuberosity. The intersection of these lines forms the Q angle. A normal angle is 13° in men and 18° in women. One theory that seeks to explain this difference in angles between men and women suggests that it is because women have a wider pelvis than men; however, there is little evidence to support this. An angle of greater than 15° to 20° is thought to contribute to knee extensor mechanism dysfunction and is regarded as an anatomical risk factor in the development of lateral patella malpositioning (Herrington et al., 2004).

Although the Q angle is an important factor in patellar mistracking, it is not the only factor. Numerous clients who have patellofemoral problems have normal Q angles, and some clients have angles that should cause dysfunction but do not. Discrepancies over what constitutes "normal" anatomy, as well as the accuracy of the measurements and the fact that the Q angle is a static measurement, demonstrate that patellofemoral functioning is based on a cluster of findings from a number of factors that contribute to the overall extensor mechanism.

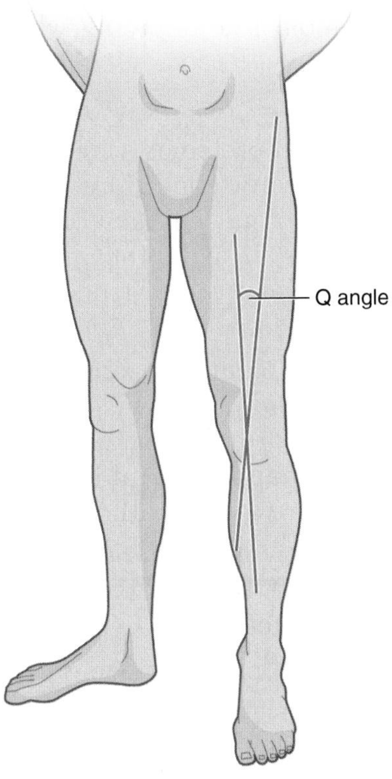

Chondromalacia patella and patellar tendonosis are two of the more common pathologies associated with patellofemoral dysfunction. **Chondromalacia patella** is the result of prolonged exposure to excessive compressive forces or abnormal shear forces due to patellar mistracking. These forces result in a softening and degeneration of the articular cartilage of the patella. Chondromalacia has four stages of progression:

Stage I: The cartilage softens.

Stage II: The cartilage starts to crack, and fissures develop.

Stage III: The cartilage is characterized by fibrillation, a fraying of the cartilage, which gives it an appearance similar to crabmeat.

Stage IV: The cartilage reveals defects so large that the subchondral bone is exposed. Even though there is a change in the tissue itself, it should not be looked at as a primary source of knee pain.

Figure 9-28 The Q angle.

quadriceps angle (Q angle) A measurement that is used to determine the patellofemoral mechanics and is a reasonable estimate of the force between the quadriceps group and the patellar tendon.

chondromalacia patella A condition that is the result of prolonged exposure to excessive compressive forces or abnormal shear forces due to patellar mistracking. These forces result in a softening and degeneration of the articular cartilage of the patella.

Practical Tip

The pain present in chondromalacia arises not from the cartilage but from the surrounding tissue.

patellar tendonosis Tendon degeneration (or failed healing), with or without symptoms or histologic signs of inflammation in the patellar tendon. This condition commonly stems from an overuse of the patellar tendon, resulting in a cycle of continued insults to the tendon with unsuccessful healing that causes the continued degeneration of the tissue.

The articular cartilage is not innervated, so the presence of degeneration is confirmed only through arthroscopy. Pain may arise directly from other biomechanical factors and the irritation of the surrounding tissues.

Patellar tendonosis is also associated with patellofemoral dysfunction. The term *tendonosis* was first used in the 1940s; its current use refers to tendon degeneration (or failed healing), with or without symptoms or histologic signs of inflammation. This condition commonly stems from an overuse of the patellar tendon, resulting in its acute version, patellar tendonitis. Over time, tendonitis becomes chronic, and a cycle of continued insults to the tendon with unsuccessful healing leads to the continued degeneration of the tissue.

Patellar tendonosis is commonly referred to as "jumper's knee" because of its associations with running and jumping. Pain initially occurs after activity at the inferior pole of the patella or the distal attachment of the tendon at the tibial tubercle. As the condition progresses, pain presents before activity, subsides after warm-up, and then returns following activity. Pain occurs while walking up or down stairs, with passive flexion beyond 120°, and during any resisted knee extension. The progression continues, and an increasing number of activities cause discomfort, eventually preventing the individual from participating at all.

Assessment

Patellofemoral dysfunction can result from a variety of factors acting together or individually. These factors can be static or dynamic and can involve more than one region of the body. It is important to conduct a thorough assessment of the area to ensure that all contributing factors are addressed. This section treats patellofemoral dysfunction as an umbrella pathology and addresses specifics for the two conditions discussed as necessary.

Condition History Therapists should inquire about the following when taking the client's history:

Question	*Significance*
What was the mechanism of injury?	Patellofemoral problems typically arise from chronic conditions with no memorable mechanism of injury; however, if a distinct event caused the injury, other structures may be involved, as well.
Are there any sounds associated with motion?	Crepitus is a common symptom of patellofemoral problems, especially in chondromalacia. Audible popping or snapping sounds may indicate a more severe pathology.
Is there a history of knee injury?	An acute injury that has occurred in the past can develop into patellofemoral problems.
Is there pain? If so, where?	Patellofemoral pain is generally felt over the anterior knee. Patellar tendonitis presents with pain over the inferior pole of the patella.

| When does the pain occur? | Pain is often present after activity, while going up and down stairs, during movement that requires deep knee flexion, and after periods of prolonged sitting (movie theater sign). |
| Is there any locking, catching, or giving way? | These are all common symptoms in patellofemoral conditions. |

Visual Assessment The client must be appropriately dressed so that the therapist can observe the hips, feet, and knees. Begin by checking the entire knee complex for signs of swelling, discoloration, gross deformity, and evidence of past injury such as scars. The posture of the lower extremity should be observed from anterior and lateral views in both standing and sitting positions to assess any deviations. Anteriorly, have the client stand with the feet pointing straight forward. Check for any rotation of the femur on the tibia, and note the angle between the femur and the tibia. Normally, the angle will range from 180° to 195°. An angle between the femur and the tibia of less than 180° is considered genu valgum or knock knees, and an angle greater than 195° is considered genu varum or bowlegs.

Observe patellar alignment from this position to note any abnormalities such as squinting or frog-eyed patella, described earlier in this section. Have the client contract both quadriceps, and check for any deviations in patellar tracking and the symmetry of the muscles between sides. Observe the feet for pronation or supination. From the lateral view, note whether there is any hyperextension of the knee, known as *genu recurvatum*. In this position, patella alta is easily noted from the presence of something known as the "camel sign." In patella alta, the patella rides higher in the trochlear groove, so the infrapatellar fat pad becomes more evident and a double hump is created.

Place the client in the seated position with the feet dangling off the table. Check anteriorly to see whether the tibial tubercles are directly below the inferior poles of the patellas. Excessive deviation can indicate a predisposition to tracking problems. The patellas should face forward and not demonstrate any displacement medially or laterally. From the side, assess the position of the patella for patella alta. In this position, the patella should be perpendicular to the floor. In patella alta, it will be at a 45° angle to the ground.

Palpation Check for the presence of swelling, point tenderness, deformity, spasm, crepitus, and temperature differences. Begin with the structures listed earlier in the chapter, and expand the area as necessary.

Orthopedic Tests Several physical assessments can help determine the presence of patellofemoral dysfunction. As discussed earlier in the chapter, discrepancies in leg length are a component of patellofemoral dysfunction because they can affect the orientation of the knee during gait. There are two types of leg-length discrepancy: true and functional.

- *To determine a true leg-length discrepancy:* Place the client in the supine position, and place the legs parallel to each other, 4 to 8 inches apart. Take a measurement from the ASIS to the medial malleolus on each leg, and then compare the measurements. A difference of ½ to 1 inch is considered normal.

- *To determine a functional leg-length difference:* Begin with the client in the same position, and measure from the umbilicus to the medial malleolus. This information is useful only when the results of the true leg-length test are negative.

⭑Practical Tip
Make sure the knee is in full extension when checking patellar mobility.

The next assessment involves determining the mobility of the patella. With the client in the supine position, grasp the patella and move it medially. This will test the restrictions in the lateral restraints, such as the lateral retinaculum. Move the patella laterally. This will test restrictions in the medial restraints, such as the medial retinaculum. The patella should move about half its width medially and laterally. Any more motion in either direction is referred to as a *hypermobile patella;* less motion is a *hypomobile patella.*

Measure the Q angle, as described earlier, by drawing a line from the anterior superior iliac spine through the midpoint of the patella. Draw the other line from the midpoint of the patella through the tibial tuberosity; the angle is created by the intersection of the two lines. An angle of greater than 18° or fewer than 13° is considered abnormal and is a predisposing factor to patellar dysfunction.

There is no specific test for patellar tendonitis other than the presence of pain at the inferior pole of the patella on palpation; however, there are two tests specific to chondromalacia, as shown in Table 9-6.

Soft Tissue Treatment

A variety of factors contribute to patellofemoral dysfunction. From a soft tissue standpoint, the focus should be to balance the musculature around the knee and then address any related imbalances in other areas.

Connective Tissue Patellofemoral dysfunction is primarily the result of chronic mistracking problems, which cause some of the involved structures to become fibrous. Thus the condition lends itself to the benefits of connective tissue work.

Prone Position Begin by assessing the superficial tissue of the hamstrings in all directions. Move into any restrictions until they release, speeding up the process by incorporating active engagement of the muscles. Once the superficial tissue has been released, strip out and define each hamstring to ensure that the hamstrings are not hindering any motion at the pelvis and knee. Move to the calf, and treat the superficial tissue of the gastrocnemius after assessing it in various directions. Define each of the heads, and separate the gastrocnemius from the deeper muscle, the soleus.

Supine Position Although the focus is on the knee, it is important to treat the entire length of the muscles. Assess the superficial tissue of the quadriceps and adductors, moving into any restrictions until they release. Once the superficial tissue has been addressed, move into the deeper layers by separating the individual muscles in the quadriceps and adductors, focusing on the distal attachments. Flex the knee to about 30°, using a bolster to

Table 9-6 Orthopedic Tests for Chondromalacia

Orthopedic Test	How to Perform
Patella compression (grind) test 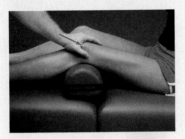 *Note:* This test is used to assess subchondral bone irritation.	Client is in either a supine or a seated position with the leg straight out on the table. Place a bolster under the knee, flexing the knee to about 20°, and compress the patella into the trochlear groove. Pain or grinding on compression is a positive sign for pathology of the patellar articular cartilage. Since different parts of the patella articulate with the trochlea at different points during movement, repeat the test at various angles of knee flexion.
Clarke sign 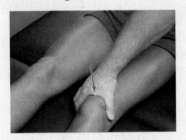	Client is in the seated position with the knee at 0° of flexion. Place the web space of the hand just proximal to the superior pole of the patella. Apply a small amount of pressure, and ask the client to slowly contract the quadriceps. The test is positive if the client experiences pain and is unable to hold the contraction. *Note:* If the pressure is significant enough, this test will be positive on a normal individual; therefore, it is imperative to perform the test several times, using increasing amounts of pressure and repeating it at 30°, 60°, and 90° of knee flexion.

> **Practical Tip**
>
> Be careful not to use too much pressure during the Clarke sign test as doing so can cause a lot of pain.

help lock the patella in place. This will enhance the effectiveness of the treatment when you are working on the tissue that surrounds the patella. Strip out the lateral quadrant around the patella and lateral joint line both generally and specifically to remove connective tissue restrictions. These areas can be quite fibrous, so incorporating movement is beneficial.

Side-Lying Position In this position, the lateral aspect of the knee is facing up, enabling easy access to the structures in the area. The iliotibial band can be directly addressed in this position. Ensure that tension is removed, especially at its distal end, where fibers attach directly to the patella. Small stripping strokes to the lateral structures of the knee help remove restrictions and release the area. Include any techniques from the previous sections in the chapter to address the hip structures, if necessary.

Tissue Inconsistencies Since this condition has many variables and can involve the entire lower limb, it is important to address the trigger points of the muscles listed earlier in the chapter. Begin with the muscles that attach directly to the patella, and expand outward from there. Remember to keep the intensity at 7 out of 10 on a pain scale, and use movement to increase the treatment's effectiveness.

Muscle Concerns

Patellofemoral dysfunction is caused by the contribution of both static and dynamic factors, so movement should be an integral component of the treatment. Again, the focus should be to balance the musculature around the patella and address any contributing factors at other joints. This condition is chronic, so the treatment process may be involved.

Prone Position Begin by warming up the hamstrings before using a forearm stroke to affect the deeper tissues. Active motion with perpendicular compressive effleurage and deep parallel stripping is effective on the hamstrings. To perform perpendicular compressive effleurage, place the heels of the hands on the middle of the muscle. Slide the hands apart as the client slowly flexes the knee. Complete the stroke when the client finishes the contraction. Start at the distal end, and work toward the proximal end.

For deep parallel stripping, have the client flex the knee to 90°. Place either the fist or the thumbs on the hamstrings at the knee, applying pressure in a proximal direction. As the client slowly extends the leg, move up the muscle a short distance. Repeat this process until the entire muscle is covered.

Supine Position Thoroughly warm up the quadriceps using a variety of strokes before applying a forearm or loose fist to work into the deeper layers of the muscle. Incorporate movement by hanging the client's leg off the side of the table at the knee. Use both perpendicular compressive effleurage and deep parallel stripping as described for piriformis syndrome, and position yourself so that you do not get kicked as the client extends the leg. Effective methods for removing tension in the area before performing the stroke include applying friction around the iliotibial band, patella, and lateral joint line while pulling the skin taut.

Side-Lying Position This position is ideal for treating the lateral knee as well as the hip and lateral thigh. Address the entire lateral thigh by performing a forearm stroke to the hip and lateral thigh as described for iliotibial band friction syndrome. Another direct way to treat the lateral thigh is to stand at the client's knee and perform strokes from the knee toward the hip. Compression broadening is effective in this position. Defining strokes to the distal ITB and lateral knee while the client flexes and extends the knee will release any restrictions in the area.

Stretching

The stretches performed for patellofemoral dysfunction should always include the entire lower extremity, since the dysfunction is such a global condition. Begin with all the stretches discussed previously in order to restore balance to the musculature (see Figs. 9-18 to 9-24).

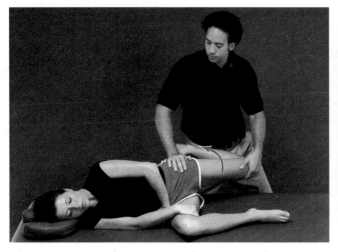

Figure 9-29 Quadriceps stretch—proximal aspect.

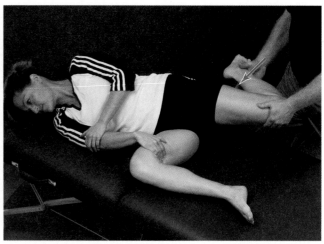

Figure 9-30 Quadriceps stretch—distal aspect.

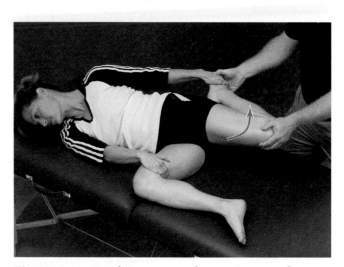

Figure 9-31 Quadriceps stretch—entire muscle.

Quadriceps Stretch One stretch that is specific to the quadriceps is also useful. Place the client in a side-lying position with the bottom knee pulled up to the chest (Fig. 9-29). Make sure that the hips are aligned on top of each other or "stacked." This stretch is performed in three parts to address all the aspects of the muscle group:

- In the first phase, the client's top knee should be at 90° of flexion. Support the top leg as the client takes a deep breath, and extend the thigh while the client exhales. Assist at the end of the range of motion, and repeat for one set of 8 to 10 repetitions. This stretch focuses on the proximal rectus femoris.

- The second phase addresses the distal quadriceps and is performed with the client in the side-lying position (Fig. 9-30). Extend the client's top hip so that it is in line with the torso, and flex the knee to 90° while supporting it. Instruct the client to take a deep breath and flex the heel toward the buttocks while exhaling. Assist at the end of the movement, and return to the starting position after 2 seconds. Isolate the vastus lateralis by lowering the top leg across the midline 15° to 20° and repeating the stretch. Both positions should be repeated for two sets of 10 repetitions.

- The last phase is the most intense and addresses the entire muscle group. Begin in the side-lying position, and ask the client to grasp the ankle of the top leg with his or her hand or a rope if necessary (Fig. 9-31). Be sure that the client keeps the bottom leg up against the chest to prevent hyperextending the back. Instruct the client to extend the thigh as he or she exhales. Assist in the same direction, supporting the knee, and repeat for two sets of 10 repetitions. For maximum results, be sure the client always contracts the muscle opposite the one being stretched.

SUMMARY

This chapter presented additional examples of the interrelationships among different regions of the body. When dysfunction occurs in an area, it is important to investigate all the involved factors to ensure that the proper treatment is given.

The anatomical review at the beginning of the chapter described the relationships between the hip and the knee. The section on palpation reinforced the concept that several structures span both regions. The sections on range of motion assessment, manual muscle testing, dermatomes, and myotomes described how to put the information to use for each of the different pathologies covered. Finally, various treatments were discussed to help effectively treat the problem.

REVIEW QUESTIONS

1. How large are the forces that the hip is subjected to during locomotion?
2. What is the angle of inclination?
3. What is the purpose of a labrum in the joint?
4. What is the strongest ligament in the body?
5. What is the function of the ligamentum teres?
6. What are the functions of the menisci?
7. What are the six orientations of the sciatic nerve in relation to the piriformis?
8. What is a classic symptom of iliotibial band friction syndrome?
9. What is the "movie theater sign"?
10. What is the difference between true and functional leg-length discrepancies?
11. Why does the degeneration of the articular cartilage in chondromalacia not cause pain?
12. What is the Q angle, and how is it measured?

CRITICAL-THINKING QUESTIONS

1. Explain the screw-home mechanism.
2. How does genu recurvatum contribute to patellar instability?
3. Why is it important to keep the hips stacked when performing Ober's test?
4. What is the importance of a correct firing pattern in the quadriceps?
5. How does a large Q angle lead to patellar tracking problems?
6. Explain the failed healing response and its contribution to tendon degeneration.

Bony Structures of the Hip

Iliac crest	Place the palms of your hands in the flank area just below the ribs, and press down and in. You should feel the top of the crests.
Iliac tubercle	From the top of the crests, move anteriorly to find this tubercle. It is the widest point on the crests.
Anterior superior iliac spine (ASIS)	This is the most anterior part of the crest. Have the client lie supine, and place the palms of your hands on the front of his or her hips.
Anterior inferior iliac spine (AIIS)	From ASIS, move inferiorly about ½ inch. You won't be able to directly palpate this structure.
Posterior superior iliac spine (PSIS)	This is the most posterior aspect of the iliac crest. It is commonly referred to as the "dimple" in the low back. It is located at the level of S2.
Sacrum	Using the PSIS, move medially onto the sacrum. Once you are on the bone, use your fingertips to trace its lateral edge in an inferior direction.
Pubic crest	Place your fingertips in the umbilicus. Rest your hand in an inferior direction on the abdomen. Slowly press down and in; the heel of your hand will hit a bony ledge.
Pubic symphysis	Once you find the crest, there is a joint directly in the middle.
Anterior femoral head	The head of the femur lies at the midpoint of the inguinal ligament. Using the palm of your hand, press just inferior to the midpoint of the ligament until you feel a hard end-feel.
Greater trochanter of the femur	Have the client lie in the prone position, and place the palm of your hand over his or her lateral hip. Bend the client's knee to 90°, press in on the hip, and rotate the leg medially and laterally. You should feel a large, bony structure rotating under your hand.
Ischial tuberosity	This structure is on the inferior ischium and is the common origin for the hamstrings. Using the gluteal fold, place the web of your hand, with the thumb pointing medially, along the fold. Press in; your thumb should be on the tuberosity.
Greater sciatic notch	Draw a line between the posterior superior iliac spine on the side opposite the notch you are trying to locate and the greater trochanter on the same side as the notch you are trying to locate to find the midpoint. Press in, and you should be in a depression, which is the notch.
Trochanteric bursa	This bursa is generally not palpable. Using the greater trochanter, palpate just posterior and behind the trochanter.
Gluteal fold	This fold is formed by the thigh as it meets the hip. Have the client lie in the prone position, and locate the fold at the base of the gluteus maximus muscle and the top of the hamstrings.
Sacrotuberous ligament	Using the ischial tuberosity, move superior and medial and press in. To make sure you are on the ligament, have the client cough; the ligament will tighten.

Soft Tissue Structures of the Hip

Inguinal ligament	Located on a line between the ASIS of the ilium and the pubic tubercles, this ligament is the inferior edge of the oblique abdominal muscles.
Femoral triangle	This is the anterior hip where the thigh meets the trunk. Have the client bend the hip and knee and place the foot across the opposite knee and let the knee fall out. The triangle is bound superiorly by the inguinal ligament, laterally by the sartorius, and medially by the adductor longus muscle.
Femoral nerve/artery/vein	These structures lie in the femoral triangle and appear in this order: lateral—nerve, middle—artery, medial—vein. To locate the structures, find the artery (the easiest to palpate) and then move laterally to find the nerve and medially to find the vein.
Superficial inguinal lymph nodes	These nodes consist of two chains. The horizontal chain runs just inferior to the inguinal ligament from lateral to medial. The vertical chain starts at the medial edge of the horizontal chain and runs inferior along the lateral border of the adductor longus.
Lateral femoral cutaneous nerve	This nerve lies inferior to the ASIS and medial to the tensor fascia latae. It is approximately around the origin tendon for the rectus femoris muscle.
Trochanteric bursa	This bursa is generally not palpable. Using the greater trochanter, palpate just posterior and behind the trochanter. This structure is generally tender.
Gluteal fold	This fold is formed by the thigh as it meets the hip. Have your client lie in the prone position, and locate the fold at the base of the gluteus maximus muscle and the top of the hamstrings.
Sacrotuberous ligament	This ligament runs between the ischial tuberosity and the inferior lateral angle of the sacrum. Using the ischial tuberosity, move superior and medial and press in. To make sure you are on the ligament, have your client cough; the ligament will tighten.
Cluneal nerves	These nerves are located along the iliac crest. Locate the PSIS and the iliac tubercles. Find the midpoint along the iliac crest, and palpate these vertically oriented nerves in a transverse direction.

Bony Structures of the Knee

Patella	This bone is better known as the *kneecap* and lies dead center on the anterior knee. It has a superior and inferior pole and is encased by the patellar tendon. Use the palm of the hand on the anterior knee to locate, and then trace its borders with your fingers.
Tibial tuberosity	This large, bony prominence lies about 1 to 1½ inches distal to the inferior pole of the patella on the tibia. It can be quite large in some people.
Lateral tibial tubercle (Gerdy's tubercle)	Locate the tibial tuberosity, and move in a lateral direction until you find a smaller bony prominence. This is the insertion for the iliotibial band.
Tibial crest	Trace from the tibial tuberosity down the midline of the tibia. This is a relatively sharp edge of bone and can be tender.
Medial joint line	Have your client sit with the knee flexed to 90°. Locate the midpoint of the patellar tendon, and move off medially until you fall into a depression.
Medial tibial plateau	This area of the knee is located just below the medial joint line. Locate the joint line, and move distally about ½ inch, staying above the concavity of the tibia.
Pes anserine region	This area on the tibia is the insertion for the sartorius, gracilis, and semitendinosus. To locate this area, use the medial tibial plateau and move inferior into the concavity of the tibia. The pes anserine bursa lies between the tendons and the tibia.
Medial condyle of the femur	Locate the middle of the patellar tendon. Move medially just off the tendon into the joint space. Press up and in just medial to the patella. You will be pressing on the condyle.
Medial epicondyle of the femur	Move up from the medial joint line along the medial side of the knee. You will feel the femur start to dip in toward the midline. This is the epicondyle.
Adductor tubercle of the femur	Continue upward from the epicondyle as the femur dips inward. There is a bony prominence deep on the femur. It is one of the attachments of the adductor magnus.
Lateral joint line	Have your client sit with the knee flexed to 90°. Locate the midpoint of the patellar tendon, and move off laterally until you fall into a depression.
Lateral femoral condyle	Locate the middle of the patellar tendon. Move laterally just off the tendon into the joint space. Press up and in just lateral to the patella. You will be pressing on the condyle. It is more prominent than the medial one.
Lateral femoral epicondyle	Move up from the lateral joint line along the lateral side of the knee. You will feel the femur start to dip in toward the midline. This is the epicondyle.
Head of the fibula	This bone part sits just below the lateral joint line of the tibia. Palpate inferior to the lateral joint line, and feel for the bone.
Fibula (shaft)	Trace from the fibular head down the lateral side of the leg to the lateral malleolus. You may or may not be able to palpate the bone directly. This bone serves as an attachment point for muscles and has no weight-bearing function.

Soft Tissue Structures of the Knee

Quadriceps tendon	This tendon attaches the quadriceps to the patella. Move superior just off the superior pole of the patella, and palpate the tendon.
Patellar ligament	This is the tendon of insertion for the quadriceps muscles and lies between the inferior pole of the patella and the tibial tuberosity. Have your client flex the knee to 90°, and palpate between these two points.
Medial collateral ligament (MCL)	Using the joint line, move in a medial direction until you are directly on the middle of the joint. The ligament runs in a vertical fashion, so palpate in a transverse direction. This structure is not always easily palpated.
Lateral collateral ligament (LCL)	This is directly on the lateral side of the knee. Have the client bend the hip and knee and place the foot across the opposite knee and let the knee fall out. Locate the lateral joint line, and palpate laterally until you find a very distinct cordlike structure.
Medial meniscus	Locate the medial joint line. Press in deep, and have your client internally rotate the tibia. The meniscus will move into your thumb. It will move away during external tibial rotation.
Lateral meniscus	Locate the lateral joint line. Press in deep, and have your client externally rotate the tibia. The meniscus will move into your thumb. It will move away during internal tibial rotation.
Peroneal nerve	This nerve sits just behind the head of the fibula. Locate the head of the fibula, and have your client rotate the tibia inward. Palpate behind the head to feel for the nerve.

Muscles of the Hip, Thigh, and Knee

Muscle	Origin	Insertion	Action	How to Palpate
Hip				
Gluteus maximus	Posterior iliac crest, sacrum, sacrotuberous and sacroiliac ligaments	Gluteal tuberosity of femur, Gerty's tubercle by way of the iliotibial tract	Extends thigh at hip; laterally rotates thigh at hip; extends leg at knee while standing; extends trunk at hip when standing; abducts thigh at hip	Prone position; palpate during hyperextension of thigh at the hip
Gluteus medius	Iliac crest and lateral surface of the ilium	Greater trochanter of the femur	Abducts, flexes, and medially rotates hip; stabilizes pelvis on the hip during gait	Side-lying position; palpate between greater trochanter and iliac crest during abduction of thigh
Gluteus minimus	Posterior ilium between the middle and inferior gluteal lines	Anterior aspect of the greater trochanter	Abducts, medially rotates, and flexes hip	Side-lying position; palpate between greater trochanter and 1 inch inferior to the iliac crest during abduction at the hip
Piriformis	Greater sciatic notch and the anterior surface of the sacrum	Greater trochanter of the femur (medial aspect)	Laterally rotates and abducts thigh at the hip	Side-lying position; palpate between greater trochanter and sacrum during lateral rotation of thigh
Tensor fascia latae	Anterior iliac crest, posterior to the anterior superior iliac spine	Gerty's tubercle by way of the iliotibial tract	Abducts thigh at the hip; flexes thigh at the hip; medially rotates thigh at the hip; extends leg at the knee	Side-lying position; palpate between greater trochanter and anterior iliac crest; have client medially rotate and abduct thigh at the hip

Chapter 9 Conditions of the Hip and Knee   393

Muscle	Origin	Insertion	Action	How to Palpate
Anterior Thigh and Knee				
Sartorius ("tailors muscle")	Anterior superior iliac spine	Proximal medial shaft of the tibia at the pes anserine region	Flexes, abducts and laterally rotates thigh at the hip; flexes and medially rotates leg at the knee	Supine position; have client flex knee and externally rotate thigh; have client lift leg off the table to make more prominent
Pectineus	Superior ramus of the pubis	Line between the lesser trochanter of the femur and the linea aspera	Adducts and medially rotates thigh at the hip; flexes thigh at the hip	Supine position; flex thigh to 45° and laterally rotate so that the knee falls out. Have client adduct thigh, and locate adductor longus. Move lateral to longus in the femoral triangle; palpate in a vertical direction for a feel similar to corduroy
Adductor longus/ brevis	Pubic tubercle	Middle third of the linea aspera	Adducts and medially rotates thigh at the hip; flexes thigh at the hip	Supine position; flex leg to 90° and laterally rotate hip so that knee falls out; resist adduction, and muscle will pop out in a triangular shape; most prominent adductor muscle
Adductor magnus	Inferior pubic ramus, ischial tuberosity, and ramus of ischium	Linea aspera and adductor tubercle	Adducts, medially rotates, and extends hip; assists hip flexion	Prone position; palpate just medial to hamstring origin but lateral to gracilis
Gracilis	Inferior pubis	Proximal medial shaft of the tibia at the pes anserine region	Adducts and medially rotates thigh at the hip; flexes leg at the knee and medially rotates the flexed knee	Supine position; flex leg to 90°; dig heel into the table; will become prominent directly up the inseam

Muscle	Origin	Insertion	Action	How to Palpate
Anterior Thigh and Knee (Continued)				
Iliopsoas	Iliac crest and fossa; anterior vertebral bodies T12-L5	Lesser trochanter of the femur	Flexes hip	Supine position; on a line between ASIS and umbilicus; press down into iliac fossa for iliacus; press down and in at lateral edge of rectus abdominus for psoas
Rectus femoris	Anterior inferior iliac spine and above the acetabulum	Tibial tuberosity by way of the patellar tendon	Flexes thigh at the hip; extends leg at the knee	Supine position; palpate between patella and just inferior to ASIS; have client extend leg; runs directly up the center of the anterior thigh
Vastus medialis	Medial linea aspera and intertrochanteric line	Tibial tuberosity by way of the patellar tendon	Extends leg at the knee; pulls patella medial	Supine position with the thigh in slight external rotation; have client extend knee, and locate the teardrop-shaped muscle just medial to the rectus femoris
Vastus intermedius	Anterior shaft of the femur	Tibial tuberosity by way of the patellar tendon	Extends leg at the knee	Supine position; palpate deep to the rectus femoris
Vastus lateralis	Linea aspera and greater trochanter of the femur	Tibial tuberosity by way of the patellar tendon	Extends leg at the knee; pulls patella lateral	Supine or side-lying position; have client extend knee, and locate the large muscle on the lateral thigh

Muscle	Origin	Insertion	Action	How to Palpate
Posterior Thigh and Knee				
Semimembrano-sus	Ischial tuberos-ity	Posterior medial condyle of the tibia	Extends thigh at the hip; medi-ally rotates hip and flexed knee;flexes leg at the knee	Prone position; bend leg to 90°, and resist knee extension; locate the semitendino-sus tendon, and relax the leg; move medial and press in
Semitendinosus	Ischial tuberos-ity	Proximal medial shaft of the tibia at the pes anser-ine region	Extends thigh at the hip; medi-ally rotates hip and flexed knee; flexes leg at the knee	Prone position; bend leg to 90°, and resist knee flexion; large tendon will be-come prominent medial to the popliteal space
Biceps femoris	Ischial tuberos-ity (long head) and linea aspera of the femur (short head)	Head of the fibula	Extends thigh at the hip; later-ally rotates hip and flexed knee; flexes leg at the knee	Prone position; bend leg to 90°, and resist knee flexion; large tendon will be-come prominent lateral to the popliteal space
Gastrocnemius	Lateral epicon-dyle (lateral head) and me-dial epicondyle (medial head) of the femur	Calcaneus bone by way of the Achilles tendon	Plantar-flexes foot at the ankle; flexes leg at the knee	Prone position; plantar-flex the foot; muscle will become promi-nent on the pos-terior lower leg

Trigger Points of the Hip and Knee

Muscle	Trigger-Point Location	Referral Pattern	Chief Symptom
Gluteus maximus	1. Lateral edge of the sacrum, halfway down 2. Just superior to ischial tuberosity 3. Medial to ischial tuberosity	1. Semicircle up along the sacrum and natal cleft to sacroiliac joint (SIJ); down along the gluteal fold 2. Entire buttock, both superficially and deep; just under the iliac crest 3. Coccyx	Pain and restlessness after long periods of sitting; pain while walking uphill and swimming the crawl stroke
Gluteus medius	1. Inferior to posterior iliac crest, near SIJ 2. Inferior to iliac crest, midway along length 3. ASIS, inferior to crest	1. Along the crest up into the SIJ and lumbar spine 2. Midgluteal region; may extend to the upper lateral thigh 3. Along crest; encompasses the lower lumbar and sacral region	Pain on walking and sitting in a slumped position; difficulty sleeping on the affected side
Gluteus minimus	1. One below the other, inferior to the anterior iliac crest 2. Superior edge of the muscle	1. Lower lateral buttock down the lateral thigh, along the peroneals, sometimes to the ankle 2. Most of the buttock down the back of the thigh into calf	Hip pain that can affect gait; difficulty lying on the affected side; difficulty standing after prolonged sitting
Piriformis	1. Just lateral to the sacrum 2. Just before the greater trochanter	1. Sacroiliac region 2. Posterior hip joint	Pain and numbness in the low back, groin, buttock, hip, and posterior thigh and leg
Tensor fascia latae	Proximal third of the muscle	To the greater trochanter and down the anterolateral aspect of the thigh	Deep hip pain exacerbated during movement of the hip; aware primarily of pain around the greater trochanter; cannot tolerate long periods of sitting with the hips flexed to 90° or more; pain prevents client from walking at a rapid pace and from lying on the side where trigger points are located

Trigger Points of the Hip and Knee *(Continued)*

Muscle	Trigger-Point Location	Referral Pattern	Chief Symptom
Sartorius	Superficially throughout length of the muscle	Up and down the thigh and knee region	Burst of superficial sharp or tingling pain
Pectineus	Just distal to the superior pubic ramus in proximal portion of muscle	Anteromedial thigh	Deep-seated groin pain just distal to the inguinal ligament that may continue to the anteriomedial thigh; in addition to pain, may notice a limitation in abduction
Adductor longus/ brevis	1. Proximal portion of muscle 2. Distal portion of muscle	1. Proximally and distally deep into the groin and upper thigh 2. Upper medial knee and spillover onto the tibia	Typically only noticed with vigorous activity or overload and not at rest
Adductor magnus	1. Midportion of muscle 2. Proximal portion of muscle just below the ischial tuberosity	1. Proximally into the groin and distally over the anteromedial aspect of the thigh almost to the knee 2. Proximally to the pelvis	Deep groin pain that may be misconstrued as pelvic pain; generalized internal pelvic pain but may include the pubic bone, vagina, or rectum; difficulty finding a comfortable position for the leg while sleeping
Gracilis	Midbelly of muscle	Locally around points in a proximal and distal direction	Superficial, hot, stinging pain in the medial thigh
Rectus femoris	Proximal end of muscle just under the anterior inferior iliac spine	Distal end of the muscle at the knee around the patella and sometimes deep in the joint	Pain in front of the knee that will awaken client at night; inability to find a comfortable position
Vastus medialis	1. Distal aspect of muscle 2. Proximal end of muscle	1. Front of the knee 2. Anteromedial aspect of the thigh in linear distribution	Initial deep ache in the knee that will often interrupt sleep; over several weeks or months, pain replaced by inhibition in muscle
Vastus intermedius	Proximal end of muscle, near its origin	Distally over the thigh almost to the knee, with the most intense pain at the midthigh	Pain and difficulty extending the knee, especially after being immobile for extended periods; pain occurs during movement and rarely at rest

Trigger Points of the Hip and Knee *(Continued)*

Muscle	Trigger-Point Location	Referral Pattern	Chief Symptom
Vastus lateralis	1. Anterior aspect of distal end of muscle 2. Posterior aspect of distal end of muscle 3. Midthigh level on posterolateral aspect of muscle 4. Directly on lateral aspect of thigh 5. Proximal attachment at greater trochanter	1. Down the lateral aspect and into the knee (This point can cause the patella to become immobilized.) 2. Lateral knee but primarily up the lateral thigh and down the lateral lower leg 3. Lateral half of the popliteal space 4. Severe pain over the entire length of the lateral thigh as high as the iliac crest 5. Locally around point	Pain during walking and difficulty lying on the involved side, which subsequently disturbs sleep
Semimembranosus	Distal portion of muscle	Upward to the gluteal fold and may spill over down the medial thigh to the medial calf	Pain on walking, which may cause limping; pain over the posterior proximal thigh, buttock, and back of the knee when sitting
Semitendinosus	Distal portion of muscle	Upward to the gluteal fold and may spill over down the medial thigh to the medial calf	Pain on walking, which may cause limping; pain over the posterior proximal thigh, buttock, and back of the knee when sitting
Biceps femoris	Distal portion of both heads of the muscle	Back of knee, with spillover distally below the lateral calf and proximally to the lateral thigh	Pain on walking, which may cause limping; pain over the posterior proximal thigh, buttock, and back of the knee when sitting
Gastrocnemius	1&2. Just proximal to middle of medial and lateral heads 3&4. Behind knee, near medial and lateral attachment points of femoral condyles	1&2. Medial point: Instep of the ipsilateral foot and spillover down the medial aspect of the calf Lateral point: A pattern around the point 3&4. General location around the point	Calf cramping at night and posterior knee pain

Orthopedic Tests for the Hip and Knee

Condition	Orthopedic Test	How to Perform	Positive Sign
Piriformis syndrome	Piriformis test	Client is in side-lying position. Flex the top hip to 60°, and flex the knee so that the foot of the top leg rests on the knee of the bottom leg. Stand at the knee of the client, and stabilize the hip with one hand; then press the bent knee down toward the floor.	If the piriformis is tight or is entrapping the sciatic nerve, this test will either increase the pain or re-create the symptoms, both of which indicate a positive test.
Iliotibial band friction syndrome	Ober test *Note:* First described in 1936, this test is widely accepted for this condition (Gajdosik et al., 2003). It is used to determine the length of the iliotibial band, which can predispose a client to developing pathology in the area or can exacerbate an existing condition.	Place the client on his or her side with the bottom hip and knee bent to 90° for stability. Stand behind the client. With the hand closest to the client's head, stabilize the client's hip so that he or she does not roll anteriorly or posteriorly and the iliums are on top of or "stacked" on each other. Instruct the client to bend the top knee to 90°. Support the client's leg at the knee with the other hand. Keep the leg parallel to the table, and passively extend the client's hip slightly. While keeping the client's hips stacked, slowly lower the top leg.	The client's leg should drop below horizontal. If it doesn't, this is an indication of tightness in the iliotibial band and constitutes a positive test.
	Noble compression test *Note:* This is a pain provocation test and is used to determine involvement at the knee.	Place the client in a supine position with the hip flexed to 45° and the knee flexed to 90°. Apply pressure with the thumb either to the lateral epicondyle of the client's femur or about ½ inch above the epicondyle. Passively extend the client's leg while maintaining pressure.	When the leg approaches about 30° of flexion, the client will report feeling pain similar to that which occurs during activity. This indicates a positive test.
Patellofemoral syndrome	Patella compression (grind) test *Note:* This is used to assess subchondral bone irritation.	Client is in either a supine or a seated position with the leg straight out on the table. Place a bolster under the knee, flexing the knee to about 20°, and compress the patella into the trochlear groove.	Pain or grinding on compression is a positive sign for pathology of the patellar articular cartilage.

Condition	Orthopedic Test	How to Perform	Positive Sign
		Since different parts of the patella articulate with the trochlea at different points during movement, repeat the test at various angles of knee flexion.	
	Clarke sign	Client is in the seated position with the knee at 0° of flexion.	The test is positive if the client experiences pain and is unable to hold the contraction.
		Place the web space of the hand just proximal to the superior pole of the patella.	
		Apply a small amount of pressure, and ask the client to slowly contract the quadriceps.	
		Note: Be aware that if the pressure is significant enough, this test will be positive on a normal individual; therefore, it is imperative to perform the test several times, using increasing amounts of pressure and repeating it at 30°, 60°, and 90° of knee flexion.	

chapter 10

Conditions of the Lower Leg, Ankle, and Foot

chapter outline

chapter objectives

At the conclusion of this chapter, the reader will understand:

- the bony anatomy of the region
- how to locate the bony landmarks and soft tissue structures of the region
- where to find the muscles, and the origins, insertions, and actions of the region
- how to assess movement and determine the range of motion for the region
- how to perform manual muscle testing to the region
- how to recognize dermatome patterns for the region
- trigger-point locations and referral patterns for the region
- the following elements of each condition discussed:
  - background and characteristics
  - specific questions to ask
  - what orthopedic tests should be performed
  - how to treat the connective tissue, trigger points, and muscles
- flexibility concerns

KEY TERMS

Achilles tendonitis

Fick angle

medial tibial stress syndrome (MTSS)

plantar fasciitis

Sharpey's fibers

tarsal tunnel syndrome

tendonosis

windlass mechanism

Introduction The ankle and foot are two of the most important structures in the body and are, in fact, biological masterpieces, considering that the average person takes between 8000 and 10,000 steps per day, walking places one and a half times the body's weight on the feet, and running can place up to four times the body's weight on the feet. Given these facts, it's easy to understand how the ankle and foot are both highly susceptible to injury. Approximately 75% of Americans will experience some sort of foot or ankle problem in their lifetime; moreover, ankle injuries are the most common type of injury to the region and are among the most common joint injuries seen by physicians.

> ★**Practical Tip**
>
> Walking places one and a half times the body's weight on the feet, while running places up to four times the body's weight on the feet.

The ankle and foot are intricate structures, containing 26 bones, 107 ligaments, and 19 muscles and tendons that hold them together and allow them to function. They are formed by the piecing together of numerous individual bones, much like a three-dimensional puzzle. Because of the numerous structures involved, true one-on-one articulations between bones are rare in this region. Instead, most bones have several articulations between surrounding structures. Even though these bones and their articulations are often discussed separately, they have a unique relationship with each other and come together to function as a unit. They form the terminal portion of the kinetic chain of the lower extremity and are essential in all locomotive activities.

The lower leg, ankle, and foot have two principal functions:

- *Support:* The foot provides a base that acts as a rigid structure; it supports the entire body and facilitates upright posture with minimal effort during standing.
- *Locomotion:* The ankle and foot act like a flexible lever that provides adaptability to the environment, accommodates shock absorption, and offers a base from which the foot can push off.

These functions distribute and dissipate the forces acting on the body when the feet make contact with the ground. Any change in structure or mobility of the ankle and/or foot can lead to the transmission of abnormal stresses through the body and ultimately lead to the dysfunction of those structures.

An in-depth study of the biomechanics and dysfunction of the ankle and foot is beyond the scope of this text. This chapter provides a clear, basic understanding of this region of the body and how its functions relate to the rest of the body. Because of its significance, the therapist must be able to properly assess this region of the body. In addition to reviewing the structures, this chapter discusses:

- Specific bony landmarks for palpation
- Soft tissue structures, including the muscles of the region
- The movements of the region, and the basic biomechanics of the ankle and foot
- Manual muscle tests for the ankle and foot
- Dermatome and trigger-point referral patterns for the involved muscles
- Some common causes of dysfunction and how to assess and treat them using soft tissue therapy

ANATOMICAL REVIEW

Bony Anatomy of the Lower Leg, Ankle, and Foot

When discussing the anatomy of the ankle and foot, it is helpful to divide the structures into three regions: the hindfoot, midfoot, and forefoot (Fig. 10-1).

Hindfoot

Technically, the hindfoot consists of the calcaneus and the talus, but it is also necessary to include the tibia and fibula in the discussion because of their relationships to the hindfoot. The previous chapter discussed the features of the proximal tibia and fibula; this chapter focuses on the distal aspects. The tibia is the major weight-bearing bone of the lower leg. It has a distinct ridge running down its anterior aspect known as the *tibial crest.* As the bone travels distally, it narrows slightly and its medial edge terminates in a large bony prominence called the *medial malleolus.* On the inferior distal end is the articular surface, covered in hyaline cartilage, for the superior aspect of the talus bone, which is discussed later. The final aspect of the tibia is on the distal, lateral surface of the bone and is a notch known as the *fibular notch.* The fibular notch accommodates the distal end of the next bone in the region, the fibula. The fibula does not contribute any significant weight-bearing function to the lower leg and is primarily a site for muscle attachments. The distal end of the fibula extends from the shaft and flares slightly, terminating in a structure called the *lateral malleolus.* Moving distally to the true hindfoot, the calcaneus is the largest bone in the foot and forms the heel. It serves as a very im-

Figure 10-1 Skeletal and surface anatomy structures of the lower leg, ankle, and foot.

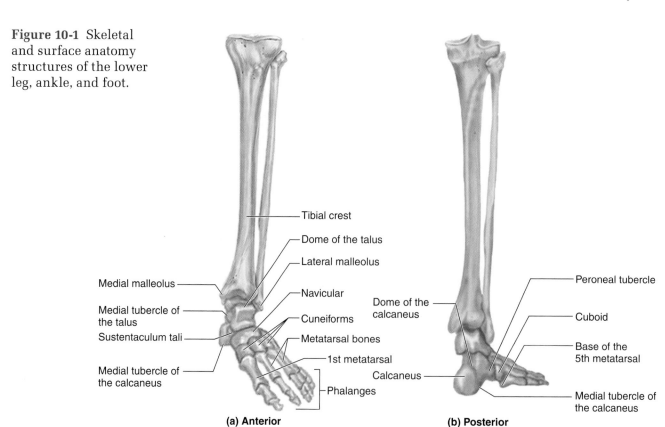

Tibial crest

Dome of the talus

Lateral malleolus

Medial malleolus

Navicular

Medial tubercle of the talus

Cuneiforms

Sustentaculum tali

Metatarsal bones

1st metatarsal

Medial tubercle of the calcaneus

Phalanges

(a) Anterior

Dome of the calcaneus

Peroneal tubercle

Cuboid

Base of the 5th metatarsal

Calcaneus

Medial tubercle of the calcaneus

(b) Posterior

portant attachment site for various muscles and ligaments. Sitting on top of the calcaneus is the second-largest and most superior bone of the foot, the talus. It has five functional articulations:

- Superiorly with the tibia
- Inferiorly with the calcaneus
- Medially with the medial malleolus
- Laterally with the lateral malleolus
- Anteriorly with the navicular

Midfoot

The midfoot consists of the navicular, the cuboid, and the three cuneiforms (see Fig. 10-1). The navicular, which derives its name from its resemblance to a ship, sits on the medial side of the foot, just distal to the talus. It articulates posteriorly with the talus and anteriorly with the three cuneiform bones. Lateral to the navicular and distal to the calcaneus is the cuboid. It articulates laterally with the 3rd cuneiform, distally with the 4th and 5th metatarsals, and proximally with the calcaneus. The last bones of the midfoot lie distal to the navicular and are known as the *cuneiform bones.* They are named for their positions medial to lateral as follows: 1st (medial), 2nd (intermediate), and 3rd (lateral) cuneiforms.

Forefoot

The forefoot comprises the 5 metatarsals and 14 phalanges (see Fig. 10-1). Each metatarsal can be looked at as a miniature long bone with a base at the proximal end, a shaft, and a head at the distal end. The metatarsals form the sole of the foot and are numbered 1 through 5, medially to laterally. The first three articulate with the cuneiforms, and the 4th and 5th articulate with the cuboid. Each toe has three phalanges (proximal, middle, and distal) with the exception of the great or first toe, which has only two (proximal and distal).

Bony Structures and Surface Anatomy of the Lower Leg, Ankle, and Foot

Palpation of this region can be more difficult than it first appears. The compact nature of the structures and the immobility of the segments can create a challenge when it comes to identifying the structures. Using movement and some massage techniques to loosen up the foot will dramatically help isolate the structures of the area. Begin at the distal tibia and fibula and work systematically into the various portions of the foot. The foot is again separated into the three regions.

> **Practical Tip**
>
> Because the foot supports a lot of weight, the structures can be very tight, so using movement to help with palpation is a good idea.

Hindfoot

The *tibial crest* runs vertically down the anterior aspect of the tibia and is often referred to as the *shin* (see Figure 10-1). At the distal medial tip of the tibia is the *medial malleolus*, commonly referred to as the *medial ankle bone.* It is very prominent and easy to palpate, making it a good landmark to use as a reference point.

Opposite the medial malleolus is the *lateral malleolus* or lateral ankle bone. This prominent landmark is the distal tip of the fibula and is found by tracing the fibula to its distal end. Between the medial and lateral malleoli sits the talus. Most of the bone is hidden in the joint, but certain aspects can be palpated.

The *dome of the talus* is found by passively placing the foot into slight plantar flexion and palpating at the midpoint between the distal tips of the malleoli in the soft spot.

Another structure on the talus is the *medial tubercle of the talus.* With the foot in neutral, move from the posterior/inferior medial malleolus in an inferior direction about a half-inch at a 45° angle until you feel a small bony prominence. This is an insertion point for a portion of the deltoid ligament, which is discussed later in the chapter.

The *calcaneus* is on the posterior foot and is commonly known as the *heel.* A variety of structures are palpable on this bone. To find the *peroneal tubercle,* locate the lateral malleolus and move distally about a half-inch; then feel for a small bony nodule. It separates the tendons of the peroneus longus (below) and the peroneus brevis (above). Moving to the medial side of the bone, find the *sustentaculum tali* by placing the foot in neutral and moving directly inferior from the medial malleolus about 1 inch until you feel a bony prominence. This is the insertion for the calcaneonavicular or "spring" ligament. Moving around to the back of the heel, the *dome of the calcaneus* is the posterior one-third of the bone and is found by pressing in and down just anterior to the Achilles tendon insertion.

The last structure on the calcaneus is the *medial tubercle* and serves as one attachment point for the plantar fascia. With the client in the prone position, palpate at the medial plantar surface of the calcaneus. Since this structure is deep and covered by thick tissue, a fair amount of pressure may be required. An alternate method is to dorsiflex the foot, extend the toes, and then trace the plantar fascia to the medial calcaneus and press in.

Midfoot

This section on the midfoot discusses the structures from medial to lateral (see Figure 10-1). The *navicular* sits just anterior to the talus and is typically very prominent on the medial aspect of the foot at the peak of the medial longitudinal arch. To locate this bone, move off the distal tip of the medial malleolus at a 45° angle; this area is the navicular. Alternatively, use the hand opposite the foot being palpated, and place the web space of the hand over the Achilles tendon; run the index finger along the medial side of the foot, inferior to the medial malleolus. The tip of the finger should be on the navicular.

The *medial* or *1st cuneiform* is found using the navicular as a starting point and moving in a distal direction until you find a joint line. The next bone distal to the joint line is the 1st cuneiform. It may be necessary to passively pronate and supinate the foot to help in locating the joint line.

The *2nd* and *3rd cuneiforms* are more difficult to palpate. They are found by using the 1st cuneiform and moving laterally, one bone at a time. They may also be located by starting with the cuboid and moving medially.

The last bone of the midfoot is the *cuboid;* it sits distal to the calcaneus. Begin at the lateral malleolus, and draw a line between the lateral malleolus and the base of the 5th metatarsal. Pick a point in the middle, and press in to feel the bone. The cuboid can also be located by moving in an anterior inferior direction off the malleolus and pressing in.

Forefoot

There are two prominent bones of this region that are easy to identify (see Figure 10-1). The *1st metatarsal* runs along the medial foot; it is found by moving proximally from the great toe onto the foot or by using the cuneiform as a starting point and moving distally until the joint line is found and continuing onto the bone. Using movement will help identify the joint space.

On the lateral side of the foot, the *base of the 5th metatarsal* is very prominent and flares out at the middle of the foot; it is often a site of injury. Begin at the anterior inferior lateral malleolus and move distally at a 45° angle to the lateral foot, moving distally from the base to trace the bone. Find the *metatarsals* by squeezing in the middle of the foot to locate each bone, tracing proximally and distally to define each one's edges. Lastly, identify the *phalanges* by palpating each of the toe bones.

Soft Tissue Structures of the Lower Leg, Ankle, and Foot

This section discusses the soft tissue structures in the region and the various joints that compose the area (Fig. 10-2). There are three different divisions of the area; however, a tremendous amount of interdependence exists among the divisions. Isolated movements of a single joint in a single plane typically do not occur.

Hindfoot

Three joints are located in this division:

1. The *tibiofibular joint* is a fibrous syndesmosis joint between the distal ends of the tibia and fibula. It comprises the anterior tibiofibular, posterior tibiofibular, and inferior transverse ligaments. It allows a minimal amount of spreading during dorsiflexion to accommodate the wider anterior surface of the talus and allows some rotation of the fibula during ankle motion.

2. The *talocrural* or *ankle joint* is a modified synovial hinge joint formed by the medial malleolus of the tibia, the

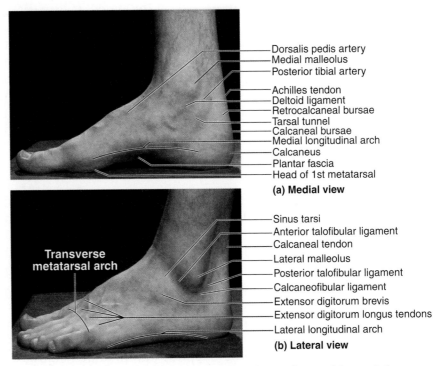

Dorsalis pedis artery
Medial malleolus
Posterior tibial artery
Achilles tendon
Deltoid ligament
Retrocalcaneal bursae
Tarsal tunnel
Calcaneal bursae
Medial longitudinal arch
Calcaneus
Plantar fascia
Head of 1st metatarsal

(a) Medial view

Transverse metatarsal arch

Sinus tarsi
Anterior talofibular ligament
Calcaneal tendon
Lateral malleolus
Posterior talofibular ligament
Calcaneofibular ligament
Extensor digitorum brevis
Extensor digitorum longus tendons
Lateral longitudinal arch

(b) Lateral view

Figure 10-2 Soft tissue structures of the lower leg, ankle, and foot.

lateral malleolus of the fibula, and the talus. This joint allows only 1° of freedom of movement: dorsiflexion and plantar flexion. It is surrounded by a thin joint capsule but is supported by strong ligaments.

- On the medial side of the joint, the *deltoid ligament* is made up of four separate bands and is extremely strong. These bands are the:
- *Anterior tibiotalar (ATT) ligament:* Runs from the anteromedial aspect of the medial malleolus to the superior portion of the medial talus.
- *Tibiocalcaneal (TC) ligament:* Connects the apex of the medial malleolus to the calcaneus.
- *Posterior tibiotalar ligament (PTT):* Runs from the posterior aspect of the medial malleolus to the posterior talus
- *Tibionavicular (TN) ligament:* Deep to the ATT, runs to the medial navicular to prevent lateral translation and lateral rotation of the tibia on the foot.

Laterally, only three ligaments support the joint:

- *Anterior talofibular (ATF) ligament:* Runs from the anterolateral surface of the lateral malleolus to the talus, near the sinus tarsi. It is taut during plantar flexion and resists inversion and anterior translation of the talus on the tibia.
- *Calcaneofibular (CF) ligament:* Runs vertically and slightly posteriorly from the distal tip of the lateral malleolus of the calcaneus. It is the primary restraint for inversion when the ankle is in neutral and during midrange.
- *Posterior talofibular (PTF) ligament:* Runs in an inferior and posterior direction from the posterior aspect of the lateral malleolus to the talus and calcaneus. The strongest of the three ligaments, its primary job is to limit the posterior displacement of the talus on the tibia.

3. The last joint of the hindfoot is the *subtalar* or *talocalcaneal joint.* As indicated by the name, it is an articulation between the superior surface of the calcaneus and the inferior surface of the talus. It allows 1° of freedom of movement: supination and pronation. No muscles attach to the talus, so its stability comes from several small ligaments and bony restraints. The interosseous talocalcaneal ligament is the primary stabilizer of the joint. It divides the joint into two cavities and provides an axis for talar tilt. The other support comes from four small talocalcaneal ligaments, the CF ligament, and portions of the deltoid ligament.

Midfoot

Individually, the joints of the midfoot do not allow for a lot of movement, but as a unit they offer a significant amount of movement that enables a variety of positions (see Figure 10-2). The midtarsal joint comprises two side-by-side articulations that create the junction between the hindfoot and the midfoot. The talocalcaneonavicular (TCN) is on the medial side. It is so-named because the talus moves simultaneously on the navicular and calcaneus. This joint is a modified ball-and-socket joint and allows both gliding and rotation. Three ligaments support this joint, with the most important being the plantar calcaneonavicular or "spring" ligament, which supports the medial longitudinal arch. The other two ligaments are the deltoid ligament and the bifurcate ligament.

The second joint is known as the calcaneocuboid (CC) joint and is a saddle-shaped joint that allows only gliding. It is supported by the long plantar ligament, the dorsal and plantar calcaneocuboid ligaments, and the bifurcate ligament. The last set of joints in this division includes those between the TCN and CC joints and the various articulations of the three cuneiform bones. These joints are held together with various ligaments and allow rotation and gliding to help the midfoot accommodate to various surfaces to increase stability.

Forefoot

This region begins at the tarsometatarsal joints between the five metatarsals and the bones of the midfoot (see Figure 10-2); it allows gliding. The five metatarsals are held together by various ligaments and terminate at the metatarsophalangeal joints, which are condyloid articulations allowing flexion, extension, and small amounts of adduction and abduction. The final joints of the foot are the interphalangeal joints between each of the phalanges, which are hinge joints allowing only flexion and extension.

A few additional structures in the area are important to identify (see Fig. 10-2). The lower leg is divided into four compartments—anterior, lateral, superficial posterior, and deep posterior—which are summarized in Table 10-1. These compartments are formed by fascial linings and contain both muscles and neurovascular components, so any injury to the area can increase pressure within the compartment and result in significant damage.

Table 10-1 Compartments of the Lower Leg

Compartment	Structures
Anterior	Tibialis anterior Extensor hallucis longus Extensor digitorum longus Peroneus tertius *Note:* The major nerve in the compartment is the deep peroneal nerve; the major vessel is the anterior tibial artery.
Lateral	Peroneus longus Peroneus brevis Superficial peroneal nerve Peroneal artery
Superficial posterior	Triceps surae group: • Gastrocnemius • Soleus Plantaris
Deep posterior	Tibialis posterior Flexor digitorum longus Flexor hallucis longus Tibial nerve Posterior tibial artery

The *sinus tarsi* is a region of the midfoot. This depression is located just anterior to the lateral malleolus and becomes more prominent during ankle inversion. The *tarsal tunnel* is on the medial side of the ankle and is formed by the flexor retinaculum. It runs from the medial malleolus to the calcaneus, creating a tunnel with several structures traveling through it.

In palpating the structures transversely, superior to inferior, the posterior tibialis tendon is the first structure, which is felt by having the client plantar-flex and invert the foot. Flexing the toes will bring out the next structure, the flexor digitorum longus. The tibial artery and nerve are the next two structures and are easily palpated. The last structure, the flexor hallucis longus, is palpated by having the client flex the great toe.

On the posterior ankle, the *Achilles tendon* can be palpated just proximal to the calcaneus; it is a prominent cordlike structure. At its attachment to the calcaneus, the *retrocalcaneal bursa* may be palpated on the anterior side of the tendon, but typically only if it is inflamed. The *calcaneal bursa* lies between the calcaneus and the skin on the posterior aspect of the bone. It is palpable only if there is a problem in the area. The *plantar fascia* is found by placing the client in the prone position and dorsiflexing the foot and extending the toes. The fascia is a very prominent cordlike structure running from the medial aspect of the calcaneus to the heads of the five metatarsals.

There are two pulses that are important to locate. The *dorsalis pedis artery* is found by palpating the top of the foot just lateral to the extensor hallucis longus tendon. The *posterior tibial artery* is located in the tarsal tunnel just behind the medial malleolus. The last structures of the region are the three arches of the foot. The medial longitudinal, lateral longitudinal, and transverse metatarsal arches primarily serve to absorb shock as the body moves, but they also function to increase the flexibility of the foot. Normally, the arches are more prominent in the non-weight-bearing position, with the medial longitudinal arch being the most noticeable. When engaged in weight bearing, the arches flatten as they support the weight of the body. The foot contacts the ground at three points: at the heads of the 1st and 5th metatarsals and at the calcaneus. The calcaneus, talus, navicular, 1st cuneiform, and 1st metatarsal form the *medial longitudinal arch*. These bones are supported by various soft tissue structures, including the calcaneonavicular or spring ligament, long plantar ligament, deltoid ligament, and plantar fascia. During static weight bearing, there is little or no contribution by the muscles in supporting the arch; however, once gait begins, the tibialis anterior, flexor digitorum longus, flexor hallucis longus, abductor hallucis, flexor digitorum brevis, and tibialis posterior help to pull the arch upward and proximal.

The *lateral longitudinal arch* is lower and stiffer than its medial counterpart and comprises the calcaneus, cuboid, and 5th metatarsal, with soft tissue support from the peroneus longus, peroneus brevis, peroneus tertius, abductor digiti minimi, flexor digitorum brevis, and plantar fascia. The last arch is the *transverse metatarsal arch* and is formed by the lengths of the metatarsals and tarsals, with soft tissue support from the tibialis posterior, tibialis anterior, peroneus longus, and plantar fascia. Problems with these arches can result in various dysfunctions, some of which are addressed later in the chapter.

⟩Practical Tip

Use repetitive movements of the structures to help with palpation.

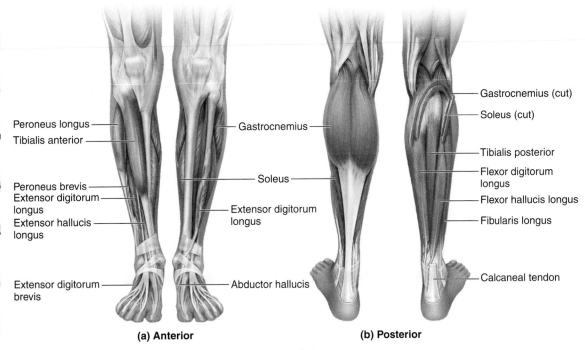

Peroneus longus

Tibialis anterior

Peroneus brevis

Extensor digitorum
longus

Extensor hallucis
longus

Extensor digitorum
brevis

Gastrocnemius

Soleus

Extensor digitorum
longus

Abductor hallucis

(a) Anterior

Gastrocnemius (cut)

Soleus (cut)

Tibialis posterior

Flexor digitorum
longus

Flexor hallucis longus

Fibularis longus

Calcaneal tendon

(b) Posterior

Figure 10-3 Muscles of the lower leg, ankle, and foot.

Muscles of the Lower Leg, Ankle, and Foot

The muscles of the lower leg, ankle, and foot are shown in Fig. 10-3. Refer
to the Quick Reference Table "Muscles of the Lower Leg, Ankle, and Foot"
at the end of this chapter (page 445).

MOVEMENT AND MANUAL MUSCLE TESTING
OF THE REGION

To ascertain whether there is dysfunction in this area, the therapist
must gather information, using the tools discussed below, to establish a
baseline for the client.

Movements of the Region

Assess the movements of this region in both the weight-bearing and non-
weight-bearing capacities, performing the most painful motions last. For
the purposes of this section, dorsiflexion and plantar flexion are the motions that occur at the talocrural joint; supination and pronation occur at
the subtalar joint. The motions at the foot and ankle are:

- Dorsiflexion
- Plantar flexion
- Pronation
- Supination
- Toe extension and flexion
- Toe abduction and adduction

> **Practical Tip**
>
> Dorsiflexion and
> plantar flexion occur
> at the talocrural
> joint; supination and
> pronation occur at the
> subtalar joint.

For weight-bearing assessment, place the client in a standing position and perform the following movements:

- *Plantar flexion:* The client should be able to raise up on the toes.
- *Dorsiflexion:* The client should be able to raise the forefoot off the ground and stand on the heels.
- *Pronation:* The client should be able to stand on the medial edge of the foot.
- *Supination:* The client should be able to stand on the lateral side of the foot.
- *Toe flexion:* The client should be able to lift the toes off the ground.
- *Toe extension:* The client should be able to curl the toes.

For non-weight-bearing range-of-motion assessment, place the client in either a supine or a seated position with the legs out straight. Stabilize the thigh and lower leg, and have the client perform the following movements:

- *Dorsiflexion:* Instruct the client to pull the foot and toes toward the body. The normal range for this is 20°.
- *Plantar flexion:* Instruct the client to point the toes and press the foot down as if pushing on a pedal. The normal range is 50°.
- *Supination:* This motion is a combination of inversion, adduction, and plantar flexion. Have the client turn the foot toward the big toe as if trying to look at the bottom of the foot. The normal range is between 45° and 60°.
- *Pronation:* This is a combination of eversion, abduction, and dorsiflexion. Instruct the client to turn the foot away from the big toe and toward the outside of the foot. The normal range is 15° to 30°.
- *Toe flexion and extension:* Instruct the client to flex and extend the toes. Compare the sides bilaterally. The great toe will have a greater range in both flexion and extension than the four small toes.
- *Toe abduction and adduction:* Have the client spread the toes and bring them back together. Compare the sides using the 2nd toe as midline.

Passive Range of Motion

As with other joints, if active full range of motion is available, a moderate amount of overpressure can be applied during this assessment to negate the need to perform passive assessments. If passive assessments are indicated, perform them with the client in a non-weight-bearing position, usually the supine position, while stabilizing the leg. Each movement will have a distinct end-feel as follows:

- *Plantar flexion:* Stabilize the leg just above the ankle with one hand, and apply force on the top of the foot with the other, moving it into plantar flexion. The end-feel will be a soft tissue stretch.
- *Dorsiflexion:* Perform this test with the knee bent and straight to assess gastrocnemius tightness. Cup the heel and rest the foot on your forearm while stabilizing just above the ankle with the other hand. Apply pressure with the forearm, and move the foot into dorsiflexion. The normal end-feel is a tissue stretch for both positions.

- *Inversion:* Grasp the foot from the bottom across the medial longitudinal arch, and stabilize the leg with the other hand. Move the foot into inversion, being careful to move only the subtalar joint. The end-feel will be firm, secondary to the tissue stretch of the ligaments and peroneus brevis and longus.
- *Eversion:* Grasp the foot the same way as that for inversion. Move the foot into eversion, being careful to move only the subtalar joint. There will be a hard end-feel secondary to the fibula contacting the calcaneus or the tissue stretch of the capsule.
- *Toe flexion and extension:* Stabilize the foot with one hand and grasp each toe, moving it into flexion and extension. The end-feel will be a soft tissue stretch.

Manual Muscle Testing

After determining the range of motion available, determine the strength of the region. Perform an isometric contraction, and instruct the client to resist the motion, resulting in an eccentric load being placed on the muscle. Test the client in the supine or seated position with the legs straight out and the foot hanging off the end of the table in the anatomical position.

- *Plantar flexion:* Place one hand on the shin just above the ankle and the other on the ball of the foot. Move the foot into dorsiflexion while the client resists.

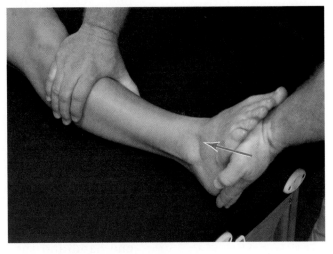

- *Dorsiflexion:* Stabilize the shin just above the ankle with one hand, and place the other on the top of the client's foot. Move the foot into plantar flexion while the client resists.

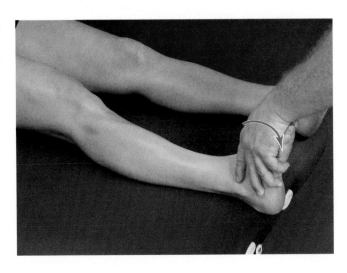

- *Inversion:* Stabilize the lower leg just above the ankle, and place the other hand along the distal medial side of the foot. Move the foot into eversion while the client resists.

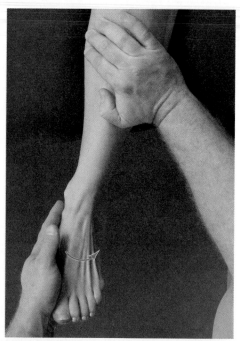

- *Eversion:* Place one hand above the ankle to stabilize the leg and the other along the distal lateral side of the foot. Move the foot into inversion while the client resists.

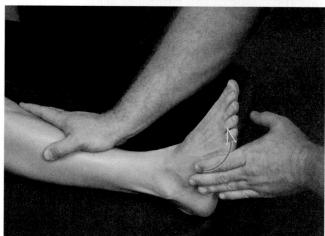

- *Toe flexion:* Grasp the foot with one hand and the toes with the other. Move the toes into extension while the client resists. This can also be performed in isolation on the great toe or the four small toes.

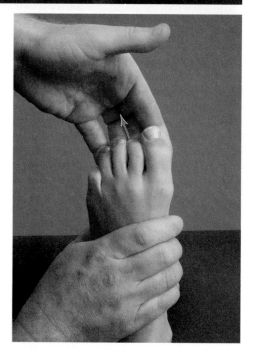

- *Toe extension:* Stabilize the foot with one hand, and place the other hand on the dorsal surface of the toes. Have the client resist as the toes are flexed. This can be performed on individual toes as well.

To ensure that there is no neurologic origin to any deficits in strength, test the myotomes of the area. Perform these specific tests in the same way as the general muscle tests:

- *L4—ankle dorsiflexion:* Place the foot in neutral, and stabilize the leg just above the ankle with one hand. Place the other hand on the top of the foot. Move the foot into plantar flexion while the client resists.
- *L5—great-toe extension:* Stabilize the foot with one hand. Press down on the top of the great toe with the other hand while the client resists.
- *S1—ankle plantar flexion:* Place the foot in neutral, and stabilize the leg just above the ankle. Press into the ball of the foot, and move it into dorsiflexion while the client resists.

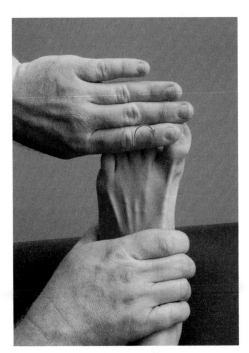

DERMATOMES FOR THE LOWER LEG, ANKLE, AND FOOT

To provide information on sensory changes in an area, assess the dermatomes for the region (Fig. 10-4). Any differences bilaterally can indicate dysfunction in the sensory nerve root. Keep in mind that there is a great deal of variability in the distribution patterns, and remember to stay in the middle of the dermatome to avoid overlap of the areas. Use a blunt

Figure 10-4 Dermatomes of the lower leg, ankle, and foot.

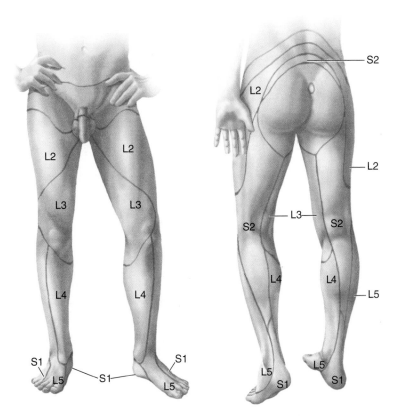

object, and touch the dermatome lightly. Ask the client whether there are any discrepancies between the sides of the body. Discrepancies can indicate pathology. The dermatomes for the ankle and foot are summarized in Table 10-2.

Table 10-2	Dermatomes of the Lower Leg, Ankle, and Foot
L3	Back, upper gluteal along iliac crest; front of thigh, knee, and medial lower leg
L4	Inner gluteal; lateral thigh, running to medial lower leg below knee; top of foot on great-toe side, including toes
L5	Gluteal; back and side of thigh; lateral aspect of lower leg; top of foot on lateral side, including toes; distal medial sole of foot including first three toes
S1	Gluteal; back of thigh and lateral lower leg; distal lateral sole of foot, including last two toes
S2	Same as S1

TRIGGER-POINT REFERRAL PATTERNS FOR MUSCLES OF THE REGION

This section examines some of the common muscles involved in lower leg, ankle, and foot pain, as well as the location and symptoms of corre-

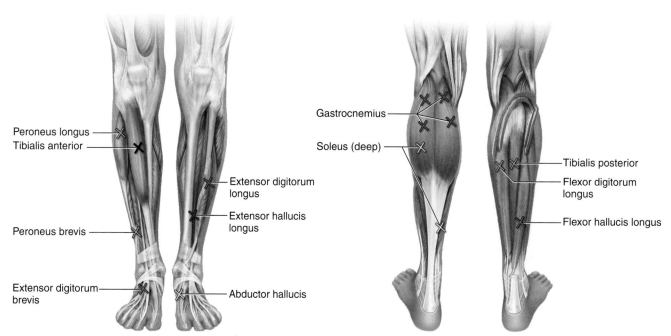

Figure 10-5 Trigger-point locations for the peroneus longus, peroneus brevis, tibialis anterior, extensor digitorum brevis, extensor digitorum longus, extensor hallucis longus, and abductor hallucis.

Figure 10-6 Trigger-point locations for the gastrocnemius, soleus (deep), tibialis posterior, flexor digitorum longus, and flexor hallucis longus.

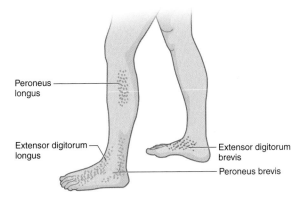

Figure 10-7 Trigger-point referrals for the peroneus longus, extensor digitorum longus, peroneus brevis, and extensor digitorum brevis.

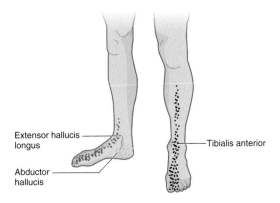

Figure 10-8 Trigger-point referrals for the extensor hallucis longus, abductor hallucis, and tibialis anterior.

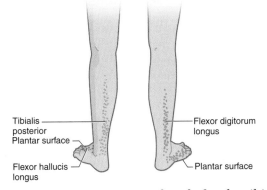

Figure 10-9 Trigger-point referrals for the tibialis posterior, flexor hallucis longus, and flexor digitorum longus.

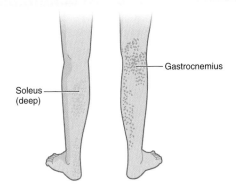

Figure 10-10 Trigger-point referrals for the soleus and the gastrocnemius.

sponding myofascial trigger points, which can arise as a result of postural issues, acute trauma, poor body mechanics, and repetitive stress. As with other muscles, trigger points in this region can mimic other conditions, so it is important to use all the information obtained during the assessment to help ensure that proper treatment is administered.

Tibialis Anterior

The *tibialis anterior* contains trigger points that are typically located in the taut bands in the upper third of the muscle (see Figs. 10-5 and 10-8). These points refer pain primarily to the anteromedial ankle and the dorsal and medial great toe. If the point is extremely irritated, there may be spillover from the point down to the ankle. Clients will complain of pain on the anteromedial ankle and big toe, as well as weakness in dorsiflexion. There is usually no pain at night even if the ankle is in sustained plantar flexion. Trigger points in this muscle are more likely the result of a traumatic incident than of simple overuse and often occur in conjunction with points in the peroneus longus due to their relationship.

Peroneus Longus and Brevis

The *peroneus longus* and *peroneus brevis* refer pain and tenderness to the area above, behind, and below the lateral malleolus and may continue a short distance into the lateral aspect of the foot (see Figs. 10-5 and 10-7). There also may be spillover in the middle third of the lateral aspect of the lower leg if the point is bad enough. Points in these muscles will result in complaints of "weak ankles," as well as pain and tenderness in the ankle and over the lateral malleolus. Such patients tend to incur ankle sprains more frequently than individuals without trigger points in the area. In the peroneus longus, the most common point is at the proximal end of the muscle about an inch distal to the head of the fibula on the shaft. For the peroneus brevis, the point is located near the transition point of the middle and lower thirds of the leg over the fibula.

Gastrocnemius

Moving to the posterior lower leg, we find the *gastrocnemius* muscle, which was discussed earlier in the text (see Figs. 10-6 and 10-10). There are trigger points in each head that tend to cluster in four locations. The first two points are located just proximal to the middle of the medial and lateral heads of the muscle. The medial point is the most common and refers primarily to the instep of the same-side foot and will spill over down the medial aspect of the calf if the point is bad enough. The lateral point refers in a general pattern around the point, and both points are associated with calf cramping at night. The other two points refer to the general location around the point and behind the knee near the medial and lateral attachment points of the femoral condyles.

Soleus

Deep to the gastrocnemius, trigger points in the *soleus* occur in two primary locations (see Figs. 10-6 and 10-10). The most common point is located just inferior to the lower border of the muscle belly of the gastrocnemius, or about 5½ inches above the heel, slightly medial to midline. It refers pain to the posterior aspect and plantar surface of the foot and to the distal Achilles tendon. This point can spill over to the region of the trigger point and into the instep. The second point is less common and located high on the lateral side of the calf. It refers diffuse pain in the upper half of the calf. A very rare third point is located just proximal and lateral to the first point. It refers to the ipsilateral sacroiliac joint in an area about 1 inch in diameter. Complaints from these points include pain in the heel that makes placing weight on the heel unbearable. Additionally, points in the upper portion of the muscle can result in symptoms of edema in the foot and ankle, as well as pain. Clients will also complain of limitations in dorsiflexion, which restrict the ability to use proper lifting mechanics. This leads to increased low-back pain in individuals who have soleus trigger points due to improper lifting.

Tibialis Posterior

The most deeply located muscle in the calf, the *tibialis posterior*, has trigger points that are accessible only indirectly through other muscles (see

Figs. 10-6 and 10-9). Tenderness can be elicited by pressing deeply between the posterior border of the tibia and the soleus near the proximal end of the bone. To ensure that the tenderness is actually associated with the tibialis posterior, be sure that the surrounding muscles are free from points as well. The points refer pain that concentrates over the Achilles tendon just proximal to the heel and may spill over from the point down the middle of the calf to the entire plantar surface of the foot. Clients will complain of severe pain in the sole of the foot and Achilles when walking or running, particularly on an uneven surface that requires additional stabilization of the foot.

Extensor Digitorum Longus

On the lateral side of the leg, the *extensor digitorum longus* refers pain over the dorsal surface of the foot and toes (see Figs. 10-5 and 10-7). This pain may concentrate over the ankle and spill over from the ankle to the point. The point is located about 3 inches distal to the fibular head between tibialis anterior and peroneus longus. Clients may complain of persistent pain over the dorsum of the foot and night cramps.

Extensor Hallucis Longus

The *extensor hallucis longus* is also located on the lateral side of the leg but refers pain to the distal aspect of the 1st metatarsal and great toe, as well as the dorsum of the foot (see Figs. 10-5 and 10-8). It may spill over up the leg as far as the point. These points are located just distal to the junction between the middle and distal thirds of the leg, just anterior to the fibula. The client will also complain of night cramps and persistent dorsal foot pain.

Flexor Digitorum Longus

The *flexor digitorum longus* lies on the posterior surface of the tibia and refers pain to the middle of the plantar surface of the forefoot, just proximal to the toes, with spillover to the toes and the medial side of the ankle and calf (see Figs. 10-6 and 10-9). The point is located at the proximal end of the muscle. To locate it, have the client lie on the affected side and apply pressure between the tibia and the gastrocnemius and soleus complex. The client will complain of pain in the feet when walking on the sole of the forefoot and on the plantar surface of the toes.

Flexor Hallucis Longus

The *flexor hallucis longus* refers to the plantar surface of the great toe and 1st metatarsal head; clients will complain of pain and occasional cramping in the toes (see Figs. 10-6 and 10-9). The point is located in the distal third of the leg on the posterior side. Palpate just lateral to midline in the distal third of the calf, against the posterior surface of the fibula. Address any points in the overlying muscles to ensure the most effective treatment is provided.

Extensor Digitorum Brevis and Abductor Hallucis

The *extensor digitorum brevis* has points located in the belly of the muscle around and just distal to the sinus tarsi (see Figs. 10-5 and 10-7). It refs to the instep and produces cramps in the foot. The *abductor hallucis* muscle refers pain to the medial side of the heel and can spill over to the instep and back of the heel (see Figs. 10-5 and 10-8). The points are located in the belly of the muscle along the medial heel into the arch, and they may require deep pressure to access. Refer to the Quick Reference Table "Trigger Points of the Lower Leg, Ankle, and Foot" at the end of this chapter (page 447).

SPECIFIC CONDITIONS

The lower leg, ankle, and foot are vital components in the kinetic chain of the lower extremity. Although pathology may cause pain, discomfort, or other symptoms at a specific site, interdependence between the parts provides foundational support, propulsion for locomotion, shock absorption, and the ability to adapt to the terrain; therefore, it is necessary to assess the entire lower extremity. Combine the results of the assessments discussed in the previous chapters that are relevant to the individual situation, keeping in mind that the pathology is unique to the person. While an extensive discussion of all the pathologies that affect this region is beyond the scope of this text, this section addresses some common sources of dysfunction and the various components of assessment and treatment.

Lower Leg: Medial Tibial Stress Syndrome

Background

medial tibial stress syndrome (MTSS) Pain along the posteromedial aspect of the distal third of the tibia arising from an overuse injury.

"Medial tibial stress syndrome (MTSS) is one of the most common causes of exercise related leg pain" (Kortebein et al., 2000). It is described as pain along the posteromedial aspect of the distal third of the tibia arising from an overuse injury. Often, the term "shin splints" is used to describe this pathology, but this term has been problematic in the medical community since it is not very descriptive and can be somewhat confusing.

The term *shin splints* was coined in 1982, but the condition itself was first described in 1913 as "spike soreness" in runners (Thacker et al., 2002). The origins of the term are not known, but it ultimately became a medical diagnosis through common use. Its controversial use spurred the American Medical Association (AMA) to define it in 1966, but it still has not been accepted universally. According to the AMA, shin splints are defined as "pain and discomfort in the leg from repetitive activity on hard surfaces, or due to forceful, excessive use of foot flexures. The diagnosis should be limited to musculoskeletal inflammations excluding stress fractures or ischemic conditions" (Thacker et al., 2002). Despite its controversy, most authors will agree that the term refers to pain in the leg between the tibial tuberosity and the ankle. For the purposes of this section, the term *shin splints* is not appropriate and the condition will instead be called *medial tibial stress syndrome,* which refers to a pathology that specifically affects the distal medial tibia. Despite narrowing down the location of the pathology, the causes of the pain can still arise from multiple sources. When pain occurs along the medial distal tibia, it is stemming from one of three etiologies:

1. *Stress fractures of the tibia:* Tibial stress fractures are beyond the scope of this text, but some of the indicators for this pathology include pain along the lower third of the tibia solely on the bone. The pain tends to be very localized, and individuals are generally unable to "work through the pain."

2. *Chronic compartment syndrome of the deep posterior compartment:* Posterior compartment syndrome is less common than anterior compartment syndrome, but it can be just as damaging. Chronic compartment syndromes are usually induced by exercise and have a gradual onset. They are commonly bilateral and do not respond well to conservative treatment. The pain generally presents in the center of the muscle rather than along the tibia, and clients will complain of tightness in the muscle. Pain is caused by increased compartmental pressure, which restricts blood flow and results in tissue ischemia. Another differentiating characteristic of compartment syndromes is the presence of sensory and motor deficits.

3. *Chronic periostitis (soleus syndrome):* This is the most likely etiology of medial tibial stress syndrome. The soleus attaches along the posterior tibia, and its medial attachment is to deep fascia, which is termed the "soleus bridge." It functions to plantar-flex and invert the foot, and excessive or prolonged foot pronation, especially eccentrically, will increase stress on this fascial insertion. This increased stress will cause the rupture of **Sharpey's fibers** and the loosening or disruption of the periosteum from the tibial cortex.

In the early stages, pain from this periostitis begins along the distal medial tibia. It is a dull ache that subsides promptly with rest. As the condition worsens, the pain becomes more persistent and can be debilitating. Both intrinsic factors, such as anatomical abnormalities or problems with the support structures of the foot, and extrinsic factors, such as overtraining or changing training surfaces or equipment, have been implicated in causing medial tibial stress syndrome.

Sharpey's fibers Direct extensions of dense, irregular connective tissue from the periosteum into compact bone. The fibers function to anchor tendons to bone.

Assessment

Medial shin pain can arise from several different sources, some of which are indications for referral to other health care practitioners. Include the entire lower extremity if necessary to ensure that all the factors are taken into consideration.

Condition History Therapists should inquire about the following while taking the client's history:

Question	Significance
Where does the pain occur?	The location of the pain can narrow down the structures that may be involved.
What is the nature of the pain?	Injuries to different types of tissues produce different types of pain.
What was the mechanism of injury?	MTSS typically does not result from an isolated incident but has a more gradual onset.

What are the client's normal pastimes and activities?	Any sudden changes in activity level or the undertaking of new activities can lead to MTSS.
What is the client's occupation?	Jobs that require long periods of standing can lead to MTSS.
Is there any history of previous injury?	This will help determine the involved structures.

Visual Assessment Since the etiology of MTSS can arise from numerous sources, it is important to assess the entire lower limb. Combine the visual assessment from the previous chapter with the components of this section to get an overall picture of the region. When assessing the lower leg, ankle, and foot, remember to observe them in both weight-bearing and non-weight-bearing postures.

The weight-bearing postures will provide information about how the body compensates for structural abnormalities. Observe clients from anterior, posterior, and lateral views.

Anterior View

1. Make sure the hips and trunk are not rotated, as rotation will affect the position of the foot.
2. Check the alignment of the tibias, noting any differences. Excessive internal rotation will result in a posture referred to as "pigeon toes." This can result from internal rotation at the hip as well, but it is more common at the tibia.
3. Note any excessive supination or pronation of the foot. Supination will cause the medial longitudinal arch to be more prominent, while pronation will make it less prominent.
4. Take care to note the **Fick angle**, which is an important observation. (Fig. 10-11). A normal angle is about 12° to 18° from the sagittal axis of the body. Any deviation will alter gait and can result in the formation of pathology.
5. Check for swelling, edema, or vasomotor changes, such as loss of hair, varicose veins, or changes in color in the lower legs, ankles, and feet.

Posterior View

1. Compare the size of the calves bilaterally, and note any differences.
2. Check the alignment of the Achilles tendons to see whether there is any calf deviation from a straight line. If the tendon bends medially, it might indicate a calcaneal valgus (rearfoot valgus), which pronates the foot. If the tendon bends laterally, it may be caused by a calcaneal varus (rearfoot varus), which supinates the foot.
3. Check for any abnormal discoloration, swelling, obvious deformity, and thickening of the Achilles tendon.

Lateral View Observe the longitudinal arches of the foot. There are two general deviations in the arches:

1. *Pes cavus (hollow foot):* Pes cavus will present as high longitudinal arches and is considered a congenital foot deformity. The soft tissues

Fick angle The angle that is created by the foot and the sagittal axis of the body. It measures how much the foot toes out (increased angle) or toes in (decreased angle). The normal range is 12° to 18°.

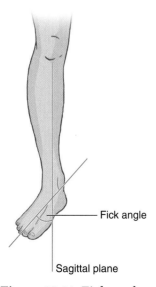

Fick angle

Sagittal plane

Figure 10-11 Fick angle.

are abnormally short, giving the foot an overall shortened appearance; this affects the foot's ability to absorb shock and adapt to stress.

2. *Pes planus (flat feet):* Pes planus can arise from a congenital source but can also occur as a result of a trauma, muscle weakness, or ligament laxity. It typically develops gradually.

There are also two types of flatfoot deformities:

1. *Rigid (congenital flatfoot):* Characterized by the absence of the medial longitudinal arch in both weight-bearing and non-weight-bearing postures; this condition is relatively rare.

2. *Acquired (flexible flatfoot):* Characterized by the arch disappearing only during weight bearing and is often corrected through the use of orthotics. As with the other views, check for any swelling, discoloration, or deformity.

It is important to determine whether any asymmetry noted is functional or anatomical. To assess this, the talus must be placed in the neutral position. Have the client stand with the feet relaxed so that the position is normal for the individual. Testing one foot at a time, palpate on either side of the dome of the talus and have the client slowly rotate the trunk to the right and then left. When the talus does not feel as though it is bulging out to one side or the other, it is considered to be in the neutral position. If the asymmetry is present only in a normal standing position, it is considered to be functional. If the asymmetry remains after the talus has been placed in neutral, it is also anatomical in nature and is probably the result of a structural deformity.

In the non-weight-bearing position, check for any abnormalities such as calluses, warts, scars, blisters, swelling, bruising, or obvious deformity. Note whether the arches are present, and check to see whether there are calluses over the metatarsal heads, which is an indication of a fallen metatarsal arch.

Palpation Include the entire lower leg when palpating the area. Focus on the structures in the distal medial tibia but include all the structures listed earlier in the chapter, as well. Check for differences in tissue temperature, tone, deformity, point tenderness, and swelling between the sides. Expand the palpation to related areas as needed.

Orthopedic Tests There are no specific orthopedic assessments for medial tibial stress syndrome; however, tests are typically administered to rule out other conditions. While manual muscle testing, and dermatome and myotome assessments, should be performed, this pathology is largely determined by the location of the pain during palpation in combination with the mechanism, history, and observations. Firm palpation over the posterior medial border of the tibia will produce pain, and in chronic cases there may be a nodular thickening of the tissue.

Soft Tissue Treatment

Unless there are structural abnormalities, this condition is largely caused by an imbalance of the soft tissues in the area. Removing any restrictions and restoring the normal mechanics to the area can be very beneficial to the treatment of this pathology. This section focuses on the lower leg and should be combined with the soft tissue treatment sections of Chapter 9 to create an overall plan.

Connective Tissue Two of the primary causes of this condition are directly related to the connective tissue in the area. The medial origin of the soleus attaches to a fibrous bridge that connects it to the tibia. Removing any restrictions in this attachment can relieve tension in the area. A posterior compartment syndrome can also cause this condition, so creating space within the connective tissue compartment will be beneficial.

Prone Position The posterior structures of the lower leg can be treated very effectively in this position. Assess the superficial tissue of the calf in various directions, and move into any restrictions until they release. Be aware of the client's tolerance level, as the calf is often tight. Perpendicular compressive effleurage works well on the calf to remove any restrictions. Move into the deeper layers, and strip out in between the gastrocnemius, soleus, and each head of the gastrocnemius to create space between the two muscles. Thumb stripping to the musculotendinous junction of the gastrocnemius and to the distal Achilles tendon is effective at releasing those areas.

Supine Position This position is used primarily to treat the tibialis anterior, but it can also be used to treat the lateral compartment. Assess the muscles in various directions, and move into any superficial restrictions. Separate the individual muscles, and work on any specific restrictions found within the individual muscles. It is best to work the anterior extensor retinaculum across the front of the ankle and the dorsal surface of the foot. Thumb strokes are also effective at releasing any tension in the area.

Side-Lying Position There is no clinical advantage to placing the client in this position unless the client specifically requests it or it is warranted by other factors. It can be used to have a slightly better mechanical advantage when working on the lateral compartment; however, be careful not to apply too much pressure directly on the fibula.

Tissue Inconsistencies Trigger points in this region can be hard to access depending on which muscle is being treated. Remove any points in the superficial muscles first to ensure that the most effective treatment possible for the deeper muscles is administered. To treat some of the deeper muscles, place the client in the side-lying position so that the medial aspect of the tibia of the bottom leg is accessible. Focus on the soleus and tibialis posterior, but treat the entire lower leg because of the interdependence of the muscles.

Muscle Concerns

Focus treatment on the posterior, superficial, and deep compartments, although it is important to address the entire lower leg as well. Incorporating movement is beneficial to the treatment's effectiveness.

Prone Position Warm up the muscles in the lower leg using a variety of strokes. Strip out the borders between the various muscles and the two heads of the gastrocnemius using the thumbs. Perpendicular compressive effleurage with active engagement is effective on the gastrocnemius and soleus. As the client slowly plantar-flexes the ankle, perform the stroke so that the end range is reached at the same time the stroke is completed.

> **Practical Tip**
>
> To incorporate movement in the foot and ankle, either hang the foot off the edge of the table or abduct the leg so that the foot is off the side of the table.

Cross-fiber fanning to the gastrocnemius is effective for removing restrictions between muscle fibers. Start at the musculotendinous junction and work proximally. Longitudinal thumb stripping can be performed with either a broad or a specific surface by having the client plantar-flex the ankle; deliver the stroke as the client dorsiflexes the ankle. Repeat until the entire length of the muscle is covered.

Friction to the Achilles tendon is an effective technique and can be done by flexing the knee and dorsiflexing the foot to remove slack in the tendon. Pinch the tendon, and move the tissue up and down. These strokes can be repeated using more pressure to affect the deeper muscle, taking care to stay within the client's tolerance level.

Supine Position The focus in this position is the lateral compartment. Warm up the muscles, and perform thumb strokes up the bellies of the muscles to release the tissue. A great stroke to this area is cross-fiber effleurage performed using a loose fist:

- Stand on the side of the client, and place one hand on the shin.
- Make a loose fist with the other hand, and grasp the thumb of the hand on the shin.
- Hook the knuckles of the fist into the tissue just lateral to the tibial crest, and perform a slow stroke toward the table (Fig. 10-12). Grasping the thumb of the hand on the shin increases the control of the stroke, allowing the application of more pressure. The hand on the shin can also function to rotate the lower leg to access different parts of the muscle.

Longitudinal thumb stripping can be effectively applied to the tibialis anterior in this position by having the client dorsiflex the foot and then plantar-flex as the stroke is delivered. Treat the dorsal surface of the foot by stripping out in between each metatarsal and applying friction around the tarsal and metatarsal joints. This will help create a more mobile foot, which may help with any biomechanical dysfunction in the area.

Side-Lying Position There is no clinical advantage to placing the client in this position unless the client specifically requests it or it is warranted by other factors. It can be used to have a slightly better mechanical advantage when working on the medial border of the tibia or the lateral compartment; however, be careful not to apply too much pressure directly on the fibula.

When treating the medial aspect of the leg in this position, longitudinal thumb stripping is very effective. Begin at the distal end of the leg, and apply force proximally just medial to the tibia. Have the client plantar-flex the foot. Move up the client's leg as he or she dorsiflexes. Repeat this process until the entire length of the tibia is covered.

Stretching

This condition is primarily caused by soft tissue dysfunction in the lower leg. Chronic tightness of the muscles in the area is a major contributor to

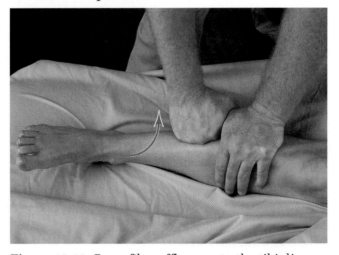

Figure 10-12 Cross-fiber effleurage to the tibialis anterior.

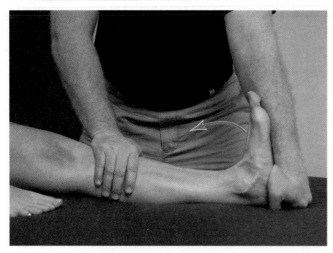

Figure 10-13 Gastrocnemius stretch.

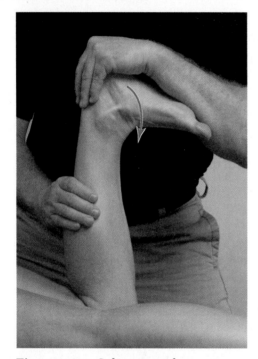

Figure 10-14 Soleus stretch.

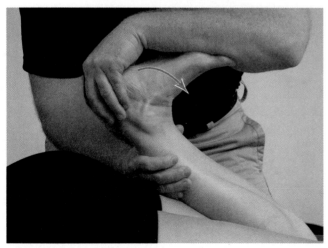

Figure 10-15 Achilles stretch.

the pathology. Stretching the various muscles in the area will remove any restrictions in the tissue and help restore normal functioning to the area.

Gastrocnemius Place the client in the supine or seated position with the knee fully extended (Fig. 10-13). Stand on the client's lateral side. Cup the heel with the hand closest to the foot, and place your forearm along the sole. Stabilize the client's leg with the other hand. Instruct the client to take a deep breath and dorsiflex the foot while exhaling. Once the client has reached the end range, use your body weight and lean to assist in the same direction. Hold for 2 seconds and return to the starting position. Repeat for one to two sets of 10 repetitions.

Soleus The soleus is related to the gastrocnemius and is stretched with the client in the prone position. Have the client bend the knee to 90° (Fig. 10-14). Place the hand over the client's heel and the forearm along the sole of the client's foot. Instruct the client to dorsiflex the ankle as he or she exhales. At the end range, assist in the same direction by leaning with the forearm, using your body weight to apply the force. Hold the stretch for 2 seconds, and repeat for 1 to 2 sets of 10 repetitions.

Achilles Tendon The Achilles tendon serves both the gastrocnemius and the soleus. It is stretched with the client in the prone position. Have the client flex the knee as far as possible to prevent the gastrocnemius or soleus from becoming involved (Fig. 10-15). Cup the heel, and place the forearm along the client's sole as in the previous stretch. Have the client dorsiflex his or her foot as far as possible while exhaling. Assist in the same direction at the end range by applying pressure to the sole with your forearm. Keep the client's knee flexed as far as possible during the entire stretch. Repeat for two to three sets of 10 repetitions.

Foot Evertors Stretch the evertors of the foot by placing the client in the seated or supine position with the knee fully extended (Fig. 10-16). Cup the heel with one hand, and place the other on the midfoot. Keep the client's foot positioned at 90°, and have the client invert the foot as far as possible while exhaling. Assist in the same direction with both hands at the end range. Repeat for one to two sets of 10 repetitions.

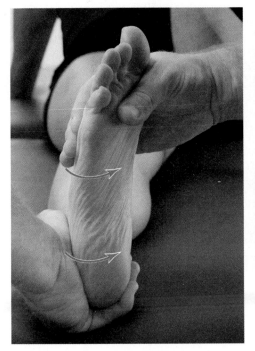

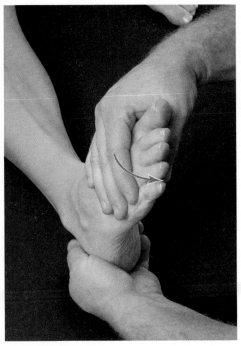

Figure 10-16 Foot evertor stretch.   Figure 10-17 Foot pronator stretch.

Foot Pronators Stretch the foot pronators in a similar manner. Begin in the same position as that for the evertor stretch, but secure the heel so that it does not move (Fig. 10-17). Place the foot into slight plantar flexion, and instruct the client to move the foot inward as far as possible without moving the heel. Hold the stretch for 2 seconds. Repeat for one to two sets of 10 repetitions.

Foot Invertors For the invertors of the foot, begin in a supine or seated position with the knee straight and the foot positioned at 90° (Fig. 10-18). Cup the client's heel with one hand, and grasp the midfoot with the other. As the client exhales, instruct him or her to evert the foot as far as possible. Using both hands, assist the client in the same direction, and hold the stretch for 2 seconds. Repeat for one to two sets of 10 repetitions.

Foot Supinators Stretch the foot supinators beginning in the position used for the invertors except with the foot positioned in slight plantar flexion (Fig. 10-19). Secure the heel so that it does not move, and have the client move the foot

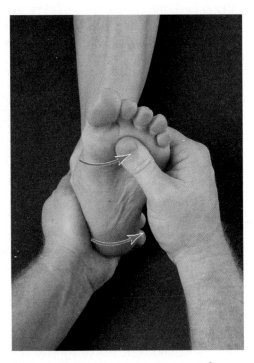

Figure 10-18 Foot invertor stretch.

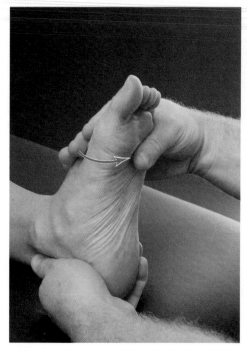

Figure 10-19 Foot supinator stretch.

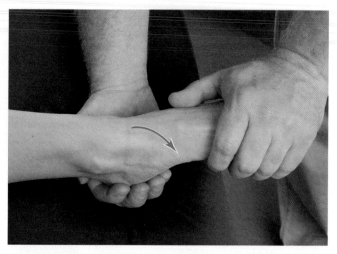

Figure 10-20 Dorsal foot stretch.

out as far as possible while exhaling. Hold the stretch for 2 seconds, and repeat for one to two sets of 10 repetitions.

Dorsal Surface of Foot For the dorsal surface of the foot, place the client in a seated or supine position with the leg fully extended (Fig. 10-20). Cup the heel with one hand, and have the client plantar-flex the foot as far as possible while exhaling. Assist in the same direction with the other hand on the top of the foot, and hold the stretch for 2 seconds. Repeat for one to two sets of 10 repetitions. There are two other variations of this stretch, one beginning with the foot in an inverted position and one with the foot in an everted position. Perform the stretches in the same way, and repeat for one to two sets of 10 repetitions.

Toe Flexors Moving into the foot, stretch the toe flexors with the client in the supine or seated position and the leg fully extended (Fig. 10-21). Support the foot, and instruct the client to extend the toes while exhaling. At the end of the range, assist in the same direction, stretching one toe at a time and holding each stretch for 2 seconds. Repeat for two to three sets of 10 repetitions each.

Toe Extensors Stretch the toe extensors by placing the client in the seated or supine position with the leg extended (Fig. 10-22). Support the foot, and instruct the client to plantar-flex and curl the toes as far as possible while exhaling. Assist in the same direction at the end of the range, stretching one toe at a time. Hold the stretch for 2 seconds for two to three sets of 10 repetitions.

Great Toe The last stretches are specifically for the great toe. For the flexors of the great toe, place the client in the seated position with the bottom of the foot on the table (Fig. 10-23). Stabilize just above the 1st metatarsal phalangeal joint, and instruct the client to extend the great toe while exhaling. Assist with the other hand at the end of the range. Hold

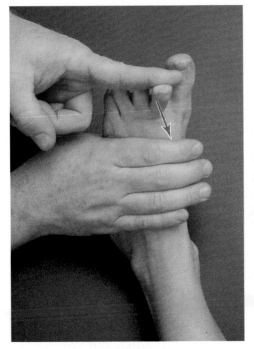

Figure 10-21 Toe flexor stretch.

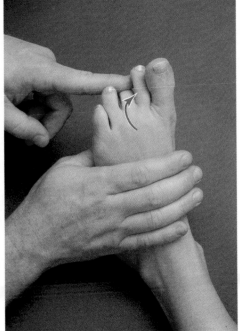

Figure 10-22 Toe extensor stretch.

for 2 seconds, and repeat for one to two sets of 10 repetitions. Repeat this stretch, instructing the client to extend the great toe up and out at a 45° angle. Assist at the end of the range. Stretch the extensors of the great toe with the client in the seated or supine position and the leg fully extended (Fig. 10-24). Stabilize just proximal to the 1st metatarsal phalangeal joint, and instruct the client to flex the great toe while exhaling. Assist in the same direction at the end of the range. Hold the stretch for 2 seconds, and repeat for one to three sets of 10 repetitions.

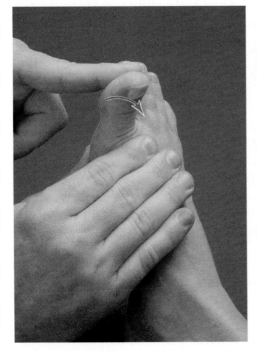

Figure 10-23 Great-toe flexor stretch.

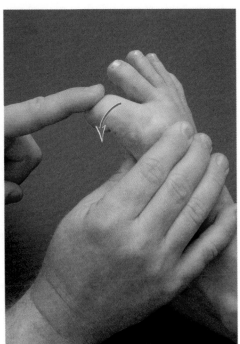

Figure 10-24 Great-toe extensor stretch.

Chapter 10 Conditions of the Lower Leg, Ankle, and Foot

Ankle: Achilles Tendonitis

Background

The Achilles tendon is the tendon of insertion for the gastrocnemius and soleus muscles, and it is the strongest tendon in the body. It is surrounded by a peritendinous membrane that is not a true synovial membrane, and it has a high capacity to withstand tensional forces during movement. Problems with the tendon tend to be multifactorial, involving both intrinsic and extrinsic factors:

- *Intrinsic components:* Leg-length discrepancies, lower extremity malalignments, muscle imbalances, decreased flexibility, and weight issues
- *Extrinsic components:* Overtraining, changing equipment, and training environment

Achilles tendonitis is an acute tendon condition and is the most common form of tendonitis. It accounts for 30% to 50% of all sports-related injuries and is becoming more common in the inactive population as well (Jarvinen et al., 2001).

The condition is characterized by pain, inflammation, and swelling in the tendon and occurs most often from a sudden increase in activity level, especially the eccentric loading of the tendon; however, a direct blow to the tendon can also cause the condition. It is thought that inflammation does not occur in the tendon itself but in the peritendinous tissue. As the condition becomes increasingly chronic, it is reclassified as another condition discussed previously, tendonosis.

Tendonosis is characterized by a degeneration of the tendon and a breakdown of the collagen structures due to repeated strain injuries, thereby disturbing the normal healing process. Tendons respond poorly to overuse, resulting in slow and incomplete healing (Cook et al., 2002). This failed healing response does not follow the normal triphasic (inflammatory, repair, remodeling) process and ultimately leaves the tendon defective and vulnerable to further injury. A hypovascular region on the tendon approximately 2 centimeters above the insertion of the Achilles is especially vulnerable to injury.

Both the acute and the chronic phases of this condition are characterized by pain that develops gradually. It is also associated with an increase in activity. In the acute phase, there is often swelling around the tendon, as well as burning or aching in the posterior heel that increases with passive dorsiflexion or resisted plantar flexion. Point tenderness is greatest in the middle third of the tendon. As the condition becomes chronic, the tendon may thicken and develop nodules along its length; crepitus may also be present. With both phases, pain occurs only during activity and quickly subsides with rest; however, it returns as soon as activity is resumed. As the condition progresses, the pain worsens and may eventually become constant.

Assessment

Achilles tendonitis is one of the more straightforward pathologies to assess; however, it is important to thoroughly assess each person individu-

📖 **Achilles tendonitis** An inflammation of the Achilles tendon that typically arises from overuse. It is characterized by pain and inflammation over the tendon.

📖 **tendonosis** A degeneration of the collagen matrix within the tendon caused by a cycle of repeated insults and partial healing that leads to an overall breakdown of the tissue.

ally because many conditions can mimic Achilles tendonitis. These include problems with the soleus, dislocation of the peroneal tendons, tarsal tunnel syndrome, and problems with the sural nerve. Although clinically it may be easy to assess this condition, include associated areas as necessary, as the factors causing the injury may stem from other regions.

Condition History Therapists should inquire about the following while taking the client's history:

Question	Significance
Where is the pain?	The classic location of the pain in this condition is over the tendon.
What is the nature of the pain?	Injuries to different types of tissue produce different types of pain.
What is the normal activity level for the client?	Any changes or increases in activity levels can be an important factor in this pathology.
Has the client changed the equipment used to participate in activities?	Changes in things such as shoes or training surfaces can lead to this condition.
What was the mechanism of injury?	Typically the onset of this condition is gradual, but it can also result from a direct blow to the tendon.
Is there a history of previous injury?	This will help determine the etiology.

Visual Assessment Observe the client in both weight-bearing and non-weight-bearing postures. Begin with the weight-bearing posture, which will show how the body compensates for any structural abnormalities. View primarily from the posterior aspect, and note the contours of the calf, comparing sizes and shapes bilaterally. The Achilles tendon should be in line with the gastrocnemius. Any deviation could be the result of calcaneal varus or valgus and can result in abnormal forces on the tendon. Check for any swelling, thickening, bruising, or deformity in the area.

Assess the client from the anterior and lateral views, as discussed for medial tibial stress syndrome. This will help identify any underlying biomechanical factors that may be causing or exacerbating this condition. In the non-weight-bearing position, check for any swelling, bruising, or obvious deformity as well as abnormalities such as calluses, warts, scars, and blisters.

Palpation While the primary location for palpation is the Achilles tendon and the immediate area, palpate the entire lower limb using the structures listed earlier in the chapter. Check for nodules in the tendon, point tenderness, temperature differences, and swelling in and around the area.

Orthopedic Tests There are really no specific tests for this condition other than direct palpation of the tendon. In addition to the results of the baseline assessments performed on the region, positive indications of this pathology include point tenderness over the tendon, the presence of nodules along the tendon, and crepitus on movement.

Soft Tissue Treatment

Treating this condition depends on identifying the underlying etiological factors and addressing them. Treatment can be difficult, however, since factors can be intrinsic, extrinsic, or both. Soft tissue treatment is a definite component to an overall strategy and can be very effective in both the acute and the chronic phases.

Connective Tissue Since this condition involves the tendon, connective tissue work directly to the tendon as well as to the surrounding structures is very beneficial.

Prone Position Assess the superficial tissue of the calf in various directions, and move into any restrictions until they release. Be aware of the client's tolerance level, as the calf is often tight. Perpendicular compressive effleurage works well to loosen up the various compartments of the posterior lower leg. Move into the deeper layers, and strip out in between the gastrocnemius and the soleus, as well as each head of the gastrocnemius, to create space between the two muscles. Stand at the base of the table, and place the client's foot on your stomach, covering it with a towel. Dorsiflex the foot just enough to take the slack out of the tendon, and perform thumb stripping to the tendon, treating all sides.

Supine Position This position is used to treat the anterior and lateral lower leg to address any contributing factors in this area. Assess the muscles in various directions, and move into any superficial restrictions. Separate the individual muscles, and work on any specific restrictions within the muscles themselves. Thumb strokes to this tissue are effective in releasing tension in the area.

Side-Lying Position There is no clinical advantage to placing the client in this position unless the client specifically requests it or it is warranted by other factors. This position can be used to access the medial and lateral sides of the Achilles tendon more directly.

Tissue Inconsistencies Because of their intimate relationship to the Achilles tendon, the two primary muscles that should be treated are the gastrocnemius and soleus. Remove any points in the superficial gastrocnemius first to ensure that the most effective treatment for the deeper soleus is administered. The entire lower leg should also be addressed because of the interdependence of the muscles.

Muscle Concerns

The focus of the treatment should be on the gastrocnemius and soleus, although the entire lower leg should be addressed because of the relationships between the structures in the area. Incorporating movement in this area is easy and adds tremendously to the effectiveness of treatment.

Prone Position After warming up the muscles in the lower leg, focus on the superficial posterior compartment by using the thumbs to strip out the borders between the various muscles and the two heads of the gastrocnemius. Perpendicular compressive effleurage with active engagement

Practical Tip

Take the slack out of the tendon by slightly dorsiflexing the foot. This will increase the effectiveness of the treatment.

is very effective on the gastrocnemius and soleus. As the client slowly plantar-flexes the ankle, perform the stroke so that the end of the range is reached at the same time the stroke is completed. Cross-fiber fanning to the gastrocnemius is effective at removing restrictions between the fibers. Longitudinal thumb stripping is also an effective stroke for this area and can be performed with either a broad or a specific surface. Have the client plantar-flex the ankle, and apply force proximally up the muscle. As the client dorsiflexes the ankle, your thumb or fist will slowly inch up the muscle. Repeat the plantar-flexion/dorsiflexion cycle until the entire muscle is covered. This is an invasive stroke and should be applied only during the later stages of healing and within the client's comfort level.

Friction to the Achilles tendon can be applied by flexing the knee and dorsiflexing the foot to remove slack in the tendon. Pinch the tendon, and move the tissue up and down; or secure one side of the tendon, and apply friction to the other side to access different parts of the tendon.

Supine Position The focus in this position should be on addressing any of the muscles in the lateral compartment that may be contributing to the condition. The techniques used for treating medial tibial stress syndrome can also be applied here.

Side-Lying Position There is no clinical advantage to placing the client in this position unless the client specifically requests it or it is warranted by other factors.

Stretching

Lengthening the muscles in this area will help take improper stresses off the involved muscles. The primary focus should be the gastrocnemius and soleus, but all of the stretches used for medial tibial stress syndrome should also be performed here to ensure that the entire region is balanced (see Figs. 10-13 to 10-24).

Tarsal Tunnel Syndrome

Background

Tarsal tunnel syndrome is another condition that falls under the broader umbrella of nerve entrapment syndromes. Specifically, it is caused by the entrapment of the posterior tibial nerve or one of its branches as it passes under the fibrous roof of the tarsal tunnel. This tunnel is formed by both bony and soft tissue structures. The tunnel floor is formed by the distal-medial aspect of the tibia, the superior aspect of the calcaneus, and the medial wall of the talus. The fibrous roof is formed by the flexor retinaculum, also known as the *laciniate ligament,* which spans between the medial malleolus and the calcaneus. Several structures in addition to the posterior tibial nerve pass through the tunnel. From superior to inferior, they are the:

- Tibialis posterior
- Flexor digitorum longus
- Posterior tibial artery
- Posterior tibial nerve
- Flexor hallucis longus

tarsal tunnel syndrome A nerve entrapment syndrome that affects the posterior tibial nerve as it passes through the tarsal tunnel.

Koppell and Thompson were the first to describe tarsal tunnel syndrome, but the term itself was first used by Keck and Lam in 1962. This condition can arise from a variety of factors, so many, in fact, that only 60% of clients that present with clinical signs have an identifiable specific cause (Jerosch et al., 2006). These factors can be extrinsic, such as:

- External trauma to the area
- Stretch injury
- Fractures
- Compression injuries
- Overuse injuries

Intrinsic factors include:

- Space-occupying lesions
- Bony abnormalities
- Varicosities
- Cysts
- Nerve tumors

Another common etiology is the presence of hindfoot deformities, which lead to either excessive eversion, thereby causing an increased tension on the tibial nerve, or excessive inversion, which can contribute to nerve compression.

Clients who have tarsal tunnel syndrome will present with symptoms that have occurred spontaneously. Bilateral involvement is not typical. The most common complaint is pain that is difficult to pinpoint but is described as burning in the medial ankle and plantar aspect of the foot that is increased by weight bearing. In addition to burning pain, there are often complaints of numbness or paresthesia, motor disturbances, and gait abnormalities.

Assessment

This condition can be elusive in its etiology and often involves multiple components. To ensure that proper treatment is administered, it is important to perform a thorough assessment. Be sure to include any related areas, and remember the possibility of the double-crush phenomenon occurring in the lower extremity as well.

Condition History Therapists should inquire about the following while taking the client's history:

Question	Significance
What is the client's occupation?	Jobs that require standing for long periods of time can exacerbate this condition, especially if there is a hindfoot deformity.
Was there an injury? If so, what was the mechanism?	Injuries such as severe ankle sprains or crush injuries can damage the structures in the tunnel.

What is the progression of the symptoms?	Are the symptoms getting better, getting worse, or staying the same?
Are there any changes in sensation?	Sensory changes are a sign of nerve involvement.
Where is the pain located?	Pain is typically located along the medial ankle into the foot.
Is there a history of previous injury?	This will help determine the etiology.

Visual Assessment Since there are a variety of causes for this condition, evaluate the biomechanics of the lower extremity to determine their involvement. Observe the client in both weight-bearing and non-weight-bearing postures, paying special attention to the posterior view of the hindfoot. Perform the same visual assessments as for medial tibial stress syndrome, as these encompass all aspects of the lower limb.

Palpation Begin by assessing the lower limb for overall tension and consistency in the muscles. Check for swelling, especially over the tarsal tunnel, obvious deformity, bruising, and the presence of nodules in the structures running through the tunnel. For completeness, include all the structures that were discussed earlier in the chapter.

Orthopedic Tests The information gathered from the history, visual assessment, palpation, and range-of-motion testing should give the therapist a good baseline from which to start. Only one orthopedic test is specific to this condition. It is the test described in Chapter 8 for a similar nerve compression pathology, carpal tunnel syndrome. Table 10-3 shows the test and how to perform it.

Table 10-3 Orthopedic Test for Tarsal Tunnel Syndrome

Orthopedic Test	How to Perform
Tinel test 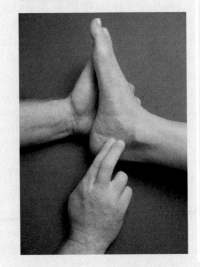	Client is in the seated position with the leg supported. Place the ankle into slight dorsiflexion and eversion to take the slack out of the tissue Tap, using the index and middle fingers, just inferior and distal to the medial malleolus. Any tingling or paresthesia indicates a positive sign.

Practical Tip
Take the slack out of the tissue by slightly dorsiflexing and everting the foot to increase the effectiveness of the test.

Soft Tissue Treatment

Typically, this condition arises after an injury to the area or as a result of improper biomechanics of the foot. These etiologies will cause an imbalance in the soft tissues of the region; therefore, soft tissue treatment is extremely beneficial. Most of the benefit will come from treating the structures that run through the tarsal tunnel indirectly. Any tension in the muscles will cause the tendons to be tight, also making them more susceptible to irritation in the tunnel. Direct work over the tunnel itself must be done with caution so that the irritated structures are not made worse; however, this work should not necessarily be avoided.

Connective Tissue The tarsal tunnel is created partly from the flexor retinaculum, which is a continuation of the deep fascia of the leg; therefore, connective tissue work is beneficial.

Prone Position Begin by assessing the superficial tissue of the calf. Locate any restrictions, and move into them. Since the structures that run through the tarsal tunnel are located in the deep posterior compartment, the overlying tissues must be thoroughly released to provide the most effective access to the deeper layers. Strip out in between the gastrocnemius and the soleus using the thumbs to separate the muscles as well as each head of the gastrocnemius. Once space has been created between the individual muscles, remove any restrictions within the bellies themselves.

Supine Position Removing restrictions to the anterior connective tissue will benefit the overall functioning of the area and contribute to the restoration of proper mechanics. Assess the superficial tissue and release any restrictions, being sure to include the dorsal surface of the foot and the extensor retinaculum. Once the superficial restrictions have been addressed, separate the individual muscles and remove any restrictions in the bellies.

Side-Lying Position There is no clinical advantage to placing the client in this position unless the client specifically requests it or it is warranted by other factors. It can be used to have a slightly better mechanical advantage when working on the medial aspect of the ankle directly on the flexor retinaculum. Dorsiflex the client's foot slightly to remove any slack in the tissue, and perform light strokes both parallel and perpendicular to the retinaculum. These strokes should be firm enough to create change in the tissue but light enough not to exacerbate the condition. This position can also be effective in accessing the muscles of the deep posterior compartment in the bottom leg.

Tissue Inconsistencies The superficial posterior compartment must be thoroughly treated and its points removed to have the greatest effect on the deeper muscles. Once the superficial points are treated, the client can be put in the side-lying position, which will allow direct access to some of the points in deeper muscles. The focus should be on the deep posterior compartment; however, the entire lower leg should also be treated.

Muscle Concerns

Focus on removing any tension in the muscle tissue to the entire lower leg. This will remove imbalances and help with problems caused by the tendons running through the tunnel. Once again, this treatment will be less direct for this pathology.

Prone Position This position is effective for treating the posterior compartments of the lower leg. Warm up the area with a variety of strokes so that the superficial tissues are sufficiently released. Perform the strokes that were used for both medial tibial stress syndrome and Achilles tendonitis.

Address the plantar aspect of the foot, as well. Support the dorsal aspect of the foot either with a bolster or by cradling it in your hand. Because the tissues are typically thicker on the bottom of the foot, perform effleurage using a loose fist to loosen up the area. Treat the deeper muscles by stripping them out with the thumbs, moving in both a parallel and a perpendicular direction. One effective technique is to make a fist and roll the wrist around in circles, working on the tissue with the knuckles. These strokes will help address the insertions for the muscles in the deep posterior compartment.

Supine Position The focus in this position should be on addressing the muscles in the lateral compartment that may be contributing to the condition. The techniques used for treating medial tibial stress syndrome and Achilles tendonitis can also be applied here. Stripping out between the metatarsals and treating the joints of the foot will help with any biomechanical dysfunction in the area.

Side-Lying Position There is no clinical advantage to placing the client in this position unless the client specifically requests it or it is warranted by other factors. It can be used to have a slightly better mechanical advantage when accessing the muscles of the deep posterior compartment in the bottom leg. Longitudinal thumb stripping, as described for medial tibial stress syndrome, is an effective technique to treat the deeper muscles of the area.

Stretching

Improving the flexibility of the lower leg will help take the pressure off any structures running through the tarsal tunnel. Perform all the stretches for the lower leg (see Figs. 10-13 to 10-24), paying special attention to the ones that focus on the deep posterior compartment (see Figs. 10-13 to 10-19).

Foot: Plantar Fasciitis

Background

Plantar fasciitis is considered the most common cause of inferior heel pain in adults. It is estimated that up to 2 million people are treated for this condition each year, accounting for up to 15% of physician visits

plantar fasciitis An inflammation of the plantar fascia caused by either an individual traumatic incident or repeated micro-traumas over a period of time. It is characterized by sharp pain with the first few steps in the morning or after a long period of non-weight bearing.

for foot pain (Roxas, 2005). This pathology is known by several other names, including:

- Heel spur syndrome
- Calcaneodynia
- Subcalcaneal pain
- Painful heel syndrome

Despite the frequency of this pathology, little is known about the physiologic process in its development (Juliano et al., 2004). This is another pathology that can change classifications as it moves from the acute stage to the chronic stage. The word *fasciitis* implies that it is an inflammatory condition, and initially it is. This inflammation can arise from a single traumatic event but is more commonly the result of repeated stress. As the condition progresses to the chronic stage, repeated insults to the plantar fascia without the ability to heal fully create a degenerative process similar to tendonosis.

The plantar fascia is a thickened fibrous sheet of connective tissue that has multiple layers. It runs from the medial calcaneal tuberosity to the heads of the five metatarsals to help form the medial longitudinal arch. It serves to support the structures of the longitudinal arch and acts as a dynamic shock absorber for the foot and leg (Roxas, 2005). When a person is engaged in weight-bearing activity, the foot contacts the ground in three main spots: at the heel and at the heads of the 1st and 5th metatarsals. The plantar fascia helps support the foot through a principle called the **windlass mechanism**.

The foot and its ligaments have been described as a triangular truss formed by the calcaneus, midtarsal joint, and metatarsals (Bolgla et al., 2004). The vertical forces created by the body's weight, coupled with the ground forces pressing up into the foot, tend to cause the medial arch to collapse. The attachments of the plantar fascia act as the tie-rod between these structures and prevent the foot from collapsing by virtue of its anatomical orientation and tensile strength. The windlass effect is the tightening of a rope or cable (Bolgla, 2004). During dorsiflexion of the foot and toes, the plantar fascia is wound around the heads of the metatarsals. This shortens the distance between the attachment points of the plantar fascia, lifting and supporting the medial arch. This also creates a great amount of tension in the plantar surface of the foot, resulting in a rigid lever arm to aid in propulsion during gait.

The etiology of plantar fasciitis is poorly understood and can be undetermined in as many as 85% of cases (Roxas, 2005). This condition is likely the result of multiple factors that can be divided into three categories:

- *Anatomical:* Can include sudden weight gain, long-term obesity, leg-length discrepancies, and pes planus or pes cavus
- *Biomechanical:* Can include muscle weakness, clubfoot, improper footwear, excessive pronation, and limited dorsiflexion
- *Environmental:* Can include trauma, prolonged weight bearing, atrophy due to inactivity, walking barefoot, and lack of flexibility

Some of the factors that have more of a significant contribution to this condition are described in greater detail below.

Pes cavus creates an environment in the foot that results in the foot's inability to dissipate forces. This decreased mobility increases the tension

📖 **windlass mechanism** A mechanical model that provides an explanation of how the plantar fascia supports the foot during weight-bearing activities. As the foot moves into dorsiflexion and the toes extend during gait, the plantar fascia is wound around the heads of the metatarsals. This shortens the plantar fascia and elevates the medial longitudinal arch.

at the insertion point of the plantar fascia at the medial calcaneus. Two other characteristics of a cavus foot are a decreased distance between the calcaneus and the metatarsal heads, and a rigid 1st ray, both of which increase the tension on the fascia.

At the other end of the spectrum, overpronation can be just as problematic. It is reported that 81% to 86% of individuals with symptoms of plantar fasciitis overpronate (Roxas, 2005). This pronation can originate from a pes planus foot, Achilles tendon tightness, or muscle weakness. As the foot overpronates, additional stress is placed on the middle band of the fascia; this leads to dysfunction.

While these factors may be difficult to address, there is one factor that is easily remedied. The lack of dorsiflexion can lead to the development of plantar fasciitis because of its relationship with the Achilles tendon. The nature of the attachment points of the two structures creates a "tug of war" on the calcaneus, with the plantar fascia pulling down while the Achilles is pulling up. A lack of flexibility, as little as a 10° decrease in dorsiflexion, will place an increased and prolonged tensile load on the plantar fascia both in static weight bearing and during movement, dramatically increasing the chances of developing a problem.

The last factor involves prolonged weight bearing. Certain occupations or any situation that requires prolonged weight bearing can lead to plantar fasciitis as a result of the repetitive loading of the fascia, which can be directly related to sudden gains in weight or chronic obesity.

Clients who have plantar fasciitis will present with classic pain in the medial plantar heel that is at its worst with the first few steps in the morning or after long periods of non-weight bearing. The pain tends to resolve after a few minutes as the tissue warms up. The pain is also present after prolonged periods of standing and can extend along the length of the plantar fascia. Paresthesia and pain at night are not common complaints with this condition and should be investigated for other causes. Constant irritation of the plantar fascia can result in the formation of an exostosis of the medial calcaneal tuberosity. This bone spur formation does not guarantee that a painful condition will develop, and there is no correlation between heel spurs and plantar fasciitis. Surgical removal of the spur may have no effect on the condition and in certain instances may make it worse.

> **Practical Tip**
>
> A classic presentation of plantar fasciitis is sharp pain with the first few steps out of bed.

Assessment

This condition can be multifactorial in its etiology and is not well understood. To ensure that proper treatment is administered, a thorough assessment of all possible contributing factors should be performed.

Condition History Therapists should inquire about the following while taking the client's history:

Question	Significance
Where is the pain located?	The pain presentation for this condition is very identifiable.
When does the pain occur?	This condition will cause a classic pattern of pain with the first few steps in the morning.
Has there been any change in weight?	Rapid weight gains can lead to increased stress on the fascia.

Has there been a change in activity levels?	Increases in activity levels can increase the stress on the tissues.
What is the client's occupation?	Prolonged periods of standing can increase the tension on the fascia.
Was there an injury? If so, what was the mechanism?	While this condition is primarily chronic in nature, blunt trauma to the tendon can cause problems as well.

Visual Assessment Observe the client in weight-bearing and non-weight-bearing postures, paying special attention to the position of the subtalar joint. Perform the same visual assessments as those for medial tibial stress syndrome. The arches can easily be visualized and assessed from the lateral view. For the non-weight-bearing posture, check for swelling, primarily over the plantar fascia, along with thickening, bruising, or deformity in the area.

Palpation Assess the muscles in the area for consistencies and imbalances. Check for bruising, obvious deformity, and swelling, especially over the plantar fascia. Complete the palpation of the area by including all the structures that were discussed earlier in the chapter.

Orthopedic Tests There are no specific tests for this condition, and assessment is based largely on the client's history and the findings during palpation. The two most identifiable signs are that the pain is most severe during the first few steps in the morning and that it is located at the medial calcaneal tuberosity. Any findings should be coupled with manual muscle, dermatome, myotome, and range-of-motion tests, as well as the other components of the assessment, to provide an overall picture.

Soft Tissue Treatment

Balancing the muscles of the lower leg and those that support the arches plays a key part in the treatment of this condition. The gastrocnemius and soleus should be an area of focus because of their relationships to this condition. This work can sometimes be slightly uncomfortable, so using cryotherapy before, during, and after treatment is beneficial.

Connective Tissue The plantar fascia is made up entirely of connective tissue, so using this type of treatment is very beneficial.

Prone Position Begin by applying the treatment techniques that were performed for the previous conditions, paying special attention to the gastrocnemius and soleus. To treat the plantar fascia directly:

1. Cover the client's toes with a towel.
2. Place the plantar fascia on your stomach or chest, and lean forward so that the foot is dorsiflexed and the toes are extended (Fig. 10-25). This will give you both hands to work with.
3. Support the heel with one hand, and perform cross-fiber thumb strokes at the proximal attachment in one direction for 2 to 3 minutes and then in the other direction for 2 to 3 minutes.

This treatment may be uncomfortable but should not be so aggressive that it is outside the client's tolerance level. Once the proximal attachment has been addressed, parallel and cross-fiber strokes can be performed along the entire length of the plantar fascia.

Supine Position Address the connective tissue of the anterior and lateral compartments of the lower leg in this position, using the techniques discussed for the previous conditions.

Side-Lying Position There is no clinical advantage to placing the client in this position unless the client specifically requests it or it is warranted by other factors. It can be utilized to treat the related tissue of the lower leg if necessary.

Tissue Inconsistencies Trigger points in the lower leg can mimic this condition, so it is important to treat the area thoroughly. Focus on the gastrocnemius, the soleus, and the muscles that help support the arch. In addition, treat the other muscles that were listed earlier in the chapter.

Muscle Concerns

While the plantar fascia is not a muscle, it is important to treat the muscles of this area to help remove any imbalances that may be contributing to the problem.

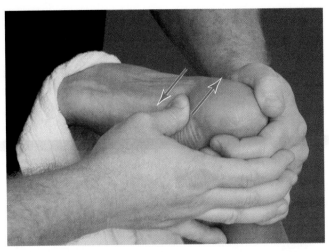

Figure 10-25 Cross-fiber thumb strokes to the plantar fascia.

Prone Position Begin by warming up the area using a variety of strokes, followed by the techniques used to treat medial tibial stress syndrome. The plantar surface of the foot can be treated effectively in this position. Support the foot with either a bolster or a hand, and use a fist to effleurage the bottom of the foot. It is also effective to support the foot with both hands and perform cross-fiber thumb strokes to the sole of the foot (Fig. 10-26). Thumb stripping the entire plantar surface and applying friction over the metatarsal heads are also beneficial.

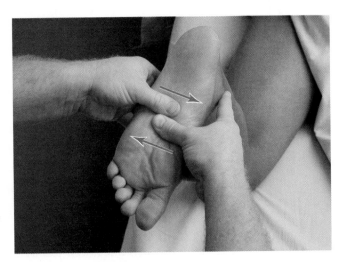

Figure 10-26 Cross-fiber effleurage to the sole of the foot.

Supine Position Utilize this position to treat the involved muscles in the area or those that may be creating imbalance in the tissue. The techniques that were used for the previous conditions can also be utilized here. One good, specific technique is to strip out between each metatarsal and traction the toes.

Side-Lying Position There is no clinical advantage to placing the client in this position unless the client specifically requests it or it is warranted by other factors.

Chapter 10 Conditions of the Lower Leg, Ankle, and Foot

Stretching

"Stretching is the single most effective method of treatment" (Dyck et al., 2004). Stretch the entire lower limb, but focus on the gastrocnemius and soleus, the great toe, and the muscles that support the arches. The stretches that were used for medial tibial stress syndrome can also be applied here (see Figs. 10-13 to 10-24).

SUMMARY

While the area of the lower leg, ankle, and foot is small compared to other regions of the body, it is a significant contributor to the kinetic chain of the lower extremity and can affect the performance of the entire body. The first section reviewed basic anatomy to give an overall picture of the structures in the area. Individual bony landmarks and soft tissue structures were identified, and assessments such as range-of-motion and manual muscle testing were explained, to give a good baseline of information for the area. Since the structures in this area are dependent on each other, the etiologies and treatments for the conditions overlap. For each condition, background information, assessment techniques, and treatment recommendations were provided.

REVIEW QUESTIONS

1. What are the two principle functions of the lower leg, ankle, and foot?
2. List the structures that are contained in the hindfoot, midfoot, and forefoot.
3. What are the names of the individual ligaments that make up the deltoid ligament?
4. What are the structures in each of the four compartments of the lower leg?
5. What is the difference between shin splints and medial tibial stress syndrome?
6. What is the most common etiology for medial tibial stress syndrome?
7. How is talar neutral found?
8. What are the structures that pass through the tarsal tunnel?
9. What is the job of the plantar fascia?
10. What is the classic symptom of plantar fasciitis?

CRITICAL-THINKING QUESTIONS

1. Explain the pathology of compartment syndrome in the lower leg.
2. How does pes planus increase the chances of developing tarsal tunnel syndrome?
3. Explain the windlass mechanism as it relates to the plantar fascia.
4. How do tight calves contribute to the formation of plantar fasciitis?
5. Explain how a heel spur forms as a result of chronic plantar fasciitis.

Part II Regional Approach to Treatment

Bony Structures of the Lower Leg, Ankle, and Foot

Tibial crest	Trace from the tibial tuberosity down the midline of the tibia. This is a relatively sharp edge of bone and can be tender.
Medial malleolus	This structure lies on the distal tip of the medial tibia. It is commonly referred to as the *medial ankle bone.* It is very prominent and easy to palpate.
Lateral malleolus	This structure lies on the distal tip of the fibula. It is commonly referred to as the *lateral ankle bone.* It extends farther distally than the medial malleolus and is very prominent and easy to palpate.
Dome of the talus	This aspect of the talus can be found by placing the foot into plantar flexion and palpating at the midpoint between the distal tips of the malleoli.
Medial tubercle of the talus	This tubercle is the insertion for a portion of the deltoid ligament. Using the posterior/inferior medial malleolus, move in an inferior direction about ½ inch at a 45° angle until you find a bony prominence.
Calcaneus	This bone is commonly referred to as the *heel* and is on the posterior foot.
Peroneal tubercle	This prominence is located on the calcaneus and is found by locating the lateral malleolus and moving distally about ½ inch. It separates the tendons of the peroneus longus (below) and the peroneus brevis (above).
Sustentaculum tali	This bone part is located on the calcaneus and is the insertion for the calcaneonavicular or "spring" ligament. Using the medial malleolus, move directly inferior about 1 inch until you find a bony prominence.
Dome of the calcaneus	This is the posterior third of the calcaneus and can be palpated at the top of the calcaneus anterior to the Achilles tendon.
Medial tubercle of the calcaneus	This tubercle is the origin of the plantar fascia. It can be palpated at the medial plantar surface of the calcaneus. A fair amount of pressure is required due to the presence of a thick fat pad on the heel. This is a common area for problems such as heel spurs and plantar fasciitis.
Navicular	This bone lies distal to the calcaneus and the talus. It typically is very prominent on the medial aspect of the foot at the peak of the medial longitudinal arch. To locate this bone, move off the distal tip of the medial malleolus at a 45° angle and you will run into the navicular. You can also use the hand opposite the foot you are trying to locate the navicular on: Place the web space of the hand over the Achilles tendon, and run your index finger along the medial side of the foot, inferior to the medial malleolus. The tip of your finger should be on the navicular.
1st cuneiform	Using the navicular as a starting point, move in a distal direction until you find a joint line. The next bone distal to the joint line is the first cuneiform. You may need to passively pronate and supinate the foot to help in locating the joint line.

Bony Structures of the Lower Leg, Ankle, and Foot *(Continued)*

Cuboid	This bone lies along the lateral foot. Draw a line between the lateral malleolus and the base of the 5th metatarsal. Pick a point in the middle, and you will be on the bone.
1st metatarsal	This bone runs along the medial foot and can be found by moving proximally from the great toe onto the foot or using the cuneiform as a starting point and moving distally.
Base of the 5th metatarsal	This bone is on the lateral aspect of the foot. It typically is easy to find the base, which flares out, at the middle of the foot.
Metatarsals	These are the bones of the feet. They have a head, which is at the "ball" of the foot and a base, which articulates with the tarsals.

Soft Tissue Structures of the Lower Leg, Ankle, and Foot

Lateral collateral ligaments	There are three ligaments of the ankle. The anterior talofibular ligament runs at a 45° angle from the anterior fibula to the talus. The calcaneofibular ligament runs distally from the tip of the fibula to the calcaneus. The posterior talofibular ligament runs at a 45° angle from the posterior distal fibula to the talus.
Sinus tarsi	This depression is located just anterior to the lateral malleolus, and it becomes larger during ankle inversion.
Tarsal tunnel (tibialis posterior, flexor digitorum longus, posterior tibial artery and nerve, flexor hallucis longus)	This tunnel is formed by the flexor retinaculum and can be the source of tarsal tunnel syndrome. Palpating transversely, starting from superior to inferior, the posterior tibialis tendon can be felt by plantar-flexing and inverting the foot. Flexing the toes brings out the flexor digitorum longus, and the tibial artery and nerve can be palpated relatively easily. The last structure, the flexor hallucis longus, can be brought out by flexing the great toe.
Achilles tendon	This is the tendon of insertion for both the gastrocnemius and soleus muscles. It starts midway down the lower leg and inserts on the calcaneus.
Retrocalcaneal bursa	This bursa lies between the calcaneus and the anterior border of the Achilles tendon
Calcaneal bursa	This bursa lies between the Achilles and the skin on the posterior calcaneus.
Plantar fascia	This thick aponeurosis runs from the medial calcaneal tubercle to the heads of the five metatarsals. It can be made more prominent by passively dorsiflexing the foot and extending the toes and palpating in a transverse direction.
Dorsalis pedis artery	This pulse is found on the top of the foot just lateral to the extensor hallucis longus tendon.

Muscles of the Lower Leg, Ankle, and Foot

Muscle	Origin	Insertion	Action	How to Palpate
Gastrocnemius	Lateral epicondyle (lateral head) and medial epicondyle (medial head) of femur	Calcaneus bone by way of Achilles tendon	Plantar-flexes foot at ankle; flexes leg at knee	Prone position; plantar-flex the foot, and the muscle will become prominent on the posterior lower leg
Soleus	Soleal line of tibia; head and proximal third shaft of fibula	Calcaneus via Achilles tendon	Plantar-flexes foot at ankle	Prone position; plantar-flex the foot with the leg flexed at the knee; under the gastrocnemius
Tibialis posterior	Posterior tibia; proximal fibula; interosseous membrane	Navicular, cuneiform, cuboid, base of 2nd–4th metatarsals	Inverts foot; assists plantar flexion	Supine position; palpate the tendon just behind the medial malleolus in the tarsal tunnel during action
Tibialis anterior	Lateral condyle, proximal half of lateral shaft of tibia; interosseous membrane	1st cuneiform bone and 1st metatarsal bone	Dorsiflexes; inverts; supports medial longitudinal arch	Supine position; dorsiflex the foot at the ankle, and invert the foot at the lower ankle; tendon prominent at the anterior ankle
Peroneus longus	Lateral condyle of tibia; head and proximal two-thirds of shaft of fibula	1st cuneiform and 1st metatarsal	Everts; assists plantar flexion; supports lateral longitudinal arch	Side-lying position; evert the foot; between the soleus and the extensor digitorum longus
Peroneus brevis	Distal two-thirds of fibular shaft	Base of 5th metatarsal	Everts foot; assists plantar flexion	Supine position; palpate between the peroneal tubercle and the lateral malleolus during action of the muscle
Flexor hallucis longus	Posterior fibula	Distal phalanx of great toe	Flexes first toe; assists plantar flexion	Supine position; palpate the tendon in the tarsal tunnel during action

Muscles of the Lower Leg, Ankle, and Foot *(Continued)*

Muscle	Origin	Insertion	Action	How to Palpate
Flexor digitorum longus	Posterior tibia	Plantar surface of distal lateral four toes	Flexes four small toes at distal interphalangeal joint; assists in plantar flexion	Supine position; palpate the tendon in the tarsal tunnel during action
Extensor digitorum brevis	Dorsal surface of calcaneus	Four small toes via extensor digitorum longus	Extends four small toes	Supine position; palpate in the sinus tarsi during action
Extensor digitorum longus	Lateral condyle of tibia; proximal two-thirds shaft of fibula	Dorsal surface of four small toes	Extends four small toes at metatarsophalangeal joint; dorsiflexes; everts	Supine position; dorsiflex and evert the foot; dorsiflex the four small toes; in the ditch between the tibialis anterior (medial) and the peroneus longus (lateral)
Extensor hallucis longus	Anterior shaft of fibula; interosseous membrane	Distal phalanx of great toe	Extends great toe; assists in dorsiflexion	Supine position; extend the great toe, and palpate the tendon lateral to the tibialis anterior tendon
Abductor hallucis	Calcaneus	Base of proximal phalanx of great toe	Abducts great toe; assists in flexion of great toe	Supine position; base of medial arch; palpate during resisted great-toe flexion

Trigger Points of the Lower Leg, Ankle, and Foot

Muscle	Trigger-Point Location	Referral Pattern	Chief Symptom
Gastrocnemius	1&2. Just proximal to middle of medial and lateral heads 3&4. Behind knee near medial and lateral attachment points of femoral condyles	1&2. Medial point: to instep of ipsilateral foot and spillover down medial aspect of calf Lateral point: in pattern around point 3&4. to general location around point	Calf cramping at night and posterior knee pain
Soleus	1. Just inferior to lower border of muscle belly of gastrocnemius, or about 5½ inches above heel, slightly medial to midline 2. High on lateral side of calf	1. Pain to posterior aspect and plantar surface of foot and distal Achilles tendon; can spill over to region of trigger point and into instep 2. Diffuse pain in upper half of calf	Pain in the heel that makes it unbearable to put weight on it; points in the upper portion of the muscle can result in edema in the foot and ankle as well as pain; complaints of limitations in dorsiflexion, which result in restrictions in the use of proper lifting mechanics
Tibialis posterior	Pressing deeply between posterior border of tibia and soleus, near proximal end of the bone	Pain that concentrates over Achilles tendon just proximal to heel; may spill over from point down middle of calf to entire plantar surface of foot	Severe pain in the sole of the foot and Achilles when walking or running, especially on uneven surface
Tibialis anterior	Taut bands in the upper one-third of muscle	Pain primarily to anteromedial ankle and dorsal and medial great toe; spillover from point down to ankle	Pain on the anteromedial ankle and big toe as well as weakness in dorsiflexion; usually no complaint of pain at night even if the ankle is in sustained plantar flexion
Peroneus longus	Proximal end of muscle about 1 inch distal to head of fibula on shaft	Pain and tenderness to area above, behind, and below lateral malleolus; may continue a short distance into lateral aspect of foot; may be spillover in middle third of lateral aspect of lower leg	Complaints of "weak ankles" and pain and tenderness in the ankle and over the lateral malleolus

Trigger Points of the Lower Leg, Ankle, and Foot *(Continued)*

Muscle	Trigger-Point Location	Referral Pattern	Chief Symptom
Peroneus brevis	Near transition point of middle and lower thirds of leg, over the fibula	Pain and tenderness to area above, behind, and below lateral malleolus; may continue a short distance into lateral aspect of foot; may be spillover in middle third of lateral aspect of lower leg	Complaints of "weak ankles" and pain and tenderness in the ankle and over the lateral malleolus
Flexor hallucis longus	In distal third of leg on posterior side	Plantar surface of great toe and 1st metatarsal head	Pain and occasional cramping in the toes
Flexor digitorum longus	At proximal end of muscle; found by having client lie on affected side	Pain to middle of plantar surface of forefoot, just proximal to toes, with spillover to toes and medial side of ankle and calf	Complaints of pain in the feet when walking on the sole of the forefoot and the plantar surface of the toes
Extensor digitorum brevis	Located in belly of muscle around and just distal to sinus tarsi	Instep of foot	Cramps in the foot
Extensor digitorum longus	About 3 inches distal to fibular head in between tibialis anterior and peroneus longus	Pain over dorsal surface of foot and toes; may concentrate over ankle and spill over from ankle to point	Persistent pain over the dorsum of the foot and night cramps
Extensor hallucis longus	Just distal to junction between middle and distal thirds of leg just anterior to fibula	Pain to distal aspect of 1st metatarsal and great toe as well as dorsum of foot; spillover up leg as far as point	Night cramps and persistent dorsal foot pain
Abductor hallucis	In belly of muscle along medial heel into arch	Pain to medial side of heel; spillover to instep and back of heel	Pain to the medial side of the heel

Orthopedic Tests for the Lower Leg, Ankle, and Foot

Condition	Orthopedic Test	How to Perform	Positive Sign
Medial tibial stress syndrome	None	Tests are typically administered to rule out other conditions. While manual muscle testing, and dermatome and myotome assessments, should be performed, pathology is largely determined by the location of the pain during palpation in combination with the mechanism, history, and observations.	Firm palpation over the posterior medial border of the tibia will produce pain, and in chronic cases there may be a nodular thickening of the tissue.
Achilles tendonitis	None	Use direct palpation of the tendon.	Positive indications of this pathology include point tenderness over the tendon, the presence of nodules along the tendon, and crepitus on movement.
Tarsal tunnel syndrome	Tinel test	Client is in the seated position with the leg supported. Place the ankle into slight dorsiflexion and eversion to take the slack out of the tissue. Tap, using the index and middle fingers, just inferior and distal to the medial malleolus.	Any tingling or paresthesia indicates a positive sign.
Plantar fasciitis	None	Assessment is based largely on the client's history and the findings during palpation. Any findings should be coupled with manual muscle, dermatome, myotome, and range-of-motion tests, as well as the other components of the assessment, to provide an overall picture.	The two most identifiable signs are that the pain is the most severe during the first few steps in the morning and the pain is located at the medial calcaneal tuberosity.

chapter outline

chapter objectives

At the conclusion of this chapter, the reader will understand:

- the significance of treating a condition or injury through an indirect approach
- techniques used to treat a condition during the different phases of healing
- how postural distortions develop, the different types of distortions, and treatment strategies for each using the treatment framework described in the text
- two types of tension pattern syndromes, how they occur, what structures are involved, and treatment strategies for each
- various characteristics—including what the conditions are, the tissues involved, the mechanism of injury, and any assessments (if applicable)—and treatment strategies for the following:
  - contusions
  - strains
  - sprains
  - joint injuries
  - tendonopathies
  - bursitis
  - nerve entrapment syndromes

KEY TERMS

kyphosis

lordosis

lower-crossed syndrome

myositis ossificans

scoliosis

upper-crossed syndrome

Introduction Previous chapters have discussed one region of the body and examined various orthopedic conditions specific to that area. Several conditions, syndromes, and injuries, however, are not isolated to one part of the body; yet the involved types of tissues are the same, and therefore treatment involves adapting equivalent techniques to the specific location. Other conditions may involve structures that are not directly accessible. In these cases, the therapist's job becomes more supportive in nature and requires addressing the injury indirectly by treating compensatory conditions. Finally, there are conditions intricately related to posture that affect the entire body. These patterns can lead to myriad localized problems but are effectively treated only if the underlying postural dysfunctions are addressed.

This chapter looks at a variety of pathologies, injuries, and conditions that encompass several different tissues, structures, and locations. These may relate to a global postural syndrome or a specific type of injury that can occur in multiple locations in the body. Some or all of the following characteristics are discussed for each pathology:

- What is the nature of the condition?
- How or why does the condition occur?
- What structures are involved?
- What are the applicable assessments for the condition?
- What are the available treatment strategies?

SPECIFIC CONDITIONS

Postural Distortions

As humans have evolved and assumed an upright bipedal posture, there have been both positive and negative consequences. On the positive side, the posture has enabled humans to have free use of their hands and to visualize their surroundings by changing the line of sight. However, disadvantages accompany these advantages, including an increase in the amount of stress placed on the spine and lower ribs, as well as potential difficulties in respiration and circulation to the brain due to the effects of gravity. The human body is in a constant battle against gravity, and over time people develop pathologies as a result.

The goal of correct posture is to allow the body to interact with gravity as efficiently as possible. Overall, posture is a composite of the position of the body's joints at one specific time, with the orientation of one joint affecting that of the next. When the body assumes correct posture, the stresses on the joints are minimized. If the body is unable to assume efficient posture, the effects of gravity will increase the stresses on the joints. Individuals who adjust their posture constantly are not as affected by these stresses as those who do not or cannot. Faulty posture can result in the development of a variety of pathologies depending on the location of the deviation. Generally, these pathologies arise as the result of the cumulative effect of numerous repeated insults over a long period of time or a continual stress on the body that occurs over a shorter duration.

> **Practical Tip**
> The goal of correct posture is to allow the body to interact with gravity as efficiently as possible.

Improper posture can arise from functional or structural causes, and the causes can occur individually or together. If they occur simultaneously, one will enhance the problems of the other. Functional posture problems involve positional factors, with the most common cause stemming from nothing more than poor postural habits: Regardless of the reasons, the individual does not maintain correct posture. This typically occurs in individuals who have to maintain certain positions for long periods of time. Children commonly display poor postural habits for a number of reasons, two of which are growth spurts and attempts to hide their body's development during adolescence.

The muscles that control posture must remain strong, flexible, and adaptable to the environment. The inability of the muscles to combat the forces of gravity will eventually lead to dysfunction in the area. Muscle imbalance, compensation from pain, respiratory conditions, and general weakness or spasm can all lead to poor postural habits. The primary tissues involved in functional posture problems are connective and muscle tissues. Over a period of time, the connective tissue in the area will adapt to its new arrangement and hold the body in that particular position, subsequently causing the muscles to shorten on one side and lengthen and weaken on the other.

Structural factors stem from changes in the anatomical makeup as a result of a congenital condition, trauma, disease, or developmental problem. It is important to note that a functional deviation can result in structural change through an adaptive process if it has been present for a long period of time. Such types of postural deviations are often not easily reversed without invasive interventions, but the symptoms can often be managed successfully.

Treatment Strategies

Regardless of whether the postural distortion is structural or functional, some general assessment and treatment strategies can be applied:

1. The posture must be assessed and compared to what is considered "normal." Recall from Chapter 4 that normal posture is assessed by having the client stand in front of a plumb line and viewing the client from the anterior, the posterior, and both lateral sides. Have the client stand with the feet equidistant from the line when assessing from the front or back. When assessing from the lateral view, line the plumb bob up just anterior to the lateral malleolus. For each position, compare the client's posture to what is considered "ideal posture," listed here:

Anterior (Fig. 11-1)

- The head should sit squarely on the shoulders.
- The tip of the nose should be in alignment with the manubrium, xiphoid process, and umbilicus, which together form what is known as the *anterior line of reference.*
- The contour of the trapezius should appear equal bilaterally. Check for unusually prominent bony areas.
- The shoulders, clavicles, and acromioclavicular joints should appear to be equal.
- The tops of the iliac crests should appear level.
- The arms should face the same direction.

- The anterior superior iliac spine (ASIS) should appear level bilaterally.
- The pubic bones should appear level.
- The patellae should face forward.
- The knees should appear straight.
- The malleoli should appear to be equal.
- The arches on both sides of the feet should be checked, noting any pes planus or cavus.

Lateral (Fig. 11-2)
- Check the lateral line of assessment, which is the line from the earlobe to the tip of the shoulder. It continues through the highest point on the iliac crest, slightly anterior to the axis of the knee joint and slightly anterior to the lateral malleolus.
- Determine whether the back has excessive curvature. Look at each spinal segment in relation to the sacrum.
- Check the musculatures of the back, abdominal, and chest regions. They should have good tone with no obvious deformity.
- Determine whether the pelvis appears level.
- Look for visible trunk rotation.
- Determine whether the knees are flexed, straight, or hyperextended (in recurvatum).

Posterior (Fig. 11-3)
- Determine whether the head and neck sit squarely on the shoulders, matching the anterior view.

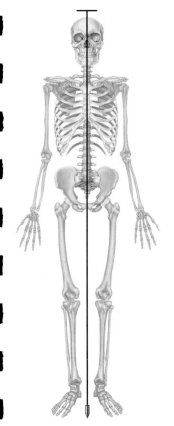 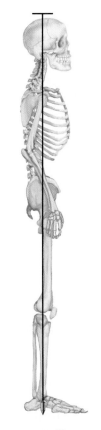 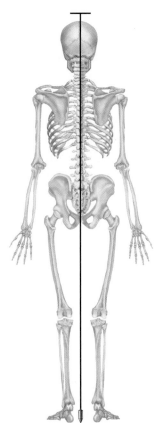

Figure 11-1 Correct posture from the anterior view.

Figure 11-2 Correct posture from the lateral view.

Figure 11-3 Correct posture from the posterior view.

- Check the scapulae. They should be positioned similarly on both sides. Note the rotation and tilt, the levels of the superior and inferior angles, and whether the scapulae sit flat on the rib cage.
- Look for lateral curves on the spine.
- Look for atrophy of the posterior musculature.
- Look for equal space between the elbows and the trunk.
- Determine whether the ribs are symmetrical.
- Check the posterior superior iliac spine (PSIS). It should appear level bilaterally.
- Determine whether the tops of the iliac crests and gluteal folds appear equal.
- Check the backs of the knees. They should appear level.
- Note whether the Achilles run vertical on both sides.
- Determine whether the heels are straight. Check for valgus or varus positioning.

2. Once any deviations have been identified, determine which structures are responsible by defining the position of the joint. It is important to determine whether deviations are structural or functional. This may be difficult and require more advanced procedures.

3. The general treatment strategy is to reverse restrictions that are causing the deviations through the application of the techniques discussed in earlier chapters, depending on where the deviations are located in relation to the treatment framework discussed in Chapter 4.

Common Postural Distortions

Lordosis

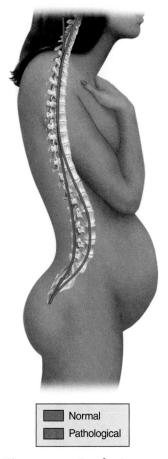

lordosis An exaggeration of either of the two secondary curves in the spine that are located in the lumbar and cervical regions.

Lordosis is an exaggeration of either of the two secondary curves in the spine that are located in the lumbar and cervical regions (Fig. 11-4). This can be caused by structural abnormalities such as spondylolisthesis, spinal segment malformations, and congenital hip dislocations; functional pathologies such as weak muscles (especially the abdominals), excess weight, and hip flexor contractures; and compensatory mechanisms from another deformity.

In the cervical spine, lordosis is often characterized by a forward head, rounded shoulders, and a sunken chest, a posture pattern that typically develops as a result of poor habits. This repetitive movement pattern reinforces any poor postural habits. As the shoulders begin to round forward, the head shifts forward, changing the line of sight to the ground so that the head must extend to level the eyes with the

Normal
Pathological

Figure 11-4 Lordosis.

horizon. This increases the lordotic cervical curve, illustrating how deviation in one part of the body leads to deviation in another part.

For the lumbar spine, an increase in the lordotic curve also tilts the pelvis forward, increasing the pelvic angle from the normal 30° to as much as 40°. This posture pattern is also created primarily through poor habits and the chronic shortening of the hip flexors, tensor fascia latae. Other behaviors that can lead to lumbar lordosis include activities that require repeated lumbar hyperextension such as gymnastics, figure skating, or football. While poor posture patterns are a major cause of lordosis, structural changes such as spinal deformities and spondylolisthesis are also common etiologies.

Assessing lordosis in both the lumbar spine and the cervical spine is easiest from the lateral view. For the lumbar spine, begin by checking the levels of the static landmarks such as the iliac crests, ASIS, and PSIS, which should be level with each other. An exaggerated curve in the lumbar spine tilts the pelvis forward, causing an angle to form with the front of the thigh and making the gluteals more prominent. In the cervical spine, the head will be forward of the ideal posture line, and the shoulders will be rounded forward.

To effectively treat these patterns, it is necessary to determine the root of the deviation and then release the shortened muscles using techniques described in earlier chapters. In addition, weakened muscles should be strengthened to help reverse the pattern.

Kyphosis

An increase in the normal thoracic curve is known as **kyphosis;** it can arise from both poor postural behaviors and congenital pathologies (Fig. 11-5).

kyphosis An increase in the normal thoracic curve.

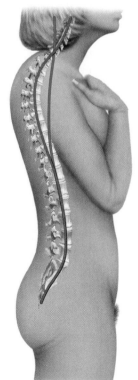

A forward-head and rounded-shoulder posture, or a muscle imbalance between the anterior and posterior thoracic muscles, will exacerbate a kyphosis. Congenital abnormalities such as a malformation of the vertebral bodies or various vertebral elements will result in a kyphosis. Certain pathologic conditions cause structural deviations. For instance, Scheuermann's disease, which occurs idiopathically during adolescence, results in the development of one or more wedge-shaped vertebra stemming from abnormal epiphyseal plate activity. It affects around 10% of the population and occurs most commonly between T10 and L2.

There are three main presentations for kyphosis:

1. *Round back* is a longer, rounded curve that shifts the body weight forward so that the pelvis rotates posteriorly to compensate; this reduces the lumbar curve.

2. *Humpback* or *gibbus* is characterized by an isolated sharp posterior angulation in the thoracic spine.

Figure 11-5 Kyphosis.

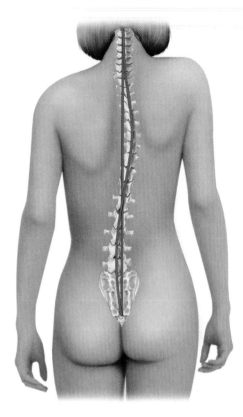

Figure 11-6 Scoliosis.

📖 scoliosis Any lateral curvature of the spine; often characterized by either a C or an S curve, depending on which and how many regions of the spine are involved.

3. *Dowager's hump* is often seen in the elderly because it is caused by the development of osteoporosis and results in the thoracic vertebra taking on a wedge-shaped appearance.

To assess for kyphosis, observe posture from the lateral view. Kyphosis is typically accompanied by a forward head and is not usually hard to discern. Treatment involves releasing the tight anterior musculature and performing stretches that increase thoracic extension. Use the techniques discussed in earlier chapters.

Scoliosis

Scoliosis is generally the most visible deviation in the spine, especially when it is severe. It is considered to be any lateral curvature of the spine and is often characterized by either a C or an S curve, depending on which and how many regions of the spine are involved (Fig. 11-6).

The two types of scoliosis, structural and nonstructural, are described in Table 11-1. Assessment of both types of scoliosis is best performed from the posterior view. Have the client forward-flex the trunk, and look for any deviation in the spine or a muscular prominence on one side of the spine. The structures on the concave side are compressed, and those on

Table 11-1 Types of Scoliosis

Type	Characteristics
Structural scoliosis *Note:* Despite the numerous etiologies for structural scoliosis, 70% to 90% are considered to be idiopathic and occur between the ages of 10 and 13.	Involves bony abnormalities that are either congenital or developmental, such as wedge-shaped vertebra or the incomplete formation of the vertebra. Can stem from neural lesions, persistent joint contractures, tumors, or inflammatory conditions. The constant forces on the vertebra from these conditions will change the structural shape of the bone over time. The key discerning characteristics of structural scoliosis are that lateral flexion is asymmetric and the curve does not disappear during flexion of the trunk.
Nonstructural scoliosis	Can stem from postural problems, muscle spasms, and compensatory patterns from other conditions, such as leg-length discrepancies. There is no bony abnormality, lateral flexion is symmetrical, and the deviation in the curve disappears during trunk flexion.

the convex side are stretched. If the curves are bad enough, they can affect lung capacity, as well as compress the organs. Treatment involves lengthening the shortened structures and strengthening the lengthened tissue to help maintain a more functional postural position.

TENSION PATTERN SYNDROMES

Muscle movement is controlled through the impulses of the nervous system. Part of this process involves input from the surrounding environment through sensory receptors. These receptors collect information and relay it to the central nervous system so that it can be processed and adjustments can be made to the musculoskeletal system in response to the input. In the 1950s and 1960s, Vladimir Janda, a physiatrist and neurologist from the Czech Republic, concluded that the sensory and motor systems of the body could not be separated with respect to human movement (Page, 2005). The "sensorimotor system," as he referred to it, functions as one unit, and changes in one component will result in adaptations in another part of the system. He applied this principle to his extensive work on muscle imbalance and proper firing patterns of muscles, and he discerned that the most important aspect of coordinated movement was proprioception (Page, 2005).

In applying these principles to chronic musculoskeletal pain, Janda took the approach that there are two types of muscle groups, postural and phasic, which perform different roles and respond differently to dysfunction. *Postural muscles* are so-named because they function primarily to support the body against the forces of gravity. *Phasic muscles* are designed to provide movement. These classifications are based on the muscles' primary role, but muscles can switch back and forth depending on the individual situation. These two groups also respond differently when dysfunction is present. Generally, postural muscles react to dysfunction with increased tightness, whereas phasic muscles react by becoming weaker.

These responses to dysfunction are present in many of the posture patterns that were discussed in the previous section. Over time, the motor programming to these muscles changes in response to the chronic patterns, and communication to change the pattern becomes inhibited, thereby creating a perpetual cycle.

Two primary muscle imbalance syndromes result from the pattern between postural and phasic muscles: upper-crossed syndrome and lower-crossed syndrome.

- **Upper-crossed syndrome** (Fig. 11-7) involves the head, neck, and upper trunk and is often accompanied by a forward-head and rounded-shoulder posture; moreover, it can contribute to kyphosis in the thoracic spine. These poor postural habits change the way gravity runs through the cervical spine and create imbalance in the muscles of the area. Some of the postural muscles that become hypertonic are the

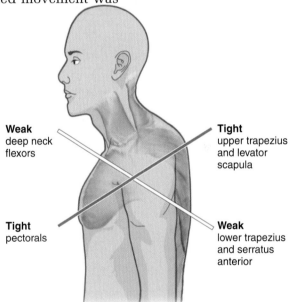

Weak deep neck flexors

Tight upper trapezius and levator scapula

Tight pectorals

Weak lower trapezius and serratus anterior

Figure 11-7 Upper-crossed syndrome.

📖 **upper-crossed syndrome** A postural dysfunction that involves the head, neck, and upper trunk and is often accompanied by a forward-head and rounded-shoulder posture. Moreover, it can contribute to kyphosis in the thoracic spine.

upper trapezius, levator scapula, and suboccipitals on the posterior side and the pectoralis major, pectoralis minor, and sternocleidomastoid on the anterior side. Some of the phasic muscles that become weakened are the deep neck flexors in the front and the lower trapezius, rhomboids, and serratus anterior on the back.

- **Lower-crossed syndrome** (Fig. 11-8) involves the lumbar spine, hips, and pelvis; it follows the pattern of imbalance between postural and phasic muscles and is often accompanied by an anteriorly tilted pelvis. On the posterior side, some of the involved postural muscles are the quadratus lumborum and erector spinae; on the anterior side, the iliopsoas. Some of the involved phasic muscles are the gluteus maximus and minimus posteriorly and the abdominals (particularly transverse abdominus) anteriorly.

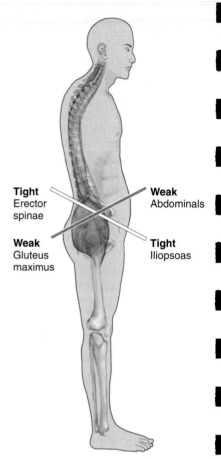

Tight Erector spinae

Weak Gluteus maximus

Weak Abdominals

Tight Iliopsoas

Figure 11-8 Lower-crossed syndrome.

While these are separate syndromes, they often occur together as part of an overall response of the body to maintain a proper center of gravity. Assess these conditions using the postural assessment tools described at the beginning of the chapter. Once the pattern is recognized, treatment involves releasing the shortened postural muscles and strengthening the weakened phasic muscles. In addition to relieving the soft tissue restrictions, include movement reeducation in the treatment process to correct dysfunctional motor programming.

CONTUSIONS

A *contusion* is a relatively common musculoskeletal injury that is caused by blunt trauma to the soft tissue. It is characterized by pain, localized tenderness, swelling, loss of strength and range of motion, and ecchymosis. Contusions are graded according to how impaired the range of motion is:

- *First-degree contusions* cause few or no limitations.
- *Second-degree contusions* produce a noticeable change in range of motion.
- *Third-degree contusions* cause severe restrictions in range of motion.

The primary result of a contusion is the formation of a *hematoma,* or local accumulation of blood, in the tissue space because of the biomechanical failure of the muscle and connective and vascular tissues.

lower-crossed syndrome A postural dysfunction that involves the lumbar spine, hips, and pelvis and follows the pattern of imbalance between postural and phasic muscles. It is often accompanied by an anteriorly tilted pelvis.

There are two types of hematomas that can form, depending on the severity of the trauma:

- *Intramuscular hematomas* are less severe and consist of damage only to the muscle tissue, with the connective tissue sheath remaining intact, thus localizing the symptoms.
- *Intermuscular hematomas* are more severe and involve the muscle. They occur when fascia is damaged and bleeding spreads, expanding the area of injury.

Treatment of a contusion will be similar regardless of where the injury is located, but each individual situation must be taken into consideration. The primary goal is to remove the excess blood and fluid from the area as quickly as possible to provide the optimal environment for healing. Because soft tissue heals in three stages, treatment is different in each stage. As discussed in Chapter 4, the initial stage of healing is the inflammatory stage; it can last up to 6 days and has familiar signs and symptoms, including heat, redness, swelling, pain, and loss of function.

> ⋆Practical Tip
>
> The primary goal in treating contusions is to remove the excess blood and fluid from the area as quickly as possible to provide the optimal environment for healing.

Inflammatory Phase

In the case of a contusion, inflammation is acute and usually brief in duration; it generates swelling called *exudate* through a process of initial vasoconstriction, secondary vasodilation, and an increase in the permeability of the vessels. The exudate that is created is important to the overall healing process. In addition to diluting toxins in the area, it provides the cells necessary to remove damaged tissue and enable reconstruction. These two factors cause swelling in the area and form what is known as the *zone of primary injury.* While this swelling process is beneficial to the overall healing process, it also can be detrimental to the area. If excess fluids, damaged tissues, chemical mediators, and white blood cells remain in the area for too long, the environment may become hypoxic. This will result in the expanded death of those tissues and create the *zone of secondary injury,* which will continue to expand until the initial inflammation is under control and the tissue returns to its normal metabolism.

Direct manual techniques are contraindicated during this phase; the area is better treated using other modalities such as ice and compression treatment. Once the swelling is under control, meaning that any activity or therapy does not create additional swelling, massage in conjunction with other modalities can be used to hasten the healing process. This may take 1 day or several days, depending on the severity. To treat during this phase:

1. Apply ice to the contusion for 10 to 20 minutes, using a barrier between the ice and the skin.
2. After the ice has sufficiently cooled the area, apply gentle effleurage strokes, radiating out from the center.
3. Once the tissue starts to warm up, reapply the ice and repeat the process two to three times, applying the ice last, followed by a compression wrap.

If additional swelling is generated from this treatment, the injury has not sufficiently begun to heal and only ice and compression should be continued. By expanding the surface area of the hematoma, it is reabsorbed more quickly and less residual scar tissue remains.

Proliferative Phase

The next phase of healing is the proliferative phase and can overlap the latter part of the inflammatory phase. Sometimes referred to as the *repair and regeneration phase,* it includes the development of new blood vessels, fibrous tissues, and epithelial tissues. Treatment during this phase involves the application of the same radiating strokes over the contusion to expand the surface area. Ice may be necessary only after the massage is performed, but each situation will be different. During this phase of healing, new tissue is laid down; therefore, the goal is to facilitate the proper amount and orientation of the new tissue. Because new-tissue formation begins when the hematoma reduces in size, early treatment will lead to faster healing. The accumulated formation of connective tissue and blood vessels is a highly vascularized mass and is transformed into the necessary structures in the third and final phase of healing.

Maturation Phase

The maturation phase is the final phase of healing; it is sometimes known as the *remodeling phase.* The newly formed mass from the repair phase is transformed into scar tissue in a process that includes decreased fibroblast activity, increased organization in the matrix, reduced vascularity, and a return to normal histochemical activity. Since scar tissue is less elastic, more fibrous, and less vascular than the original tissue, the focus of the treatment should be on creating a functional scar. This can be done using techniques from previous chapters, depending on the location of the contusion.

A therapist may encounter a contusion in any of these stages of healing. It is important to determine what phase it is in by performing a thorough assessment so that appropriate treatment is administered.

One major contraindication is **myositis ossificans**. The exact cause of this condition is unknown, but it can appear following severe contusions. It is characterized by the deposition of calcium within the muscle fibers or the formation of a spur on the underlying bone. It is generally found through palpation and x-ray, and it can permanently limit range of motion and function.

MUSCLE STRAINS

Recall from Chapter 4 that muscle strain typically occurs due to excessive tensile force. The force that stretches the muscle past its elastic region is commonly caused by an excessive eccentric load. Muscle strains are graded into one of three degrees, depending on severity and the extent of damage:

1. *First-degree strains* are the mildest type, characterized by only a few torn muscle fibers. Symptoms include mild weakness and spasm, mild swelling, but no palpable defect in the muscle. Pain occurs on both contraction and stretching, and range of motion is decreased.
2. *Second-degree strains* are moderate injuries with nearly half of the muscle fibers torn, resulting in the formation of a hematoma and bruising or ecchymosis. Spasm, swelling, and loss of function are moderate

to severe, but there is still no palpable defect. Pain is worse with contraction and stretching, and there is decreased range of motion.

3. *Third-degree strains* are the most severe and result in the total rupture of the muscle. Swelling, weakness, and spasm are severe, and some bruising may occur; however, pain is mild to nonexistent due to the rupture of the nerves in the area. Loss of function is significant, and there is a palpable defect in the muscle.

When assessing a muscle strain, first identify the location of the injury and what muscles are in the area. Palpate the area to check for swelling, spasm, and obvious defects, and observe the area for any bruising. Check the range of motion in the area to detect any deficits. Lastly, perform manual muscle tests on the involved muscles bilaterally and compare the results. Use the grading scale discussed in Chapter 4. Strains to muscles will heal differently depending on what part of the muscle is injured and the muscle's function and location. Injuries in the belly of the muscle tend to heal better than those located near the tendon because the bellies have a better blood supply and are more vascular than the tissue near the tendons.

If the injured muscle performs a function that is involved in multiple movements and is unable to sufficiently rest, the healing time will be longer. Muscles such as the intercostals and abdominals are involved in just about every move the body makes, so it is hard to rest these muscles to allow them to heal.

Muscle strains follow the three-phase healing process of other soft tissue injuries, as discussed in the contusion section; therefore, treatment is similar.

Inflammatory Phase

The focus is on removing any excess fluid to limit secondary tissue damage and prevent excessive connective tissue from forming. Gentle effleurage in the direction of the lymphatic vessels in the area will help with fluid movement and enhance the delivery of nutrients and the removal of waste products. Use ice as part of the treatment, and wait until the swelling is under control before administering manual techniques.

Repair and Regeneration Phase

Focus on creating a functional scar. Use gentle stretching in conjunction with massage techniques, such as friction, to help facilitate the alignment of the new scar tissue.

Remodeling Phase

The focus is on increasing the functionality of the scar, and removing adhesions that are restricting motion is important. Techniques such as deep parallel thumb stripping with active engagement are very effective during this phase.

In all phases, it is important to treat the whole muscle to remove any tension that may be pulling on the injury site. Contraindications for working on strains include beginning the work too soon, before the swelling is under control, or being too aggressive and creating more trauma in the area. Good communication and follow-up are important to monitor the progress of the treatment.

SPRAINS

A *sprain* occurs when a joint is stretched beyond its normal anatomical limits and damage to the ligaments and/or joint capsule occurs. Ligaments contain a slightly larger percentage of elastin fibers, so they can withstand tensile forces a little better than tendons can. However, if the stress is great enough, the tissue will move beyond the elastic region into the plastic region and cause permanent deformation and even rupture. Some ligaments are nothing more than a thickening of the joint capsule; others are more distinct and separate from the capsule. Sprains are classified in three degrees that are very similar to the degrees of strains:

1. *First-degree sprains* have only a few of the fibers torn, with no recognizable joint instability, and a firm end-feel is present. Mild weakness and loss of function, as well as mild swelling and decreased range of motion, may also be present.
2. *Second-degree sprains* are more severe, with almost half of the fibers torn. Some joint laxity occurs, but there is still a definite end point with mild to moderate weakness. Symptoms include loss of function, swelling, and decreased range of motion.
3. *Third-degree sprains* are the most severe and result in the total rupture of the ligament. There is gross joint instability, which results in an absent end point with moderate weakness. Because the joint has lost its stability, loss of function is severe and there is marked swelling. Range of motion may increase due to the instability or decrease due to swelling.

Assessment of a sprain begins by determining which joint is involved and what movements the ligaments around the joint are preventing. The rate of healing depends on where the ligament is located, how much force is required to injure it, and the blood supply in the area.

Syndesmotic joints, such as those in the tibiofibular joints, are very strong, require a large amount of force to be injured, and heal slower in comparison to the lateral ankle, whose ligaments are not as strong and are commonly injured. Check the area for swelling, pain on palpation, joint instability (if practical), discoloration, and obvious deformity.

Treatment of sprains is similar to that of strains.

Inflammatory Phase

The focus is on removing any excess fluid to limit the secondary tissue damage. Remember to wait until the swelling is under control, and use ice as part of the treatment to prevent any increase in swelling. Strokes such as light effleurage should be used to clear out the area. Start at the proximal end of the limb and work toward the injury, administering strokes in the direction of the heart. This will help with fluid movement and enhance the delivery of nutrients and removal of waste products.

Practical Tip

The rate of healing depends on where the ligament is located, how much force is required to injure it, and the blood supply in the area.

Repair and Regeneration Phase

Techniques such as light friction can be used to help create a functional scar during connective tissue formation. Use gentle stretching to facilitate alignment of the new scar tissue.

Remodeling Phase

Techniques such as deep transverse and multidirectional friction are effective. Remember to treat the whole muscle to remove any tension surrounding the joint. As with strains, to prevent causing more trauma to the area, avoid treating too aggressively.

Assessments for Specific Locations

Shoulder

Acromioclavicular Joint Chapter 7 discussed the anatomy of the acromioclavicular joint, which is formed by the lateral end of the clavicle and the acromion process of the scapula. It is considered a diarthrodial joint and has limited motion in all three planes. There is a thin capsule surrounding the joint with a fibrocartilaginous disk between the two articulating surfaces. The joint is stabilized by the strong superior and inferior acromioclavicular ligaments, with a third ligament running between the coracoid process and the acromion process. It is called the *coracoacromial ligament,* and it supports the overall position of the joint and the coracoclavicular ligament, which runs from the clavicle to the coracoid process.

While chronic conditions can affect this joint, injury is more commonly caused through an acute mechanism. Typically, the mechanism results in the acromion being driven away from the clavicle, or vice versa. This can be caused by what is termed a *FOOSH (fall-on-an-outstretched-hand) injury,* in which the client lands on a forward-flexed outstretched arm or the point of the elbow, which subsequently drives the humerus up into the underside of the acromion. Another mechanism is a lateral blow to the shoulder, such as from an impact or a fall on the tip of the shoulder, which causes the joint to separate. Regardless of the mechanism, this injury is commonly referred to as a "separated shoulder," even though it is actually a sprain.

Acromioclavicular joint sprains are classified into three categories depending on the severity of the injury:

- *Type I sprains* are first-degree injuries with no tearing of the ligaments of the joint, minimal swelling, pain, and some discomfort with abduction past 90°.
- *Type II sprains* are more severe and involve some tearing of the acromioclavicular ligaments, but the coracoacromial and coracoclavicular ligaments are intact. This often results in a noticeable displacement of the joint called a *step deformity,* in which the shoulder drops down to create an obvious step-off. There is swelling, and pain is increased when the clavicle is moved. The client is unable to abduct or horizontally adduct the arm without pain.

- *Type III sprains* involve a total rupture of the acromioclavicular and coracoclavicular ligaments. This causes sagging of the acromion, which creates a very prominent clavicle and results in something called the "piano key sign," wherein the lateral clavicle bobs up and down when depressed, causing severe swelling, pain, and a definite step deformity. The range of motion is limited in abduction and horizontal adduction, with greater pain than that in Type II.

Assessments for this condition are designed to create movement in the joint in an effort to re-create the pain. The two main assessments for an acromioclavicular sprain are discussed in Table 11-2.

Table 11-2 Orthopedic Tests for Acromioclavicular Sprains

Orthopedic Test	How to Perform
Acromioclavicular distraction test 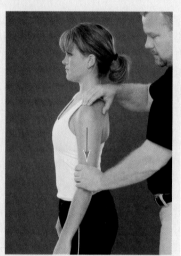	Client is in a standing position. Standing at the side of the client, grasp the arm just proximal with one hand and palpate the joint with the other. Apply a downward traction to the arm. Pain and/or joint motion is a sign of a positive test.
Crossover (acromioclavicular) compression test 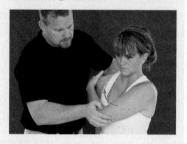	Client is in a standing or seated position. Standing to the side, horizontally adduct the client's arm across the chest and compress it into the body. Pain at the joint is a positive sign.

Treatment for an acromioclavicular sprain will vary depending on the severity of the injury. Because of the significance of the joint in overall shoulder motion, addressing compensatory reductions in range of motion by using the techniques discussed in Chapter 7 is an important component of the treatment process. If the sprain is severe enough and causes significant joint instability, the mechanics of the shoulder will become permanently altered, resulting in chronic problems.

As the sprain moves through the three healing phases, the treatment process is similar to that for other ligament injuries. In the initial phases, the focus is on facilitating the removal of excess swelling and creating an optimal healing environment. As the repair phase begins, techniques such as friction over the joint can help prevent excessive scar tissue formation. In the remodeling phase, the focus should be on removing any restrictions around the various joints of the shoulder girdle, using friction and stripping. Increasing range of motion should be a focus in all the stages of healing.

Knee

Anterior Cruciate Ligament As discussed in Chapter 9, the anterior cruciate ligament (ACL) is attached to the anterior tibia and passes posteriorly through the intercondylar notch of the femur to attach on the posterior lateral femoral condyle. Its purpose is threefold, as it serves to:

- Prevent anterior translation of the tibia on the femur
- Prevent hyperextension of the knee
- Prevent excessive rotation of the tibia on the femur

Injury to this ligament can cause severe joint instability at the knee. The primary cause of injury to the ACL is mechanical overload, which can occur from a direct blow that forces the tibia anteriorly. A more common cause, however, is a non-contact-related rotational injury. One example of this occurs when an individual is running or moving in one direction, plants his or her foot, and then turns quickly. This can cause a rotational force at the joint that can injure the ligament. Sudden deceleration can also cause an ACL injury by creating a tremendous eccentric load from the quadriceps. Another mechanism arises from hyperextending the knee through a direct blow or something such as stepping in a shallow hole while walking or landing from a jump improperly, causing the knee to snap back.

When discussing the injury, the client will often describe a rotational mechanism, along with popping, snapping, or tearing sensations accompanied by pain and immediate loss of knee function. Rapid swelling often occurs within 3 hours due to the associated injury of the ACL's blood supply, the medial geniculate artery. The client will complain that during weight bearing the knee feels like it will "give way" or is unstable or it "just doesn't feel right." ACL injuries are rarely isolated; therefore, it is necessary to conduct a thorough assessment of the other structures in the area.

Often, the medial collateral ligament or the menisci are involved as well. If the medial collateral ligament and the medial meniscus are both involved along with the ACL, this is termed the "unhappy triad" injury.

The incidence of ACL injuries is higher in women than in men, and there are several theories on why this occurs, including intrinsic factors, such as the width of the intercondylar notch, limb alignment due to a greater Q angle, and hormone-related ligament laxity, and extrinsic factors, such as styles of play and muscle imbalances between the hamstrings and the quadriceps.

There are two primary tests for an ACL sprain, both of which are designed to test stability of the ligament, as shown in Table 11-3.

> **Practical Tip**
>
> ACL injuries are rarely isolated; therefore, it is necessary to conduct a thorough assessment of the other structures in the area.

Table 11-3 Orthopedic Tests for ACL Injury

Orthopedic Test	How to Perform
Anterior-drawer test 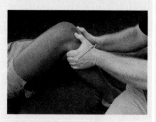 *Note:* This test is not the most accurate and has several shortcomings that can result in the masking of a positive result.	Have the client lie supine on the table while flexing the hip to 45° and the knee to 90°. Sit on the table and place the client's foot that is on the table under his or her thigh to keep it from moving. Place the thumbs on either side of the patellar tendon in the joint line and the fingers in the popliteal fossa to palpate the hamstring tendons; make sure they do not contract. While palpating the joint line with the thumbs, apply an alternating anterior and posterior force on the proximal tibia. Check for any translation of the tibia, which can be either seen from the lateral view or felt with the thumbs. Compare the amount of movement to that on the uninvolved side, and make a determination relative to laxity. Repeat the test with the foot internally and externally rotated to assess different parts of the ligament.
Lachman's test 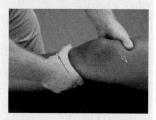 *Note:* This test is more reliable than the anterior-drawer test.	Place the client in the supine position. Flex the client's knee to 20° with one hand, and stabilize the distal femur with the other. *Note:* It is important for the client to remain as relaxed as possible to prevent any guarding of the muscles, which will render the test results inaccurate. Apply an anterior force to the tibia while either stabilizing or applying a slight posterior force to the femur. *Note:* If the client's leg is too large or the therapist's hand is too small to stabilize the femur, a small towel or bolster may be used to keep the knee at the proper angle. A positive test is determined by the lack of a solid end-feel and a "mushy" feeling compared to the uninvolved side.

Since the ligament is inside the knee joint, treatment focuses on restoring the normal biomechanics of the muscles surrounding the joint that are in spasm from guarding the area. This will begin with assisting the removal of swelling during the initial phases of healing and will continue through postsurgical range-of-motion improvement and scar tissue remodeling.

Posterior Cruciate Ligament The posterior cruciate ligament (PCL) is intimately related to the ACL inside the knee and attaches to the posterior aspect of the tibia, which runs anteriorly past the ACL to the anterolateral aspect of the femur. Its functions are the opposite of the ACL's functions and include preventing posterior translation of the tibia on the femur and providing lateral rotational stability. The PCL has been described as the primary stabilizer of the knee.

Unlike injuries to the ACL, the primary mechanism of injury to the PCL is direct trauma. Because the PCL is thicker and shorter, the incidence of trauma to the PCL is less than that to the ACL. The most common mechanism of injury is a direct blow to the proximal tibia when the knee is flexed, which drives the tibia posteriorly. This can occur as a result of falling with the ankle in dorsiflexion, which causes the proximal tibia to hit the ground first, or being in a car accident in which bent knees strike the dashboard. Another mechanism is hyperextension of the knee, which can occur when the heel steps in a hole. Isolated injuries to the posterior cruciate ligament do occur, but it is more common for injuries to occur in multiple structures in the knee.

Injuries to the PCL result in less knee instability than injuries to the ACL, so they are often not surgically repaired unless other structures are involved. Depending on the severity, the client may describe the familiar "pop" when discussing the injury. In milder cases, symptoms may be hard to determine and may mimic a medial head gastrocnemius strain. Over time, range-of-motion deficits and hamstring weakness may be evident and be accompanied by pain. In total ruptures, swelling is rapid and range of motion is limited due to the effusion. In a PCL injury, the extensor mechanism of the knee is affected, increasing pressure on the patellofemoral joint. There is also an increase in the loading of the joint due to the posterior displacement of the tibia; this may also increase the likelihood of patellofemoral pain.

The two tests for PCL injuries seek to determine the amount of posterior displacement of the tibia on the femur compared to the uninjured side, as shown in Table 11-4.

As with injuries to the ACL, treatment for PCL injuries consists of supportive care to address the compensatory issues that arise as a result of the change in joint stability. Depending on the severity, there may be swelling or spasm in the area. Address patellofemoral problems using the techniques described in Chapter 9.

Medial Collateral Ligament

Running from the medial condyle of the femur to the medial side of the proximal tibia, just posterior to the pes anserine tendons, the medial collateral ligament (MCL) provides stability to the medial side of the knee. All the fibers are taut in full extension, but the ligament can be isolated from the other medial stabilizing structures such as the ACL and the medial capsule by flexing the knee to 15°. Also known as the *tibial collateral ligament,* its primary function is to resist valgus forces to the knee, but it also serves to counteract rotational forces, particularly medial rotation of the femur on the tibia.

Table 11-4 Orthopedic Tests for PCL Injury

Orthopedic Test	How to Perform
Posterior-drawer test 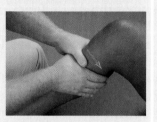	Have the client lying supine on the table with the hip bent to 45° and the knee at 90°.
	Sit on the client's foot to hold the tibia in a neutral position; grasp the proximal tibia and push it posteriorly.
	Compare the amount of movement to that on the uninvolved side; if it moves more or there is a soft or mushy end-feel, the test is considered positive.
Godfrey's (posterior-sag) test 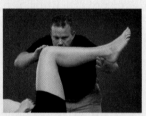 *Note:* This test uses gravity to accentuate the posterior movement of the tibia.	Have the client lie supine and flex the hips and knees to 90° so that they are parallel to the table.
	Support the client's lower legs, and visualize the levels of the tibial tuberosities, looking for differences in posterior displacement.
	A difference in displacement on the involved side indicates a positive test.

> **Practical Tip**
>
> Because it is not isolated, any injury to the MCL should trigger an assessment of the capsule and meniscus.

A valgus force from something like a blow to the lateral knee when the foot is planted is the most common mechanism of injury for the MCL, but trauma can also arise from rotational forces such as planting the foot and turning quickly. The MCL is not an isolated structure. It has fibrous attachments to both the medial joint capsule and the medial meniscus. Any injury to the ligament should trigger an assessment of the capsule and meniscus as well.

Clients will describe either a valgus force or a rotational mechanism along with immediate pain over the medial knee. Complaints may include hearing or feeling a pop, weakness, swelling, and loss of function. There are three degrees of MCL injuries, which are classified the same way as other ligament injuries:

1. *First-degree sprains* are characterized by a tearing of less than one-third of the fibers, mild swelling and pain over the ligament, normal range of motion, and normal to slightly diminished strength with no joint laxity.
2. *Second-degree sprains* are more severe and include more intense pain and swelling, a feeling of instability and an inability to walk with the heel on the ground, decreased range of motion, and visible joint laxity on a stress test.
3. *Third-degree sprains* are the most severe; they are characterized by an initial sharp pain that subsides relatively quickly. Symptoms also include more severe diffuse swelling, joint instability, significant loss of

range of motion, substantial visible laxity, and no end-feel of the joint during a stress test.

There is one test for a medial collateral ligament sprain, as shown in Table 11-5.

Table 11-5 Orthopedic Test for MCL Injury

Orthopedic Test	How to Perform
Valgus stress test 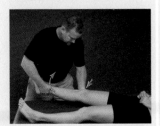	Have the client lie supine on the table with both legs straight.
	Support the involved leg, and place one hand on the lateral aspect of the joint line and the other hand on the medial distal tibia.
	Be sure that the client is relaxed, and push medially on the lateral joint line while pulling laterally at the medial ankle.
	Perform the test both in full extension to test all the medial stabilizing structures and in 15° to 25° of knee flexion to isolate the MCL.
	A positive test is indicated by pain over the ligament and/or joint gapping or a mushy end-feel.

Since the ligament is external to the joint, direct treatment is indicated. Depending on the severity, treatment will vary from swelling control to assisting healthy scar tissue formation. Techniques such as light effleurage over the medial knee aid in removing excess swelling during the initial healing phases. Make sure that the inflammation is under control to avoid exacerbating the condition. Once the healing reaches the later stages, perform friction, along with the other advanced techniques discussed in Chapter 3, over the injury site to encourage the formation of a functional scar. During all stages of healing, utilize strokes such as parallel thumb stripping, cross-fiber fanning, and perpendicular compressive effleurage to remove any biomechanical imbalances in the muscles surrounding the knee.

Lateral Collateral Ligament Unlike the MCL, the lateral collateral ligament (LCL) is a separate structure and has no fibrous connections to the joint capsule or lateral meniscus. Also known as the *fibular collateral ligament,* this cordlike structure arises from the lateral condyle of the femur and attaches to the head of the fibula. It is separated from the capsule and meniscus by a small fat pad, and the ligament is significantly smaller than its medial counterpart. It serves as the primary restraint to varus forces on the knee between 0° and 30° of flexion and as a secondary restraint to external rotation of the tibia on the femur.

Injuries to the LCL occur primarily from a true varus force on the knee, which can occur as a result of a lateral blow to the medial side of the knee when the foot is firmly planted. Often the less stable lateral ankle will invert and become injured before the knee. Rotational force can also damage the ligament. Even though it is a separate structure, injury to the ligament is rarely isolated. The biceps femoris tendon, iliotibial band, and lateral capsule all provide lateral stability to the knee and can be injured in addition to the LCL.

Clients will describe a varus or rotational mechanism of injury. They may describe a pop and sharp pain at the site of the injury. There are three degrees of LCL sprains, and they follow the same classifications associated with MCL sprains. Swelling will be less severe than that of an MCL injury because the LCL is not attached to the capsule or meniscus; moreover, instability will be subtle since there are several other supportive structures involved.

The test for an LCL injury is very similar to the one used for a medial collateral ligament sprain, as shown in Table 11-6.

Table 11-6 Orthopedic Test for LCL Injury

Orthopedic Test	How to Perform
Varus stress test 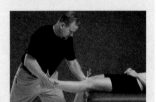	Client is in the supine position with the legs straight out. *Note:* To maintain proper body mechanics, position the client at the edge of the table or at the end of the table. With the client at the bottom of the table, stand between the client's legs and support the involved leg by placing one hand at the medial joint line and the other at the distal lateral tibia. With the knee in full extension, push laterally on the medial joint line and medially on the lateral ankle. Repeat the test with the client's knee in 30° of flexion to better isolate the ligament. A positive test is indicated by pain over the ligament and/or joint gapping or a mushy end-feel.

As with the MCL, the LCL is superficial and direct treatment is indicated. The goals are the same as those for treating an MCL sprain and include removing excess swelling during the initial stages of healing and using techniques that promote the formation of a healthy, functional scar in the later stages. In all stages, keeping the surrounding muscles functioning properly and removing any imbalances or restrictions will help the overall recovery process. The techniques mentioned in treating MCL injuries are appropriate here.

Ankle

Lateral (Inversion) Sprains "The ankle is one of the most common sites for acute musculoskeletal injuries, and sprains account for 75% of ankle injuries" (Wolfe et al., 2001). Three ligaments support the lateral ankle:

1. The *anterior talofibular (ATF) ligament* is the weakest of the three and runs between the anterior distal tip of the fibula and the talus; it re-

sists inversion during plantar flexion and the anterior translation of the talus on the tibia.

2. The *calcaneofibular (CF) ligament* is stronger than the ATF and connects the distal tip of the fibula to the calcaneus. It resists inversion of the talus during the midrange of the ankle.

3. The *posterior talofibular ligament (PTF)* is the strongest of the three; it connects the posterior distal tip of the fibula to the talus and prevents posterior translation of the talus on the tibia.

Because it is the weakest, the ATF is the most frequently injured, followed by the CF. The PTF is rarely injured unless trauma is severe.

Injuries to the lateral ankle occur as a result of excessive inversion force, especially when the foot is in plantar flexion. These injuries can occur from activities such as landing from a jump, pushing off during running, stepping off a curb, or cutting when changing direction. Inversion sprains occur at a higher rate than eversion sprains due to several factors:

- The medial malleolus does not extend down as far as the lateral malleolus, creating a fulcrum that allows for easier inversion.
- The ligaments on the lateral ankle are not as strong as those on the medial side of the ankle.
- Hypertension in the gastrocnemius and soleus prevent optimal dorsiflexion during gate, which leaves the foot in slight plantar flexion and places it in a vulnerable position for inversion.

Clients will describe an inversion mechanism that causes a sharp pain on the lateral side of the ankle. Determine the position of the foot at the time of the injury to help identify which ligaments are involved. The client may describe a cracking, popping, or tearing sound, as well as a possible loss of function after the injury. Expanding on the general signs and symptoms of sprains covered in Chapter 3, lateral ankle sprains are characterized in three degrees:

1. *First-degree sprains* are mild and can involve both the ATF and the CF ligaments. Pain and swelling are minimal and located on the anterolateral aspect of the lateral malleolus, and individuals are often able to bear weight immediately after the injury. Point tenderness is located over the ATF ligament.

2. *Second-degree sprains* often include a tearing or popping sensation. The pain and swelling are more severe and extend to the inferior aspect of the lateral malleolus. Both the ATF and the CF ligaments are involved and both are point tender. Weight bearing is still possible, although it will not be full and there will be decreased function.

3. *Third-degree sprains* are classified as a total rupture of the ATF and CF with a partial to full tearing of the PTF ligaments. There is definitely a tearing or popping sensation over the lateral aspect of the ankle and rapid diffuse swelling over the entire lateral ankle. Bruising may be present, and the individual will not be able to bear weight and will have substantial instability and loss of function. It is important to have third-degree sprains evaluated for possible fracture because of the severity of the trauma.

In assessing inversion ankle sprains, other structures can be involved depending on the degree of the injury. Avulsion fractures to the base of

> **Practical Tip**
>
> Because it is the weakest, the ATF is the most frequently injured followed by the CF.

the 5th metatarsal, lateral malleolus, and other attachment sites of the ligaments are possible. Because the muscles of the lateral leg contract eccentrically to prevent excessive inversion, they can be strained to various degrees. Pain up the lateral leg after an ankle sprain is an indication of this. The individual may experience pain and bruising on the medial side of the ankle if the inversion is extensive enough because the tissue can become compressed and pinched and cause damage.

There are two primary tests to determine the extent of a lateral ankle sprain, as shown in Table 11-7.

Treatment for ankle sprains follows the same pattern as for other sprains. After the inflammation is under control, the focus should be to remove excess swelling. As the injury moves into the later stages of healing, focus on creating a functional scar and preventing any unwanted adhesions from forming between adjacent structures. Edema in ankle sprains tends to linger longer than other types of sprains, and massage is extremely effective at removing it. A great technique is to "milk" the ankle by placing the client in the prone position and flexing the knee to 90°:

- Start at the foot and effleurage toward the knee, conforming to the ankle.
- Adjust the pressure to the client's tolerance level, but pressure should never cause excessive discomfort.
- Swelling that has been lingering can become thick, so some more direct techniques with fingertips and thumbs may be needed to soften it before it can be moved out.
- Use the thumbs to trace the malleoli, helping to define them, and on either side of the Achilles tendon, to prevent the swelling from collecting in the area.

Remember that the techniques should not be so aggressive as to cause an increase in swelling. In the later stages, friction to the involved ligaments will help with scar tissue remodeling. Address the entire lower leg to prevent imbalances from occurring. Depending on the length of time since the injury and its severity, the treatment area may need to be expanded to address any compensation that has taken place.

Medial (Eversion) Sprains While sprains to the medial ankle are much less common than those to the lateral ankle, they can still occur. The deltoid ligament provides the major stability for the medial ankle and consists of the anterior tibiotalar, tibiocalcaneal, posterior tibiotalar, and tibionavicular ligaments. This group of ligaments serves to prevent excessive eversion of the ankle. The frequency of eversion sprains is small, mostly due to the strength of the deltoid ligament. Another factor is that the deltoid ligament receives help from the distal fibula. The distal tip of the fibula extends farther than the tibia. While this may increase the risk of inversion sprains, it acts as a bony block that helps prevent eversion injuries.

Because of the strength of these ligaments, the amount of force required to cause damage is much higher; therefore, the severity of injury tends to be greater.

Excessive eversion force is one mechanism of injury, and individuals with pronated feet have a greater risk. This type of injury occurs from a high-impact trauma, such as a car accident, or the application of a valgus force to the lateral ankle on a foot that is planted. Two other mechanisms

✳Practical Tip

Because of the strength of the deltoid ligament, the amount of force required to cause damage is much higher; therefore, the severity of injury tends to be greater.

Table 11-7 Orthopedic Tests for Lateral Ankle Sprains

Orthopedic Test	How to Perform
Ankle-drawer test 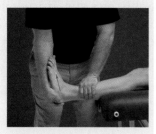 *Note:* This test focuses on the anterior talofibular ligament, and it has several variations.	Client is in the seated position with the distal lower leg off the table. Stand to the lateral side of the involved leg, and cup the heel with the bottom hand while resting the client's foot along the forearm and holding it at a 90° angle. With the other hand, stabilize the distal tibia and apply an upward force to the heel. *Note:* Make sure that the client is relaxed to optimize the accuracy of the test. Clients will have a tendency to actively dorsiflex the ankle. To ensure the client relaxes, let his or her toes rest on your forearm. Pain over the lateral ankle or anterior translation of the talus compared to the uninvolved side is considered a positive test. *Note:* Remember that with third-degree sprains, there may be minimal pain because of the total rupture of the ligament; however, there will be significant translation.
Talar tilt test 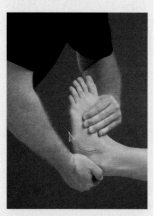 *Note:* This test isolates the calcaneofibular ligament.	Client is in the seated position with the distal lower leg off the table. Stand at the bottom of the client's foot, and cup the heel with the hand on the lateral side. Grasp the foot with the other hand, keeping the thumb on the plantar aspect. Instruct the client to relax. With the hand that is on the foot, dorsiflex the ankle so that it is at 90°; with the hand cupping the heel, invert the foot to stress the CF ligament. Keep the ankle at 90° when inverting it to keep the emphasis on the calcaneofibular ligament. Pain over the ligament or a lack of a firm end-feel compared to the uninvolved side is considered a positive test.

of injury are excessive dorsiflexion of the foot and external rotation of the talus in the ankle mortise.

Clients will describe an eversion, rotational, or hyperdorsiflexion mechanism of injury. The client will initially feel pain over the medial ankle, but if the injury is not severe, the pain will subside once the joint is returned to its normal position. Swelling and bruising will be evident and will vary depending on the severity of the injury. Loss of function will also depend on the degree of the injury, and passive range of motion may elicit pain only with dorsiflexion. Severe eversion sprains must be assessed for fractures to the malleoli. The medial malleolus can suffer an avulsion fracture, while the lateral malleolus can sustain what is described as a "knock-off" fracture, wherein the talus breaks off the tip of the fibula. There is a primary test to determine the extent of a medial ankle sprain, as shown in Table 11-8.

Table 11-8 Orthopedic Test for a Medial Ankle Sprain

Orthopedic Test	How to Perform
Talar tilt test 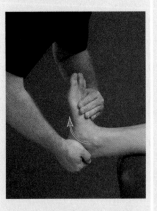 *Note:* This test is used to assess the integrity of the deltoid ligament; it can also be used to determine whether an eversion injury has occurred.	Client is in the seated position with the distal lower leg off the table. Stand at the bottom of the client's foot, and cup the heel with the hand on the medial side of the client. Grasp the foot with the other hand, and keep the thumb on the plantar aspect. Instruct the client to relax. Using the hand that is on the foot, passively dorsiflex the ankle so that it is at 90°; use the hand that is cupping the heel to evert the foot, stressing the deltoid ligament. Pain over the ligament or a lack of a firm end-feel compared to the uninvolved side is considered a positive test.

Treating medial ankle sprains follows the progression used for treating lateral sprains. Milking the ankle is effective for eversion sprains and will dramatically improve healing rates. Friction to the medial structures helps facilitate proper scar tissue formation. Always treat the entire lower leg to address any muscular imbalance issues.

Syndesmosis Sprain Syndesmosis injuries are less common than the other two types of ankle sprains; moreover, they are often overlooked and undetected, which can prolong recovery time and lead to greater disability. There are three main stabilizers to the distal syndesmosis joint at the ankle. The most commonly injured is the anterior inferior tibiofibular ligament, which connects the anterior distal fibula to the tibia. The least injured is the posterior inferior tibiofibular ligament, which connects the posterior distal fibula to the tibia. The last supporting structure is the distal portion of the interosseous membrane. These structures primarily function to hold the two bones together; this composes the ankle mortise.

The distal syndesmosis joint is extremely strong; therefore, great force is necessary to cause an injury. One mechanism of injury is the extreme dorsiflexion of the foot. The anterior inferior portion of the talus is wider than the rest of the bone, so when there is hyperdorsiflexion, the wider portion of the talus is forced into the mortise and separates the fibula and tibia. This can happen when an individual steps into a hole or is fallen on from behind when the foot is planted. Another mechanism of injury is the external rotation of the talus within the mortise. The talus rotates and separates the tibia and fibula, causing damage to the ligaments. This can occur when a person makes a plant-and-pivot movement or is fallen on and sustains external rotation of the foot.

The client will generally describe an incident with one of the above mechanisms, which results in pain that is not in the traditional place for a lateral ankle sprain. The pain and swelling for a syndesmosis sprain tend to be above the lateral malleolus, and thus the injury is nicknamed "high-ankle" sprain. There is a higher degree of instability in the ankle with this type of sprain than with lateral ankle sprains, as well as increased functional limitations, especially with weight bearing, since the mortise spreads apart with each step. Because of the amount of force necessary to cause the initial injury, recovery time tends to be longer than that of more common inversion and eversion sprains.

There is a primary test to determine the extent of a syndesmosis sprain, as shown in Table 11-9.

Practical Tip
Because of the amount of force necessary to cause the initial injury, recovery time tends to be longer than that of more common inversion and eversion sprains.

Table 11-9 Orthopedic Test for a Syndesmosis Sprain

Orthopedic Test	How to Perform
Dorsiflexion test 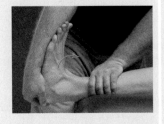	Client is in the seated position with the distal lower leg off the table. Stabilize the lower leg with one hand, and passively dorsiflex the foot with the other hand to its end range; apply additional pressure to stress the joint. Pain over the distal ankle syndesmosis is considered a positive sign.

Since this injury tends to take longer to heal, any techniques that can speed up the process are advantageous. To help remove excess swelling, milk the ankle once the swelling is under control. In the later stages of healing, friction over the involved ligaments is beneficial to help with both scar tissue remodeling and increased circulation to speed healing. As with the other sprains, treat the entire lower leg to address any compensatory issues.

JOINT INJURIES

Meniscus Injuries

Recall that the menisci are disks of fibrocartilage that are attached to the tibial plateau. They serve to deepen the articulation and fill in the gaps during movement, as well as provide lubrication and shock absorption and increase joint stability. They are thicker on the periphery and thinner on the medial edge. The blood supply is restricted to the lateral margins, and the medial portions get their nutrients from the synovial fluid. The lateral meniscus is almost a complete circle and is much more mobile than its medial counterpart. The medial meniscus is C-shaped and less mobile due to its attachments to the joint capsule and MCL.

As the body ages, the pliability of the menisci decreases, making them more susceptible to injury. The highest incidence of injury seems to occur in men between the ages of 21 and 40 and in women between 11 and 20. The primary mechanism of injury is excessive compressive force, which can arise from the normal wear and tear of walking or running; however, the chance of a meniscus injury dramatically increases with the addition of a rotational component. The shear forces that are generated from a plant-and-twist movement can easily result in a tear. The four classifications of meniscal tears are summarized in Table 11-10.

Table 11-10 Meniscal Tears

Classification	Characteristics
Longitudinal	Occurs when the foot is fixed and there is a twisting motion at the knee
Bucket handle	Occurs when the entire longitudinal segment of the tear is displaced medially; can cause locking of the knee at 10° of flexion
Horizontal	Occurs because of tissue degeneration and the cumulative effects of wear and tear
Parrot beak	Consists of two horizontal tears in the middle of the lateral meniscus

The tearing or cracking of the meniscus can cause a piece to dislodge and float freely within the joint. This "joint mouse," as it is called, can become temporarily lodged between the tibia and the femur, resulting in the temporary locking of the joint.

The client will describe feeling a pop or click while performing a movement that caused a sharp pain in the knee. Because the menisci are not innervated, pain can be hard to pinpoint and is often seen along the joint line and near the collateral ligaments. Swelling will occur from the onset of the trauma to several hours postinjury. Extreme flexion will cause discomfort, and there may be periods of knee buckling or locking. If the tear is mild, functional limitation may be minimal, with problems occurring only when the flap from the tear catches on something.

There are two tests to assess for a meniscal tear, as shown in Table 11-11.

Treatment for meniscus injuries is similar to that for ACL and PCL injuries in the sense that the structures are internal and not directly accessible. Focus on removing any muscle imbalances that were caused as a result of compensation, using any of the techniques described in Chapter 9.

Table 11-11　Orthopedic Tests for Meniscal Tears

Orthopedic Test	How to Perform
Apley's compression test 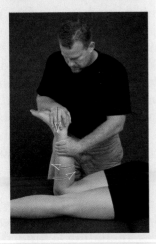	Client is in the prone position with the knee flexed to 90°. Apply a downward force to the heel while attempting to drive the leg into the table. Rotate the tibia internally and externally, compressing the tibial plateau into the femoral condyles. Pain in the knee is considered a positive sign.
Apley's distraction test 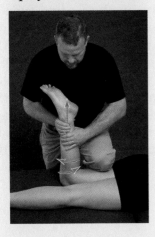 *Note:* This test is performed only if the Apley's compression test is positive.	Client is in the prone position with the knee flexed to 90°. Place one knee on the back of the client's thigh to stabilize it, and grasp the lower leg with both hands. Lift the lower leg while rotating it medially and laterally. Pain during the Apley's compression test but not during the Apley's distraction test is an indication of a meniscal injury.

Osteochondral Defects

Damage to the articular cartilage of a joint is referred to as an *osteochondral defect*. The articular cartilage provides joint surfaces with a low-friction environment that is necessary to perform repetitive movements without symptoms (Scopp et al., 2005). In addition to reducing friction, the articular cartilage serves to protect the subchondral bone from compressive forces.

Injuries to the chondral surface result from two causes:

1. A *high-force trauma* that directs an axial or rotational load on the joint surfaces, resulting in the tearing away of the cartilage
2. *Repetitive micro-traumas* leading to a progressive degeneration of the cartilage

Progressive loss begins as chondropenia (loss of cartilage volume), which leads to defects that will elevate joint contact pressures and further joint degeneration. Defects can be classified as full thickness or partial thickness. *Full-thickness defects* penetrate the cartilage and move into the subchondral bone, while *partial-thickness defects* affect only the cartilage. As the depth of the defect increases, the corresponding stress on the underlying bone increases, leading to greater disability.

The client may describe a traumatic mechanism, such as landing on straight legs from a fall, or may report that the joint has become sore and swollen with no recollection of any injury. The joint will typically be swollen and painful, with tenderness along the joint line. Weight bearing may be difficult due to pain, and range of motion is diminished secondary to swelling.

Another type of osteochondral injury known as *osteochondritis dissecans* is characterized by a piece of subchondral bone and cartilage that becomes dislodged from the articular surface. It is classified as either stable, wherein the articular cartilage remains in its anatomical position, or unstable, wherein the fragment becomes dislodged. Such injuries can occur from trauma, repetitive micro-traumas, or a loss of vascularity to the bone. In an unstable injury, the fragment, once dislodged, can become caught in the joint, causing it to periodically lock. The injury presents with similar symptoms to that of chondral defects, including aching, diffuse pain, swelling, and a loss of function.

Treatment of osteochondral injuries usually involves some type of surgery to either repair the defect or initiate a healing response. If the defect is not in an area of high contact between surfaces, just managing the symptoms may be an option. Using glucosamine sulfate and chondroitin sulfate has shown to be effective in minimizing the symptoms associated with these injuries. These substances do not repair or regenerate the articular surface, but they work to reduce inflammation in the area. Massage therapy helps support these functions, as well. Pain during weight bearing will result in compensation to the area, so techniques that balance the surrounding musculature will be beneficial.

TENDONOPATHIES

Any disease or dysfunction of a tendon falls under the broad umbrella of various conditions classified as *tendonopathies.* Recall that tendons are made up of collagen fibers arranged in a parallel fashion so that they can withstand tremendous tensile forces. Several muscles are especially prone to developing pathologies in the tendons, including the:

- Biceps brachii
- Quadriceps
- Hamstrings
- Achilles
- Elbow flexors and extensors
- Triceps

However, any tendon can develop problems.

Three primary pathologies can affect tendons: tendonitis, tenosynovitis, and tendonosis. Treatment for tendonopathies is similar regardless of the injury's location. Using techniques that will relieve tension on the involved muscle will help take the pressure off the tendon. Friction is a valuable stroke with all three types of conditions, but the focus is different with each. Table 11-12 lists and describes the three primary pathologies.

Table 11-12 Pathologies of Tendons

Condition	Description	Symptoms	Treatment
Tendonitis	Inflammation of a tendon. Can be caused by a single traumatic event, but is generally caused by repetitive overuse.	Pain and swelling. Tendon may begin to thicken if the condition has been present for a period of time.	Use friction to prevent any unwanted adhesion formation around the tendon itself. Take slack out of the tendon by placing it in a lengthened position.
Tenosynovitis	Tendons pass through a sheath, which reduces friction to the tendon. Overuse and chronic irritation can cause the formation of adhesions between the tendon and the sheath, reducing its ability to slide back and forth.	Similar to tendonitis, except pain is more localized and there is a distinct crepitus sound with movement.	Use friction to break up adhesions that have already formed between the synovial sheath and the tendon sliding through it. Take slack out of the tendon by placing it in a lengthened position.
Tendonosis	Differs from tendonitis and tenosynovitis in that there are no inflammatory cells. A degeneration of the collagen matrix within the tendon exists, causing an overall breakdown of the tissue. Can arise from a single incident but is more likely caused by repeated insults to the tendon.	A failed healing response with a repeated cycle of insults and partial healing that leads to degeneration of the tissue over time.	Use friction to initiate a mild inflammatory state, which will stimulate fibroblast production. Take slack out of the tendon by placing it in a lengthened position.

BURSITIS

Inflammation of the bursa regardless of location is termed *bursitis.* Bursae are fluid-filled sacs located under muscles, tendons, ligaments, and other structures that are exposed to friction. They serve to reduce friction between surfaces and allow for smooth motion. In the body, there are certain places where bursae are more common, such as over the patella and olecranon process, but bursae can actually develop where they are needed. Under normal conditions bursae are not palpable, but they can become inflamed, making them more prominent.

Injury to the bursa can occur from direct force that causes an inflammatory response; however, it is more likely to occur as a result of repetitive friction or compression. Depending on the location of the bursa, varying degrees of dysfunction can occur. A subcutaneous bursa may swell, but it will stay contained within the sac and not cause a great degree of dysfunction; however, a bursa located beneath a tendon or ligament can generate a tremendous amount of pain during movement, subsequently leading to significant dysfunction.

There are no specific assessments to determine whether the bursa is involved; however, performing active and passive movements helps determine whether the involved tissue is contractile or not:

- Pain with active motion can be an indicator of bursitis, but it can also indicate tendon involvement.
- Pain on passive movement indicates that only noncontractile tissues, such as the bursa, are involved.
- Pain on active motion but not on passive motion probably indicates a tendon-related problem.
- Pain on active and passive motion may indicate a bursa-related problem.

To treat bursitis appropriately, it is necessary to identify the structures around the inflamed bursa and determine their respective roles. If the bursa is immediately subcutaneous, massage cannot do much more than help relieve irritation of the surrounding tissues. If inflammation to the bursa is the result of excessive tension or compression, the involved muscles need to be released to relieve the pressure on the bursa. For example, if the bursa that lies under the distal end of the iliotibial band as it crosses the lateral femoral condyle is inflamed, it is likely due to the fact that the iliotibial band is tight and compressing the bursa. Work to the gluteus maximus, tensor fascia latae, and iliotibial tract to remove the tension in the area; this will lessen the pressure on the bursa.

NERVE ENTRAPMENT SYNDROMES

Nerve entrapment syndromes occur when a nerve becomes "trapped" due to changes in the tissue through which the nerve passes (Schoen, 2002). These syndromes are not an uncommon problem and tend to occur more frequently in the upper extremities. Some common locations include:

- Pectoralis minor
- Cubital tunnel

Practical Tip

Use movement to help determine whether the bursa is involved.

- Thoracic outlet
- Carpal tunnel

Nerve entrapment can be caused by chronic conditions such as repeated micro-traumas, but it can also arise as a result of hypertrophied muscles, fibrous bands, tumors, injuries, blunt traumas, and bone prominences.

These entrapments develop because as the nerve travels its course, it has to pass through various narrow anatomical passageways. The passageways create a vulnerable environment, and since the nerve is the softest structure in the area, they become compressed. This pressure diminishes blood flow to the nerve, and the ischemic portion does not repolarize normally; this results in a conduction delay, causing a vague aching in the area of the compression. Other signs and symptoms include:

- Pain
- Numbness
- Paresthesia
- Muscle weakness
- Tingling
- Burning
- A "pins and needles" feeling

There are two terms used to describe this pathology, depending on the location of the entrapment. A compression that occurs at the nerve root, such as a herniated disk, is called a *radiculopathy*. Injury along the length of the nerve, such as thoracic outlet syndrome, is termed a *neuropathy*.

A condition known as the *double-crush phenomenon* occurs when more than one region of the nerve is being compressed at the same time. The proximal entrapment creates a nutritional deficiency along the distal nerve, making it more sensitive to compression; this explains why individuals may have simultaneous symptoms from two different conditions.

Treatment should focus on addressing the structures that are causing the entrapment. Locate the affected nerve, and determine which surrounding structures may be involved. Treat the structures to remove pressure on the nerve, taking care not to work on the nerve directly as this may exacerbate the condition.

SUMMARY

This chapter took on a different appearance than the previous chapters and addressed conditions that encompass different tissues, structures, and locations or that are not isolated to one region of the body. The conditions ranged from isolated structures that are both accessible and inaccessible to global posture patterns that involve the entire body. The various characteristics of the conditions—including what they are, the tissues involved, the mechanism of injury, and any assessments (if applicable)—and soft tissue treatment strategies were discussed.

REVIEW QUESTIONS

1. What is the goal of correct posture?
2. Where are the two locations where lordosis can occur?
3. What are the three presentations of kyphosis?
4. What is the difference between structural and nonstructural scoliosis?
5. Name the two types of hematomas that can occur from a contusion, and describe each.
6. What is a FOOSH injury?
7. Describe the three types of AC joint sprains.
8. What is the purpose of the ACL?
9. What is the function of the meniscus?
10. What are the two mechanisms of osteochondral defect injuries?
11. What is the purpose of a bursa?
12. What is the difference between a neuropathy and a radiculopathy?

CRITICAL-THINKING QUESTIONS

1. Discuss the development of upper- and lower-crossed syndromes.
2. Describe why lateral ankle sprains are the most common.
3. Discuss why syndesmotic ankle sprains are the most severe.
4. Discuss the difference between tendonitis, tenosynovitis, and tendonosis.
5. Discuss how the use of motion can help assess a bursa injury.

Orthopedic Tests for General Conditions

Condition	Orthopedic Test	How to Perform	Positive Sign
Acromiocla-vicular sprain	Acromioclavic-ular distraction test	Client is in standing position. Standing at the side of the client, grasp the arm just proximal with one hand and palpate the joint with the other. Apply a downward traction to the arm.	Pain and/or joint motion is a sign of a positive test.
	Crossover (acro-mioclavicular) compression test	Client is in standing or seated position. Standing to the side, horizontally adduct the client's arm across the chest and com-press it into the body.	Pain at the joint is a positive sign.
Anterior cruci-ate ligament sprain	Anterior-drawer test *Note:* This test is not the most ac-curate and has several short-comings that can result in the masking of a positive result.	Have the client lie supine on the table while flexing the hip to 45° and the knee to 90°. Sit on the table, and place the client's foot that is on the table under his or her thigh to keep it from moving. Place the thumbs on either side of the patellar tendon in the joint line and the fingers in the popliteal fossa to palpate the hamstring tendons; make sure they do not contract. While palpating the joint line with the thumbs, apply an alternating anterior and posterior force on the proximal tibia. Repeat the test with the foot internally and externally rotated to assess different parts of the ligament.	Check for any translation of the tibia, which can be either seen from the lateral view or felt with the thumbs. Compare the amount of move-ment to that on the uninvolved side, and make a determination relative to laxity.
	Lachman's test *Note:* This test is more reliable than the anterior-drawer test.	Place the client in the supine position. Flex the client's knee to 20° with one hand, and stabilize the distal femur with the other. *Note:* It is important for the client to remain as relaxed as possible to prevent any guarding of the muscles, which will render the test results inaccurate. Apply an anterior force to the tibia while either stabilizing or applying a slight pos-terior force to the femur. *Note:* If the client's leg is too large or the therapist's hand is too small to stabilize the femur, a small towel or bolster may be used to keep the knee at the proper angle.	A positive test is determined by the lack of a solid end-feel and a "mushy" feeling compared to the uninvolved side.

Orthopedic Tests for General Conditions *(Continued)*

Condition	Orthopedic Test	How to Perform	Positive Sign
Posterior cruciate ligament sprain	Posterior-drawer test	Have the client lying supine on the table with the hip bent to 45° and the knee at 90°. Sit on the client's foot to hold the tibia in a neutral position; grasp the proximal tibia and push it posteriorly.	Compare the amount of movement to that on the uninvolved side; if it moves more or there is a soft or mushy end-feel, the test is considered positive.
	Godfrey's (posterior-sag) test *Note:* This test uses gravity to accentuate the posterior movement of the tibia.	Have the client lie supine and flex the hips and knees to 90° so that they are parallel to the table. Support the client's lower legs, and visualize the levels of the tibial tuberosities, looking for differences in posterior displacement.	A difference in displacement on the involved side indicates a positive test.
Medial collateral ligament sprain	Valgus stress test	Have the client lie supine on the table with both legs straight. Supporting the involved leg, place one hand on the lateral aspect of the joint line and the other hand on the medial distal tibia. Be sure that the client is relaxed, and push medially on the lateral joint line while pulling laterally at the medial ankle. Perform the test both in full extension to test all the medial stabilizing structures and in 15° to 25° of knee flexion to isolate the MCL.	A positive test is indicated by pain over the ligament and/or joint gapping or a mushy end-feel.
Lateral collateral ligament sprain	Varus stress test	Client is in the supine position with the legs straight out. *Note:* To maintain proper body mechanics, position the client at the edge of the table or at the end of the table. With the client at the bottom of the table, stand between the client's legs, and support the involved leg by placing one hand at the medial joint line and the other at the distal lateral tibia.	A positive test is indicated by pain over the ligament and/or joint gapping or a mushy end-feel.

Orthopedic Tests for General Conditions *(Continued)*

Condition	Orthopedic Test	How to Perform	Positive Sign
		With the knee in full extension, push laterally on the medial joint line and medially on the lateral ankle. Repeat the test with the client's knee in 30° of flexion to better isolate the ligament.	
Lateral ankle sprain	Ankle-drawer test *Note:* This test focuses on the anterior talofibular ligament, and it has several variations.	Client is in the seated position with the distal lower leg off the table. Stand to the lateral side of the involved leg, and cup the heel with the bottom hand while resting the client's foot along the forearm and holding it at a 90° angle. With the other hand, stabilize the distal tibia and apply an upward force to the heel. *Note:* Make sure that the client is relaxed to optimize the accuracy of the test. Clients will have a tendency to actively dorsiflex the ankle. To ensure the client relaxes, let his or her toes rest on your forearm.	Pain over the lateral ankle or anterior translation of the talus compared to the uninvolved side is considered a positive test. *Note:* Remember that with third-degree sprains, there may be minimal pain because of the total rupture of the ligament; however, there will be significant translation.
	Talar tilt test *Note:* This test isolates the calcaneofibular ligament.	Client is in the seated position with the distal lower leg off the table. Stand at the bottom of the client's foot, and cup the heel with the hand on the lateral side. Grasp the foot with the other hand, keeping the thumb on the plantar aspect. Instruct the client to relax. With the hand that is on the foot, dorsiflex the ankle so that it is at 90°; with the hand cupping the heel, invert the foot to stress the CF ligament. Keep the ankle at 90° when inverting it to keep the emphasis on the calcaneofibular ligament.	Pain over the ligament or a lack of a firm end-feel compared to the uninvolved side is considered a positive test.

Orthopedic Tests for General Conditions *(Continued)*

Condition	Orthopedic Test	How to Perform	Positive Sign
Deltoid ligament sprain	Talar tilt test *Note:* This test is used to assess the integrity of the deltoid ligament; it can also be used to determine whether an eversion injury has occurred.	Client is in the seated position with the distal lower leg off the table. Stand at the bottom of the client's foot, and cup the heel with the hand on the medial side of the client. Grasp the foot with the other hand, and keep the thumb on the plantar aspect. Instruct the client to relax. Using the hand that is on the foot, passively dorsiflex the ankle so that it is at 90°; use the hand that is cupping the heel to evert the foot, stressing the deltoid ligament.	Pain over the ligament or a lack of a firm end-feel compared to the uninvolved side is considered a positive test.
Ankle sydesmosis sprain	Dorsiflexion test	Client is in the seated position with the distal lower leg off the table. Stabilize the lower leg with one hand, and passively dorsiflex the foot with the other hand to its end range; apply additional pressure to stress the joint.	Pain over the distal ankle syndesmosis is considered a positive sign.
Meniscus tear	Apley's compression test	Client is in the prone position with the knee flexed to 90°. Apply a downward force to the heel while attempting to drive the leg into the table. Rotate the tibia internally and externally, compressing the tibial plateau into the femoral condyles.	Pain in the knee is considered a positive sign.
	Apley's distraction test *Note:* This test is performed only if the Apley's compression test is positive.	Client is in the prone position with the knee flexed to 90°. Place one knee on the back of the client's thigh to stabilize it, and grasp the lower leg with both hands. Lift the lower leg while rotating it medially and laterally.	Pain during the Apley's compression test but not during the Apley's distraction test is an indication of a meniscal injury.

State-by-State Requirements

Note: *State requirements for curriculum hours, licensure, and registration or certification are constantly changing. For this reason, we ask that you check with your individual state and the AMTA or NCBTMB for current data. The information listed below can be found on individual state, AMTA, or NCBTMB websites.*

Alabama Massage Therapy Board
610 S. McDonough St.
Montgomery, AL 36104
Ph: (334) 269-9990
www.almtbd.state.al.us
Educational requirements: 1000 (or 650) hours from accredited massage therapy school
Fees: application, $25; licensing, $100; renewal, $100; exam, $160
Reciprocity: On a state-by-state basis
Continuing education: 16 hours biennially
Exam: NCETMB

Arizona
http://MassageTherapy.az.gov or massageboard.az.gov
Educational requirements: 500 hours from an accredited massage therapy school
Fees: license, $250; renewal (biennial), $250
Continuing education: 25 hours biennially
Exam: NCETMB

Arkansas State Board of Massage Therapy
103 Airways
Hot Springs, AR 71903-0739
Ph: (501) 520-0555
www.state.ar.us or arkansasmassagetherapy.com
Educational requirements: 500 hours from an accredited massage therapy school
Fees: registration, $75; exam, $25; renewal (annual), $30
Reciprocity: On a state-by-state basis
Continuing education: 6 hours annually
Exam: NCETMB

California
www.californiahealthfreedom.com
Freedom of access

Connecticut
Massage Therapy Licensure
Department of Public Health
410 Capitol Ave., MS#12 APP
P.O. Box 340308
Hartford, CT 06134-0308
Ph: (860) 509-7573
www.dph.state.ct.us
Educational requirements: 500 hours from a COMTA-approved school
Fees: application, $300; renewal, $200
Reciprocity: No
Continuing education: 24 hours every 4 years
Exam: NCETMB

Delaware Board of Massage and Bodywork
Cannon Building
861 Silver Lake Blvd., #203
Dover, DE 19904
Ph: (302) 744-4506
www.state.de.us
Educational requirements: for CMT, 200 hours plus CPR; for LMT, 500 hours
Fees: application, pro-rated depending on how many months are left in the license period; renewal: You are notified at the time of renewal.
Reciprocity: Yes
Continuing education: for LMT, 24 hours biennially; for CMT, 12 hours biennially
Exam: NCETMB

Government of the District of Columbia
Department of Health Board of Massage Therapy
717 14th Street N.W., Suite 600
Washington, DC 20005
Ph: (202) 724-4900

www.dcra.org or www.doh.dc.gov
Educational requirements: 500 hours
from a board-approved school
Fees: application, $65; license, $111; renewal, $111;
verification of records, $26
Reciprocity: No
Continuing education: 12 hours biennially
Exam: NCETMB

Florida Board of Massage Therapy
Department of Health
2020 Capital Cir. S.E.
Bin #C09
Tallahassee, FL 32399-3259
Ph: (850) 488-0595
www.doh.state.fl.us/mqa/massage
Educational requirements: 500 hours
from a board-approved school plus 3 hours HIV/AIDS
Fees: application, $205; renewal: $155
Reciprocity: No
Continuing education: 24 hours biennially and a course
in HIV/AIDS
Exam: NCETMB

State of Hawaii
Board of Massage Therapy
DCCA
P.O. Box 3469
Honolulu, HI 96801
Ph: (808) 586-3000
www.state.hi.us or hawaii.gov
Educational requirements: 570 hours—must spend a
minimum of 6 months at an AMTA or Rolf Institute school
Fees: application, $50; exam, $120; renewal (biennial), $20
Reciprocity: No
Continuing education: No
Exam: State exam

Idaho
Freedom of access

Illinois
Ph: (217) 782-8556
www.ildpr.com
Educational requirements: 500 hours from an accredited
school
Fees: license, $100; renewal, $175
Continuing education: 24 hours biennially

Iowa Department of Public Health
Iowa Board of Massage Therapy
321 E. 12th St.
Des Moines, IA 50319
Ph: (515) 281-6959
www.idph.state.ia.us/licensure
Educational requirements: 500 hours
from an accredited school
Fees: application, $120; license, $120; renewal, $60
Reciprocity: Yes

Continuing education: 24 hours biennially
Exam: NCETMB

**Kentucky Finance and Administration Cabinet Board
of Licensure for Massage Therapy**
P.O. Box 1360
Frankfort, KY 40602
Ph: (502) 564-3296
http://finance.ky.gov/bmt
Educational requirements: 600 hours from an accredited
school
Fees: application, $50; license, $125; renewal, $100
Reciprocity: Yes
Continuing education: 24 hours biennially
Exam: NCETMB

Louisiana Board of Massage Therapy
12022 Plank Road
Baton Rouge, LA 70811
Ph: (225) 771-4090
Fax: (225) 771-4021
www.lsbmt.org
Educational requirements: 500 hours from an accredited
school
Fees: application, $75; license, $125; renewal, $125
Reciprocity: Yes
Continuing education: 12 hours annually
Exam: NCETMB plus oral exam

Maine Board of Massage Therapy
Department of Professional and Financial Regulation
35 State House Station
Augusta, ME 04333-0035
Ph: (207) 624-8613
www.maine.gov/pfr/professionallicensing/professions/
massage
Educational requirements: 500 hours from an accredited
school plus CPR and first aid
Fees: application, $25; license, $25; criminal record (SBI)
check, $15; renewal (annual), $25
Reciprocity: Yes
Continuing education: No
Exam: NCETMB or a transcript that outlines a course
of training consisting of 500 hours

Maryland Board of Chiropractic Examiners
Massage Therapy Advisory Committee
4201 Patterson Ave., 5th floor
Baltimore, MD 21215-2299
Ph: (410) 764-4738
www.mdmassage.org
Educational requirements: for CMT, 500 hours
from a COMTA school plus 60 hours of college; for RMT,
500 hours plus 60 college credits
Fees: application, $100; registration/certification, $200;
jurisprudence/state exam, $50; renewal (biennial), $200
Reciprocity: Yes
Continuing education: 24 hours biennially

Exam: NCETMB, NCETM, or NCCAOM plus jurisprudence/state exam

Minnesota
Ph: (800) 657-3957
Freedom of access

Mississippi State Board of Massage Therapy
P.O. Box 12489
Jackson, MS 39236-2489
Ph: (601) 919-1517
www.msbmt.state.ms.us
Educational requirements: 700 hours from an accredited school
Fees: application, $50; renewal (2 years): $192
Reciprocity: Yes
Continuing education: 12 hours from a CEU board-approved program plus CPR annually
Exam: NCETMB, NCCAOM, or similar exam approved by board

Missouri Board of Therapeutic Massage
3605 Missouri Blvd.
P.O. Box 1335
Jefferson City, MO 65102
Ph: (573) 522-6277
www.pr.mo.gov/massage.asp or massagether@pr.mo.gov
Educational requirements: 500 hours from a board-approved school
Fees: application, $200; renewal, $200
Reciprocity: Yes
Continuing education: 12 hours biennially
Exam: NCETMB, NCCAOM, or exam approved by the board

Nebraska Massage Therapy Board
Health and Human Services Credentialing Division
301 Centennial Mall South
14th and M Streets, 3rd Floor
Lincoln, NE 68509
Ph: (402) 471-2115
www.state.ne.us or www.hhs.state.ne.us
Educational requirements: 1000 hours
Fees: license, $25 and Licensee Assistance Program fee of $1 for each year remaining during the current biennial renewal period; renewal (biennial), $25 and Licensee Assistance Program fee of $2; certification, $25
Reciprocity: Yes
Continuing education: 18 hours biennially, approved by state board
Exam: NCETMB

New Hampshire Office of Program Support
Board of Massage Therapy
Health Facilities Administration
129 Pleasant St.
Concord, NH 03301-6527
Ph: (603) 271-5127
www.dhhs.state.nh.us or www.dhhs.nh.gov
Educational requirements: 750 hours plus CPR and first aid

Fees: application, $125; renewal, $100
Reciprocity: Yes
Continuing education: 12 hours biennially
Exam: NCETMB and NH Massage Therapy Practical Examination

New Jersey Board of Nursing
Massage, Bodywork & Somatic Therapy Examining Committee
124 Halsey Street, 6th Floor
P.O. Box 45048
Newark, NJ 07101
Ph: (973) 504-6430
www.NJConsumerAffairs.gov/medical/nursing.htm
Educational requirements: 500 hours
Fees: application, $75; certification, $120; criminal history/background check, $78; renewal (biennial), $120
Continuing Education: 20 hours biennially

New Mexico Massage Therapy Board
2550 Cerrillos Road
Santa Fe, NM 87505
Ph: (505) 476-4870
www.rld.state.nm.us/b&c/massage
Educational requirements: 650 hours
Fees: application, $75; initial license (pro-rated), $5 per month; renewal (biennial), $125
Reciprocity: No
Continuing education: 16 hours biennially, approved by board
Exam: NCETMB and jurisprudence exam

New York State Board of Massage Therapy
Division of Professional Licensing Services
Massage Therapy Unit
89 Washington Avenue
Albany, NY 12234-1000
Ph: (518) 474-3817, ext. 270
www.op.nysed.gov/massage.htm
Educational requirements: 1000 hours from a New York school program or equivalent
Fees: license: $100; exam, $115; renewal (3 years), $50
Reciprocity: Yes
Continuing education: No
Exam: New York State Massage Therapy Examination

North Carolina Board of Massage and Bodywork Therapy
P.O. Box 2539
Raleigh, NC 27602
Ph: (919) 546-0050
www.bmbt.org
Educational requirements: 500 hours from a board-approved school
Fees: application, $20; license, $150; renewal, $100
Reciprocity: No
Continuing education: 25 hours biennially
Exam: NCETMB

North Dakota State Board of Massage
P.O. Box 218
Beach, ND 58621
Ph: (701) 872-4895
www.health.state.nd.us or www.ndboardofmassage.com
Educational requirements: 750 hours
from a COMTA-approved school
Fees: application, $150; renewal (annual), $50
Reciprocity: Yes
Continuing education: 18 hours per year
Exam: NCETMB

Ohio Massage Therapy Board
77 South High St., 17th floor
Columbus, OH 43215-6127
Ph: (614) 466-3934
www.state.oh.us/med or www.med.ohio.gov
Educational requirements: 750 hours
from a board-approved school
Fees: application, $35; exam, $250; renewal, $50
Reciprocity: Case by case
Continuing education: No
Exam: State exam

Oregon Board of Massage Therapists
748 Hawthorne Ave N.E.
Salem, OR 97301
Ph: (503) 365-8657
www.oregonmassage.org
Educational requirements: 500 hours
Fees: application, $50; exam, $100; renewal, $100
Reciprocity: Certain states
Continuing education: 25 hours biennially plus current CPR
Exam: NCETMB and jurisprudence exam

Rhode Island Department of Health
Professional Regulation
3 Capitol Hill, Room 104
Providence, RI 02908-5097
Ph: (401) 222-2827
www.health.state.ri.us
Educational requirements: 500 hours from a COMTA school
Fees: license: $31.25
Reciprocity: Endorsement approved
Continuing education: No
Exam: NCETMB

South Carolina Board of Massage/Bodywork Therapy
P.O. Box 11329
Columbia, SC 29211-1329
Ph: (803) 896-4490
www.llr.state.sc.us
Educational requirements: 500 hours
from an accredited school
Fees: application, $50; license, $100; renewal, $175
Reciprocity: Yes
Continuing education: 12 hours biennially
Exam: NCETMB

South Dakota Board Massage Therapy
Great Plains Solutions, LLC
107 W. Missouri
P.O. Box 7251
Pierre, SD 57501
Ph: 605-224-8005
www.state.sd.us/doh/massage
Educational requirements: 500 hours and CPR
Continuing education: 16 hours biennially
Fees: application: $100; license, $200; renewal
(biennial), $200
Exam: NCETMB

Tennessee Massage Licensure Board
227 French Landing, Suite 300
Heritage Place Metro Center
Nashville, TN 37243
Ph: (615) 532-3202, ext. 32111
www.state.tn.us
Educational requirements: 500 hours
from a state-approved school
Fees: application: $110; renewal (biennial), $100
Reciprocity: Yes
Continuing education: 25 hours biennially
Exam: NCETMB and criminal background check

Texas Department of State Health Services
Massage Therapy Licensing Program
Texas Department of State Health Services MC-1982
1100 West 49th St.
Austin, TX 78756-3183
Ph: (512) 834-6616
www.dshs.state.tx.us/massage/default.shtm
Educational requirements: 300 hours
from a state-approved school
Fees: application, $117; written exam, $87; practical
exam, $100; renewal (biennial), $106
Reciprocity: No
Continuing education: 12 hours biennially
Exam: State exam (Written is offered in specific cities
throughout Texas; practical, only in Austin.)

State of Utah Department of Commerce
Board of Massage Therapy
P.O. Box 146741
Salt Lake City, UT 84144-6741
Ph: (801) 530-6964
www.commerce.state.ut.us or www.dopl.utah.gov
Educational requirements: for LMT, 600 hours
from a COMTA-approved school; for AMT,
1000 hours
Fees: application, $75; FBI fingerprint fee, $24; renewal
(biennial), $52
Reciprocity: Yes
Continuing education: No
Exam: NCETMB and Utah Massage Law and Rule
Examination

Virginia Board of Nursing
6603 W. Broadway St., 5th floor
Richmond, VA 23230-1717
Ph: (804) 662-9909
www.vdh.state.va.us or www.dhp.virginia.gov
Educational requirements: 500 hours
from a board-approved school
Fees: application and certification (biennial), $105;
renewal, $70
Reciprocity: Yes
Continuing education: 25 hours biennially
Exam: NCETMB

Washington State Department of Health
Health Professions Quality Assurance
P.O. Box 47865
Olympia, WA 98504-7865
Ph: (360) 236-4700
www.doh.wa.gov/massage/default.htm
Educational requirements: 500 hours
from a board-approved school
Fees: license, $50; exam, $150; renewal (annual), $10
Reciprocity: Yes
Continuing education: 16 hours biennially
Exam: NCETMB

State of West Virginia Board of Massage Therapy
704 Bland Street, Suite 308
P.O. Box 107
Bluefield, WV 24701
Ph: (304) 325-5862
www.wvmassage.org
Educational requirements: 500 hours
from a COMTA-approved school
Fees: application, $25; license (2 years), $200; renewal
(2 years), $100
Reciprocity: Yes
Continuing education: 25 CEUs biennially
Exam: NCETMB

Wisconsin Department of Regulation and Licensing
Massage Therapy Board
1400 E. Washington Ave., Room 173
Madison, WI 53703
Ph: (608) 266-0145
www.wisconsin.gov
Educational requirements: 600 hours
Fees: initial credential, $53; exam, $57; renewal
(biennial), $53
Reciprocity: Yes
Continuing education: None
Exam: NCETMB

appendix B

References and Resources

Chapter 1

Basu S, et al: Competence in the musculoskeletal system: assessing the progression of knowledge through an undergraduate medical course. *Medical Education* 2004; 38: 1253–1260.

Benson B: The massage tapestry: our first decade, an era of growth. *Massage and Bodywork* 2002; 27(5): 16–22.

Billis EV, et al: Reproducibility and repeatability: errors of three groups of physiotherapists in locating spinal levels by palpation. *Manual Therapy* 2003; 8(4): 223–232.

Comeaux Z, et al: Measurement challenges in physical diagnosis: refining inter-rater palpation, perception and communication. *Journal of Bodywork and Movement Therapies* 2001; 5(4): 245–253.

DiCaprio MR, et al: Curricular requirements for musculoskeletal medicine in American medical schools. *Journal of Bone and Joint Surgery* 2003; 85(5): 565–567.

DiFabio R: Efficacy of manual therapy. *Physical Therapy* 1992; 72(12): 853–863.

Field T: Massage therapy. *Medical Clinics of North America* 2002; 86(1): 163–171.

Hippocrates: *Hippocrates, Vol. III: On Wounds in the Head. In the Surgery. On Fractures. On Joints.* Mochlicon, Cambridge, Harvard University Press, 1928.

Integrating prevention into health care. *Journal of Advanced Nursing* 2003; 41(6): 524–525.

Jacob T: AMMA releases guidelines for medical massage curriculum. *Massage Today* 2002; 2(9).

Jull G, Moore, A: Are manipulative therapy approaches the same? *Manual Therapy* 2002; 7(2): 63.

Lawton GT: Medical massage therapy: the search for definition. *Massage Today* 2002; 2(1).

Lowe W: Exploring orthopedic assessment. *Massage Today* 2001; 1(1).

———: How accurate is that test? *Massage Today* 2001; 1(9).

———: Clinical reasoning skills. *Massage Today* 2004; 4(3).

———: Essentials of assessment: how should we teach assessment? *Massage Today* 2005; 5(4).

Moore A, Jull G: Reflections on the musculoskeletal therapists' multifaceted role and influences on treatment outcomes. *Manual Therapy* 2002; 7(3): 119–120.

Ramsey S: Holistic manual therapy techniques. *Primary Care* 1997; 24(4): 759–784.

Rivett D: Manual therapy cults. *Manual Therapy* 1999; 4(3): 125–126.

Salvo S: *Massage Therapy: Principles and Practice*, 2nd ed. St. Louis, Saunders, 2003.

Chapter 2

Andrade CK, Clifford P: *Outcome-Based Massage.* Baltimore, Lippincott Williams & Wilkins, 2001.

Beck M: *Theory and Practice of Therapeutic Massage*, 3rd ed. New York, Milady, 1999.

Salvo S: *Massage Therapy: Principles and Practice*, 2nd ed. St. Louis, Saunders, 2003.

Tappan F, Benjamin P: *Tappan's Handbook of Healing Massage Techniques: Classic, Holistic, and Emerging Methods*, 3rd ed. Stamford, Appleton and Lange, 1998.

Chapter 3

Akbayrak T, et al: Manual therapy and pain changes in patients with migraine—an open pilot study. *Advances in Physiotherapy* 2001; 3: 49–54.

Arnheim DD, Prentice WE: *Principles of Athletic Training*, 8th ed. St. Louis, Mosby, 1993.

Bailey-Lloyd C: Myofascial release. *Ezine Articles,* www.ezinearticles.com (9/6/2005).

Barnes J: Mind and body. *PT/OT Today* 5(40) on *Myofascial Release*, www.myofascialrelease.com/articles/article_pain.asp?wss=F61DC1450D5F4D48BEB718B0B82420E5&nav=mfr (7/11/2003).

———: Myofascial release: the "missing link" in your treatment. *Myofascial Release*, www.myofascialrelease. com/articles/article_missinglink.asp?wss=F61DC1450 D5F4D48BEB718B0B82420E5&nav=mfr (7/11/2003).

Brattberg G: Connective tissue massage in the treatment of fibromyalgia. *European Journal of Pain* 1999; 3: 235–245.

Comerford MJ, Mottran SL: Movement and stability dysfunction—contemporary developments. *Manual Therapy* 2001; 6(1): 15–26.

Farina D, et al: Experimental muscle pain decreases voluntary EMG activity but does not affect the muscle potential evoked by transcutaneous electrical stimulation. *Clinical Neurophysiology* 2005; 116: 1558–1565.

Feland JB, et al: Acute changes in hamstring flexibility: PNF versus static stretch in senior athletes. *Physical Therapy in Sport* 2001; 2: 186–193.

Ferber R, et al: Effect of PNF stretch techniques on knee flexor muscle EMG activity in older adults. *Journal of Electromyography and Kinesiology* 2002; 12: 391–397.

Fernandez C, et al: Manual therapies in myofascial trigger point treatment: a systematic review. *Journal of Bodywork and Movement Therapies* 2005; 9: 27–34.

Ford GS, et al: The effect of 4 different durations of static hamstring stretching on passive knee-extension range of motion. *Journal of Sports Rehabilitation* 2005; 14: 95–107.

Fritz S: *Sports and Exercise Massage: Comprehensive Care in Athletics, Fitness, and Rehabilitation.* St. Louis, Mosby, 2005.

Fryer G, et al: The effect of manual pressure release on myofascial trigger points in the upper trapezius muscle. *Journal of Bodywork and Movement Therapies* 2005; 2: 1–8.

Graven-Nielsen T, et al: Effects of experimental muscle pain on muscle activity and co-ordination during static and dynamic motor function. *Electroencephalography and Clinical Neurophysiology* 1997; 105: 156–164.

Halbertsma JPK, et al: Sport stretching: effect on passive muscle stiffness of short hamstrings. *Archives of Physical Medicine and Rehabilitation* 1996; 77: 688–692.

———: Repeated passive stretching: acute effect on the passive muscle moment and extensibility of short hamstrings. *Archives of Physical Medicine and Rehabilitation* 1999; 80: 407–414.

History of Rolfing. *About Rolfing,* www.rolf.org/about/history.html (9/6/2005).

Holey EA: Connective tissue manipulation: towards a scientific rationale. *Physiotherapy* 1995; 81(12): 730–739.

———: Connective tissue zones: an introduction. *Physiotherapy* 1995; 81(7): 366–368.

———: Connective tissue massage: a bridge between complementary and orthodox approaches. *Journal of Bodywork and Movement Therapies* 2000; 4(1): 72–80.

Huguenin LK: Myofascial trigger points: the current evidence. *Physical Therapy in Sport* 2004; 5: 2–12.

Jenson MG: Reviewing approaches to trigger point decompression. *Physician Assistant* 2002; 26(12): 37–41.

Juett T: An introduction for the patient. *Myofascial Release*, www.myofascialrelease.com/articles/article_for-patient.asp?wss=0CA0D102EBDA4385833F39F865F6F0 A6&nav=mfr (7/11/2003).

Kizuka T, et al: Relationship between the degree of inhibited stretch reflex activities of the wrist flexor and reaction time during quick extension movements. *Electroencephalography and Clinical Neurophysiology* 1997; 105: 302–308.

Knutson GA, Owens EF: Active and passive characteristics of muscle tone and their relationship to models of subluxation/joint dysfunction, part II. *Journal of the Canadian Chiropractic Association* 2003; 47(4): 269–283.

Lowe W: *Orthopedic Massage: Theory and Technique.* New York, Mosby, 2003.

Lucas KR, et al: Latent myofascial trigger points: their effects on muscle activation and movement efficiency. *Journal of Bodywork and Movement Therapies* 2004; 8: 160–166.

Madeleine P, Arendt-Nielsen L: Experimental muscle pain increases mechanomyographic signal activity during sub-maximal isometric contractions. *Journal of Electromyography and Kinesiology* 2005; 15: 27–36.

Marke SM, et al: Acute effects of static and proprioceptive neuromuscular facilitation stretching on muscle strength and power output. *Journal of Athletic Training* 2005; 40(2): 94–103.

Matre DA, et al: Experimental muscle pain increases the human stretch reflex. *Pain* 1998; 75: 331–339.

Mattes A: *Active Isolated Stretching: The Mattes Method.* Sarasota, Aaron Mattes, 2000.

McAtee RE: An overview of facilitated stretching. *Journal of Bodywork and Movement Therapies* 2002; 6(1): 47–54.

Meinders M, et al: The stretch reflex response in the normal and spastic ankle: effect of ankle position. *Archives of Physical Medicine and Rehabilitation* 1996; 77: 487–492.

Myers T: *Anatomy Trains: Myofascial Meridians for Manual and Movement Therapists.* St. Louis, Churchill Livingstone, 2002.

———: Structural integration—developments in Ida Rolf's "recipe," part 1. *Journal of Bodywork and Movement Therapies* 2003; 8 (2): 131–142.

———: Structural integration—developments in Ida Rolf's "recipe," part 2. *Journal of Bodywork and Movement Therapies*: 2004; (8): 189–198.

———: Structural integration—developments in Ida Rolf's "recipe," part 3. *Journal of Bodywork and Movement Therapies* 2004; 8(4): 249–264.

———: The anatomy trains "recipe." *Massage and Bodywork* 2004; June/July.

———: The three-ring circus: a fond farewell. *Massage and Bodywork* 2004; Oct/Nov.

Myofascial release therapy: what is it? (2000). www.wholehealthmd.com/print/view/1,1560,SU_10156,00.html (9/6/2005).

Ogiso K, et al: Stretch-reflex mechanical response to varying types of previous muscle activities. *Journal of Electromyography and Kinesiology* 2002; 12: 27–36.

Rolfing: what is it? (2000). www.wholehealthmd.com/refshelf/substances_view/1,1525,732,00.htm (9/6/2005).

Roozeboom H: Connective tissue massage—a review. *Journal of the Hong Kong Physiotherapy Association* 1986; 8: 26–29.

Rudolf A: Dr. Rolf, Rolfing and Structural Integration. www.positivehealth.com/permit/Articles/Bodywork/rudol56.htm (9/6/2005).

Saladin KS: *Human Anatomy.* New York, McGraw-Hill, 2005.

Salvo S: *Massage Therapy, Principles and Practice*, 2nd ed. St. Louis, Saunders, 2003.

Schulte E, et al: Experimental muscle pain increases trapezius muscle activity during sustained isometric contractions of arm muscles. *Clinical Neurophysiology* 2004; 115: 1767–1778.

Shumway-Cook A, Woolacott MH: *Motor Control: Theory and Applications*, 2nd ed. Baltimore, Williams and Wilkins, 2001.

Simons DG: Understanding effective treatments of myofascial trigger points. *Journal of Bodywork and Movement Therapies* 2002; 6(2): 81–88.

———: Review of enigmatic MTrPs as a common cause of enigmatic musculoskeletal pain and dysfunction. *Journal of Electromyography and Kinesiology* 2004; 14: 95–107.

———, Mense S: Understanding and measurement of muscle tone as related to clinical muscle pain. *Pain* 1998; 75: 1–17.

Sohn, MK, et al: Effects of experimental muscle pain on mechanical properties of single motor units in human masseter. *Clinical Neurophysiology* 2004; 115: 76–84.

Stone, JA: Proprioceptive neuromuscular faciliation. *Athletic Therapy Today*, 2000; 5(1): 38–39.

Threlkeld AJ: The effects of manual therapy on connective tissue. *Physical Therapy* 1992; 72(12): 893–902.

Travell JG, Simons DG, Simons LS: *Myofascial Pain and Dysfunction: The Trigger Point Manual, Vol. I: Upper Half of Body,* 2nd ed. Baltimore, Williams and Wilkins, 1999.

Weldon SM, Hill RH: The efficacy of stretching for prevention of exercise-related injury: a systematic review of the literature. *Manual Therapy* 2003; 8(3): 141–150.

What is myofascial release. *Myofascial Release,* www.myofascialrelease.com/mfr/mfr_what.asp?wss=24F3FD180A1346E0A377D3F1DC996C00 (7/11/2003).

What is Rolfing? www.vanderbilt.edu/AnS/psychology/health_psychology/rolfing.html (9/6/2005).

Whitridge P: *Myofascial Componenets of Low Back and Leg Pain.* Ft. Pierce, FL, Whitridge, 2001.

———: *Myofascial Components of Neck and Shoulder Pain.* Ft. Pierce, FL, Whitridge, 2001.

Zakas A: The effect of stretching duration on the lower-extremity flexibility of adolescent soccer players. *Journal of Bodywork and Movement Therapies* 2005; 9: 220–225.

———, et al: Effects of stretching exercise during strength training in prepubertal, pubertal and adolescent boys. *Journal of Bodywork and Movement Therapies* 2002; 6(3): 170–176.

Chapter 4

Anderson MK, Hall SJ, Martin M: *Sports Injury Management,* 2nd ed. Baltimore, Lippincott Williams and Wilkins, 2000.

———, et al: *Foundations of Athletic Training: Prevention, Assessment, and Management,* 3rd ed. Baltimore, Lippincott Williams and Wilkins, 2005.

Arnheim DD, Prentice WE: *Principles of Athletic Training,* 8th ed. St. Louis, Mosby, 1993.

Bitner, Joe: Bloom's taxonomy of educational objectives. www.selu.edu/Academics/Faculty/jbitner/etec620/bloom_taxmy.htm (8/16/2005).

Curran N, Brandner B: Chronic pain following trauma. *Trauma* 2005; 7: 123–131.

Garrett B: Student nurses' perceptions of clinical decision-making in the final year of adult nursing studies. *Nurse Education in Practice* 2005; 5: 30–39.

Goodman C, Synder T: *Differential Diagnosis in Physical Therapy, Musculoskeletal and Systemic Conditions.* Philadelphia, W.B. Saunders, 1990.

Griffiths H, Phillips N: A case study of lateral epicondyle pain in a cricketer: a clinical reasoning approach to management. *Physical Therapy in Sport* 2003; 4: 192–198.

Gurney B, et al: Effects of limb-length discrepancy on gait economy and lower-extremity muscle activity in older adults. *Journal of Bone and Joint Surgery* 2001; 83A(6): 907–915.

Hoppenfeld S: *Physical Examination of the Spine and Extremities.* Norwalk, Appleton-Century-Crofts, 1976.

Jones M: Clinical reasoning and pain. *Manual Therapy* 1995; 1: 17–24.

Kendall FP, et al: *Muscles: Testing and Function with Posture and Pain.* Baltimore, Lippincott Williams and Wilkins, 2005.

Kraft, G.H: Neck pain: perspectives and strategies for the new millennium. *Physical Medicine and Rehabilitation Clinics of North America* 2003; 14(3): xi-xiii.

Lowe W: *Functional Assessment in Massage Therapy,* 3rd ed. Bend, OMERI, 1997.

———: *Orthopedic Massage: Theory and Technique.* New York, Mosby, 2003.

Magee DJ: *Orthopedic Physical Assessment*, 3rd ed. Philadelphia, W.B. Saunders, 1997.

McCarberg B: Contemporary management of chronic pain disorders. *Journal of Family Practice Supplement* 2004; 53(10): 11–22.

Mense S, et al: *Muscle Pain: Understanding Its Nature, Diagnosis, and Treatment*. Baltimore, Lippincott Williams and Wilkins, 2001.

Myers J, et al: The wheel of wellness counseling for wellness: a holistic model for treatment planning. *Journal of Counseling and Development* 2000; 78: 251–266.

Saladin KS: *Human Anatomy*. New York, McGraw-Hill, 2005.

Starkey C, Ryan J: *Evaluation of Orthopedic and Athletic Injuries*. Philadelphia, F.A. Davis, 1996.

Suebnukarn S, Haddawy P: *Clinical-Reasoning Skill Acquisition Through Intelligent Group Tutoring*. Asian Institute of Technology: Computer Science and Information Management Program 2005.

Yeager MP: Glucocorticoid regulation of the inflammatory response to injury. *Acta Anaesthesiologica Scandinavica* 2004; 48: 799–813.

Chapter 5

Anderson MK, Hall SJ, Martin M: *Sports Injury Management*, 2nd ed. Baltimore, Lippincott Williams and Wilkins, 2000.

Atasoy E: Thoracic outlet compression syndrome. *Orthopedic Clinics of North America* 1996; 27(2): 265–303.

Banerjee R, Palumbo MA, Fadale PD: Catastrophic cervical spine injuries in the collision sport athlete, part 1. *American Journal of Sports Medicine* 2004; 32(4): 1077–1087.

Brantigan CO, Roos DB: Diagnosing thoracic outlet syndrome. *Hand Clinics* 2004; 20: 27–36.

———, et al: Etiology of neurogenic thoracic outlet syndrome. *Hand Clinics* 2004; 20: 17–22.

Brismee JM, et al: Rate of false positive using the Cyriax release test for thoracic outlet syndrome in an asymptomatic population. *Journal of Manual and Manipulative Therapy* 2004; 12(2): 73–81.

Casbas L, et al: Post-traumatic thoracic outlet syndrome. *Annals of Vascular Surgery* 2005; 19: 25–28.

Cheng JCY, et al: Clinical determinants of the outcome of manual stretching in the treatment of congenital muscular torticollis in infants. *Journal of Bone and Joint Surgery* 2001; 83-A(5): 679–687.

Childs SG: Cervical whiplash syndrome: hyperextension-hyperflexion injury. *Orthopedic Nursing* 2004; 23(2): 106–110.

Clay JH, Pounds DM: *Basic Clinical Massage Therapy: Integrating Anatomy and Treatment*. Baltimore, Lippincott Williams and Wilkins, 2003.

Cleland J, Palmer J: Effectiveness of manual physical therapy, therapeutic exercise, and patient education on bilateral disc displacement without reduction of the temporomandibular joint: a single-case study design. *Journal of Orthopaedic and Sports Physical Therapy* 2004; 34: 535–548.

DeBar LL, et al: Use of complementary and alternative medicine of temporomandibular disorders. *Journal of Orofacial Pain* 2003; 17(3): 224–236.

Ferrari R: Myths of whiplash. *Surg J R Coll Surg Edinb Irel* 2003; 1: 99–103.

Gilman S, et al: Denny-Brown's views on the pathology of dystonia. *Journal of the Neurological Sciences* 1999; 167: 142–147.

Gremillion HA, et al: Psychological consideration in the diagnosis and management of temporomandibular disorders and orofacial pain. *General Dentistry* 2003; Mar/Apr: 168–171.

Irnich D, et al: Randomized trial of acupuncture with conventional massage and "sham" laser acupuncture for the treatment of chronic neck pain. *BMJ* 2001; 322: 1–6.

Ito S, et al: Soft tissue injury threshold during simulated whiplash. *Spine* 2004; 29(9): 979–987.

Jaye C: Managing whiplash injury. *Emergency Nurse* 2004; 12(7): 28–33.

Johansson A, et al: Gender difference in symptoms related to temporomandibular disorders in a population of 50-year-old subjects. *Journal of Orofacial Pain* 2003; 17: 29–35.

Jurch S: *Surface Anatomy: A Therapist's Guide to Palpation*. Charleston, Wellness Education and Research Alliance, 2005.

Kubota T, Miyata A: Successful use of shakuyaku-kanzo-to, a traditional herbal medicine, for intractable symptoms of thoracic outlet syndrome: a case report. *Journal of Anesthesia* 2005; 19: 157–159.

Luther BL: Congenital muscular torticollis. *Orthopaedic Nursing* 2002; 21(3): 21–28.

Magee DJ: *Orthopedic Physical Assessment*, 3rd ed. Philadelphia, W.B. Saunders, 1997.

Manchikanti L, et al: Prevalence of facet joint pain in chronic spinal pain of cervical, thoracic, and lumbar regions. *BMC Musculoskeletal Disorders* 2004; 5(15).

Mattes A: *Active Isolated Stretching: The Mattes Method*. Sarasota, Aaron Mattes, 2000.

McLain RF: Determining treatment of lumbar disk protrusion and disk extrusion. *Journal of Musculoskeletal Medicine* 2005; 22: 21–28.

Novak CB, Mackinnon SE: Thoracic outlet syndrome. *Orthopedic Clinics of North America* 1996; 27(4): 747–762.

Pearson AM, et al: Facet joint kinematics and injury mechanisms during simulated whiplash. *Spine* 2004; 29(4): 390–397.

Raphael KG, et al: Complementary and alternative therapy use by patients with myofascial temporomandibular disorders. *Journal of Orofacial Pain* 2003; 17: 36–41.

Rayan GM: Thoracic outlet syndrome. *Journal of Shoulder and Elbow Surgery* 1998; 7: 440–451.

Ritter A, et al: Thoracic outlet syndrome: a review of the literature. *Journal of Dental Hygiene* 1999; 73(4): 205–207.

Saladin KS: *Human Anatomy.* New York, McGraw-Hill, 2005.

Sanders RJ, Hammond SL: Etiology and pathology. *Hand Clinics* 2004; 20: 23–26.

Schoen DC: Upper extremity nerve entrapments. *Orthopaedic Nursing* 2002; 21(2): 15–33.

Simons DG, Travell JG, Simons LS: *Myofascial Pain and dysfunction: The Trigger Point Manual, Vol. 1.* Baltimore, Williams and Wilkins, 1999.

Starkey C, Ryan J: *Evaluation of Orthopedic and Athletic Injuries.* Philadelphia, F.A. Davis, 1996.

Stemper BD, et al: Gender and region-dependent local facet joint kinematics in rear impact. *Spine* 2004; 29(16): 1764–1771.

Sterner Y, Gerdle B: Acute and chronic whiplash disorders—a review. *Journal of Rehabilitative Medicine* 2004; 36: 193–210.

Taylor JR: The pathology of whiplash: neck sprain. *BC Medical Journal* 2002; 44(5): 252–256.

Treleaven J, Jull G, Sterling M: Dizziness and unsteadiness following whiplash injury: Characteristic features and relationship with cervical joint position error. *Journal of Rehabilitative Medicine* 2003; 35: 36–43.

Vaughn BF: Integrated strategies for treatment of spasmodic torticollis. *Journal of Bodywork and Movement Therapies* 2003; 7(3): 142–147.

Vazquez-Delgado E, et al: Psychological and sleep quality differences between chronic daily headache and temporomandibular disorders patients. *Cephalgia* 2004; 24: 446–454.

Velickovic M, Benabou R, Brin MF: Cervical dystonia pathophysiology and treatment options. *Drugs* 2001; 61(13): 1921–1943.

Virani SN, Ferrare R, Russell AS: Physician resistance to the late whiplash syndrome. *Journal of Rheumatology* 2001; 28(9): 2096–2099.

Winkelstein BA, et al: The cervical facet capsule and its role in whiplash injury. *Spine* 2000; 25(10): 1238–1246.

Chapter 6

Adams M, Dolan P: Spine biomechanics. *Journal of Biomechanics* 2005; 38: 1972–1983.

Anderson MK, Hall SJ, Martin M: *Sports Injury Management*, 2nd ed. Baltimore, Lippincott Williams and Wilkins, 2000.

———, et al: *Foundations of Athletic Training: Prevention, Assessment, and Management*, 3rd ed. Baltimore, Lippincott Williams and Wilkins, 2005.

Cavanaugh J, et al: Lumbar facet pain: biomechanics, neuroanatomy and neurophysiology. *Journal of Biomechanics* 1996; 29(9): 1117–1129.

Chen A, Spivak J: Degenerative lumbar spinal stenosis. *The Physician and Sportsmedicine* 2003; 31(8).

Cibulka MT: Understanding sacroiliac joint movement as a guide to the management of a patient with unilateral low back pain. *Manual Therapy* 2002; 7(4): 215–221.

Clay JH, Pounds DM: *Basic Clinical Massage Therapy: Integrating Anatomy and Treatment.* Baltimore, Lippincott Williams and Wilkins, 2003.

Cook C, et al: Rehabilitation for clinical lumbar instability in a female adolescent competitive diver with spondylolisthesis. *Journal of Manual and Manipulative Therapy* 2004; 12(2): 91–99.

Dickson RA: Spine: spondylolisthesis. *Current Orthopedics* 1998; 12: 273–282.

DonTigny R: Critical analysis of the sequence and extent of the result of the pathological failure of self-bracing of the sacroiliac joint. *Journal of Manual and Manipulative Therapy* 1999; 7: 173–181.

Exelby L: The locked lumbar facet joint: intervention using mobilizations with movement. *Manual Therapy* 2001; 6(2): 116–121.

Ferrara L, et al: A biomechanical assessment of disc pressures in the lumbosacral spine in response to external unloading forces. *Spine Journal* 2005; 5: 548–553.

Frank A: Low back pain. *BMJ* 1993; 306(6882): 901–910.

Gard G, et al: Functional activities and psychosocial factors in the rehabilitation of patients with low back pain. *Scandinavian Journal of Caring Science* 2000; 14: 75–81.

Hoppenfeld S: *Physical Examination of the Spine and Extremities.* Norwalk, Appleton-Century-Crofts, 1976.

Jackson J, Browning R: Impact of national low back pain guidelines on clinical practice. *Southern Medical Journal* 2005; 98(2): 139–143.

Jurch S: *Surface Anatomy: A Therapist's Guide to Palpation.* Charleston, Wellness Education and Research Alliance, 2005.

Laslett M: Diagnosis of sacroiliac joint pain: validity of individual provocation tests and composites of tests. *Manual Therapy* 2005; 10: 207–218.

Liebenson C: The relationship of the sacroiliac joint, stabilization musculature, and lumbo-pelvic instability. *Journal of Bodywork and Movement Therapies* 2004; 8: 43–45.

Lively M, Bailes J: Acute lumbar disk injuries in active patients: making optimal management decisions. *The Physician and Sportsmedicine* 2005; 33(4).

Magee DJ: *Orthopedic Physical Assessment*, 3rd ed. Philadelphia, W.B. Saunders, 1997.

Maluf K, et al: Use of a classification system to guide nonsurgical management of a patient with chronic low back pain. *Physical Therapy* 2000; 80: 1097–1111.

Mattes A: *Active Isolated Stretching: The Mattes Method.* Sarasota, Aaron Mattes, 2000.

McGeary D, et al: Gender-related differences in treatment outcomes for patients with musculoskeletal disorders. *Spine Journal* 2003; 3: 197–203.

McGrath MC: Clinical considerations of sacroiliac joint anatomy: a review of function, motion and pain. *Journal of Osteopathic Medicine* 2004; 7(1): 16–24.

McKinley M, O'Loughlin V: *Human Anatomy.* New York, McGraw-Hill, 2006.

McLain R: Determining treatment of lumbar disk protrusion and disk extrusion. *Journal of Musculoskeletal Medicine* 2005; 22: 21–28.

McNeely M, et al: A systematic review of physiotherapy for spondylolysis and spondylolisthesis. *Manual Therapy* 2003; 8(2): 80–91.

O'Sullivan P: Diagnosis and classification of chronic low back pain disorders: maladaptive movement and motor control impairments as underlying mechanism. *Manual Therapy* 2005; 10(4): 256–269.

Peace S, Fryer G: Methods used by members of the Australian osteopathic profession to assess the sacroiliac joint. *Journal of Osteopathic Medicine* 2004; 7(1): 25–32.

Pool-Goudzwaard A, et al: The iliolumbar ligament: its influence on stability of the sacroiliac joint. *Clinical Biomechanics* 2003; 18: 99–105.

Prather H, Hunt D: Sacroiliac joint pain. *Disease-A-Month* 2004; 50: 670–683.

Prentice WE: *Arnheim's Principles of Athletic Training: A Competency-Based Approach*, 11th ed. New York, McGraw-Hill, 2003.

Riddle D, et al: Evaluation of the presence of sacroiliac joint region dysfunction using a combination of tests: a multicenter intertester reliability study. *Physical Therapy* 2002; 82: 772–781.

Rumball J, et al: Rowing injuries. *Sports Medicine* 2005; 35(6): 537–555.

Saladin KS: *Human Anatomy.* New York, McGraw-Hill, 2005.

Salvo S: *Massage Therapy: Principles and Practice,* 2nd ed. St. Louis, Saunders, 2003.

Saunders HD, Saunders R: *Evaluation, Treatment and Prevention of Musculoskeletal Disorders, Vol. 1: Spine*, 3rd ed. Chaska, Saunders Group, 1993.

Simons DG, Travell JG, Simons LS: *Myofascial Pain and Dysfunction: The Trigger Point Manual, Vol. 1.* Baltimore, Williams and Wilkins, 1999.

Snijders C, et al: The influence of slouching and lumbar support on iliolumbar ligaments, intervertebral discs and sacroiliac joints. *Clinical Biomechanics* 2004; 19: 323–329.

Starkey C, Ryan J: *Evaluation of Orthopedic and Athletic Injuries.* Philadelphia, F.A. Davis, 1996.

Thompson B, et al: Sacroiliac joint dysfunction: introduction and case study. *Journal of Bodywork and Movement Therapy* 2001; 5(4): 229–234.

Travell JG, Simons DG: *Myofascial Pain and Dysfunction: The Trigger Point Manual, Vol. 2.* Baltimore, Williams and Wilkins, 1999.

Verrills P, Vivian D: Interventions in chronic low back pain. *Australian Family Physician* 2004; 33(6): 421–426.

Warren P: Management of a patient with sacroiliac joint dysfunction: a correlation of hip range of motion asymmetry with sitting and standing postural habits. *Journal of Manual and Manipulative Therapy* 2003; 11(3): 153–159.

Wong E: Discuss the part played by facet joint in low back pain syndromes. *Journal of the Hong Kong Physiotherapy Association* 1984; 6: 7–11.

Wong L: Rehabilitation of a patient with a rare multi-level isthmic spondylolisthesis: a case report. *Journal of the Canadian Chiropractic Association* 2004; 48(2): 142–151.

Chapter 7

Albritton M, et al: An anatomic study of the effects on the suprascapular nerve due to retraction of the supraspinatus muscle after a rotator cuff tear. *Journal of Shoulder and Elbow Surgery* 2003; 12(5): 497–500.

Anderson MK, Hall SJ, Martin M: *Sports Injury Management*, 2nd ed. Baltimore, Lippincott Williams and Wilkins, 2000.

————, et al: *Foundations of Athletic Training: Prevention, Assessment, and Management*, 3rd ed. Baltimore, Lippincott Williams and Wilkins, 2005.

Beall D, et al: Association of biceps tendon tears with rotator cuff abnormalities: degree of correlation with tears of the anterior and superior portions of the rotator cuff. *American Journal of Radiology* 2003; 180: 633–639.

Beam JW: Athletic trainer response. *Journal of Bodywork and Movement Therapies* 2000; 4(1): 4–13.

Beltran J, et al: Shoulder: labrum and bicipital tendon. *Topics in Magnetic Resonance Imaging* 2003; 14(1): 35–50.

Bennett WF: Specificity of the Speed's test: arthroscopic technique for evaluating the biceps tendon at the level of the bicipital groove. *Arthroscopy: The Journal of Arthroscopic and Related Surgery* 1998; 14(8): 789–796.

Boyles RE, et al: Manipulation following regional interscalene anesthetic block for shoulder adhesive capsulitis: a case series. *Manual Therapy* 2005; 10: 164–171.

Bunker TD: Frozen shoulder. *Current Orthopedics* 1998; 12: 193–201.

Burke WS, et al: Strengthening the supraspinatus: a clinical and biomechanical review. *Clinical Orthopaedics and Related Research* 2002; 402: 292–298.

Chen CH, et al: Incidence and severity of biceps long-head tendon lesion in patients with complete rotator cuff tears. *Journal of Trauma Injury, Infection, and Critical Care* 2005; 58(6): 1189–1193.

Clarnette RG, et al: Clinical exam of the shoulder. *Medicine and Science in Sports and Exercise* 1998; 30(4): 1–6.

Clay JH, Pounds DM: *Basic Clinical Massage Therapy: Integrating Anatomy and Treatment.* Baltimore, Lippincott Williams and Wilkins, 2003.

Cohen RB, et al: Impingement syndrome and rotator cuff disease as repetitive motion disorders. *Clinical Orthopaedics and Related Research* 1998; 351: 95–101.

Diwan DB, et al: An evaluation of the effects of the extent of capsular release and of postoperative therapy on the temporal outcomes of adhesive capsulitis. *Arthroscopy: The Journal of Arthroscopic and Related Surgery* 2005; 21(9): 1105–1113.

Duckworth DG, et al: Self-assessment questionnaires document substantial variability in the clinical expression of rotator cuff tears. *Journal of Shoulder and Elbow Surgery* 1999; 8(4): 330–333.

Favorito PJ, et al: Complete arthroscopic examination of the long head of the biceps tendon. *Arthroscopy: The Journal of Arthroscopic and Related Surgery* 2001; 17(4): 430–432.

Galatz LM, et al: Delayed repair of tendon to bone injuries leads to decreased biomechanical properties and bone loss. *Journal of Orthopaedic Research* 2005; 23: 1441–1447.

Gerber C, et al: Classification of glenohumeral joint instability. *Clinical Orthopaedics and Related Research* 2002; 400: 65–76.

Halder AM, et al: Dynamic contributions to superior shoulder stability. *Journal of Orthopaedic Research* 2001; 19: 206–212.

Hannafin, JA, et al: Adhesive capsulitis: a treatment approach. *Clinical Orthopaedics and Related Research* 2000; 372: 95–109.

Hashimoto T, et al: Pathologic evidence of degeneration as a primary cause of rotator cuff tear. *Clinical Orthopaedics and Related Research* 2003; 415: 111–120.

Healey JH, et al: Biomechanical evaluation of the origin of the long head of the biceps tendon. *Arthroscopy: The Journal of Arthroscopic and Related Surgery* 2001; 17(4): 378–382.

Heers G, et al: Gliding properties of the long head of the biceps brachii. *Journal of Orthopaedic Research* 2003; 21: 162–166.

Holtby R, et al: Accuracy of the Speed's and Yergason's tests in detecting biceps pathology and SLAP lesions: comparison with arthroscopic findings. *Arthroscopy: The Journal of Arthroscopic and Related Surgery* 2004; 20(3): 231–236.

Hoppenfeld S: *Physical Examination of the Spine and Extremities.* Norwalk, Appleton-Century-Crofts, 1976.

Jett PL, et al: Solving a common shoulder problem. *American Journal of Physical Medicine and Rehabilitation* 2005; 84(8): 648.

Jobe CM: Superior glenoid impingement: current concepts. *Clinical Orthopaedics and Related Research* 1996; 330: 98–107.

Jurch S: *Surface Anatomy: A Therapist's Guide to Palpation.* Charleston, Wellness Education and Research Alliance, 2005.

Kim TK, et al: Internal impingement of the shoulder in flexion. *Clinical Orthopaedics and Related Research* 2004; April: 112–119.

Laska T, et al: Physical therapy for spinal accessory nerve injury complicated by adhesive capsulitis. *Physical Therapy* 2001; 81(3): 936–944.

Levy AS, et al: Function of the long head of the biceps at the shoulder: electromyographic analysis. *Journal of Shoulder and Elbow Surgery* 2001; 10(3): 250–255.

Levy O, et al: Traumatic soft tissue injuries of the shoulder girdle. *Trauma* 2002; 4: 223–235.

Lowe WW: Orthopaedic assessment skills in bodywork care of rotator cuff injury. *Journal of Bodywork and Movement Therapies* 1997; 1(2): 81–86.

Lyons PM, et al: Rotator cuff tendinopathy and subacromial impingement syndrome. *Medicine and Science in Sports and Exercise* 1998; 30(4): 12–17.

Magee DJ: *Orthopedic Physical Assessment,* 3rd ed. Philadelphia, W.B. Saunders, 1997.

Mattes A: *Active Isolated Stretching: The Mattes Method.* Sarasota, Aaron Mattes, 2000.

McKinley M, O'Loughlin V: *Human Anatomy.* New York, McGraw-Hill, 2006.

Mitsch J, et al: Investigation of a consistent pattern of motion restriction in patients with adhesive capsulitis. *Journal of Manual and Manipulative Therapy* 2004; 12(3): 153–159.

Morag Y, et al: MR arthrography of rotator interval, long head of the biceps brachii, and biceps pulley of the shoulder. *Radiology* 2005; 235(1): 21–30.

Onga T, et al: Case report: biceps tendinitis caused by an osteochondroma in the bicipital groove: a rare cause of shoulder pain in a baseball player. *Clinical Orthopaedics and Related Research* 2005; 431: 241–244.

Pagnani MJ, et al: Role of the long head of the biceps brachii in glenohumeral stability: a biomechanical study in cadavera. *Journal of Shoulder and Elbow Surgery* 1996; 5(4): 255–262.

Parentis MA, et al: Disorders of the superior labrum: review and treatment guidelines. *Clinical Orthopaedics and Related Research* 2002; 400: 77–87.

Pearsall AW, et al: Frozen shoulder syndrome: diagnostic and treatment strategies in the primary care setting. *Medicine and Science in Sport and Exercise* 1998; 30(4): 33–39.

Pfahler M, et al: The role of the bicipital groove in tendopathy of the long biceps tendon. *Journal of Shoulder and Elbow Surgery* 1999; 8(5): 419–424.

Prentice WE: *Arnheim's Principles of Athletic Training: A Competency-Based Approach*, 11th ed. New York, McGraw-Hill, 2003.

Richards DP, et al: Relation between adhesive capsulitis and acromial morphology. *Arthroscopy: The Journal of Arthroscopic and Related Surgery* 2004; 20(6): 614–619.

Rundquist PJ, et al: Shoulder kinematics in subjects with frozen shoulder. *Archives of Physical Medicine and Rehabilitation* 2003; 84: 1473–1479.

————: Patterns of motion loss in subjects with idiopathic loss of shoulder range of motion. *Clinical Biomechanics* 2004; 19: 810–818.

Saladin KS: *Human Anatomy*. New York, McGraw-Hill, 2005.

Salvo S: *Massage Therapy: Principles and Practice,* 2nd ed. St. Louis, Saunders, 2003.

Simons DG, Travell JG, Simons LS: *Myofascial Pain and Dysfunction: The Trigger Point Manual, Vol. 1*. Baltimore, Williams and Wilkins, 1999.

Sizer PS, et al: Diagnosis and management of the painful shoulder, part 2: examination, interpretation, and management. *Pain Practice* 2003; 3(2): 152–185.

Smith SP, et al: The association between frozen shoulder and Dupuytren's disease. *Journal of Shoulder and Elbow Surgery* 2001; 10(2): 149–151.

Starkey C, Ryan J: *Evaluation of Orthopedic and Athletic Injuries*. Philadelphia, F.A. Davis, 1996.

Trojian T, et al: What can we expect from nonoperative treatment options for shoulder pain? *Journal of Family Practice* 2005; 54(3): 216–223.

Tuoheti Y, et al: Attachment types of the long head of the biceps tendon to the glenoid labrum and their relationships with the glenohumeral ligaments. *Arthroscopy: The Journal of Arthroscopic and Related Surgery* 2005; 21(10): 1242–1249.

Tytherleigh-Strong G, et al: Rotator cuff disease. *Current Opinion in Rheumatology* 2001; 13: 135–145.

Wiffen F: What role does the sympathetic nervous system play in the development or ongoing pain of adhesive capsulitis? *Journal of Manual and Manipulative Therapy* 2002; 10(1): 17–23.

Wilson C: Rotator cuff versus cervical spine: making the diagnosis. *Nurse Practitioner* 2005; 30(5): 45–50.

Woodward TW, et al: The painful shoulder, part I: clinical evaluation. *American Family Physician* 2000; 61(10): 3079–3088.

————: The painful shoulder, part II: acute and chronic disorders. *American Family Physician* 2000; 61(11): 3291–3300.

Yamaguchi K, et al: Biceps activity during shoulder motion. *Clinical Orthopaedics and Related Research* 1997; 336: 122–129.

Chapter 8

Ahn D-S: Hand elevation: a new test for carpal tunnel syndrome. *Annals of Plastic Surgery* 2001; 46: 120–124.

Anderson J: Carpal tunnel syndrome: common ailment, many treatments. *Journal of Controversial Medical Claims* 2005; 12(3): 7–14.

Anderson MK, Hall SJ, Martin M: *Sports Injury Management*, 2nd ed. Baltimore, Lippincott Williams and Wilkins, 2000.

————, et al: *Foundations of Athletic Training: Prevention, Assessment, and Management*, 3rd ed. Baltimore, Lippincott Williams and Wilkins, 2005.

Bland J: Carpal tunnel syndrome. *Current Opinion in Neurology* 2005; 18: 581–585.

Chumbley EM, et al: Evaluation of overuse elbow injuries. *American Family Physician* 2000; 61(3): 691–700.

Clay JH, Pounds DM: *Basic Clinical Massage Therapy: Integrating Anatomy and Treatment*. Baltimore, Lippincott Williams and Wilkins, 2003.

Daniels J, et al: Hand and wrist injuries, part I: nonemergent evaluation. *American Family Physician* 2004; 69(8): 1941–1948.

Davis E, et al: The Tinel sign: a historical perspective. *Plastic and Reconstructive Surgery* 2004; 114(2): 494–499.

Fairbank SM, et al: The role of the extensor digitorum communis muscle in lateral epicondylitis. *Journal of Hand Surgery* 2002; 27B(5): 405–409.

Feinberg E: Nerve entrapment syndromes about the elbow. *Topics in Clinical Chiropractic* 1999; 6(4): 20–32.

Field L, et al: Common elbow injuries in sport. *Sports Medicine* 1998; 26(3): 193–205.

Field T, et al: Carpal tunnel syndrome symptoms are lessened following massage therapy. *Journal of Bodywork and Movement Therapies* 2004; 8: 9–14.

Gabel, G: Acute and chronic tendinopathies at the elbow. *Current Opinion in Rheumatology* 1999; 11(2): 138–148.

Holm G, et al: Carpal tunnel syndrome: current theory, treatment, and the use of B6. *Journal of the American Academy of Nurse Practitioners* 2003; 15(1): 18–22.

Hong, QN, et al: Treatment of lateral epicondylitis: where is the evidence? *Joint Bone Spine* 2004; 71: 369–373.

Hoppenfeld S: *Physical Examination of the Spine and Extremities*. Norwalk, Appleton-Century-Crofts, 1976.

Ingram-Rice B: Carpal tunnel syndrome: more than a wrist problem. *Journal of Bodywork and Movement Therapies* 1997; 1(3): 155–162.

Jurch S: *Surface Anatomy: A Therapist's Guide to Palpation*. Charleston, Wellness Education and Research Alliance, 2005.

Kuhlman K, et al: Sensitivity and specificity of carpal tunnel syndrome signs. *American Journal of Physical Medicine and Rehabilitation* 1997; 76(6): 451–457.

Love C: Carpal tunnel syndrome. *Journal of Orthopaedic Nursing* 2003; 7: 33–42.

Magee DJ: *Orthopedic Physical Assessment*, 3rd ed. Philadelphia, W.B. Saunders, 1997.

Marx RG, et al: The reliability of physical examination for carpal tunnel syndrome. *Journal of Hand Surgery* 1998; 23B(4): 499–502.

Mattes A: *Active Isolated Stretching: The Mattes Method*. Sarasota, Aaron Mattes, 2000.

McKinley M, O'Loughlin V: *Human Anatomy*. New York, McGraw-Hill, 2006.

Moore S: De Quervain's tenosynovitis: stenosing tenosynovitis of the first dorsal compartment. *Journal of Occupational and Environmental Medicine* 1997; 39(10): 990–1002.

Piza-Katzer H: Carpal tunnel syndrome: diagnosis and treatment. *European Surgery* 2003; 35(4): 196–201.

Prentice WE: *Arnheim's Principles of Athletic Training: A Competency-Based Approach*, 11th ed. New York, McGraw-Hill, 2003.

Rettig AC: Elbow, forearm and wrist injuries in the athlete. *Sports Medicine* 1998; 25(2): 115–130.

Saladin KS: *Human Anatomy*. New York, McGraw-Hill, 2005.

Salvo S: *Massage Therapy, Principles and Practice*, 2nd ed. St. Louis, Saunders, 2003.

Schoen DC: Injuries of the wrist. *Orthopaedic Nursing* 2005; 24(4): 304–307.

Seivier TL, et al: Treating lateral epicondylitis. *Sports Medicine* 1999; 28(5): 375–380.

Simons DG, Travell JG, Simons LS: *Myofascial Pain and Dysfunction: The Trigger Point Manual, Vol. 1*. Baltimore, Williams and Wilkins, 1999.

Starkey C, Ryan J: *Evaluation of Orthopedic and Athletic Injuries*. Philadelphia, F.A. Davis, 1996.

Stasinopoulos D: Cyriax physiotherapy for tennis elbow/ lateral epicondylitis. *British Journal of Sports Medicine* 2004; 38: 675–677.

———, et al: 'Lateral elbow tendinopathy' is the most appropriate diagnostic term for the condition commonly referred to as lateral epicondylitis. *Medical Hypotheses* 2006; 67(6): 1400–1402.

Viera AJ: Management of carpal tunnel syndrome. *American Family Physician* 2003; 68(2): 265–272.

Watts AC, et al: Carpal tunnel syndrome in men. *Current Orthopaedics* 2006; 20(4): 294–298.

Wilson JK, et al: A review of treatment for carpal tunnel syndrome. *Disability and Rehabilitation* 2003; 25(3): 113–119.

Zepf B: Computer use and carpal tunnel syndrome. *American Family Physician* 2004; 69(3): 643–647.

Chapter 9

Adkins SB, et al: Hip pain in athletes. *American Family Physician* 2000; 61(7): 2109–2018.

Amis AA, et al: Anatomy and biomechanics of the medial patellofemoral ligament. *The Knee* 2003; 10: 215–220.

Anderson MK, Hall SJ, Martin M: *Sports Injury Management*, 2nd ed. Baltimore, Lippincott Williams and Wilkins, 2000.

———, et al: *Foundations of Athletic Training: Prevention, Assessment, and Management*, 3rd ed. Baltimore, Lippincott Williams and Wilkins, 2005.

Arendt E: Anatomy and malalignment of the patellofemoral joint. *Clinical Orthopaedics and Related Research* 2005; 436: 71–75.

Beatty R: The piriformis muscle syndrome: a simple diagnostic maneuver. *Neurosurgery* 1994; 34(3): 512–514.

Bellemans J: Biomechanics of anterior knee pain. *The Knee* 2003; 10: 123–126.

Benzon H, et al: Piriformis syndrome. *Anesthesiology* 2003; 98: 1442–1448.

Birrell F, et al: Defining hip pain for population studies. *Annals of the Rheumatic Diseases* 2005; 64: 95–98.

Byrd JWT: Piriformis syndrome. *Operative Techniques in Sports Medicine* 2005; 13: 71–79.

Donell S: Patellofemoral dysfunction–extensor mechanism malalignment. *Current Orthopaedics* 2006; 20: 103–111.

Dye S: The pathophysiology of patellofemoral pain. *Clinical Orthopaedics and Related Research* 2005; 436: 100–110.

Farahmand F, et al: The contribution of the medial retinaculum and quadriceps muscles to patellar lateral stability—an in-vitro study. *The Knee* 2004; 11: 89–94.

Farrell K, et al: Force and repetition in cycling: possible implications for iliotibial band friction syndrome. *The Knee* 2003; 10: 103–109.

Fredericson M, et al: Quantitative analysis of the relative effectiveness of 3 iliotibial band stretches. *Archives of Physical Medicine and Rehabilitation* 2002; 83: 589–592.

———: Iliotibial band syndrome in runners. *Sports Medicine* 2005; 35(5): 451–459.

———: Physical examination and patellofemoral pain syndrome. *American Journal of Physical Medicine and Rehabilitation* 2006; 85: 234–243.

Gajdosik R, et al: Influence of knee positions and gender on the Ober test for length of the iliotibial band. *Clinical Biomechanics* 2003; 18: 77–79.

Gerbino P, et al: Patellofemoral pain syndrome. *Clinical Journal of Pain* 2006; 22: 154–159.

Green ST: Patellofemoral syndrome. *Journal of Bodywork and Movement Therapies* 2005; 9: 16–26.

Grelsamer R, et al: The biomechanics of the patellofemoral joint. *Journal of Orthopaedic and Sports Physical Therapy* 1998; 28(5): 286–298.

Hamilton B, et al: Patellar tendinosis as an adaptive process: a new hypothesis. *British Journal of Sports Medicine* 2004; 38: 758–761.

Hansen P, et al: Mechanical properties of the human patellar tendon, in vivo. *Clinical Biomechanics* 2006; 21: 54–58.

Herrington L, et al: Q-angle undervalued? The relationship between q-angle and medio-lateral position of the patella. *Clinical Biomechanics* 2004; 19: 1070–1073.

———: The relationship between patella position and length of the iliotibial band as assessed using Ober's test. *Manual Therapy* 2006; 11: 182–186.

Holmes SW, et al: Clinical classification of patellofemoral pain and dysfunction. *Journal of Orthopaedic and Sports Physical Therapy* 1998; 28(5): 299–306.

Hoppenfeld S: *Physical Examination of the Spine and Extremities.* Norwalk, Appleton-Century-Crofts, 1976.

Jurch S: *Surface Anatomy: A Therapist's Guide to Palpation.* Charleston, Wellness Education and Research Alliance, 2005.

Katchburian MV, et al: Measurement of patellar tracking: assessment and analysis of the literature. *Clinical Orthopaedics and Related Research* 2003; 412: 241–259.

Kaufmann P, et al: New insights into the soft-tissue anatomy anterior to the patella. *Lancet* 2004; 363: 586.

Khaund R, et al: Iliotibial band syndrome: a common source of knee pain. *American Family Physician* 2005; 71(8): 1545–1550.

Lee EY, et al: MRI of piriformis syndrome. *American Journal of Roentgenology* 2004; 183: 63–64.

Livingston L: The quadriceps angle: a review of the literature. *Journal of Orthopaedic and Sports Physical Therapy* 1998; 28(2): 105–109.

———, et al: Bilateral Q angle asymmetry and anterior knee pain syndrome. *Clinical Biomechanics* 1999; 14: 7–13.

Magee DJ: *Orthopedic Physical Assessment,* 3rd ed. Philadelphia, W.B. Saunders, 1997.

Mattes A: *Active Isolated Stretching: The Mattes Method.* Sarasota, Aaron Mattes, 2000.

McCrory P, et al: Nerve entrapment syndromes as a cause of pain in the hip, groin, and buttock. *Sports Medicine* 1999; 27(4): 261–274.

McKinley M, O'Loughlin V: *Human Anatomy.* New York, McGraw-Hill, 2006.

Nemeth W, et al: The lateral synovial recess of the knee: anatomy and role in chronic iliotibial band friction syndrome. *Arthroscopy: The Journal of Arthoscopy and Related Surgery* 1996; 12(5): 574–580.

Nicholls RA: Intra-articular disorders of the hip in athletes. *Physical Therapy in Sport* 2004; 5: 17–25.

Paluska SA: An overview of hip injuries in running. *Sports Medicine* 2005; 35(11): 991–1014.

Pedowitz RN: Use of osteopathic manipulative treatment of iliotibial band friction syndrome. *Journal of the American Osteopathic Association* 2005; 105(12): 563–567.

Prentice WE: *Arnheim's Principles of Athletic Training: A Competency-Based Approach,* 11th ed. New York, McGraw-Hill, 2003.

Saladin KS: *Human Anatomy.* New York, McGraw-Hill, 2005.

Salvo S: *Massage Therapy: Principles and Practice,* 2nd ed. St. Louis, Saunders, 2003.

Simons DG, Travell JG, Simons LS: *Myofascial Pain and Dysfunction: The Trigger Point Manual, Vol. 2.* Baltimore, Williams and Wilkins, 1999.

Starkey C, Ryan J: *Evaluation of Orthopedic and Athletic Injuries.* Philadelphia, F.A. Davis, 1996.

Wilson T, et al: Is the Q-angle an absolute or a variable measure? *Physiotherapy* 2002; 88(5): 296–302.

Chapter 10

Alfredson A, et al: Chronic Achilles tendinosis: recommendations for treatment and prevention. *Sports Medicine* 2000; 29(2): 135–146.

Allen MJ, et al: Exercise pain in the lower leg: chronic compartment syndrome and medial tibial syndrome. *Journal of Bone and Joint Surgery* 1986; 68B(5): 818–823.

Anderson MK, Hall SJ, Martin M: *Sports Injury Management,* 2nd ed. Baltimore, Lippincott Williams and Wilkins, 2000.

———, et al: *Foundations of Athletic Training: Prevention, Assessment, and Management,* 3rd ed. Baltimore, Lippincott Williams and Wilkins, 2005.

Astrom M, et al: Chronic Achilles tendinopathy: a survey of surgical and histopathologic findings. *Clinical Orthopaedics and Related Research* 1995; 316: 151–164.

Barrett SJ, et al: Plantar fasciitis and other causes of heel pain. *American Family Physician* 1999; 59(8): 2200–2206.

Bolgla LA, et al: Plantar fasciitis and the windlass mechanism: a biomechanical link to clinical practice. *Journal of Athletic Training* 2004; 39(1): 77–82.

Cook JL, et al: Achilles tendinopathy. *Manual Therapy* 2002; 7(3): 121–130.

Donatelli RA: *The Biomechanics of the Foot and Ankle,* 2nd ed. Philadelphia, F.A.Davis, 1996.

Dyck DD, et al: Plantar fasciitis. *Clinical Journal of Sports Medicine* 2004; 14(5): 305–309.

Finch PM: Chronic shin splints: a review of the deep posterior compartment. *The Foot* 1998; 8: 119–124.

Hoppenfeld S: *Physical Examination of the Spine and Extremities.* Norwalk, Appleton-Century-Crofts, 1976.

Jarvinen T, et al: Achilles tendon injuries. *Current Opinion in Rheumatology* 2001; 13: 150–155.

Jerosch J, et al: Results of surgical treatment of tarsal tunnel syndrome. *Foot and Ankle Surgery* 2006; 12: 205–208.

Juliano PJ, et al: Plantar fasciitis, entrapment neuropathies, and tarsal tunnel syndrome: current up to date treatment. *Current Opinion in Orthopaedics* 2004; 15: 49–54.

Jurch S: *Surface Anatomy: A Therapist's Guide to Palpation.* Charleston, Wellness Education and Research Alliance, 2005.

Kortebein PM, et al: Medial tibial stress syndrome. *Medicine and Science in Sports and Exercise* 2000; 32(2): S27–33.

Magee DJ: *Orthopedic Physical Assessment*, 3rd ed. Philadelphia, W.B. Saunders, 1997.

Mattes A: *Active Isolated Stretching: The Mattes Method.* Sarasota, Aaron Mattes, 2000.

Mazzone MF, et al: Common conditions of the Achilles tendon. *American Family Physician* 2002; 65(9): 1805–1810.

McBryde AM, et al: Injuries to the foot and ankle in athletes. *Southern Medical Journal* 2004; 97(8): 738–741.

McKinley M, O'Loughlin V: *Human Anatomy.* New York, McGraw-Hill, 2006.

Norkus SA, et al: The anatomy and mechanics of syndesmotic ankle sprains. *Journal of Athletic Training* 2001; 36(1): 68–73.

Persich G, et al: Tarsal tunnel syndrome. *EMedicine from Web MD,* www.emedicine.com/orthoped/topic565.htm (12/24/2006).

Prentice WE: *Arnheim's Principles of Athletic Training: A Competency-Based Approach*, 11th ed. New York, McGraw-Hill, 2003.

Read HK: Shin splints. *The Foot* 1996; 6: 82–85.

Roxas M: Plantar fasciitis: diagnosis and therapeutic considerations. *Alternative Medicine Review* 2005; 10(2): 83–93.

Saladin KS: *Human Anatomy.* New York, McGraw-Hill, 2005.

Salvo S: *Massage Therapy: Principles and Practice,* 2nd ed. St. Louis, Saunders, 2003.

Simons DG, Travell JG, Simons LS: *Myofascial Pain and Dysfunction: The Trigger Point Manual, Vol. 2.* Baltimore, Williams and Wilkins, 1999.

Singh SK, et al: The surgical treatment of tarsal tunnel syndrome. *The Foot* 2005; 15: 212–216.

Starkey C, Ryan J: *Evaluation of Orthopedic and Athletic Injuries.* Philadelphia, F.A. Davis, 1996.

Thacker SB, et al: The prevention of shin splints in sports: a systematic review of literature. *Medicine and Science in Sports and Exercise* 2002; 34(1): 32–40.

Turan I, et al: Tarsal tunnel syndrome. *Clinical Orthopaedics and Related Research* 1997; 343: 151–156.

Witt P: Neuromuscular perspective. *Journal of Bodywork and Movement Therapies* 2001; 5(1): 36–45.

Young CC, et al: Treatment of plantar fasciitis. *American Family Physician* 2001; 63(3): 467–474.

Chapter 11

Anderson MK, Hall SJ, Martin M: *Sports Injury Management*, 2nd ed. Baltimore, Lippincott Williams and Wilkins, 2000.

———, et al: *Foundations of Athletic Training: Prevention, Assessment, and Management*, 3rd ed. Baltimore, Lippincott Williams and Wilkins, 2005.

Bell SJ, et al: Chronic lateral ankle instability: the Brostrom procedure. *Operative Techniques in Sports Medicine* 2005; 13: 176–182.

Franco J: Adolescent patellar tendinosis: operative treatment. Unpublished article 2006.

Friel K, et al: Ipsilateral hip abductor weakness after inversion ankle sprain. *Journal of Athletic Training* 2006; 41(1): 74–78.

Hinman MR: Comparison of thoracic kyphosis and postural stiffness in younger and older women. *Spine Journal* 2004; 4: 413–417.

Hoppenfeld S: *Physical Examination of the Spine and Extremities.* Norwalk, Appleton-Century-Crofts, 1976.

Hunt GC: Injuries of peripheral nerves of the leg, foot and ankle: an often unrecognized consequence of ankle sprains. *The Foot* 2003; 13: 14–18.

Kendall FP, et al: *Muscles: Testing and Function with Posture and Pain.* Baltimore, Lippincott Williams and Wilkins, 2005.

Liu SH, et al: Ankle sprains and other soft tissue injuries. *Current Opinion in Rheumatology* 1999; 11:132–137.

Lowe W: *Functional Assessment in Massage Therapy*, 3rd ed. Bend, OMERI, 1997.

———: *Orthopedic Massage: Theory and Technique.* New York, Mosby, 2003.

Macagno AE, et al: Thoracic and thoracolumbar kyphosis in adults. *Spine* 2006; 31(19): S161–170.

Magee DJ: *Orthopedic Physical Assessment*, 3rd ed. Philadelphia, W.B. Saunders, 1997.

Mangwani J, et al: Chronic lateral ankle instability: review of anatomy, biomechanics, pathology, diagnosis and treatment. *The Foot* 2001; 11: 76–84.

McKinley M, O'Loughlin V: *Human Anatomy.* New York, McGraw-Hill, 2006.

Otter SJ: The conservative management of lateral ankle sprains in the athlete. *The Foot* 1999; 9: 12–17.

Page P: Sensorimotor training: a "global" approach for balance training. *Journal of Bodywork and Movement Therapies* 2005; 10(1): 77–84.

Prentice WE: *Arnheim's Principles of Athletic Training: A Competency-Based Approach*, 11th ed. New York, McGraw-Hill, 2003.

Safran MR, et al: Lateral ankle sprains: a comprehensive review, part 1: etiology, pathoanatomy, histopathogenesis, and diagnosis. *Medicine and Science in Sports and Exercise* 1999; 31(7): S429–437.

Saladin KS: *Human Anatomy.* New York, McGraw-Hill, 2005.

Schoen DC: Upper extremity nerve entrapments. *Orthopaedic Nursing* 2002; 21(2): 15–33.

Scopp JM, et al: Osteochondral injury of the knee. *Hospital Physician* 2005; 2(3): 2–12.

Smith TO, et al: The physiotherapy management of muscle haematomas. *Physical Therapy in Sport* 2006; 7: 201–209.

Starkey C, Ryan J: *Evaluation of Orthopedic and Athletic Injuries.* Philadelphia, F.A. Davis, 1996.

Wolfe MW, et al: Management of ankle sprains. *American Family Physician* 2001; 63(1): 93–104.

Wright IC, et al: The effects of ankle compliance and flexibility on ankle sprains. *Medicine and Science in Sports and Exercise* 2000; 32(3): 260–265.

———: The influence of foot positioning on ankle sprains. *Journal of Biomechanics* 2000; 33: 513–519.

Glossary

Absolute contraindication A condition that would require the clearance of a physician or prohibit treatment altogether.

Acetabulum The point at which the three bones of the pelvis (ilium, ischium, and pubis) fuse. It forms the pelvic portion of the hip joint and articulates with the head of the femur.

Achilles tendonitis An inflammation of the Achilles tendon that typically arises from overuse. It is characterized by pain and inflammation over the tendon.

Acromegaly A hormonal disorder that results when the pituitary gland produces excess growth hormone.

Actin A globular structural protein that polymerizes in a helical fashion to form an actin filament that is, among its other functions, involved in muscle contraction.

Active myofascial trigger point A point that generally causes complaint. It is tender, restricts range of motion, inhibits muscle strength, re-creates pain on compression, produces a local twitch response, and refers to a general reference zone.

Active range of motion Motion performed by the client with no help from the therapist.

Acute injury An injury caused by a single force.

Adhesion A localized buildup of connective tissue within the muscle fibers that binds it together and restricts motion.

Adhesive capsulitis An insidious condition that begins with pain and progresses to a loss of motion in all planes.

Agonist A muscle that provides the desired movement.

Amalgam therapy methods Techniques that combine both energy system treatment and hands-on methods of treatment.

Angle of inclination The angle of the head of the femur in the socket. It is approximately 125° in the frontal plane, allowing the femur to angle downward medially, which brings the knees closer together to provide a better base of support.

Anisotropic Able to resist force better from one direction than another.

Antagonist A muscle that performs the motion opposite that of the agonist.

Antalgic gait A posture or gait that is assumed in order to avoid or lessen pain.

Anteversion An excessive internal rotation of the shaft of the femur in relation to the neck.

Attachment trigger point A trigger point that lies at the musculotendinous junction and is caused by the tension characteristic of the taut band produced by the central point.

Attrition tendonosis A pathology of the biceps tendon caused by a narrow bicipital groove and resulting in irritation of the extracapsular portion of the tendon.

Auscultation The act of listening to the internal sounds of the body, usually using a stethoscope.

Axonotmesis A nerve injury that disrupts the axon and myelin sheath but leaves the connective tissue covering, the epineurium, intact.

Backward thinking The process of formulating and testing a hypothesis to obtain information.

Bending The result of the combination of compression and tension that is applied perpendicular to the long axis. The side of the structure where the force is applied is compressed, while the opposite side is loaded under tension.

Biceps brachii tendonosis A pathology of the biceps brachii caused by various factors.

Bindegewebsmassage A type of connective tissue massage discovered and developed by German physiotherapist Elizabeth Dicke.

Body mechanics The proper use of postural techniques to deliver massage therapy with the highest level of efficiency while causing the least amount of strain to the practitioner.

Bruxism Clinching or grinding of the teeth.

Bursae Fluid-filled sacs located under muscles, tendons, ligaments, and other structures that are exposed to friction. They serve to reduce friction between surfaces and allow for smooth motion.

Camel sign A condition that stems from patella alta, which causes the infrapatellar fat pad to become more evident, creating the appearance of a double hump.

Capsular pattern A proportional motion restriction that is unique to every joint that indicates irritation of the entire joint.

Carpal tunnel syndrome A type of nerve entrapment injury that is brought on by increased pressure in the carpal tunnel. This can arise from two causes: a decrease in available space or an increase in the size of the tendons and other structures that pass through the tunnel. Symptoms include pain, numbness, and tingling along the median nerve distribution.

Carrying angle The angle that is formed by the long axis of the humerus and the long axis of the ulna.

Caudal A directional term referring toward the tail or away from the head.

Central myofascial trigger point A point located near the center of the muscle belly and is associated with a dysfunctional motor end plate.

Chondromalacia patella A condition that is the result of prolonged exposure to excessive compressive forces or abnormal shear forces due to patellar mistracking. These forces result in a softening and degeneration of the articular cartilage of the patella.

Chondropenia The loss of cartilage volume.

Chronic injury An injury caused by a repetitive load placed on an area.

Clinical massage The treatment of musculoskeletal conditions using a framework based on information gathered through an advanced knowledge of anatomy, proficient palpation skills, competent assessment ability, a thorough history, and visual observation.

Clinical reasoning The process of taking separate details of the subject, analyzing and evaluating the information, and organizing it into usable patterns that can be applied to the treatment.

Collagenous fiber Connective tissue fiber that is made of collagen and is extremely strong and resists stretching.

Colle's fracture A fracture of the distal radius with displacement.

Compression A force directed along the long axis of a structure that squeezes the structure together.

Concentric A contraction that occurs when the two ends of the muscle move closer together and shorten during the contraction. The angle at the joint is decreased during this type of contraction.

Congenital muscular torticollis A painless condition, usually presenting during infancy, in which a tight sternocleidomastoid muscle causes the child's head to be tilted to the tightened side.

Congenital spondylolysis A type of defect that occurs when there is a predisposed weakness in the pars interarticularis.

Connective tissue Any type of biologic tissue with an extensive extracellular matrix; often serves to support, bind together, and protect organs.

Connective tissue therapy A general system of connective tissue massage that was developed by Pete Whitridge. The focus of this work is to change the consistency of the connective tissue matrix and redistribute the fascia to its original position, creating more space in the tissue.

Continuity The flow of the strokes and the transition from one stroke to the next.

Contraction knots Knots that are formed as a result of localized contracted sarcomeres. The more sarcomeres involved, the larger the knot.

Contraindication A condition or factor that increases the risk involved in performing a certain treatment or engaging in a particular activity.

Contralateral Referring to an occurrence or a body part on the opposite side of the body.

Contranutation Anterior rotation of the ilium on the sacrum.

Convergence projection theory The theory that each sensory neuron has multiple branches. When pain arises in unexpected areas of the body, it sensitizes some of the other branches and the pain is projected to those other areas.

Cranial A directional term referring toward the head.

Cubital valgus A carrying angle that is greater than 15°.

Cubital varus A carrying angle that is less than 5°.

Cytokines Cell messengers that control fibroblast activity.

Delto-pectoral interval The natural separation that is present between the anterior deltoid and the pectoralis major.

Dense connective tissue Tissue that has a higher ratio of fibers to ground substance. It is categorized as regular and irregular.

Depth The distance traveled into the body's tissue. This stroke element is controlled by the client.

de Quervain's tenosynovitis An inflammation of the tendon on the side of the wrist at the base of the thumb, specifically the extensor pollicis longus, which lies in the 1st dorsal compartment of the wrist.

Dermatome The area of skin innervated by a single nerve root.

Developmental spondylolysis A type of defect that occurs as the result of a fracture in the pars due to continued micro-traumas, which weaken the structure. These micro-traumas can occur from a variety of sources, including postural conditions, various activities, and repetitive movement patterns.

Disk extrusion A condition in which the annulus is perforated and the nucleus material moves into the epidural space.

Disk prolapse A condition in which the annulus is not ruptured but its outermost fibers contain the nucleus.

Disk protrusion A condition in which the disk protrudes in a posterior direction but does not rupture the annulus.

Double-crush syndrome A diagnosis of a compressed or trapped nerve in one area and a second entrapment in another location, with both entrapments contributing to symptoms.

Dupuytren's disease A deforming condition of the hand caused by the contracture of the palmar fascia and resulting in one or more fingers, usually the ring finger and little finger, contracting toward the palm, often leading to functional disability.

Duration The length of time spent massaging a certain area.

Dystonia A generic term used to describe a neurologic movement disorder involving involuntary, sustained muscle contractions.

Eccentric A contraction that generates more force on the muscle than does a concentric contraction and lengthens the muscle as it is contracting. An outside force is acting on the muscle that is greater than the stimulus to contract, so lengthening takes place.

Effleurage The most widely used stroke in massage therapy. It has several uses, including applying lubricant, warming up the tissue, and assessing the condition of the tissue. Also known as *gliding stroke*.

Elastic region A region of tissue that, after being subjected to a force, will return to its original shape once the force is removed.

Elastin fiber A connective tissue fiber, made of a protein called *elastin*, that is thinner and more flexible than collagen fibers; it recoils like an elastic band.

Emollient A substance that softens the skin.

Energy therapy methods Techniques that utilize the energy systems of the body to treat dysfunction.

Ergonomics The scientific study of the relationship of anatomy and physiology to the work of humans.

Essential pain zone A region of referred pain produced by an active trigger point.

Excursion The distance traveled over the body in one stroke.

Exudate Any fluid that filters from the circulatory system into areas of inflammation. Its composition varies but generally includes water and the dissolved solutes of the blood, some or all plasma proteins, white blood cells, platelets, and red blood cells.

Facet joint syndrome Low-back pain that is caused by a dysfunction in the facet joints of the spine.

Fibroblasts Large, flat cells that produce the fibers and ground substance that form the matrix of the tissue.

Fibrocartilage Cartilage that is located between the bones and provides cushioning against compressive forces.

Fick angle The angle that is created by the foot and the sagittal axis of the body. It measures how much the foot toes out (increased angle) or toes in (decreased angle). The normal range is 12° to 18°.

Flat palpation Technique in which the fingertip is used to locate a taut band along the length of the muscle.

Flexibility The ability of a joint to move through a normal range of motion without creating an excessive amount of stress to the muscle-tendon unit.

FOOSH (fall-on-an-outstretched-hand) injury An injury in which the client lands on a forward-flexed outstretched arm or the point of the elbow, which subsequently drives the humerus up into the underside of the acromion.

Force A push or a pull that acts on the body.

Forward thinking The process of recognizing patterns without the need for hypothesis testing.

Friction The most specific Swedish stroke. The skin is secured and the tissue underneath is moved in various directions depending on the intent. It is typically used around joints, bony areas, and specific restrictions within the muscles.

Frog-eyed patella A misalignment of the patellas in which they are oriented as if they were looking away from each other even though the feet are pointed straight ahead.

Front stance A stance used when motion along a client's body is required. Feet are parallel to the table in the direction of motion and at least shoulder width apart.

Functional leg-length discrepancy Leg shortening that is typically a result of a compensation for a posture, such as scoliosis or unilateral foot pronation.

Gait cycle The sequence of motions that occur between two initial contacts of the same foot.

Ganglion cysts Localized fluid-filled sacs that often appear on or around joints and tendons in the hand.

Gate theory The theory that pain signals carried by small-diameter nerves are blocked through the overstimulation of large-diameter nerves, which carry sensory or nonpain signals.

Genu recurvatum The postural condition of hyperextension of the knee.

Genu valgum ("knock-knees") A condition in which the knees angle in toward each other when standing. This places a great amount of stress on the medial structures of the knee.

Genu varus ("bowlegged") A condition in which there is an outward bowing of the knees when standing. This places a great amount of stress on the lateral structures of the knee.

Golgi tendon organ A receptor located in the tendon that monitors the force of a contraction.

Ground substance The amorphous extracellular material in which the cells and fibers of connective tissue are embedded. Also referred to as *extracellular matrix*.

Gunstock deformity An exaggerated cubital varus that occurs as a result of trauma to the distal humerus.

Hyaline cartilage Cartilage that covers the ends of bones and provides a smooth articular surface.

Hyperesthesia An increase in sensation.

Hypoesthesia A reduction in sensation.

Hypovascular zone The portion of the supraspinatus tendon that corresponds to the most common site of rotator cuff injuries.

Idiopathic Relating to a pathology for which a recognized cause has not yet been established.

Iliotibial band friction syndrome (ITBFS) A common overuse injury caused by excessive friction between the distal iliotibial band and the lateral condyle of the femur, resulting in inflammation and pain.

Impingement tendonosis A pathology of the biceps tendon in which the intracapsular portion of the tendon is compressed against various structures.

Integrated hypothesis The theory that a central myofascial trigger point consists of several muscle fibers that are demonstrating regional sarcomere shortening due to an excessive and uninterrupted release of acetylcholine through a positive feedback loop.

Intention The desired outcome of the stroke application.

Ipsilateral Referring to the same side of the body.

Ischemia A restriction in blood supply, generally due to factors in the blood vessels, with resultant damage or dysfunction of tissue.

Isometric A contraction during which no movement takes place at the joint. The force of the muscle contraction equals the outside force.

Keystone The central, wedge-shaped stone of an arch that locks its parts together.

Kinesis Myofascial Integration A method of connective tissue treatment that was developed by Thomas Myers. This approach is based on structural relationships in the body's fascia and examines global patterns known as *anatomy trains*.

Kinetic chain The relationship among body parts and the effect of one body part on another.

Kyphosis An increase in the normal thoracic curve.

Labrum A U-shaped fibrocartilaginous structure that lies around the edge of the acetabulum, contributing to additional stability by deepening the socket of the joint.

Latent myofascial trigger point A point that demonstrates the same characteristics as an active point but exhibits pain and other symptoms only when palpated.

Lateral epicondylitis A condition considered to be a cumulative trauma injury that occurs over time from repeated use of the muscles of the arm and forearm that leads to small tears of the tendons.

Law of Facilitation Principle which states that when an impulse passes through a specific set of neurons to the exclusion of others, it generally takes the same course on a future occasion; each time it traverses this path, resistance is less.

Ligamentum teres A small ligament that runs from the femoral head to the acetabulum. It does not add stability to the joint but contains a small artery that supplies the head of the femur.

Local contraindication A condition that will require modification or adaptation of techniques in the area.

Local twitch response A contraction of localized muscle fibers in a taut band around a trigger point, in response to stimulation of that trigger point.

Loose connective tissue Tissue that has a higher ratio of ground substance to fibers. It contains all the different types of fibers and is categorized into areolar, reticular, and adipose tissue.

Lordosis An exaggeration of either of the two secondary curves in the spine that are located in the lumbar and cervical regions.

Lower-crossed syndrome A postural dysfunction that involves the lumbar spine, hips, and pelvis; it follows the pattern of imbalance between postural and phasic muscles and is often accompanied by an anteriorly tilted pelvis.

Lubricant A substance that allows minimal to unhindered glide over a client's body.

Lumbago A nonspecific diagnosis used to refer to the symptom of low-back pain.

Malocclusion The misalignment of teeth and or incorrect relation between the teeth of the two dental arches.

Manipulative therapy methods Techniques that utilize hands-on methods to treat dysfunction in the body.

Manual therapy Therapy that encompasses the diagnosis and treatment of ailments of various etiologies through hands-on intervention.

Massage therapy The manual manipulation of the soft tissues of the body for therapeutic purposes.

Mastication The process by which food is torn and/or crushed by teeth.

Matrix metaloproteinases Enzymes that act as collagenases and have the task of remodeling connective tissue.

Mechanical response Any effect of massage techniques that occurs as a direct result of the manipulation of the tissues from components such as pressure, range of motion, and the pushing, pulling, lifting, compressing, and twisting of the tissue.

Mechanoreceptor A sensory receptor that responds to mechanical pressure or distortion.

Medial epicondylitis An overuse injury affecting the flexor-pronator muscle origin at the anterior medial epicondyle of the humerus.

Medial tibial stress syndrome (MTSS) Pain along the posteromedial aspect of the distal third of the tibia arising from an overuse injury.

Medical massage A system of manually applied techniques designed to reduce pain, establish normal tissue tension, create a positive tissue environment, and normalize the movement of the musculoskeletal system.

Meralgia paresthetica A condition that arises as a result of the entrapment of the lateral femoral cutaneous nerve as it exits the pelvis. Symptoms include burning pain and paresthesias in the distribution of the nerve.

Mobilizers The muscles that have a role in generating movement.

Motor end plate The area where the terminal branch of a motor neuron contacts the skeletal muscle fiber.

Movie theater sign A term used to describe patellofemoral pain that occurs after sitting for long periods of time, as in sitting in a movie theater.

Muscle spindle fiber A receptor within the muscle belly that registers the magnitude and the velocity of a stretch.

Muscular cervical dystonia A type of torticollis that arises from the body's protective mechanism for safeguarding the neck. Its causes can vary and include trauma to the area, a sleeping position wrong for the neck, or repetitive motion of the head for extended periods of time. Often referred to as *wryneck*.

Musculotendinous junction The portion of the muscle where it transitions from muscle to tendon.

Myofascial release A system of connective tissue massage that was developed in the 1970s by osteopaths at Michigan State University. Made popular by John Barnes, this system of treatment works with the fascial network to realign and restore the balance between the body and gravity.

Myofascial trigger point (clinical definition) A hyperirritable spot in a skeletal muscle that is associated with a hypersensitive palpable nodule in a taut band. The spot is painful on compression and can give rise to referred pain, tenderness, motor dysfunction, and autonomic phenomena.

Myosin A large family of motor proteins that, together with actin, create a bond that shortens a muscle fiber.

Myositis ossificans A condition that can appear following severe contusions. It is characterized by the deposition of calcium within the muscle fibers or the formation of a spur on the underlying bone.

Myotatic stretch reflex A protective reflex that engages if a muscle is lengthened too far or too fast and results in the contraction of that muscle to resist its lengthening.

Myotomes Adjacent muscles that receive their innervation from one or two nerve roots.

Nerve entrapment syndrome A condition that occurs when a nerve becomes "trapped" due to changes in the tissue through which the nerve passes.

Neuralgia Pain associated with injury to nerves.

Neurapraxia A nerve injury in which the nerve, epineurium, and myelin sheath are stretched but still intact. There is a localized conduction block, which causes a temporary loss of sensation and motor function.

Neurologic cervical dystonia A type of dystonia that typically occurs in adults between the ages of 25 and 60 and can be secondary to a known neuropathological process such as trauma, brain tumor, stroke, or neurodegenerative disease. It can also occur as a primary disorder, with no abnormality found. Sometimes called *spasmodic torticollis*.

Neuropathy An injury along the length of a nerve.

Neurotmesis A nerve injury in which the entire nerve is disrupted.

Neutralizer A muscle that cancels out unwanted movement (since muscles typically have more than one function at a particular joint) so that only the desired action is performed.

Nociceptor A sensory receptor that sends signals that cause the perception of pain in response to a potentially damaging stimulus.

Nutation The backward rotation of the ilium on the sacrum.

Orthopedic massage Massage that involves therapeutic assessment, manipulation, and movement of locomotor soft tissues to reduce pain and dysfunction.

Osteochondritis dissecans A condition characterized by a piece of subchondral bone and cartilage that becomes dislodged from the articular surface. It is classified as either stable, wherein the articular cartilage remains in its anatomical position, or unstable, wherein the fragment becomes dislodged.

Osteoligamentous tunnel The tunnel formed by the eight carpal bones and the fibrous band of tissue called the *flexor retinaculum*.

Overpressure A force that attempts to move a joint beyond its normal range of motion.

Painful arc The arc of the shoulder that is created during abduction and goes through a phase of no pain between 0° and 45° to 60°, pain between 60° and 120°, and then no pain again after 120°.

Pallor An abnormal loss of skin color.

Paresthesia A sense of numbness, prickling, or tingling.

Pars interarticularis A thin slice of bone on the vertebra located between the inferior and superior articular processes of the facet joint.

Passive range of motion Motion performed on the client by the therapist while the client remains totally relaxed.

Patella alta A condition in which an abnormally long patellar tendon causes the patella to ride higher in the trochlea, giving the patella a greater chance of tracking abnormally.

Patella baja A condition in which an abnormally short patellar tendon causes the patella to sit lower in the trochlea, giving the patella a greater chance of tracking abnormally.

Patellar tendonosis Tendon degeneration (or failed healing), with or without symptoms or histologic signs of inflammation in the patellar tendon. This condition commonly stems from an overuse of the patellar tendon, resulting in a cycle of continued insults to the tendon with unsuccessful healing that causes the continued degeneration of the tissue.

Patellofemoral pain syndrome (PFPS) Anterior knee pain caused by abnormal motion of the patella in the trochlear groove, which results from biochemical and/or physical changes within the patellofemoral joint.

Petrissage A stroke that is applied by kneading the tissues to wring out the waste products and bring in new blood flow.

Piano key sign A condition, resulting from a grade III AC sprain, in which the lateral clavicle bobs up and down when depressed, causing severe swelling, pain, and a definite step deformity.

Piezoelectric charge The ability of an inorganic or organic substance to generate an electric charge from pure mechanical deformation.

Pincer palpation Technique in which the belly of the muscle is grasped between the thumb and the fingers and is rolled back and forth to locate the bands.

Piriformis syndrome A nerve entrapment condition that involves the compression of the sciatic nerve and its branches by the piriformis. It can arise from trauma and chronic conditions and is characterized by pain in the hip and along the distribution of the sciatic nerve.

Plantar fasciitis An inflammation of the plantar fascia caused by either an individual traumatic incident or repeated micro-traumas over a period of time. It is characterized by sharp pain with the first few steps in the morning or after a long period of non-weight bearing.

Plastic region A region of tissue in which a force will cause tissue deformation and the tissue will not return to its original shape.

Popeye deformity A deformity caused by a complete rupture of the tendon and displacement of the belly of the long head of the biceps brachii.

Postisometric relaxation A latency period that occurs after an isometric contraction and prevents the muscle from contracting again too rapidly. This is attributed to the repolarization of the muscle fibers.

Pressure The amount of force that is applied to the tissue. This stroke element is controlled by the therapist.

Primary curves The curves of the spinal column that are present at birth.

Pseudothoracic syndrome The referral pattern created when three of four muscles (pectoralis major, latissimus dorsi, teres major, and subscapularis) have active trigger points. The points refer pain that is similar to the true thoracic outlet syndrome.

Quadriceps angle (Q angle) A measurement that is used to determine the patellofemoral mechanics and is a reasonable estimate of the force between the quadriceps group and the patellar tendon.

Radiculopathy Compression that occurs at the nerve root.

Reciprocal inhibition The principle that as one muscle contracts, simultaneous inhibition of the opposing muscle on the other side of the joint occurs.

Reflex zones Skin zones discovered by Dr. Head in 1889 that occur in the dermatomes, which share the same segmental distribution as the sympathetic supply of the associated organ.

Reflexive response Any effect of massage techniques that occurs as a result of changes directed through the nervous system. When the nerves in the area are stimulated, they create a response either locally or systemically.

Release phenomenon The principle that neurovascular symptoms that present as a result of compression will change if the structures causing the compression are moved.

Repetitive motion injury An injury that results from an accumulation of micro-traumas related to inefficient biomechanics, poor posture, incorrect work habits, or constant motion.

Resting position The position of elbow flexion of 70°. This position allows the most amount of space possible within the joint.

Reticular fiber A connective tissue fiber that is a thinner, immature version of collagen fiber. It forms spongelike frameworks for different organs.

Rhythm The repetition or regularity of massage movements.

Rotator cuff tear A tear in one of the muscles of the rotator cuff.

Sacroiliac joint (SIJ) dysfunction Misalignment of the sacroiliac joint, which can result in damage to the joint and thus cause pain.

Satellite myofascial trigger point A central point induced either neurologically or mechanically by the activity of another trigger point.

Scapulohumeral rhythm The ratio of movement between the scapulothoracic and glenohumeral joints.

Scheuermann's disease Considered a form of juvenile osteochondrosis of the spine, a kyphosis that is found mostly in teenagers and presents a significantly worse deformity than postural kyphosis. In postural kyphosis, the vertebrae and disks appear normal; in Scheuermann's kyphosis they are irregular, often herniated, and wedge-shaped over at least three adjacent levels.

Scoliosis Any lateral curvature of the spine; often characterized by either a C or an S curve, depending on which and how many regions of the spine are involved.

Scope of practice As used by licensing boards for various medically related fields, a term that refers to the procedures, actions, and processes that are permitted for licensed individuals. The scope of practice is limited to practice for which the individual has received education and clinical experience and in which he or she has demonstrated competency.

Screw-home mechanism The lateral rotation of the tibia during the last few degrees of extension, which locks the joint in its most stable position.

Secondary curves The curves in the spinal column that develop as a result of adapting to the forces of gravity.

Sensitivity The percentage of subjects tested who have the condition and show a positive result.

Sequence The combination and arrangement of strokes. Sequence is based on the plan of care.

Sequestrated disk injury The most severe disk injury, with fragments from the annulus and nucleus outside the disk.

Sesmoid bone A bone that is embedded in a tendon; typically found where a tendon crosses a joint.

Sharpey's fibers Direct extensions of dense, irregular connective tissue from the periosteum into compact bone. The fibers function to anchor tendons to bone.

Shear A force that acts parallel to a plane and causes the tissues to slide past each other in opposite directions.

Signs Objective, measurable findings obtained during an assessment.

SLAP lesion A superior labrum anterior to posterior lesion. It affects the labrum and typically begins where the biceps tendon inserts into the labrum at the supraglenoid tubercle. With increasing instability comes an increase in the severity of the lesion, which eventually makes its way down the superior part of the biceps tendon.

Snapping palpation Similar to plucking a guitar string, palpation that is done by placing a fingertip at a right angle to the fiber direction of a tense band and then suddenly pressing down while drawing the finger back and rolling the band under the finger.

Specificity The percentage of subjects tested who show a negative result but do not have the condition.

Speed How fast or slow a massage movement is.

Spillover pain zone An area beyond the essential pain zone in which pain is experienced by some clients due to a greater hyperirritability of a trigger point.

Spondylolisthesis The forward slippage of one vertebra on another and the spine's inability to resist the shear force associated with this shifting.

Spondylolysis A defect or break in an area of the vertebra between the superior and inferior facets of the vertebral arch known as the *pars interarticularis*.

Sprain An injury to a ligament.

Squinting patella A misalignment of the patellas in which they are oriented as if they were looking at each other even though the feet are pointed straight ahead.

Stabilizer A muscle that fixates or supports a body part so that other muscles can perform a particular function.

Stance phase The portion of the gait cycle in which the foot is in contact with the ground. This phase makes up 60% to 65% of the cycle.

Stenosis An abnormal narrowing in a blood vessel or other tubular organ or structure.

Step deformity A condition, resulting from a grade II AC sprain, in which the tip of the shoulder drops down, creating an obvious step-off.

Straddle stance A stance used when little or no movement along the client is necessary. The therapist's feet are perpendicular to the table, at least shoulder width apart, and the knees are bent to lower the therapist to the client.

Strain An injury to a muscle or tendon.

Structural Integration A connective tissue modality that was developed by Ida Rolf. Commonly known as "Rolfing," this system utilizes 10 sessions to restore the body's balance with gravity.

Subacromial impingement syndrome A condition characterized by painful contact between the rotator cuff, the subacromial bursa, and the undersurface of the anterior acromion.

Sulcus sign A depression in the glenohumeral joint; created by a downward traction of the humerus.

Swedish Movement System Developed by Pehr Henrik Ling, a combination of massage, gymnastics, and exercise used in the treatment of disease and injury.

Swing phase The portion of the gait cycle in which the foot is suspended in the air. This phase makes up 35% to 40% of the cycle.

Symptoms Information obtained from the client during an assessment.

Tapotment A stroke that involves striking movements using various parts of the hand. Its uses include stimulating or relaxing the nervous system, increasing local blood flow, and mechanically loosening phlegm in the respiratory system. Also known as *percussion*.

Tarsal tunnel syndrome A nerve entrapment syndrome that affects the posterior tibial nerve as it passes through the tarsal tunnel.

Temporomandibular disorder (TMD) An aching in the muscles of mastication, sometimes with occasional brief, severe pain on chewing; often associated with restricted jaw movement and clicking or popping sounds.

Tendinopathy A global term encompassing a number of tendon pathologies that can be seen in isolation or in combination.

Tendonitis An inflammation of the tendon.

Tendonosis A degeneration of the collagen matrix within the tendon; caused by a cycle of repeated insults and partial healing, which leads to an overall breakdown of the tissue.

Tenosynovitis An inflammatory reaction in the sheath surrounding certain tendons.

Tensegrity system A system wherein structures stabilize themselves by balancing the counteracting forces of compression and tension.

Tension A pulling force directed along the long axis that stretches the structure.

Thoracic outlet syndrome (TOS) A compression or tension of the brachial plexus and/or subclavian vessels in the region of the thoracic outlet.

Tinnitus Ringing in the ear.

Torsion The application of torque about the long axis of a structure, thereby creating a shear stress throughout the structure.

Torticollis A type of dystonia that affects the cervical region in which the head is tilted toward one side and the chin is elevated and turned toward the opposite side.

Translation Motion of a joint along an axis.

Triangular fibrocartilage complex (TFCC) A small meniscus resting on the ulnar side of the wrist, opposite the thumb. The complex serves as a site of connection of ligaments as well as a spacer or cushion between the carpal bones and the end of the forearm.

True leg-length discrepancy Leg shortening that comes from an anatomical or structural change in the lower leg, which is either a congenital condition or the result of trauma.

Upper-crossed syndrome A postural dysfunction that involves the head, neck, and upper trunk and is often accompanied by a forward-head and rounded-shoulder posture. It can contribute to kyphosis in the thoracic spine.

Vascular hyperplasia An excessive growth of the cells that form blood vessels, causing clusters of incomplete vessels in the skin or internal organs.

Vasoconstriction   The narrowing of the lumen or opening of a blood vessel.

Vasodilation   The widening of the lumen in a blood vessel as a result of the relaxation of the smooth muscle.

Vibration   A shaking, quivering, trembling, or rocking motion applied using the hands, fingers, or tools.

Viscoelastic   Pertaining to the elastic properties of tissue, which enable a tissue to return to its original length and extensibility.

Whiplash   An acceleration-deceleration mechanism of energy transfer to the neck, resulting in a hyperextension-hyperflexion injury.

Windlass mechanism   A mechanical model that provides an explanation of how the plantar fascia supports the foot during weight-bearing activities. As the foot moves into dorsiflexion and the toes extend during gait, the plantar fascia is wound around the heads of the metatarsals. This shortens the plantar fascia and elevates the medial longitudinal arch.

Y ligament of Bigelow   The iliofemoral ligament that runs from the AIIS to the intertrochanteric line, supporting the anterior region of the joint. It is the strongest ligament in the body.

Zone of primary injury   The area of dead or damaged tissue caused by the initial injury to the tissue.

Zone of reference   The specific region of the body where the referral caused by the trigger point is observed.

Zone of secondary injury   The expanded area of damage to the tissue created by the hypoxic environment that results from the inability of the surrounding tissues to access oxygen and nutrients and remove waste products.

Index

Note: *Italic* page numbers indicate figures and tables.

extension of, 349
  manual muscle testing of, 351
  myotome testing and, 168, 354
  passive, 350
external (lateral) rotation of, 350
  manual muscle testing of, 351
  passive, 350
flexion of, 349
  manual muscle testing of,
    350–351
  myotome testing and, 168, 352
  passive, 350
internal (medial) rotation of,
  349–350
  manual muscle testing of, 351
  passive, 350
manual muscle testing of, 350–351
movements of, 349–351
muscles of, *206–207, 348,* 349, *393*
orthopedic tests for, *400–401*
palpation of, 341–342
passive range of motion of, 350
posterior, stretching of,
  184–185, *185*
soft tissue structures of,
  342, 342–344, *390*
stability of, 343
surface anatomy of, 341–342
trigger point referrals of, *397–399*
trigger points of, 356–363, *397–399*
Hip adductors, stretching of, for
  piriformis syndrome, 372, *372*
Hip bone. *see* Os coxae
Hip extensors, stretching of, for lumbar
  spine conditions, 183, *183*
Hip rotators, stretching of, for piriformis
  syndrome, *370,* 370–371, *371*
Hippocrates, 3, *3*
History
  client, in assessment, 77–79, *78*
  of uninvolved side, 77
Hold/relax, in Proprioceptive
  Neuromuscular Facilitation, 59
Hollow foot. *see* Pes cavus
HOPS method, of
  assessment, 76–77
Horse stance, 22, *23*
Humeral ligament,
  transverse, *220*
Humeroradial joint, 283, *283*
Humeroulnar joint, 283, *283*
Humerus, 215–216, *216,* 219–220, *220,*
  280–281, *281, 283*
  head of, 219, *267*
  shaft of, 219, *267*
Humpback kyphosis, 455
Hyaline cartilage, 75
Hyaluronic acid, 34
Hyoid bone, 104, *149*
Hyperesthesia, 76
Hyperextension, of knee. *see* Genu
  recurvatum
Hypermobile patella, 384
Hypermobility, 57
Hypoesthesia, 76
Hypomobile patella, 384
Hypothenar eminence, *287,*
  287–288, *329*
Hypothesis testing, 91
Hypovascular zone, of supraspinatus
  tendon, 240

IGHL. *see* Inferior glenohumeral ligament
Iliac crest, *159,* 160, *203,* 340,
  340, 341, *389*
Iliac fossa, 340
Iliac tubercle, *159,* 160, *203, 340,* 341, *389*
Iliocostalis lumborum
  trigger point referrals of, *173, 209*
  trigger points of, 170, *172, 209*
Iliofemoral ligament, *342, 343*
Iliopsoas, *348*
  action of, *208, 395*
  insertion of, *208, 395*
  and lumbar spine conditions,
    182, *182*
  origin of, *208, 395*
  palpation of, *208, 395*
  stretching of, 185, *185*
    for piriformis syndrome, 372, *372*
  trigger point referrals of, *173, 175, 210*
  trigger points of, *171, 175, 210*
Iliotibial band, *343,* 344, *348*
  stretching of, for iliotibial band
    friction syndrome, 377–379, *378*
Iliotibial band friction syndrome (ITBFS),
  373–379
  assessment of, 373–374
  condition history of, 374
  definition of, 373
  orthopedic tests for, 374, *375, 400*
  palpation of, 374
  treatment of
    connective tissue, 375
    muscle concerns, 376–377
    in prone position, 375–376, 377
    in side-lying position, 376, 377
    soft tissue, 374–376
    stretching for, 377–379
    in supine position, 376, 377
    tissue inconsistencies and, 376
  visual assessment of, 374
Ilium, 340, *340, 342*
Impingement
  primary, 242
  secondary, 242
Impingement syndrome, 240–241
  orthopedic tests for, *244*
  stage I, 241
  stage II, 241–242
  stage III, 242
  stage IV, 242
  subacromial, 240–241
Impingement tendonosis, 253
Impingement zone, 373
Inclination, angle of, 341
Inert tissue, 74
Infants, and torticollis, 128–133
Inferior articular process, of axis, *103*
Inferior fossa, 216
Inferior glenohumeral ligament (IGHL),
  220, 221
Inferior nasal concha, *96, 97*
Inferior pharyngeal
  constrictor, *107*
Inferior ramus, 341
Inflammation
  acute, 68
  chronic, 68
  contusions and, 459
  palpation and, 85

Inflammatory phase
  of contusion, 459
  of injury, 68–69
Infrahyoids
  action of, *152*
  insertion of, *152*
  origin of, *152*
  palpation of, *152*
  treatment of, for temporomandibular
    disorder, 127
  trigger point referrals of, 115, *153*
  trigger points of, 115, *153*
Infraorbital foramen, *96,* 98, *147*
Infraspinatus, *108, 164, 223, 269*
  action of, *269*
  insertion of, *269*
  origin of, *269*
  palpation of, *269*
  trigger point referrals of, *236, 272*
  trigger points of, *234, 236, 272*
Infraspinatus tendon, *220*
  and rotator cuff injuries, 240
Infraspinous fossa, *217*
Inguinal ligament, 161, *204, 343,
  343, 390*
Inguinal lymph nodes, superficial,
  343, 344, *390*
Inhibition, reciprocal, 50, 58
Inion. *see* External occipital
  protuberance
Initial swing, in gait cycle, 83, *83*
Injury(ies). *see also specific injuries*
  acute, 73
  to cartilage, 75
  chronic, 73
  compensation for, 66–67
  inflammatory phase of, 68–69
  to ligaments, 74–75
  maturation phase of, 69–70
  mechanism of, in client history, 78
  to muscles, 73
  phases of, 68–70
  proliferative phase of, 69
  subacute phase of, 73
  to tendons, 73–74
  zone of primary, 69
  zone of secondary, 69
Innominate bone. *see* Os coxae
Integrated hypothesis, of trigger points,
  47–48
Intention, of strokes, 23
Interclavicular ligament, 221
Intercondylar eminence, 345
Intermuscular hematoma, 459
Internal abdominal obliques, *164*
  action of, *207*
  insertion of, *207*
  origin of, *207*
  palpation of, *207*
  trigger points of, 175
Interosseous sacroiliac
  ligaments, 163
Interphalangeal joints, *287, 329, 409*
Intertrochanteric crest, 341
Intertrochanteric line, 341
Intertubercular groove. *see* Bicipital
  groove
Intervertebral disk, 101, *158,* 158–159
Intervertebral foramen, 102
Interview, for client history, 8
Intramuscular hematoma, 459

M

orthopedic tests for, 366, *366*, 400
palpation for, 366
treatment of
connective tissue, 367
muscle concerns, 368–370
in prone position, 367, 368–369
in side-lying position, 368, *369,*
369–370
soft tissue, 367–368
stretching for, 370–373
in supine position, 367–368, 369
tissue inconsistencies and, 368
visual assessment of, 365–366
Piriformis test, 366, *366*, 400
Pisiform, *284*, 285, 286, *328*
Pitting edema, 85
Plantar calcaneonavicular (spring)
ligament, 408
Plantar fascia, *407*, 410, *444*
Plantar fasciitis, 437–442
assessment of, 439–440
condition history of, 439–440
definition of, 437
etiology of, 438–439
orthopedic tests for, 440, *449*
palpation of, 440
treatment of
connective tissue, 440
muscle concerns, 441
in prone position, 440–441, *441*
in side-lying position, 441
soft tissue, 440–441
stretching for, *426–429*, 442
in supine position, 441
tissue inconsistencies and, 441
visual assessment of, 440
Platysma, *107*
PLL. *see* Posterior longitudinal ligament
Plumb line, 80
PNF. *see* Proprioceptive neuromuscular
facilitation
Point tenderness, 85
Positioning, 13–14
prone, 14
draping in, *15,* 15–17, *16*
side-lying, 14
draping in, 18–20, *19*
supine, 14
draping in, *17,* 17–18, *18*
Postauricular lymph nodes,
100, 100–101, *148*
Posterior arch, of atlas, 103, *103, 149*
Posterior cervical triangle, 104, *104, 149*
Posterior cruciate ligament (PCL), *347, 347*
sprain of, 467
orthopedic tests for, 467, *468, 484*
Posterior inferior iliac spine (PIIS), 340
Posterior longitudinal ligament (PLL),
102, 159
Posterior sternoclavicular ligament, 221
Posterior superior iliac spine (PSIS),
159, 163, *205,* 340, *340,* 341, *389*
Posterior talofibular (PTF) ligament,
407, 408, 471
Posterior tibial artery, *407,* 410, *444*
Posterior tibial nerve, *444*
Posterior tibialis tendon, 410
Posterior tibiotalar (PTT) ligament, 408
Posterior tubercle, of atlas, 103, *103, 149*
Posterior-drawer test, for posterior
cruciate ligament injury, *468, 484*

Posterior-sag test. Godfrey's
(posterior-sag) test
Postisometric relaxation, 58
definition of, 49
passive stretching and, 49
Postural distortions, 451–457
kyphosis, *455,* 455–456
lordosis, *454,* 454–455
scoliosis, *456,* 456–457
treatment strategies for, 452–453
Postural muscles, 457
Postural torticollis, 128
Posture
assessment of, 80–81, 452
anterior, *80,* 80–81,
452–453, *453*
lateral, 81, *81,* 453, *453*
posterior, 81, *81,* 453, 453–454
connective tissue and, 452
correct, goal of, 451
definition of, 80
incorrect, causes of, 452
muscles and, 452
upright, pros and cons of, 451
Preauricular lymph nodes,
100, 100–101, *148*
Pressure, of strokes, 23
Preswing, in gait cycle, *82,* 83
Primary curves, of spine, 80
Primary impingement, 242
Primary injury, zone of, 459
Problem-based education, 5
Prolapse, in lumbar spine
conditions, 177
Proliferative phase
of contusions, 460
of injury, 69
Pronator teres, *288*
action of, *330*
insertion of, *330*
origin of, *330*
palpation of, *330*
trigger point referrals of,
296, 299, *335*
trigger points of, *294,* 299, *335*
Prone positioning, 14
draping in, *15,* 15–17, *16*
Proprioceptive Neuromuscular
Facilitation (PNF), 59
contract/relax in, 59
hold/relax in, 59
Protein, contractile, and trigger
points, 44
Protein fibers, *33*
Proteoglycans, 34
Protrusion, in lumbar spine
conditions, 177
Proximal radioulnar joint, 283
Pseudothoracic syndrome, 232
PSIS. *see* Posterior superior
iliac spine
Pterygoid(s)
lateral
action of, *150*
insertion of, *150*
origin of, *150*
palpation of, *150*
treatment of, for temporomandibular
disorder, 127
trigger point referrals of,
113, 114, *153*

trigger points of, *112,* 114, *153*
medial
action of, *150*
insertion of, *150*
origin of, *150*
palpation of, *150*
treatment of, for temporomandibular
disorder, 127
trigger point referrals of,
114, *114, 153*
trigger points of, *112,* 114, *153*
PTF ligament. *see* Posterior talofibular
ligament
PTT. *see* Posterior tibiotalar
ligament
Pubic crest, *159,* 160, *203,* 340, 342, *389*
Pubic symphysis, *159,* 160, *203,*
340, 342, *389*
Pubic tubercle, *159,* 160, *203,* 340, 342
Pubis, 340, *340,* 341
Pubofemoral ligament, *342,* 343

Q

Q angle. *see* Quadriceps angle
Quadrant test, for facet joint syndrome,
194, 212
Quadratus lumborum
action of, *206*
insertion of, *206*
origin of, *206*
palpation of, *206*
trigger point referrals of,
170–171, *173, 209*
trigger points of, 170–171, *172, 209*
Quadriceps, stretching of
for patellofemoral joint dysfunction,
387, *387*
for spondylolysis/spondylolisthesis,
191, 191–192
Quadriceps (Q) angle, 381
Quadriceps femoris group
trigger point referrals of, 361–362
trigger points of, 361–362
Quadriceps tendon, 346, *392*

R

Radial artery, 287, *287, 329*
Radial collateral ligament, 283, 286, *287*
Radial deviation, 290, 291
Radial deviators, stretching of, for lateral
epicondylitis, 308, *308*
Radial fossa, 281
Radial nerve, *105,* 287, *287, 329*
Radial notch, 282
Radial styloid, *284,* 285, *328*
Radial tuberosity, 281, *281, 282, 326*
Radiculopathy, 481
Radiohumeral joint line, *326*
Radioulnar joint, proximal, 283
Radius, 281, *281, 283,* 285
head of, 281, *281, 282, 326*
Ramus
inferior, 341
superior, 341
Range of motion
active

condition history of, 117–118
definition of, 116
etiology of, 116
grading system of, 116
orthopedic tests for, 118
palpation of, 118
psychological aspect of, 117
symptoms of, 116–117
treatment of
    connective tissue, 118–120, *119*
    muscle concerns, 120–121
    in prone position, 119, *119*, 120–121
    in side-lying position, 120, 121
    soft tissue, 118–120
    stretching for, 121–123, *121–123*
    in supine position, 119–120, 121
    tissue inconsistencies and, 120
visual assessment of, 118
Whitridge, Pete, 40
Width, of massage tables, 13
Windlass mechanism
    definition of, 438
    and plantar fasciitis, 438
Women, draping of
    in side-lying position, 18–19, *19*
    in supine position, 17
Wrist
    bony anatomy of, *284*, 284–285
    bony structures of, 285–286, *328*

dermatomes for, 293, *293, 294*
disorders of, 314–324
extension of, 292, *292*
flexion of, 292, *292*
functions of, 280
manual muscle testing of, 291–293, *291–293*
movements of, 290–293
muscles of, 288, *288*
passive range of motion of, 291
soft tissue structures of, 286–288, *287, 329*
surface anatomy of, 285–286
Wrist extensors
    stretching of, for lateral epicondylitis, 307, *307*, 308, *308*
    trigger point referrals of, 297–299
    trigger points of, 297–299
Wrist flexors
    stretching of, for medial epicondylitis, 313, *313*
    trigger point referrals of, 299
    trigger points of, 299
Wryneck. *see* Muscular cervical dystonia

X

Xiphoid process, *216,* 217, 218, *268*

Y

Yergason's test, for biceps brachii tendonopathy, *256, 277*

Z

Z line, and trigger points, 44
Zone of primary injury, 69, 459
Zone of reference, 44
Zone of secondary injury, 69, 459
Zygapophysial joints. *see* Facet joint(s)
Zygomatic arch, 98, *107, 147*
Zygomatic bone, *96, 97,* 98, *147*
Zygomatic branch, of facial nerve, 100, *100*
Zygomatic process, *96*
Zygomaticus major, *107*
Zygomaticus minor, *107*